ISSUES and TRENDS in NURSING

ISSUES and TRENDS in NURSING

Grace DELOUGHERY, R.N., M.P.H., Ph.D.
Nurse Practitioner
Nursing Services & Resources, Inc.
La Crescent, Minnesota

THIRD EDITION

With 40 illustrations

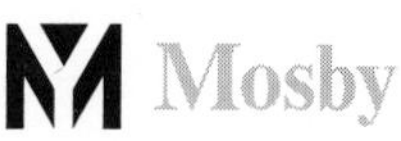

St. Louis Baltimore Boston Carlsbad Chicago Minneapolis New York Philadelphia Portland
London Milan Sydney Tokyo Toronto

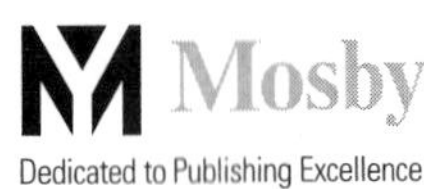

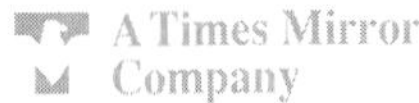

Publisher Sally Schrefer
Editor Michael S. Ledbetter
Associate Developmental Editor Lisa P. Newton
Project Manager Dana Peick
Production Editor Cindy Deichmann
Designer Amy Buxton
Manufacturing Supervisor Karen Boehme

THIRD EDITION

Printed in the United States of America
Composition by Carlisle Communications, Ltd.
Printing/binding by RR Donnelley

Mosby-Year Book, Inc.
11830 Westline Industrial Drive
St. Louis, Missouri 63146

International Standard Book Number 0-8151-2608-5

97 98 99 00 01 / 9 8 7 6 5 4 3 2 1

CONTRIBUTORS

Diane M. Billings, R.N., Ed.D., F.A.A.N.
Professor of Nursing
Indiana University School of Nursing
Indianapolis, Indiana

Luther Christman, R.N., Ph.D.
Dean Emeritus
Rush University
Chicago, Illinois;
Adjunct Professor
Vanderbilt University

M. Pat Donahue, Ph.D., R.N., F.A.A.N.
Professor
College of Nursing
The University of Iowa
Iowa City, Iowa

Judith Halstead, R.N., D.N.S.
Assistant Professor of Nursing
University of Southern Indiana
School of Nursing
Evansville, Indiana

Cheryl Hall Harris, R.N., B.S.N.
Consultant
Overland Park, Kansas

Barbara Hulsmeyer, Ed.D., M.S.N., R.N.
Assistant Professor
Bellarmine College
Louisville, Kentucky

Gladys L. Husted, R.N., Ph.D.
Professor
Duquesne University School of Nursing
Pittsburgh, Pennsylvania

James Husted
Independent Scholar
Pittsburgh, Pennsylvania

Philip Jacobs, Ph.D.
Professor, Department of Health Service
University of Alberta
Edmonton, Alberta
Canada

Kem Louie, Ph.D., R.N., C.S., F.A.A.N.
Associate Professor and Chairperson
Graduate Nursing Program
College of Mount Saint Vincent
Bronx, New York

Edwina A. McConnell, R.N., Ph.D., F.R.C.N.A.
Consultant
Medical-Surgical Nursing
Continuing Education
Medical Device Use
Madison, Wisconsin
Professor, School of Nursing
Texas Tech University Health Sciences Center
Lubbock, Texas
Research Fellow
University of South Australia
Centre for Research into Nursing and Health Care
Underdale, South Australia

Shirley M. Newberry, R.N., Ph.N., M.S.
Public Health Nurse
Assistant Professor
Winona State University
Winona, Minnesota

Linda Peterson Seppanen, R.N., B.S.N., M.S.N., Ph.D.
Associate Professor
College of Nursing and Health Science
Winona State University
Winona, Minnesota

Iris R. Shannon, R.N., Ph.D.
Associate Professor
College of Nursing
Rush University
Chicago, Illinois

Carmen Germaine Warner, M.S.N., R.N., M.Div., F.A.A.N.
Editor, Topics in Emergency Medicine;
Publishing Consultant
Minister Welcome Home Ministries
Ordained Minister
Chaplain for Women at Vista Jail and Donovan Prison
San Diego, California

Jack Antony Phillip Yensen, R.N., B.sc. (Hons), Ph.D.
Instructor
Langara College Nursing Department
Vancouver, British Columbia
Canada

Gloria Y. York, R.N., M.A. Ed.
Education Consultant
San Diego, California

Mary Jane Zusy, R.N., B.A., M.A.
Contributor Editor
The Nursing Spectrum
Kensington, Maryland

REVIEWERS

Judith Haber, R.N., Ph.D., C.S., F.A.A.N.
Visiting Professor
Division of Nursing
New York University
New York, New York
Private Practice
Stamford, Connecticut

Rita J. Lourie, R.N., M.S.N.
Assistant Professor of Nursing
Director of Community and Academic Outreach
Temple University Neighborhood Nursing Center
Philadelphia, Pennsylvania

Lorys F. Oddi, Ed.D., R.N.
Professor
School of Nursing
Northern Illinois University
DeKalb, Illinois

Mary O'Neill, M.S.N., R.N.
Faculty
Department of Nursing
State University of West Georgia
Carrollton, Georgia

Linda S. Smith, M.S.N., R.N.
Faculty
Department of Nursing
State University of West Georgia
Carrollton, Georgia

PREFACE

One generation has the responsibility to leave for the next what it has learned through extensive experience, including rewards of work well thought out and carried out and the cruel encounters from the world that is for various reasons unappreciative of contributions made. So this book passes on from the mature, seasoned practitioners of nursing in the 1990s information that may hopefully be most useful as the nursing students of today enter practice around the year 2000. The primary goal of this text is to provide the most current, most relevant information available on contemporary issues and trends that will affect all areas of nursing practice in the years to come.

Students today are of varying ages and have backgrounds that differ widely. It is difficult to address all of them without seeming to either assume that everyone has a fairly sophisticated background in the basic knowledge areas of the physical and social sciences or, on the other hand, to insult some by explaining rudimentary material. Hopefully this text will reach both so that additional resources provided in suggested readings and appendices will explain what is not clear to some and add depth for those who wish more extensive detail.

Women and men entering nursing today may enter with a financially reachable goal in mind and then extend that goal as they earn while they learn. The associate degree student may find that to pursue the baccalaureate degree is reasonable in the coming few years. However, highly skilled nurses who can conduct research, teach, and become master's or doctorally prepared practitioners in one of many areas of specialization provide hope that nursing will be an equal partner on the health care team. For the beginning student this may seem unrealistic in terms of where she or he is currently. It might be suggested that to dream is sometimes beneficial when it serves the purpose of spurring one on toward a higher goal.

To prepare the nurses of tomorrow is not to cram the same theory and practice into different levels of education. Rather it is a matter of making students aware that there are indeed incremental levels of performance and expectations. Until the levels of knowledge and performance of nurses is parallel to practitioners in the other health care professions, all those entering the field will experience negative ramifications to one degree or another.

I have come to certain conclusions after many years of education and experience; these are passed on to the readers in hopes that they may benefit as they build their own careers. Over the last few years I have developed my current nursing practice into a private home care business. This provides an opportunity to apply knowledge gained in meeting the nursing needs of many different kinds of people and problems. It is today's challenge to assist individuals with maintaining their dignity from birth through the dying process. I have had vast experience in nursing people of all ages, with even the most severe health problems, and those in the last stages of life to determine whether to be institutionalized or remain within the home setting. The home care staff that I direct serves the population of six counties in a radius of about 80 miles. I am often consulted on difficult nursing situations and problems, and my practice is based on extensive experience in clinical practice, teaching, research, supervision, and management. My view of nursing reflects what is going on in the "real world." My distinguished colleagues who have contributed to the book bring further insight and understanding to the issues confronting the nursing profession today. Because of the diverse backgrounds, belief systems, and experiences of the contributors, their statements and positions are not necessarily shared by me or by all contributors. This diversity challenges the reader to think critically and to formulate her or his own interpretations and perspectives.

Issues and Trends in Nursing is a text designed for nurses in a wide variety of undergraduate educational programs. An extensive amount of material from nurses in specific areas of expertise has been included. For more detail on any one subject, it may be necessary to consult other sources, so suggested readings are included at the ends of chapters.

The content of the book is organized into three general thematic parts. These are (1) sociohistoric, (2) nursing education, and (3) nursing practice.

The sociohistoric part includes Chapters 1 through 8. Chapters 1 and 2 present an overview of the history and evolution of nursing science and practice. A timeline has been added to enhance appreciation of the historical development of the profession. Chapters 3 through 7 present economic, social, political, cultural, legal, and ethical dynamics that interactively influence health care generally and nursing specifically.

The nursing education material is to be found mainly in Chapters 8 through 13. Chapter 8 is geared specifically to nursing education. Chapter 9 presents the subject of licensure and related issues in nursing, and Chapter 10 discusses continuing education for relicensure.

Chapter 11 presents practical ways that might be useful to nurses in order to effect change; knowing some of these ways will help make the nurse make the most of her career both personally and professionally. The potential of the nurse for making change depends on the understanding and use of the political process.

The last of the three major parts of the text present material on areas of nursing practice. Chapter 12 (urban health care problems), Chapter 13 (rural nursing), and Chapters 14, 15, 16, 17, and 18 are devoted to the special challenges of nursing today: the contribution that American nurses are making on the international level, changing image, building a nursing career that is both personally and professionally productive, understanding and use of the political process, the nurse in the computer age, and future perspectives.

Important threads are synthesized throughout the three major parts of the text and suggest directions for future growth.

The appendixes provide information about nursing organizations and state boards of nursing.

In this book, the nurse is often referred to by the feminine pronoun *she.* This is done to avoid the awkwardness and repetitiveness of *he or she* or *he/she* and because females still significantly outnumber males in the nursing profession. However, the number of men in nursing is slowly growing. Their contributions to the profession are important and certainly not to be overlooked. No offense to either male or female nurses is implied or intended.

Nurses have traditionally referred to people for whom they care as *patients.* With the new climate of “prevention,” “healthy living,” and revolutionary changes in health care, the term has to a large extent become outdated. People in the health care system are now often referred to by nurses and others as *clients.* Because of this trend and the ambiguity that using both terms would make for the reader, the term *client* is consistently used throughout this book.

ACKNOWLEDGMENTS

Four decades in the active practice of professional nursing have provided me with a historical perspective that only experience can give. Many are the memories of colleagues who shared the same workplace and persons for whom I cared in a multitude of situations along the way. With the passing time, faces and details remain vivid in mind even when names have been forgotten. I extend thanks to all those persons who have contributed to such a rich education and varied career as what I have had. Many of these persons have died either during the time we met or since. In either circumstance it has been a blessing to have been part of their lives.

So many years in nursing practice may encourage one to be all the more capable and eager to pass on one's heritage to the new generation of nurse students who will read this text. To tell the true stories of what nursing has been like during these past 40 years is not easy because it is only the extraordinarily imaginative reader who will be able to truly see the picture. It is, however, only from such a vantage point that one can see into the future and imagine the entire picture as a realistic continuum of events through which threads bind the whole together.

Many friends and supporters have watched as this project was developing, and their inquisitiveness was an encouragement. Some of my staff wondered what could be so enticing as to make me stay up late and rise early to undertake this in addition to many other responsibilities. Others gave nonverbal or verbal messages that indicated they felt there must be "more interesting things to do." Nonetheless, my secretary, Cindy Blagsvedt, caught my enthusiasm, and I wish to thank her for her perseverance as the days of preparing manuscript material sometimes became arduous and long. And the ongoing encouragement and support of the Mosby staff—Jeff Burnham, Lisa Newton, and others—was greatly appreciated.

Last but not least, I must call all future nurses to the challenge of moving the profession into the twenty-first century. It will not be easy as the changes are coming rapidly and are of horrendous magnitude. The payoff will be well worth it, since any effort applied has both potential of providing self-satisfaction and contributing to those people in tomorrow's society whose lives will be touched.

CONTENTS

■ Chapter 3: Economics of Health Care, 105

Philip Jacobs

■ Chapter 4: Social Policy and Health Care Delivery, 132

Shirley Newberry

■ Chapter 5: Cultural Influences on Nursing, 171

Kem B. Louie

■ Chapter 6: Legal Aspects of Nursing, 195

Cheryl Hall Harris

■ Chapter 9: Licensure and Related Issues in Nursing, 270

Linda Seppanen

■ Chapter 10: Continuing Education for Relicensure, 308

Gloria Y. York

■ Chapter 11: Political Awareness in Nursing, 322

Mary Jane Zusy

PART THREE *Nursing Practice, 331*

■ Chapter 12: Urban Health Care Problems, 333

Iris R. Shannon

■ Chapter 16: Nursing as a Career, 412

Grace L. Deloughery

■ Chapter 17: Computers in Nursing: Navigating the Information Superhighway, 439

Jack Yensen

■ Chapter 18: The Future: A Challenge for Nurses and Nursing, 448

Luther Christman

PART ONE

Social and Historical Aspects

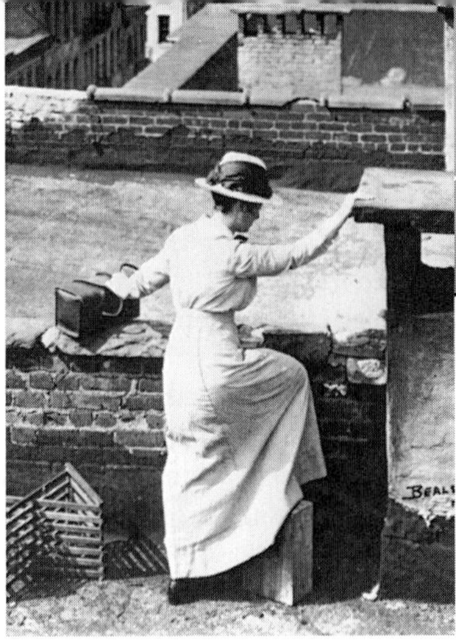

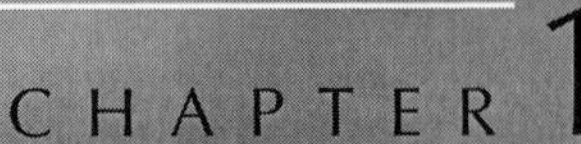

History of the Nursing Profession

Grace Deloughery

OBJECTIVES After completing this chapter the reader should be able to:

- **Describe nursing care in ancient times**
- **Summarize major events, developments, and struggles of each period in nursing history**
- **Describe how nursing today is related to the development of education for women, and when and how education for women evolved**
- **Discuss the contribution of Florence Nightingale and other leaders in nursing before the twentieth century**
- **Discuss the impact that social reform in the nineteenth century had on nursing**
- **Describe nursing in pioneer America and how it evolved through the various wars that followed**
- **List six major factors influencing health care and the provision of health and nursing services since World War II**
- **Discuss crucial health issues today and how they have affected the nursing profession. Describe how nurses can be leaders and influence the outcome of these issues and the status of nursing**

The history of nursing has and always will be linked with the issues and trends that are occurring in health care, economics, society, and cultural dynamics. These current changes occurring in the health care field are profoundly affecting the nursing profession. Economic incentives inherent in managed care are encouraging health care organizations to reduce the costs of client care more than ever before. The nursing profession continues to be integrally involved in this cost-cutting process by continuing to develop such innovations as critical pathways. As nurses face the upcoming years, they must continuously strive to maintain unity between conscience and intellect. In other words, nurses will be struggling to achieve a satisfactory balance between cutting costs and providing quality nursing care.

Important historical developments have profoundly conditioned and influenced the evolution of nursing. Primarily these are the Crusades, the Renaissance, the Reformation, the Industrial Revolution, the development of modern science and health facilities, the World Wars, various types of research in social and basic science, social welfare, rapid technologic advances, and the Equal Rights movement. Perhaps more important than any of these, the liberation of women served as a catalyst and critical component of the evolution of the nursing profession. The new freedom enabled women to develop professions and achieve recognition. Today they continue to strive for additional freedom to develop individual and professional potentials.

■ ANCIENT BEGINNINGS

Nursing dates from prehistoric times, when those who proved themselves adept in caring for the sick naturally were asked to nurse friends or acquaintances; some established a practice of nursing through reputation.

Though separate and distinct from medicine, nursing is closely allied to medical progress and practice. Just as one cannot understand modern nursing without some understanding of medicine and surgery, one cannot understand the evolution of nursing without an awareness of the primitive beginnings of medicine. Medicine progressed from its origins in witchcraft in Egypt to the rediscovery of Hippocratic principles by the English clinicians of the seventeenth century. Modern medicine rests on the physiologic principles that William Harvey (1578–1657) discovered and the correlation of symptoms with organic changes taught by Giovani Morgagni (1682–1771). When these great principles became integrated with clinical medicine, they gave it impetus under which present understanding of cure and prevention of disease continue to progress.

Egyptian Medicine

Egyptian medicine originated in the practice of magic and centered around Imhotep, chief physician to Pharaoh Zoser of the Third Dynasty (about 3000 BC). In early Egypt certain empirical knowledge regarding sickness slowly accumulated from witchcraft. The practice of medicine never entirely outgrew the superstitions that surrounded its origins. (Even well-educated clients today look to physicians for something more than the logical application of a technical science.) Medicine in Egypt reached a surprisingly advanced stage of knowledge. The custom of embalming enabled the Egyptians to become well acquainted with organs of the body. From clinical observation they learned to recognize some 250 different diseases, and to treat them they developed a number of drugs and procedures such as surgery. By about 480 BC neurosurgery in Egypt was advanced beyond the imagination of the Greeks. However, Egyptian lack of knowledge regarding normal and pathologic physiology and lack of experimental investigation limited their theories.

Greek Medicine and Hospitals

With the decline of Egyptian civilization during the last millennium BC, medicine came under Greek influence. Hippocrates (about 400 BC) changed the magic of medicine into a science of medicine. He taught physicians to use their eyes and ears and to reason from facts rather than from gratuitous assumptions. His writings on fractures and dislocations were unsurpassed until the discovery of the x-ray. The oath of Hippocrates is used today to admit many to the practice of medicine, and the Hippocratic school has been given credit for the first ethical guide on medical conduct.

In ancient Greece there were two kinds of refuges for the sick—secular and religious. Physicians directed the secular locations, which corresponded roughly to spas or health resorts of today. Some were endowed and had outpatient departments, and some were used for instruction of medical students. The secular places of healing and the sanctuaries of the gods, especially the god Aesculapius, were closely associated. Importance was placed on the role of emotions in bringing about cure; also included was the role of wholesome food, physiotherapy, and fresh air and sunshine, perhaps on porches overlooking the blue Mediterranean, while the client awaited the appearance of the god in dreams.

The first instance of women being associated with the healing arts is found in Greek mythology in relation to Aesculapius, who eventually became deified as the god of healing. One of his daughters, Hygeia, became the goddess of health, and another, Panacea (whose name came into our language as the word meaning *cure-all*), became the restorer of health. Later most Greek healing centered around shrines in which clients congregated. Attendants were *basket bearers* who looked after the sick, somewhat in the manner of nurses.

The Hippocratic Oath

Hippocrates' approach to health care, summarized in *Corpus Hippocraticum,* nearly parallels the teaching of professional nursing today. The writings of Hippocrates refer to procedures that today would be undertaken in modern hospitals by nurses but do not refer to a nursing vocation as such. He labeled the health care provider a *physician.* His use of this word should not be confused with modern usage. In fact, much of the ancient Greek physician's craft falls under what modern nurses would claim as their practice. Hippocrates showed that disease had only natural causes and believed that the treatment of disease required more than religion. He treated his clients with fresh air, proper diet, changes in climate, and attention to habits and living conditions. Emphasis was on the client—describing the problem and solving it. (In comparing his writings with those of Florence Nightingale, one is struck by the similarities of many of their philosophies and observations.)

The Hippocratic oath promotes professional loyalty (Box 1-1). Physicians even today have an ethic of mutual support of one another. Lack of similar support among nurses is one of the most damaging problems of the profession. Nurses today destroy each other with petty criticisms and jealousies and thereby damage the whole profession.

It might be appropriate for nurses to learn the Hippocratic oath and to study its components as a part of their professionalization process. It is proactive. The Nightingale Pledge is more reactive and provides less structure to the building of a strong and cohesive nursing profession. The work of both nurses and physicians is directed toward the same end. Furthermore, the Hippocratic oath speaks of teamwork and supporting colleagues.

Box 1-1 The Hippocratic Oath

I swear by Apollo, the physician, and Aesculapius and Health and All-Heal and all the gods and goddesses that, according to my ability and judgment, I will keep this oath and stipulations:

To reckon him who taught me this art equally dear to me as my parents, to share my substance with him and relieve his necessities if required; to regard his offspring as on the same footing with my own brothers, and to teach them this art if they should wish to learn it, without fee of stipulation, and that by precept, lecture, and every other mode of instruction I will impart a knowledge of the art to my own sons and to those of my teachers, and to disciples bound by a stipulation and oath, according to the law of medicine, but to none others.

I will follow that method of treatment which, according to my ability and judgement, I consider for the benefit of my patients, and abstain from whatever is deleterious and mischievous. I will give no deadly medicine to anyone if asked, nor suggest any such counsel; furthermore, I will not give to a woman an instrument to produce abortion.

With purity and with holiness I will pass my life and practice my art. I will not cut a person who is suffering from a stone, but will leave this to be done by practitioners of this work. Into whatever houses I enter I will go into them for the benefit of the sick and will abstain from every voluntary act of mischief and corruption; and further from the seduction of females or males, bond or free.

Whatever, in connection with my professional practice, or not in connection with it, I may see or hear in the lives of men which ought not to be spoken abroad I will not divulge, as reckoning that all such should be kept secret.

While I continue to keep this oath unviolated, may it be granted to me to enjoy life and the practice of the art, respected by men at all times, but should I trespass and violate this oath, may the reverse be my lot.

Early Christian Church and Hospitals

Beginning in the first centuries AD, the early Christian church and the teachings of Jesus Christ expressed the need to succor orphans, the poor, travelers, and above all the sick. The deaconesses of the early church, lay women appointed by the bishops, visited the sick much as modern visiting nurses or home health care nurses do. These appointments were highly esteemed and were given to women of good social standing.

One of the best-known deaconesses of the early Christian church was Phoebe, a Greek woman who is also remembered as the bearer of St. Paul's epistle to the Romans. Acting as visiting nurses soon became an important responsibility of these early deaconesses, and Phoebe is often referred to as the first visiting nurse, as well as the first deaconess.

In addition to being visited in their homes, clients often stayed in the bishops' houses. When this proved impractical, special facilities were set up throughout the Roman Empire through endowments. In Rome the first large hospital was established by Fabiola, a beautiful, worldly woman who thereby did penance for her second marriage. She administered this hospital so well that her death was mourned by all Rome. Separate hospitals developed for the care of lepers, children, the aged, and strangers; these were forerunners of present-day specialty institutions. A few centuries later the first hospitals immediately under the auspices of the Roman Catholic Church were founded in the Western world; these still exist. In Lyons, France, the Hôtel Dieu was established in AD 542 by Childebert; it is now the hospital with the longest record of continuous service. Detailed records were kept at the Hôtel Dieu in Paris, which was founded in AD 650 by Saint Landry, Bishop of Paris. It was enlarged in the thirteenth century by Saint Louis and was the prototype of the medieval hospital. The records of this hospital constitute a principal source of information regarding nursing in those days.

Muslim Medicine and Hospitals

During the eighth to the tenth centuries magnificent hospitals were constructed throughout the Muslim world. They were staffed by physicians superior to any in the world because of knowledge gained and preserved from their Greek counterparts. One well-endowed hospital was in Cairo and was a prized target that the Crusaders tried very hard to destroy. These Muslim structures were in marked contrast to the rather gloomy, gothic Hôtel Dieu in France of a few centuries before. Physiology and hygiene were studied by Arabian scientists, and knowledge of *materia medice* was expanded. Surgeons used various drugs as anesthetics, but Muslim belief in the uncleanliness of the dead forbade dissection.

■ MIDDLE AGES

Many of the characteristic methods of providing health care in Europe from the collapse of the Roman Empire in the fifth century to around the 1500s were applied in Sweden. The first monasteries were founded there in the 1100s. One of the orders, the Franciscans (known as "barefoot brothers"), spent much of their time helping the poor. Archeologists have found surgical instruments inside monasteries, especially instruments used for bloodletting, a good indication that health care took place there. Historians believe the nuns and monks themselves were the main recipients of such care. Books about herbal cures and healing have been found dating back to the 1400s. Charitable institutions or sanctuaries were first started in the twelfth century. They were intended mainly for the aged, sickly, and poor and were situated in the towns. Each one could hold about 20 to 25 people. The mayor would appoint a manager for the home who would be in charge of receiving gifts and donations, as well as selling private property to pay expenses. Care given to people in these facilities was mainly of a spiritual character. Those who seemed stronger and healthier cared for the weaker. Income from donations at these sanctuaries and homes was insignificant compared to the income at monasteries and churches, which included tithes.[40]

Influence of the Crusades on Nursing

The Crusades were Christian military expeditions to recapture the Holy Land, where Jesus had lived, from the inhabiting Muslims. The Crusades began shortly before AD 1100 and lasted until almost AD 1300. In 1244 about 19,000 hospitals existed throughout Western Europe. This large number was due to the spread of leprosy during the Crusades. It was strongly emphasized that hospitals existed for the poor, and those who worked in them were expected to give up everything for Christ. No type of care or nursing was mentioned in their statutes except for the spiritual care provided by masses, fasting, and prayers.[40]

For a thousand years after Christ there were no attempts to organize nursing. But as the Middle Ages advanced, three types of organizations developed that have persisted in some form to the present day and/or established certain principles still recognized as important. These organizations were the military orders, regular (religious) orders, and secular orders.

Military Orders

The most spectacular focus of this period was the Crusader, a man who purported to combine a lofty spirit devoted to the service of God with a fierce, belligerent temper and who sought to fight the Muslims in the Middle East so that the holy ground on which Christ trod might again belong to His followers. He supposedly carried the principles and the glory of knighthood to their fullest as he traveled over the continent of Europe and throughout the Mediterranean basin. When he traveled to the Near East he learned much from his enemy, including the Arabian idea of the organized hospital. Natural places for the establishment of hospitals were outposts, particularly Jerusalem, where those wounded in battle sought refuge while they recovered. The hospital had to be staffed by physicians and nurses who were members of the regular orders. Men went to battle and then retired to nurse the sick. They were called *knight hospitalers.* In later years they devoted themselves entirely to nursing. Two great influences shaped nursing practice during this period—the military and the religious. Gradually the care of the sick was considered more and more a religious duty.

Three nursing orders became preeminent: the Knights of St. John, the Teutonic Knights, and the Knights of Saint Lazarus. Corresponding to these were the three orders of women who tended female clients in special hospitals. The Order of Saint John—Italian and highly successful in its mission—originated the entire staff of two major hospitals in Jerusalem. It established an ambulance service and was a major organizer of the International Red Cross, which still carries its insignia. This order established customs that remain the heritage of nursing today. Military in character, it was steeped in the tradition of discipline. Modern nursing traces its tradition of obedience to the principles of complete and unquestioning devotion to duty held forth by the Order of Saint John.

Regular Orders

Because of the insecurity of life during the Crusades, people could not be given nursing care in their homes. Refuge behind moats and walls led to the establishment of monasteries wherein hostels, hotels, and hospices were organized to care for travelers, paupers, and the sick, particularly those with epidemic diseases. As the words *hostels, hotels,* and *hospices* imply, each served a different clientele. It was not until society became better organized and life was more stable that hospitals became separate institutions apart from monasteries.

The early hospital was called a *hôtel Dieu.* It was at the Hôtel Dieu in Paris that the Augustinian sisters in charge (the first organization of nurses) developed a record-keeping system credited with being the most complete of its time.

During the epidemics of this era, care of the sick was performed mainly by volunteers who devoted themselves to nursing. One outstanding volunteer was Saint Catherine of Siena (1347–1380). At night her lamp represented to the sick at Siena what Florence Nightingale's lamp came to mean in the Crimea 500 years later. Catherine received training in her middle-class home, staying at home to help with housework, which was the custom of the day. She later taught herself to read and write. In 1372 the plague came to Siena, and Catherine went to work night and day caring for the sick. She became well known for her work at a hospital in La Scala; it stands as a memorial to her today.

The regular orders were structured so that the sisters advanced from a stage of probationer to wearing the white robe to wearing the hood. In the beginning there was no uniform: nurses wore their regular clothes while on duty. As the Middle Ages advanced, clothes became more gaudy, and because the church secluded itself from the more worldly aspects of life, there was a tendency to adopt a uniform dress, which eventually became standardized.

Secular Orders

The disadvantages of church connections became increasingly apparent. Demands for complete and perpetual devotion to God did not always attract those best suited to care for the sick. Consequently secular orders developed that were separate lay branches of the regular holy orders but approached the effectiveness of regular orders by requiring temporary vows, uniformity in dress, and religious observances. Some of these secular orders include the Third Order of Saint Francis, the Order of Saint Vincent de Paul, and the Sisters of Charity. The Beguines were active and prolific in West Flanders, the Netherlands, France, and Germany. The Oblates evolved in Italy, and the Order of the Holy Ghost, remembered chiefly as a male nursing order, evolved in France.

■ THE RENAISSANCE

In the early 1300s a great revival of learning and art developed in Italy and spread elsewhere throughout Europe. This period is referred to as the *Renaissance.* Humanists of this time believed that by referring back to the classics—literature, history, and philosophy of ancient Greece and Rome—they could begin a new golden era of culture and human life.

One of the causes of the Renaissance was the bubonic plague* epidemic that devastated the Western world from 1347 to 1351, killing 25% to 50% of Europe's population. This relatively sudden catastrophe either caused or accelerated marked political, economic, social, and cultural changes. Mortality among men of learning was extremely high, and new ideas and doctrines had the opportunity to infiltrate traditional teachings. Many people believed that the church had let them down. Consequently there was a rise in secularism and humanism. Humanism—a philosophy emphasizing the importance of man and his place in the universe—provided the foundation for the development of modern science.

Death and disappearance of half the clergy population put a heavy strain on the momentum of the church and reduced its capacity to deal effectively with movements of protest or revolt. This helped establish the mindset that made

*Old diseases are making new appearances. In India the pneumonic plague (one of the more deadly forms of pneumonic plague) has returned with such ravaging intensity that the demand for antibiotics such as tetracycline to treat the sick and insecticides to kill the disease-carrying fleas has sometimes exceeded the supply. Hundreds of millions of people in rural India have little access to health care facilities; it is they who will probably have the worst chance of obtaining the needed treatment.

possible the Protestant Reformation of the 1500s. But the plague caused a parallel growth in religious fervor among other Europeans. The church played a strong role in the development of this period. There was concern about the large administrative structure of the Roman Catholic Church, the church's weak regard for people, and the increased stress on good works, such as giving to charity, to earn salvation. The intervention of movable type in the mid-1400s helped spread learning through printed books, which resulted in an increased number of laymen (literally, *men* outside the church structure) gaining an education.*

Contributors to the great medical developments of this period were (1) Leonardo da Vinci (1452–1519), whose anatomic studies and sketches remain classic; (2) Andreas Vesalius (1514–1564), credited with developing anatomy as a science; and (3) William Harvey (1578–1657), who is credited with founding medical science based on fact rather than tradition. The work of these sixteenth-century anatomists enabled physicians to work on a more solid basis. Ambroise Paré (1510–1590), a military surgeon, wrote a book on natural history in general and surgery in particular in which he emphasized that it was necessary to dress wounds with boiling oil and that bleeding could be controlled with ligatures as well as by red-hot cautery. He also devised artificial limbs for the victims of war. During this period nursing reached a high level of organization and efficiency in the religious and military orders.

In Sweden the Church rules of 1571 included a paragraph "on hospitals and sick houses." This paragraph was considered to be Sweden's first common hospital regulation. It said that hospitals located near churches should be able to contain 25 to 30 clients besides caregivers. Priests and bishops were to encourage the people of the community to donate to the hospital. The mayor had to appoint the manager, and special rooms and bath houses had to exist for those with contagious diseases. Each hospital was to have its own rules for how a client should behave and what his or her obligations to the hospital were to be.

In seventeenth-century Sweden the need for care of the sick and poor escalated. A new law established in 1642 stated that hospitals were to be used only for the physically or mentally ill and those who were weak, aged, or had contagious diseases. The bishop and the manager were to decide who was to be admitted. A fee was then charged, and if the client could not pay at the time he would later have to pay the town or county in which he lived. This step at least partially eliminated the use of hospitals as poor houses.[40]

Beginnings of Modern Science

William Harvey discovered circulation of the blood but contributed something even more important to medicine: he established the principle of the physiologic experiment. He received his anatomic training in Padua and returned to Saint Bartholomew's Hospital in London, where he served as demonstrator of anatomy at the Physicians' College on Amen Street. Here he completed his discovery, which he communicated in a lecture in 1616. His book was not published until 12 years later. While he was in Oxford during the reign of Charles I, London was besieged during a civil war, his home was searched, and all of his manuscripts and notes were

*The reference to *laymen* is literal here, meaning education of men, not women.

destroyed. We can only ponder the loss medicine suffered as a result, for some of the titles were of great promise, including "The Practice of Medicine Conformable in the Thesis of the Circulation of the Blood" and "Anatomy in Its Application to Medicine."

After several decades of political disturbance, which led to the ultimate beheading of Charles I in 1649, Harvey returned to London and became a scientific leader. He donated his library to the College of Physicians and established a lectureship that has continued to this day and to which is owed, among others, Sir Williams Osler's marvelous oration in 1905 on the founder himself. Harvey exhorted his fellows and members of the college to study the ways of nature by means of experiment.

Thomas Sydenham (1624–1689) was the first person to set the example of true clinical methodology. His independent and unprejudiced spirit, combined with great powers of observation, made him the prototype of the clinical investigator. Referred to as the "English Hippocrates," he resurrected the great but simple methods and principles taught by Hippocrates many centuries earlier. He emphasized the need to observe phenomena and let observations lead to logical conclusions. Puritan by birth and outlook, he expounded, "We should not imagine or think out, but find out, what nature does or produces." This sounds obvious to us now only because Sydenham succeeded to such an extent that his teaching has become commonplace. In his time medical science carried a superstructure of wanton superstitions and theories so complicated and cumbersome that it was deprived of real value. In fact, Sydenham was attacked because he made the practice of medicine too simple and easy. In modern times his name is commonly associated with his description of chorea, although his description of gout was better. His philosophy was to use probability as a guide, thus eliminating fantasies and vagaries that tend to distract the mind. Sydenham had much in common with his friend John Locke (1632–1704), the physician-philosopher and private physician to Lord Shaftsbury. Locke, a proponent of common sense and straight thinking, was the forerunner of Hume and Kant.

Sydenham's views met with great opposition. He did not participate in the activities of the Royal Society of Medicine. Even though during his lifetime he was considered one of the great physicians, the true magnitude of his accomplishments was not appreciated for several generations. Sydenham's methodic approach to medicine was ahead of his time.

During the seventeenth century London abounded in quackery of all kinds. Quacks, mountebanks, chemists, apothecaries, and even surgeons, who were not supposed to treat internal diseases in those days but nevertheless did, joined in exploiting the healing crafts. Druggists copied prescriptions they were supposed to fill and sold the drugs privately over the counter. Such a person was said to have profited a hundred times as much from a single prescription as did the physician who wrote it.

More than any time before, increased taxes, polls, and large fees for houses, servants, and entertainment were imposed on physicians. Bureaucracy was bad in those days, just as it is today. The emphasis was mostly on making money and not on compassion. In those days the main requirements for beginning a practice were to have a good understanding with a druggist and to be seen regularly at church.

It was thought that there was an overabundance of students graduating in medicine. Because labor was cheap in those days, it was considered normal for head physicians to treat newly graduated physicians as bond servants. Whoever wanted to practice in the field took a lot of abuse as an apprentice and accepted being a perpetual slave and servant to the head surgeon.

The scientific method was born when people began to ask questions to which they expected rational answers based on facts. This method of reasoning led to objective observations and to the physical and physiologic experiments that form the basis for modern natural sciences. The writings of John Locke, Roger Bacon, and Thomas Hobbes guided people's thoughts. William Gilbert of Rochester assembled knowledge pertaining to magnetism and introduced the word *electricity.* Newton invented calculus and discovered laws governing optics and the law of gravity, and Boyle introduced atomic theory. Thus, through hundreds of observations and discoveries that often gained practical importance in the most unexpected way, the foundations for sciences were established.

It was this scientific attitude that led to the discovery of steam power and the construction of the steam engine, and somewhat later to the discovery of the electromagnetism and the construction of the electric motor. Without it modern engines would not have come into being, and the Industrial Revolution would not have occurred. In the course of time, the scientific attitude laid the foundations for modern medicine; the fundamental work of Harvey and Sydenham was its direct outgrowth.

All these developments had an impact on nursing, perhaps not immediately, but in subsequent eras as nursing developed into a science and a profession using these theories as foundation for practice.

■ THE REFORMATION

The Reformation began in the early 1500s. Martin Luther (1483–1546), a monk and professor of theology, and other scholars of that time developed increasing conflict with the direction in which the church was moving. This began a long struggle in which the teachings of these leaders of the Protestant movement spread, particularly throughout Germany, Switzerland, England, and Scandinavia.

Nursing sank to its lowest levels in those countries where the Roman Catholic organizations were upset by the Reformation. Protestant states closed churches, monasteries, and hospitals. In England over a hundred hospitals were closed, and for a while there was little or no provision for the institutional care of the indigent sick. When the demand became too great to be ignored, lay persons were appointed to run the hospitals. For example, St. Bartholomew's Hospital in London, the Hospital of St. Giles in the Fields, and St. Katherine's Hospital were not run because of the principle of charity but because of social necessity. No honor was attached to running a hospital or being on its staff. At St. George's Hospital a man and his wife were engaged at the relatively small salaries of £8 and £11 per annum to be messenger and matron, respectively. The matron was in charge of the nurses. A nurse in charge of a ward or a division was called a *sister,* possibly because of the belief that the title might retain some of the devotion and dignity of the old days. However, when deprived of the dignity of the church, nursing somehow lost its social standing. Nurses were no longer recruited from the respectable classes of the community but from distinctly lower social classes or discharged patients.* The new Protestant church abhorred cloisters and religious institutions and did not feel the same responsibility to the sick as the Roman Catholic church had. Thus followed a dark period in nursing and society in Protestant countries that dates roughly from the end of the seventeenth to the middle of the nineteenth century.

The Protestant church advocated religious freedom and freedom of thought but did not champion freedom for women either in the seventeenth and eighteenth centuries or in the Victorian era. The place of the average respectable woman was in the home; a career woman would have been unthinkable in the year 1700. Men performed all teaching, secretarial work, and literary endeavors; even the work considered unsuitable for men, such as nursing, was entirely unobtainable by the average woman. Women of means hired servants to perform the heavy load of daily housework and gave their efforts entirely to the shallow and superficial life of society. The only profession available to women was acting, and that was not respectable.

So women who were faced with the necessity of earning their own living were practically forced to enter domestic service; nursing was not considered a very desirable type of domestic service. The chief duties of a nurse in those days were taking care of the physical needs of the patient to make sure of reasonable cleanliness, although this was not considered essential in early municipal hospitals. Dressings were applied by dressers or by surgeons; the dispensing of medicines was the responsibility of physicians and the apothecary.

Oppression of women has a long history and indirectly thwarted any advancement of the nursing profession for centuries. Nursing existed in a low and dismal state, without organization and without social standing. Nurses were considered the most menial of servants. They frequently worked 24 or 48 hours at a time, and their pay was insufficient to support themselves, not to mention dependents. The future for these women was bleak.

Early American Hospitals

Great discoveries in medicine and early immigration to America occurred around the same time as the Reformation, which split European nations into Catholic or Protestant states. The early Spanish and French explorers were Catholic and brought with them Dominicans, Franciscans, Jesuits, and later the nursing orders as missionaries. The care of the sick and wounded among friends and foes in the missions and the wilderness was largely their task. In the Spanish settlements, nursing was the responsibility of the monks, and a high degree of efficacy was never achieved.

English colonists organized institutions for the care of the sick and the poor after the pattern of their homeland—not so much out of Christian charity as for social

*Today many references are directed at current and potential nurses to "earn while you learn." Inherent in this phase is the implication that educational and employment recruiters are targeting lower socioeconomic groups. Put in respectable terms by academic institutions and professional organizations, this trend is referred to as "the career ladder."

convenience. After all, something had to be done with the unfortunate. In early days poorhouses and hospitals were housed under the same roof. The filth and squalor of some of the early hospitals are well documented and at the time existed in well-known hospitals that remain in existence today, such as Bellevue of New York City. Only the utterly destitute went to the hospital. Anyone who had a home or place to stay remained there when they were sick, and the mother or grandmother of the home, or trusted servants in well-to-do homes, provided nursing care. In some areas women gained a reputation for providing good nursing care and were sought to care for specific cases of sickness and confinement.

When the great European hospitals were flourishing, American hospitals were just being established. Clients included the sick, as well as casualties of the various frontier battles. People willing to accept this responsibility were usually connected with the numerous religious orders. For example, the Ursuline Sisters, who originated in France, went to Canada in 1639 to teach. They were accompanied by three Augustinian nuns who were to nurse the sick in a hospital yet to be established in the new land. However, as it turned out, nurses were needed so badly that the Ursuline Sisters gave up teaching and began nursing. Originally the hospital at which they worked was the Hôtel Dieu in Quebec, established in 1658. Although it is not known what communication took place, another group of Ursuline Sisters from France followed and came to New Orleans to assist with the rampant epidemics of yellow fever and smallpox in this seaport. The Ursuline sisters made a major contribution to nursing during such major epidemics. They established Charity Hospital of New Orleans in 1737, along with the numerous hospitals throughout the entire territory of Louisiana and up the Mississippi. A school of nursing was established at Charity Hospital, but not until 1894. Charity Hospital may be the oldest hospital in America that is still in operation. In its modern form it is known as Charity Hospital and Medical Center of Louisiana at New Orleans.

During the late 1700s and the first decades of the 1800s definite landmarks were established, namely the big "general hospitals" in Pennsylvania, New York, and Massachusetts, as well as Bellevue of New York. The Philadelphia Dispensary established in 1786 was the forerunner of the modern outpatient department and clinic for ambulatory patients. It was independent of any hospital and supported by civic-minded citizens of Philadelphia. It apparently was so successful that the idea soon spread to other American cities.

Nursing orders in eighteenth- and nineteenth-century America, such as the Sisters of Mercy, the Sisters of the Holy Cross, and the Irish Sisters of Mercy, established hospitals and practiced high standards of nursing at that time. On the other hand, American medicine in the eighteenth century was for the most part at a low ebb. Although numerous medical principles and discoveries emerged, there was a great lag between their discovery and application. Medical instruction continued along primitive lines, and physicians persisted in old habits.

Certain individuals stand out for making notable advancements. For example, Benjamin Franklin influenced American medicine not only by inventing bifocal glasses but also by preaching the use of fresh air and by helping in the foundation of the Pennsylvania Hospital. The American Medical Association, established much later, gradually brought medicine to its present standards.

■ INDUSTRIAL REVOLUTION IN THE MACHINE AGE (1700s AND 1800s)

Female Nursing Leaders

Women with social conscience and character continued to struggle against the oppression of women during this time. Social and physical ills endured by people in all the known nations of the world challenged some women to try to bring about change. Because various individuals worked on similar problems in relative isolation from those in other lands, they were unable to obtain much support from one another. One example among many is that of Mother Mary Catherine McAuley (1787–1841), the extraordinary Irish leader who founded the Sisters of Mercy, a religious order that by 1830 was increasingly emphasizing nursing. It seems unfortunate that such strong women as Mother McAuley and Florence Nightingale did not have the benefit of sharing one another's experiences. Mother McAuley's life waned in middle age from fatigue and illness contracted through her efforts to nurse the sick poor during the dreaded cholera and other epidemics. At the same time, Ms. Nightingale was still a very young woman struggling for freedom from parental and social constraints to explore a career in nursing.

The results of Mother Catherine McAuley's efforts did, however, have an impact on Ms. Nightingale's career. Mother McAuley believed that her Order needed to stand out from secular workers as little as possible to command a greater amount of respect. This did not detract from her close ties with the Roman Catholic Church and the religious expectations she had of younger women entering the Order. Members of the Sisters of Mercy were challenged to join the efforts of Ms. Nightingale during the Crimean War some 20 years after Mother McAuley's death. By this time the focus was on a new crisis, a new challenge, and new places in which to learn.

Emancipation of Women

The emancipation of women may be traced to the desire for personal freedom, which was one of the factors in the Industrial Revolution. It is part of the fight for human rights that was first audibly expressed in the eighteenth century and that became one of the principles of the French Revolution. It is a step that developed nursing from a craft into a profession as it is known today. Many attitudes of Florence Nightingale appear peculiar if one does not appreciate the difference between the social position of women at that time and the present. Therefore the emancipation of women forms part of the background required to understand the evolution of nursing.

In the United States during the seventeenth, eighteenth, and nineteenth centuries it was expected that women were to be not only excellent at housework but also expert nurses, using the folk traditions taught them by their mothers. During the nineteenth century the almost entirely male medical profession began attacking its own past, as well as traditional practices it saw as "old wives' tales," quackery, and superstitions. Recently these practices are all being reevaluated and viewed more critically in light of what is now recognized as the "natural" healing process. It has been discovered that many so-called "old wives' tales" were actually sensible and effective.

Marxist theory claims that nursing and housework were used by proponents of the capitalist mode of production to provide benefits to men and to the capitalist class. One may ask whether this male-oriented, capitalist tradition is the reason nurses have continued to be technical, doing things in a mechanical, orderly, *Hausfrau*-like fashion. By not understanding the dynamics of how nurses and women have systematically been conditioned to function in that role, it has been more difficult to get out of the old mold.

Until about 1820, the period during which the United States was first settled, the division of labor usually placed men in agriculture and women in manufacturing or some subsistence farm tasks as ways to make a living. During this period men looking for wives commonly placed greater value on physical strength than on other factors. If women went against accepted mores, for example by practicing healing, blaspheming, or breaking family discipline, they were sometimes burned as witches or banished. Early settlement of the American colonies was mainly by Protestants, whose emphasis on hard work shaped American values and is commonly referred to today as the American work ethic. In those days idleness was labeled a sin.

The American Revolution was a rebellion against the imperialistic hierarchical class system of the British. As a result, the Revolution had an impact on women. A sense of crisis helped break down traditional barriers of women's activities—women helped with boycotts, stepped into jobs when men were scarce, and organized care for sick and wounded soldiers. They remained subordinate to men, although they worked alongside men. Widows often carried on their husbands' learned craftswork, which under normal circumstances would have been unacceptable.

As inaccurate as prejudices can be, the beliefs themselves can provide insights into a society's values. During the mid-1800s there was a definite aversion by employers in the United States to hiring Irish girls for any employment, be it housework, nursing, or other jobs. Blacks were hired before Irish. The reason for this was that "colored" servants were considered more submissive than the Irish, whose reputation for docility under their English rulers was extremely questionable. One might speculate that this somewhat rebellious disposition laid the foundation for some of the recent strides made by nursing in Ireland and Scotland.

The American work ethic has undoubtedly had its effect on nursing as well and serves as the foundation for a need to be *doing* something. Many nurses today remember the time they spent fulfilling menial labor tasks, such as restocking supplies, assembling specific simple kits used daily, and cleaning and organizing work areas. Presently, nurses who step out of line with these expectations are often harshly punished, even to the extent of receiving lower ratings on performance evaluations and suggested pay increases.

Nurses like to be praised for their commitment and the jobs they perform. President Clinton did this at the American Nurses Association audience of delegates and Centennial Convention in August 1996. At this convention, a pictorial review of the ANA's first century, "Voices of the Past . . . Visions of the Future" was unveiled.* During the same year, a survey conducted by the *American*

*Ann E. Conway, "Clinton Praises Nurses for Commitment," *Nursing Matters,* P.O. Box 8056, Madison, WI, 53708 Vol. 7, No. 8, Aug. 1996, pp. 1, 12.

Journal of Nursing reported that 9 out of 10 nurses polled expressed serious concerns about the safety and quality of client care being given as a result of cost-saving measures in health care. Over a third of nurses stated that they would not recommend that their own family members receive care in the hospitals in which they themselves worked.* So while the President was praising them for their dedication, he represented a system that simultaneously was bringing the message, "We are proud that you work so hard, but you need to work harder and faster with fewer resources so that the quality of client care does not continue to decrease."

The model of nursing in Germany and, to some extent, the Scandinavian countries grew to fit into existing society and systems. Even today, training of nurses (particularly in Germany) places high focus on clinical experience and less emphasis on scholarly performance, text material, and theory testing. Rather than rebel as individuals against the system, German nurses tend to join unions to protest their wages, do their daily duties, and "roll with the punches."

Socialism and Social Legislation

By the end of the nineteenth century most men in Europe and North America had obtained the right to vote in government elections. Women's suffrage movements developed only after the male population won their rights. Social reformers of nineteenth-century Europe such as Karl Marx had a resultant effect on the United States as well. The chief enemies of the laboring class were considered to be old age, sickness, exploitation, and unemployment. Protection from these enemies had an indirect, if not direct, impact on nursing. Social legislation was built on political philosophies that reevaluated human rights and the basic premise that citizens are not chattel, that real power is not in the hands only of people with property or of men. Following this thought to a logical conclusion, women became increasingly unwilling to be "property" within the family unit or on the job. Nurses became less willing to be handmaidens of physicians or property of hospitals.

Before women could advance as a group, they had to be equal with men before the law. The original concept of the family was that of a unit led by a male household head; the change in legal concept recognized all members of the family as equivalent members of society. This change resulted from many individual laws pertaining to the franchise, permitted occupations, and the civil standing of women in the community. Some of these changes are listed as follows:

1. Women may acquire and hold property.
2. After 1925 a mother in England had the same rights of guardianship of her children as the father did.
3. Divorce laws changed in favor of the wife.†

Although changing laws gave women the same legal status of men, equal pay and positions lag behind in some fields.

The right to vote and the suffragist movement of the 1800s marked a significant advance and were accelerated by the antislavery movement. After the Civil War

*"AJN Survey Uncovers Critical Concerns Among RN's About Quality of Patient Care," *Nursing Matters,* P.O. Box 8056, Madison, WI 53708, Col. 7, No. 8, pp. 1, 16.

†Reciprocity is increasingly reflected in divorce laws. In some cases, customs changed before the law.

abolitionists pushed for a constitutional amendment granting voting rights to all male Americans except slaves. Feminist leaders such as Elizabeth Stanton interpreted the law to extend voting privileges to women but were unsuccessful at casting ballots in a subsequent election. Susan B. Anthony's arrest and trial aroused widespread public visibility and lent impetus to the feminist movement. Effort was invested at state and federal levels until the first state, Wyoming, granted women the right to vote in 1890. However, it was not until after World War I that the Nineteenth Amendment to the Constitution was ratified and became law. During this period new societies spread everywhere, public demonstrations were held, and militant tactics with parades, heckling of clergy during public appearances, marches, and hunger strikes testified to women's desire to come out of their mold and be recognized.

Education

When women were recognized equal before the law in decision making (voting), new opportunities for education opened up. Early in the nineteenth century it was difficult for women to obtain an education except through private tutoring. Such education was expensive and available to only a privileged few. Florence Nightingale was educated by her father and by travel and social contact. At that time there were no colleges to which she could have been admitted. If there had been, the evolution of nursing might have been quite different. As it is, the growth of colleges and universities for women has profoundly affected nursing education. Higher educational opportunities for women were available in women's colleges first, among them Oberlin in Ohio (1833), Wheaton in Massachusetts (1835), and Mount Holyoke in Massachusetts (1857). Many others followed in the next 30 or 40 years, outstanding among them being Vassar in New York in 1865.

During the latter part of the century, when higher education became more generally recognized, large numbers of institutions all over the country admitted women. Some of them were separate colleges for women; others were established within already existing universities, and some were coeducational. Tulane University of New Orleans and Western Reserve in Cleveland were the first universities to admit women (in 1887 and 1888, respectively), and others soon followed. The University of Chicago was established in 1893 on the basis of equal admittance of men and women. Not only did the number of women admitted to college increase during this period, but the educational standards of institutions admitting them advanced rapidly.

Following the trend of the time, the American Association of University Women was established in 1915. This organization is active in establishing fellowships for the advanced education of women, with the result that an increasing number of women have obtained the doctor of philosophy degree. Most of these women continue to pursue advanced teaching and research careers, although there are signs of more entrepreneurship among women educated at this level.

The participation of the nursing profession as a whole in the development of the education of women will be discussed in subsequent chapters. Note here that a significant number of women seeking professional education go into nursing. Thus the advances made in the education of women form an integral part of the professional evolution of nursing.

It is questionable whether the Industrial Revolution would have extended very far had it not been stimulated by new thought, which may be traced to the Reformation. In addition to the far-reaching religious aspects, the new stimulation of thought provided by freedom generated by the Reformation transformed ideas regarding government, politics, business, and philosophy. Locke and his concepts of individual prerogative, "due process," and the right to acquire and hold property led to the fundamental Protestant work ethic. In turn, the Protestant work ethic made possible the Industrial Revolution and profoundly influenced the development of nursing.

At the turn of the twentieth century, industrialism developed into the Machine Age. Because machines required manpower to operate them, increases in population were welcome and increased family size was an asset. The poverty of feudalism became a part of the past because people were no longer occupied simply with obtaining food and other basic commodities. Ample commodities were available for everyone living within Western civilization as a result of the productive power of the modern industrial structure. A new twist to this feudal system has reappeared as large companies locate in underdeveloped countries where women and child labor are used to cut costs of production. The resulting goods are then sold on the market to American consumers. Health care professionals must be genuinely concerned for the consequences of these dynamics.

However, even when there is enough to go around, poverty still exists. In industrial society, the two causes of poverty are (1) that society fails to provide an adequate distribution of its commodities or (2) the citizens at the bottom of the economic scale lack the capacity or education to acquire a reasonable share of the communal wealth.

The effects of industrialism and the Machine Age caused philosophers to question the conduct and rights of man. A concern for public health emerged as the new capitalists squeezed the workers and exploited them. Although workers were now free to hold contract and property, starvation wages made them less than free agents and they were unable to achieve a reasonable standard of living. Consequently, with the unhygienic environment of rapidly growing cities, the health of the population was jeopardized. The field of public health expanded. Organized health measures required more and better nursing; the Industrial Revolution and its collateral economic, political, and philosophical developments may be considered the soil that nurtured the growth of all the healing arts.

■ FLORENCE NIGHTINGALE

The dominant figure in the development of organized nursing is Florence Nightingale. At the time she made her mark in history, society had changed to the point that hospitals seemed amenable to a new profession, and there was a realization that the Protestant orders needed some organization similar to Catholic nursing orders, although with more freedom in various ways.

The training and organization of lay Protestant nurses began before Florence Nightingale made her contribution to nursing. But with her powerful personality, her vision, and her practical organizing ability she took the lead in the movement, placed it on a powerful foundation of organization based on sound educational principles and high ethics, and inspired it with an enthusiasm that gave to it an

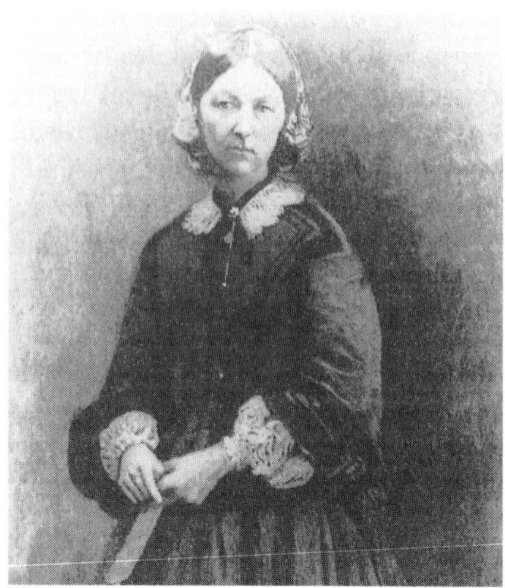

impetus under which it is still progressing. A few years before Miss Nightingale's time there was no professional nursing. At the time of her death nursing was a profession, a status that was formerly unthinkable.

Though Florence Nightingale is perhaps best known for her advancement of nursing, she also contributed to reforms in the Army and improved sanitation in India and public health in Great Britain. Her full stature cannot be comprehended unless attention is given to the following accomplishments.

Early Life and Education

Born in 1820 to Mr. and Mrs. William Edward Nightingale, Florence was their second daughter, named after the Italian city in which the family then lived. Having considerable wealth, Florence was brought up with good social standing, culture, and the best education available to children of that era. She learned French, German, and Italian, and her father personally instructed her in mathematics and the classics.

The Nightingales' permanent home was England, but they traveled extensively. Florence thrived on the many acquaintances and experiences she had as she traveled through France, Italy, and Switzerland. She was expected to enter society when she returned to England, but she desired a more satisfying life. Knowing societal attitudes about nursing, her parents discouraged her interest in pursuing such a career. Nevertheless, she persevered and planned to become a nurse at Salisbury Hospital not far from her home.

In 1844 Ms. Nightingale met the American philanthropist Samuel Gridley Howe and his wife, Julia Ward Howe, who later authored "The Battle Hymn of the Republic." The Howes stayed at the Nightingale family home and impressed Ms. Nightingale with an institution for the blind that Dr. Howe had founded in New York. In this facility he planned to make medical and nursing care available without payment to elderly and ill American citizens. At this time Florence explored the possibility of working in English hospitals much as the Catholic sisters did. However, no respectable English woman could expect to pursue such a vocation unless she were to enter the church, and Florence's family refused to discuss the matter further.

Until 1845 Florence believed that qualifications such as tenderness, sympathy, goodness, and patience were all that a nurse required. After experience in caring for some members of her family during their illnesses, she recognized that knowledge and skill were also necessary and that acquisition of these required education and training.

After a busy "social summer," Florence returned home to visit close friends of the family. This accomplished a dual purpose: (1) she explored life in a Catholic convent in preparation for nursing (though she remained deeply religious throughout her life, she was not converted to Catholicism; she remained within the Church of England) and (2) she met Mr. and Mrs. Sidney Herbert, through whom she was to go to the Crimea. The Herberts were deeply interested in hospital reform, and public opinion was shifting sufficiently to accept Ms. Nightingale's expertise regarding hospital reform, a subject about which she had collected data for a long time.

By the age of 28 Ms. Nightingale was expected to marry, but that did not happen. She continued to travel as opportunities presented themselves, and wherever she went she intently studied what she saw. After a trip to Greece and Egypt she learned about the institution in Kaiserswerth, Germany. Through some friends she received the Yearbook of the Institution of Deaconesses at Kaiserswerth in 1846. She studied it carefully and realized that here she could receive the training she wanted. Because the institution was under religious auspices and the character of the deaconesses and pastors were beyond reproach, she could go there without the stigma attached to the English hospitals.

Experience at Kaiserswerth

On one of her journeys Florence paid a visit to Kaiserswerth. She followed the visit by writing a 32-page pamphlet called *Institute of Kaiserswerth on the Rhine for the Practical Training of Deaconesses Under the Direction of the Reverend Pastor Fliedner, Embracing the Support and Care of a Hospital, Infant and Industrial Schools, and a Female Penitentiary.* She was impressed with the organization and high purpose of Kaiserswerth, but not with its training of nurses.

She assumed several administrative jobs, and each time she went back to the task of visiting hospitals and collecting data for reforming conditions for nurses. In the middle of the nineteenth century social reform was increasingly popular, and people such as the Herberts and their friends became interested in the reform of medical and social institutions. Ms. Nightingale realized that nursing reform required the organization of some type of school for the training of reliable, qualified nurses. As superintendent of nurses at King's College Hospital, among other administrative jobs, she saw the need for a new type of nurse.

Crimean War (1853–1856)

The Crimean War won Ms. Nightingale the title "Lady with the Lamp." The British, French, and Turks were fighting with the Russians, chiefly near the Black Sea and the Crimean Peninsula. There were serious problems with the handling of sick and wounded soldiers, especially by the British, and a leader was needed to organize an all-out effort to save lives of the wounded and sick. Thirty-eight nurses were recruited, some of them Roman Catholic sisters. Conditions under which these nurses worked were atrocious; even the simplest means of healthy living were absent.

At first Ms. Nightingale and the nurses did not have the respect and confidence of the physicians. This required time and evidence of what the nurses could do. Initially she and the nurses were virtually ignored by the physicians, but Florence insisted that the nurses not give help unless they were asked. Finally, as the fighting increased and wounded came in ever-increasing numbers, the physicians asked the nurses for assistance. Ms. Nightingale and her nurses set to work at once, and a hospital was established from what had been shambles. It had a staff of 125 nurses by the end of the war.

Nursing staff was expected to cooperate and not take charge. A nurse took orders from physicians only. Florence divided her time between administration and personal attention to clients. She became famous for her nightly rounds, performed after long days of work. It was during her nightly rounds with her lantern that she made her tour of inspection past the long lines of cots, with a friendly word to some, a smile for others. She inspired a feeling of comfort by sympathizing with the patients and striving to make their hard lot a little easier. Of all her activities in Scutari, these nightly rounds are perhaps the most famous and were immortalized by Longfellow in his poem *Santa Filomena,* in which he made reference to Florence Nightingale as "The Lady with a Lamp."

In addition to being a nurse, Ms. Nightingale was a social worker. She was concerned with recreational facilities for soldiers and their families and even developed a type of savings bank through which the soldiers might transmit money to relatives in England. Toward the end of the war she became ill with Crimean fever (typhoid, or typhus), from which she never fully recovered.

Two archetypal figures gained prominence at the end of the Crimean War: the common British soldier and the nurse. At the beginning of the war most British soldiers were regarded as the drunken immoral dregs of society, and the status of women in nursing was not much better. Ms. Nightingale's work in the Crimea did much to set the pattern for improvement of conditions for these two groups.

The significance of Ms. Nightingale's work in Scutari became known and understood far and wide in England; people realized that in the future nurses must be properly trained, and the nursing care of the sick must take its place beside the surgical and medical care. Accordingly, a public meeting to recognize Nightingale's work was held in London on November 25, 1855 under the presidency of the commander-in-chief, the Duke of Cambridge. As a result of the meeting, the Nightingale Endowment Fund was established for the purpose of furthering nursing education. The medical profession, which ultimately was to benefit so greatly from this undertaking, remained critical of it and did not enter it wholeheartedly.

In August 1856 Ms. Nightingale returned from Scutari, 6 months after the war ended. Her brilliant ambitions were hindered by her lack of physical strength. She did not recover from her malady and her stamina never returned. Some speculate she contracted neurasthenia. Others believe she suffered from an exhaustion neurosis because she never afforded herself sufficient rest. The amount of work she undertook with respect to her various full-time projects, including extensive army reforms, is truly staggering.

Ms. Nightingale published *Notes on Matters Affecting the Health, Efficiency and Hospital Administration of the British Army,* a volume of nearly 1000 printed pages, in 1856. Three years later, in 1859, she published a small book titled *Notes on Hospitals.* In 1860 the Nightingale School for Nurses opened as an independent educational institution funded by the Nightingale Endowment. Ms. Nightingale, devoted to the establishment of the school, chose Saint Thomas Hospital as the site and took an active interest in all details of the school for many years. In fact, this school served as the prototype for others established in the next 30 or 40 years.

Distribution of her books throughout the world enhanced her fame, and graduates of the Nightingale School disseminated her ideas. Graduates used her writings, such as *Notes on Nursing: What It Is and What It Is Not,* published in 1860, wherever they went. Graduates of the Nightingale School went to various countries of the world to practice, and many of them became head nurses in such countries as Germany, Norway, Sweden, Scotland, Canada, the United States, India, South Africa, and Australia. Her book *Notes on Nursing* was so much in demand that the year after publication two editions already existed in Sweden.

In Sweden the ideas of Florence Nightingale were imported by Emmy Rappe, a noblewoman who was sent to St. Thomas Hospital in London by the Organization for Care of the Wounded and Sick on the Field, for which she worked. After arriving back from London she was allowed to be the manageress for the education of nurses at the newly opened Uppsala Academy Hospital. Florence Nightingale's ideas became a reality in Sweden when emphasis was finally put on discipline, hygiene, and the importance of good care. The education of nurses improved the image of nursing so that well-educated women could proudly say that health care was a proper way of contributing to society.[31]

At the turn of the century Florence was nearly 80 years old; she spent the last 10 years of her life in a state of decline. She continued to be involved in health policy well into her eighties. Most official papers on Army sanitation and medical affairs were routinely sent to her for criticism. She became the first woman to receive the Order of Merit, in 1907, from the King of England. She continued to use her back bedroom in South Street, London, as the "Little War Office," as public officials referred to it, until she died quietly in her sleep on August 13, 1910. It was proposed that she be buried in Westminster Abbey, but according to her wish she was interred in the family burial place at Willows, Hampshire.

Nightingale Pledge

The Nightingale pledge (Box 1-2) has been taken by many professional nurses who are practicing today. Canadian-born Lystra Gretter, principal of the Farrand Training School for Nurses in Detroit, wrote the pledge in 1893. This pledge reflects Florence Nightingale's philosophy and style. At face value, its tone is incongruent with that of contemporary nursing. However, as stressed throughout this book, nurses must acknowledge their past to constructively plan a future in which society holds the profession, as well as those entering the field, in high esteem. As stated in the pledge, high moral and ethical standards are expected of professional nurses. The major issue that contemporary nurses may take with the

Box 1-2 The Nightingale Pledge

I solemnly pledge myself before God and in the presence of this assembly to pass my life in purity and to practice my profession faithfully. I will abstain from whatever is deleterious and mischievous, and will not take or knowingly administer any harmful drug. I will do all in my power to maintain and elevate the standard of my profession, and will hold in confidence all personal matters committed to my keeping and all family affairs coming to my knowledge in the practice of my profession. With loyalty I will endeavor to aid the physician in his work, and devote myself to the welfare of those committed to my care.

A committee of which Mrs. Lystra E. Gretter, R.N., was the chairman formulated this pledge in 1893. The 1893 graduating class of Farrand Training School, now the Harper Hospital Detroit, Michigan, was the first to take the pledge.

Nightingale oath is the expressed emphasis on "aiding the physician in his work." This does not mean subordination of nurses to physicians. In fact, all health care providers should aid each other. Nurses and physicians alike verbalize that more professional partnership is needed to provide good care from both a nursing and medical standpoint.

The implication of the pledge, however, is that nurses should assume a subservient relationship to physicians. Perhaps the old adage applies: "You become what you think about." To this day, some students admit to having to recite the Nightingale pledge as a requirement before graduation. This leads one to realize that the nursing profession will not advance if schools for nursing hold students and graduates to even "say the pledge for old times' sake." If nurses are to become what nursing leaders and organizations say they should become, they must lay claim to a more positive expression. Forward movement in nursing cannot happen if the Nightingale pledge is internalized as the prime aspiration in nursing.

Nurses in Germany, Sweden, Norway, and other European countries evolved from the Nightingale model, and conditions for them still reflect that foundation. They are primarily assistants with little latitude for independent thought. Nurses in Scotland and Ireland, on the other hand, shed many of the shackles that kept them subservient, dependent, and unable to determine their own destiny. In this way the latter group more closely resembles the American model of nursing.

▪ NURSING MOVES INTO THE TWENTIETH CENTURY

Nursing During the Early American Wars

The Red Cross, established in Italy in 1859, was inspired by the work of Ms. Nightingale during the Crimean War. It was established as an international body by diplomatic conference. In the United States the Civil War interfered with the establishment of the Red Cross; Clara Barton subsequently developed it in the United States in 1882. During the Spanish-American War (1898), American Red Cross nurses served on both land and sea.

Some Americans had heard about the Red Cross and Florence Nightingale's work in the Crimean War. When the Civil War began little organized information was available. Independent of the previous structure that existed to promote cleanliness and health, the U.S. Sanitary Commission was established in 1861. A branch of this commission opened a bureau in New York to examine and register nurses for war service; about 100 applicants were available as nurses to the federal army at that time.

When the war began this arrangement was totally inadequate, and the Surgeon General agreed to the organization of its own sanitary commission as a part of the army. The nurses were supplied by the Roman Catholic orders of the Sisters of Charity, the Sisters of Mercy, and the Sisters of Saint Vincent. Protestant nursing orders, including deaconesses, served in the war as well. But all this was not enough. It took women of great strength and insight to move nursing to a new level in a new century.

In the American army, as well as in other armies, two types of nursing developed: (1) a regular army nursing service, which was placed under the direction of Miss Dorothea Dix (1802–1887), and (2) an organization sponsored by private citizens, at first tolerated and later supported by the government. Ms. Dix was known for her crusade to improve conditions for the care of the mentally ill. In 1861 she was appointed superintendent of female nurses and proceeded to organize the first nurse corps of the U.S. Army. Ms. Dix was rigid in her standards, accepting nurses only under 30 years of age (preferably homely), requiring no uniform but insisting on black or brown dresses, and paying an allowance of $12 a month to each nurse. She herself served without pay. She found, as did Ms. Nightingale before her, that most nurses came from religious orders, both Protestant and Roman Catholic.

About 2000 nurses served in the Civil War, a number totally inadequate considering the primitive equipment and hospital conditions. Hygiene was atrocious: the approximately 6 million medical hospital admissions were mainly from epidemics and contagious diseases; only about 425,000 surgical cases were actual war casualties. In those days war claimed more victims from disease than from bullets. The war emphasized, especially in light of Ms. Nightingale's work, the desperate need for organized schools of nursing. Various such schools were accordingly initiated in New York City, Boston, and New Haven.

At the turn of the century, when trouble between America and Cuba was imminent, Congress authorized employment of nurses under contract. This was necessary because military nursing had not advanced since the Civil War and because no mechanisms existed by which the surgeon general could find nurses if needed. By 1898, when the Spanish-American War began, schools of nursing had been training young women for about 20 years. More than 500 schools of nursing graduated about 10,000 nurses by the year 1900. In 1900, 202 nurses were in the nurse corps, and the Army Reorganization Bill presented to Congress in that year provided for a permanent nurse corps as part of the medical department of the army. The Army Nurse Corps, specified as totally female, was created by law in 1901.

The International Council of Nurses (ICN), considered to be the oldest international organization of professional workers, began with an idea among nursing leaders at the Columbia Exposition in Chicago in 1893. In 1899 the ICN was founded, and a constitution was adopted the following year. The United States, Canada, Australia, New Zealand, and Denmark were some of the founding members. The number of national nursing member organizations of the ICN is around 100 and continues to increase.

The headquarters of the ICN is in Geneva, Switzerland, and the organization maintains official relationships with many international organizations such as the World Health Organization (WHO), UNICEF, the Red Cross, and others. It publishes a bimonthly official journal called *The International Nursing Review.*

Public health nursing was proposed as a Red Cross program by Lillian D. Wald as early as 1908. Public health nursing was initially confined to rural nursing, but by 1913 it extended to towns having populations as large as twenty-five thousand and became known as the Town and Country Nursing Service. In 1915 the first plan for training nurses' aides was proposed, but it did not develop fully until World War I.

Early Nursing Schools

The earliest schools of nursing in America were organized using Nightingale's criteria. First, they must be independent of hospitals. Clinical practice would occur in hospitals. Second, they must be administered by a director of nursing, preferably a nurse, with power and freedom to develop the school and a budget separate from that of the hospital. Finally, students should be housed in a facility separate from the hospital.

The schools were easily absorbed into the hospitals with which they were connected, however. An illustration of this development occurred in nineteenth-century Italy. During the 1850s sanitoriums were introduced in Pompeii and patterned after Roman convalescent homes. These were only for the wealthy. People who were poor had to resort to hospitals. During the next 50 years all of this changed radically because the use of anesthesia for surgery, germ theory, and biochemistry were all introduced in hospitals. Hospitals were becoming important as scientific laboratories. Now there were reasons for the well-to-do also to go to hospitals—because the services they needed could be obtained only there. At this point nursing became a hospital-based profession, and nurses may be credited with establishing the scientific basis of sterile technique.

Even today some would say it is nurses, not physicians, who really determine the quality of day-to-day hospital care.[48] This stage of professionalization of nurses was a prerequisite to the rise of the modern hospital. All of this made the hospital a natural place to learn, so schools of medicine and nursing developed there. Therefore the history of nursing in America is inextricably bound with the growth and development of hospitals. Contrary to the Nightingale model, which gave birth to independent schools of nursing, most of the schools at this point were created and conducted by hospitals to serve their needs; the education of the nurse became a by-product of her service to the hospital. Hospitals rapidly discovered that nursing students were a source of free or inexpensive labor under the guise of "practical experience."

In 1874, Ms. Linda Richard, America's first "trained nurse," instituted the system of keeping written records and orders, which has since become a requirement in all nursing schools. Later, uniforms were introduced. A *Manual of Nursing,* published in 1876, was the first text for nursing students and provided their first formal instruction. It was subsequently improved upon in other manuals that appeared in subsequent years.

As early as 1909, there were 1105 hospital-based diploma schools of nursing. A developing dialectic force in nursing led to the establishment of the first collegiate school of nursing at the University in Minnesota in that year. In 1917 *A Curriculum Guide for Schools of Nursing* was published, and it was revised in 1927. University standards for nursing education were refined,and modern nursing began to evolve.

Educational requirements are just one way that a profession such as nursing is distinguished from other occupations. In 1915 Dr. Abraham Flexner read a paper before the National Conference of Charities and Correction in which he set down certain criteria that have ever since formed a basis for judging whether an occupation has attained professional status. According to his interpretation of the professions, (1) they involve essentially intellectual operations accompanied by large individual responsibility; (2) they are learned in nature, and their members are constantly resorting to the laboratory and seminar for a fresh supply of facts; (3) they are not merely academic and theoretical, however, but are definitely practical in their aims; (4) they possess a technique capable of communication through a highly specialized educational discipline; (5) they are self-organized, with activities, duties, and responsibilities that completely engage their participants and develop group consciousness; and finally (6) they are likely to be more responsive to public interest than are unorganized and isolated individuals, and they tend to become increasingly concerned with an achievement of social ends.[37]

During the 1920s and 1930s, in an effort to eliminate wartime activities, the number of nurses in the army and navy was reduced. These were important years for nursing because, during this period, nurses became aware that they are a potent social power and recognized nursing as something far more comprehensive than taking care of the sick. An equal emphasis was placed on the prevention of illness. Documents by nurses of this period include *Nursing as a Profession,* prepared by Dr. Esther Lucille Brown under the auspices of the Russell Sage Foundation, published in 1936 and revised in 1940. In 1936 the National League of Nursing Education published a manual, *Essentials of Good School of Nursing.* In the same year the Council of the American Hospital Association's division of nursing and a committee of the league published *Essentials of a Good Hospital Nursing Service.* Although the profession demonstrated a desire to improve education for nurses, a major handicap was the lack of qualified nurse educators. The National League for Nursing published a manual in 1933 called *The Nursing School Faculty: Duties, Qualifications and Preparation of its Members.*

Professional nursing organizations developed to (1) control conditions of training, work, and compensation, (2) disseminate new knowledge affecting nursing, and (3) maintain communication—through alumni associations, for example. Two professional nursing organizations are the American Nurses Association and the National League for Nursing (NLN). NLN concentrates on standards of nursing education, entrance requirements of students, and accreditation of schools of nursing.

Impact of the Great Depression

Wars accelerate the need for nurses and emphasize the necessity for better nursing service; but for nursing the years between World Wars I and II were anything but quiet. The Great Depression began in the United States in 1929 and was followed by a worldwide depression in the 1930s. The New Deal, designed and implemented by President Franklin D. Roosevelt, called for measures to provide relief from the effects of the crashed economy. The Federal Emergency Relief Administration distributed funds to the needy of the nation; this distribution was accomplished at the state level and was a program in which many nurses participated. Other programs involving nurses were the Civilian Conservation Corps, designed to employ young people in reforestation and soil conservation, and the Federal Civil Works Administration, which created jobs for the unemployed. Many nurses worked in government-supported health care. Nursing made a major contribution to society and, during the Great Depression, in turn, furthered its own development not only in the United States but also internationally.

Before the economic crash the Rockefeller Foundation, because of its interest in public health and preventive medicine, financed a committee for the study of nursing education. Organized in 1918, this committee's report encompassed a study of the entire field of nursing. It was called *The Goldmark Report* (sometimes referred to as *The Winslow-Goldmark Report*), named after Josephine Goldmark, whose social research skills were used while she was secretary to the committee chairman, Professor C.E.A. Winslow of Yale University.

■ BEGINNING OF CONTEMPORARY NURSING

Shortly before World War II, curricula in schools of nursing were being readjusted to meet contemporary situations. More emphasis was placed on social sciences. The preventive and social aspects were integrated in the clinical programs, as were mental hygiene and health teaching. More community experiences were recommended for all students. In 1940 a joint committee of the NLN and the ANA published a pamphlet titled *Administrative Cost Analysis for Nursing Service and Nursing Education,* which addressed the issue of increased cost of these programs. The accrediting program of the League progressed, and collegiate programs increased in number. In 1941 the first list of schools accredited by the National League of Nursing Education was published. In the same year, through the efforts of the National Nursing Council and the Committee on Educational Policies and Resources and with the cooperation of the U.S. Public Health Service under the sponsorship of Representative Frances Payne Bolton of Ohio, Public Law 146 was introduced; it was passed by Congress in 1943. This provided the first government funds for the education of nurses for national defense. Under the terms of the act, 1000 graduate nurses were given postgraduate preparation, and 2500 nonpracticing nurses were given refresher courses. The goal was to increase enrollment in over 200 basic schools of nursing.

Early in 1942 a plan introduced the U.S. Cadet Nurse Corps, and in July the bill known as the Bolton Act became a law. The main purpose of this act was to prepare nurses in adequate numbers for the armed forces, government and civilian hospitals, health services, and war industries through appropriations to qualified institutions. The programs were supervised by a newly created Department of Nursing Education in the U.S. Public Health Service, with Lucille Petry (Leone), as chief director, responsible to the surgeon general.

Nursing During World War II

Nursing in World War II differed from nursing in any other war. Tremendous advances in medical science and the widespread activities of personnel in the different branches of the military presented a challenge and a great responsibility to the Army and Navy Nurse Corps. In World War II army and navy nurses served in every part of the world. World War II has been described as a "total war," and as such nurses had to be trained under combat conditions and had to know how to adapt techniques to meet changing conditions. The medical department worked as a team so successfully that 97% of all casualties were saved, and the death rate from diseases was reduced to 5% of what it had been in World War I. In 1944 full military recognition was given to the nurses of World War II, and they became a permanent part of the regular military force. Colonel Julie O. Flikke, superintendent of the Army Nurse Corps from 1937 to 1942, was the first woman colonel in the U.S. Army. In 1942 she was succeeded by Colonel Florence A. Blanchfield. Training for all military nursing personnel was the responsibility of the Office of the Surgeon General. Direction of the Navy Nurse Corps was under the chief of the Bureau of Medicine and Surgery.

Post–World War II Developments

World War II stimulated many new advances in medicine and nursing. Psychiatry and neurology emerged as modern specialty areas. Physiologic research related to the design of protective clothing, and individual equipment was important because soldiers were exposed to extreme climatic conditions. Examples of research in this area include the following:

1. Determining water requirements in the heat
2. Developing cold weather clothing
3. Describing processes such as acclimatization and physical conditioning
4. Ascertaining the relationship between physical anthropometry and the human engineering of vehicles

Penicillin, discovered and developed by British scientists before World War II, was first used in military campaigns by the Allies in North Africa in 1943. Atomic research led to the development of the atomic bomb and nuclear research. DDT, first synthesized in 1870, was studied by the U.S. Department of Agriculture in 1942 and field-tested by the medical department in Naples in 1943, where it stopped a typhus epidemic. The following year army malaria control teams introduced DDT to control mosquitoes in the Pacific; DDT is still the primary insecticide for malaria control, although its use is discouraged today because of its toxicity and the crusade against it by environmentalists.

The opportunity to use wounded men as human subjects in scientific studies rather than to continue hypotheses based on the use of animal subjects led to many developments in understanding blood replacements, study of shock, and the process of resuscitation. As men returned from battle with hopes of leading normal, productive lives, prosthetic research development, education, and rehabilitation were stimulated.

The Korean War, from 1950 to 1953, prompted studies of frostbite, and correlations made during this time resulted in safer and more functional military and civilian cold-weather living. By the end of the Korean War helicopters had developed as a major means of evacuating large numbers of casualties, and they became widely used as ambulances and rescue vehicles during the Vietnam War and in the civilian world.

Medical care of dependents of military personnel required an enormous number of health care professionals, many of them nurses. This program expanded and

Box 1-3 Some Early Leaders of Nursing

- Isabel Hampton Robb (1860–1910) was one of the founders of *The American Journal of Nursing.*
- Lavinia Dock (1858–1956) campaigned against male dominance and its negative impact on the nursing profession.
- Mary Mahoney (1845–1926) was the first professional black nurse in the United States.
- Mary Sewell Gardner (1870–1961) is best known for the development of the National Organization for Public Health Nursing.
- Annie Goodrich (1876–1955) became a state inspector of schools of nursing, president of the International Council of Nurses from 1912 to 1915, and, later, dean of the Army School of Nursing when it was organized in 1918.
- Mary Breckinridge (1877–1965) founded the Frontier Nursing Service and was a public pioneer in nurse-midwifery and in bringing modern nursing to rural America.
- Isabel Maitland Stewart (1878–1963) was only recently recognized for her contributions as an educator, writer, organization worker, and important figure in international nursing affairs for 40 years.

became the Civilian Health and Medical Program of Uniformed Services (CHAMPUS). A new generation of army hospitals began in 1960 with the construction of 10 new facilities over the next 5 years. Restrictions on the promotion of Army Medical Specialists Corps and Army Nurse Corps officers were removed in 1967. In 1968 Congress changed the Army Medical Service back to the earlier Army Medical Department. Colonel Anne Mae V. Hayes, chief of the Army Nurse Corps, was promoted to the grade of brigadier general in 1970. She became the first female general in the U.S. Army. In July 1975 the Army Medical Department observed the bicentennial anniversary of the beginning of health care for the American soldier.

World War II stimulated the upward mobility of women; for the first time, top ranks were achieved by women in the armed services. The wars after World War II required nursing personnel in hospital evacuation sites, behind battle lines, on ships and aircraft carrying casualties back to the States, and in veterans' hospitals providing care to the mentally and physically disabled. This period was the beginning of contemporary nursing. Early leaders who helped move nursing into the twentieth century are listed in Box 1-3.

Nursing practice over this period of time developed into the following specialized areas:

1. Private duty nursing
2. Visiting nursing
3. Settlement nursing (work among the poor)
4. School nursing
5. Nurse clinician work
6. Anesthesia
7. Industrial nursing
8. Nurse-midwifery
9. Nursing in the federal government such as in the Armed Service, Veterans Administration, Indian Services, and the U.S. Public Health Service (now a department within the Division of Health and Human Services)

Nurses played an active role in the Korean War (1950–1953) and Vietnam War (U.S. involvement, 1964–1973). During Desert Storm (1990–1991) they established field hospitals, but they had already been assuming different leadership roles in other areas of the world for some time. Nurses involved in U.S. government foreign missions have helped take care of the millions of starving people and diseased infants, women, and children in underdeveloped and war-ravaged countries. This activity is sponsored by U.S. programs of food and medical supply and is often coordinated with United Nations and WHO efforts. With the closing of military bases and a major reduction in the numbers of military personnel at the end of the Cold War has come a parallel reduction in nurses in the military.

▪ KNOWLEDGE EXPLOSION, TECHNOLOGY, AND HEALTH CARE

Major factors influencing health care and the provision of health services have developed since World War II. Recently society has been witnessing a profound shift from an industrial to an information-based society, accompanied by countless shifts in power. The technology that has enabled this major revolution has forced us to rethink our values and assumptions about health care. These vast changes are incredibly complex and have begun to effect changes in health care that will continue for some time. These changes could potentially benefit nurses and the nursing profession.

New Knowledge

A surge of new knowledge has begun within the health sciences. Diagnosis and treatment have been undergoing revolutionary changes as a result of new developments in drugs and equipment and new research findings—not only in the physical but also in the psychosocial aspects of health care. Communicable disease control and child welfare programs that reduced the incidence of contagious disease are now drastically changed. New communicable diseases such as the human immunodeficiency virus (HIV) are threatening the entire population, and published statistics regarding infant mortality and morbidity have put the United States to shame, compared with some other nations. Whether such comparisons between nations are valid will be briefly discussed in Chapter 14.

Technologic developments refine the quality of care that can be provided but make the administration of that care far more complex. Renal dialysis, heart-lung machines, monitoring devices of numerous kinds, closed-circuit television, computers, and radioactive isotopes preceded artificial organs and organ transplants. All of these developments demand rigorous scientific training of responsible health personnel.

Information is also increasingly accessible to the general public. People now expect to know more about what is wrong with them, the medications they take, and the tests they undergo. The number and availability of books, television and radio programs, and on-line computer networks support this. Health care personnel are becoming less trusted because of books such as *The Great White Lie: Dishonesty, Waste and Incompetence in the Medical Community*,[12] which describes how America's hospitals and physicians betray people's trust and endanger their lives. Even columnist Ann Landers has received letters describing the understaffing of nurses at the same hospitals that construct new buildings and actually purchase additional small hospitals rather than pay for an adequate number of nurses.[12] *In Sickness and in Wealth: American Hospitals in the Twentieth Century,*[75] describes the state of crisis of the entire hospital system/industry. Throughout this century the voluntary not-for-profit hospitals have been maximizing profit although they had been portraying themselves as charities serving communities. Not to be forgotten are the stories of unnecessary operations, especially on women.

This is an era of seeming contradictions. In an age of bottled water, no-fat foods, and vitamin-filled pet foods, young parents are not necessarily supporting the companies that promote baby foods that are "natural" and are free of added sugar, salt, and fillers. Gerber Product Company sales surpass Growing Healthy and Earth's Best Inc. Much has been done to increase child safety in past years with the development of child-resistant packages. These first came on the market almost 25 years ago. The one problem with this precautionary safety is that often the packages not easily accessed by children are also not easily accessed by older people. To eliminate the problem that older people experience with these "child-proof" containers, the bottles are often left open or the contents transferred to an easily opened container. The Consumer Product Safety Commission has credited more careful packaging with reducing the number of child fatalities from accidental poisonings, but made a change in packaging to apply more safety precautions for protecting children under 5 years of age. It added the stipulation that the package must not be difficult to open for persons ages 18 to 45, and persons ages 50 to 70 must be able to open the package within 5 minutes the first time and then within 1 minute on a second try.

Adverse Effects

New health care knowledge is introducing cost-cutting techniques that managed care companies are implementing—some of which are not in the best interest of clients. Managed-care companies are encouraging the increased use of high-dose, high-powered psychiatric drugs instead of psychotherapy to decrease costly time of the latter. Cheaper when bought in large volumes, giant-size doses of the newer psychotropics such as Prozac, Lithium, and Paxil may seem to the economist the logical approach to cost-cutting, but not to the individuals and society who must live with the unintended consequences and a culture of apparent drug abuse. This may well be the situation with which nurses will very soon be confronted. As advocate for the client, what is the nurse to do? Is it possible for a change to be brought about when the bottom line is the monetary savings and the stretching of limited health resources to all people?

There is already evidence that when HMOs say no to health coverage, more people are taking them to court. Some of us see a revolt against cost-conscious medicine. Even though it may be saving money, it is considered bad. Attorneys are being contracted either when routine care is denied or after people pay out of pocket for the needed care and sue later. Cases are often arbitrated, but others actually make it to the courts until the persons suing are satisfied with the results.

With the aging of the population, children are having to face the possibility that they may be required to care for their aging parents. Persons at about age 50, whose parents are nearing the age of 80, often learn that they have new responsibilities. With a chronic illness like Alzheimer's, the parent probably has a number of years

> **How or Why?**
>
> We often hear people giving advice on how to live longer; but they have little advice on why.

during which care will be needed. It becomes a part of the adult child's responsibility, and perhaps even budget, to contribute to the care of the parent. When the parent is receiving support from such programs as Medicaid, some states such as Arizona have already made such suggestions. Adult children with incomes over the state median (approximately $20,000 to $40,000 per year) are the most likely to be targeted for assuming the financial responsibility for care of their parents.

This is an era of food consciousness in America. It will probably go down in history as an era of eating. Eating too much is easily translated into eating way too much. The "couch potato" culture of the grade-school student and his ever-working parent is all too familiar. The popularity of the "all-you-can-eat" meals of restaurants and restaurant chains is an American eater's attraction. Both living in the land of plenty and depression because life has not doled out "plenty" can lead to the same result . . . becoming overweight. The diagnosis *morbidly obese* is a peculiarly American diagnosis.

Because of increased costs of medical care, questionable outcomes, and the "do-it-yourself" attitude that has resulted from the democratization of knowledge, some results have been less than positive. In the United States today a network of illegal pharmacies has developed, mainly dealing with drugs for AIDS (acquired immunodeficiency syndrome). This is a black market distributing useless and even dangerous drugs offered as treatment to desperate AIDS victims. These are untested and potentially harmful herbal remedies.

There seems to be a double standard on the part of the public, which on the one hand demands more stringent controls on manufactured drugs yet on the other hand supports the herbalists for substances, sold over the counter and in health-food stores, that have no standards of usefulness and safety applied. The frustration with a costly and unrelenting medical and drug system may well have driven people to a point of desperately trying anything.[48]

Basic Change in Attitude Toward Health Care

A basic attitudinal change stems from the philosophy of WHO, which defines health as more than the absence of disease, but rather as a state of physical, psychologic, and social well-being. WHO proclaims that health is a right, not a privilege, to which individuals are entitled—even though the present system in the United States often does not seem congruent with the philosophy. It is a common belief in the United States that health care should be oriented toward prevention, yet its overall focus, including resource distribution, is on treatment of disease. Modern mass media has reinforced the latter and has increased public awareness of disease and health problems, even though the information presented is sometimes inaccurate.

Although health care is provided in schools, industries, and public clinics, it is often superficial. Health maintenance organizations have not become a favorite means of obtaining necessary health care for the majority. National health insurance proposals contain inadequacies. Nursing homes have proliferated and can usually provide maintenance or skilled nursing care for the chronically ill and elderly, yet workers in these facilities often earn minimum wages while the cost to the client far exceeds personal means or even expenditures of life savings.

Our society's performance in the area of disease prevention is equally questionable. There are currently nine vaccine-preventable diseases: measles, mumps, rubella, diphtheria, tetanus, pertussis, polio, hepatitis B, and influenza type B. However, it seems that people in the United States do not place great value on using vaccines, as evidenced by a nationwide epidemic of measles in 1989 and 1990 that resulted in numerous deaths. The goal is to have 90% of children immunized by age 2. Despite the low cost and public availability of vaccines, it has been reported that only 42% of inner-city infants under age 2 are fully immunized. The United States has an overall immunization rate that is lower than that of 69 other countries, almost equaling the rate for children in Bolivia and Haiti.[19]

There is a parallel problem: children who do not get immunizations also do not get well-baby checkups, so preventive care is lacking. It takes a total of six visits to receive complete immunization against all nine vaccine-preventable diseases. The Comprehensive Child Immunization Act of 1993 addresses this need and points to establishment of a federal universal vaccine-purchasing program in 1995 to ensure that children are vaccinated on schedule.

Additionally, the American public's debate regarding whether terminally ill clients should have a right to reject medical treatment or to receive aid from their physicians in hastening their deaths has taken on a new prominence as a result of a number of developments. With the availability of new health technologies, Americans no longer die from the slew of illnesses and infirmities that were common causes of death 100 years ago. Now, however, the cost of caring for the dying and how to best enforce advance directives ("living wills") are burning issues. Americans frequently die with less dignity than they did in days when ravaging diseases typically ended their lives quickly. One result of this is the publicity surrounding a series of trials of Dr. Jack Kevorkian of Michigan for his involvement in physician-assisted suicides.

Health Care Personnel Supply and Distribution

Harry S Truman, president of the United States from 1945 to 1953, envisioned a health care team that consisted of physicians, dentists, nurses, and various allied health professionals. He recognized the need for specialization but also acknowledged that increased specialization created a need for allied workers to serve as auxiliary workers, especially in the specialized areas of prevention, psychiatry, and rehabilitation.

One difficulty in providing adequate care for everyone in the United States is that health workers and health facilities are usually located in urban centers. Better distribution of institutions and personnel is a problem that has been recognized and studied by medical, nursing, state, regional, and federal health organizations. Numerous approaches have been tried to deliver health care to underserved populations. Satellite clinics, mobile units, high-tech communication methods, and rapid means of transportation such as helicopters are used to bring client, patient, and health care professionals together. Rural health teams are an example of the cooperative system of health care delivery in which nurses play a more active part in coordinating efforts and skills of various health care professionals. To meet the needs of rural communities, the nation's first Rural Health School was opened at the University of Minnesota in 1996. Medical, pharmacy, nurse practitioner, and physician assistant trainees are beginning 3-month clinical rotations in the rural communities of New Ulm, Moose Lake, and Grand Rapids, Minnesota. These nurses specialize and at the same time continue to address the needs of the general population that they serve. In this role the nurse is challenged with much more independent practice and responsibility.

Decreased Hospitalization

Incidence of disease has changed vastly, and the emphasis of care has shifted to the home or early discharge from the hospital when hospitalization is necessary. Follow-up care is provided in clinics or by home health nurses. Long-term illness is managed through outpatient and extended care facilities.

Prevention has been a household word for a long time. The founders of Kaiser Permanente believed that prevention was indeed the answer to affordable health care. This health system was established during the late 1930s and 1940s for construction, shipyard, and steel mill workers employed by the Kaiser industrial companies. Kaiser Permanente developed public enrollment into the programs in 1945, starting clinics in California during the 1960s. Since then, many different approaches to health maintenance organizations (HMOs) may have been used, but this one continues to survive. As of 1997, Kaiser Permanente was the largest HMO in the country and served 19 states. Kaiser Permanente has served as a prototype for the burgeoning number of HMOs currently being developed for the purpose of improving accessibility to affordable health care.

Alternative Health Care

As health care costs have increased and many people have felt they could not afford to go to clinics for their various complaints and ailments, they have attempted to find their own solutions. Not unlike their grandparents before them, they rediscovered ways in which discomforts and illnesses were treated before the advent of modern technical medicine. Alternative health care is on the rise also because the traditional medical model does not always alleviate people's afflictions.

Use of alternative therapies is increasing. According to *The New England Journal of Medicine,* more than one in three Americans used some form of alternative therapy in 1990, and the trend continues without weakening. At least 25% of Americans use alternative medicine, even excluding those people who were enrolled in commercial weight loss programs or taking part in self-help groups such as Alcoholics Anonymous. In 1990 alone Americans spent $13.7 billion on unconventional therapies—more than their $12.8 billion annual out-of-pocket hospitalization expenses. For purposes of the study, unconventional medicine was defined as "medical interventions not taught widely at U.S. medical schools or generally available at U.S. hospitals."[30] Examples of such remedies include acupuncture, chiropractic, homeopathy, and herbal medicine.

The mainstreaming of alternative medicine is a global development. According to the traditional American medical viewpoint, drug therapies, surgery, psychotherapy, and recommendations about daily hygiene are considered conventional. Almost everything else is regarded as alternative medicine. This distinction has become increasingly less clear in the United States and especially in Europe. In France and Germany the most popular prescription drug is *Gingko biloba*—an extracted herb with significant research supporting its effectiveness for cerebral insufficiency, senility states, and memory loss. Homeopathic medicines* are also used quite commonly in Western Europe.

At least some correlation exists between the increasing use of alternative therapies and the increasing emphasis on health maintenance. The conventional medical model defines health as the absence of symptoms. The problem with this approach is that by the time symptoms are treated, the measures necessary to return the person to health are often more expensive and complex than preventing the disease in the first place. The alternative medical model, on the other hand, stresses that health and disease are a continuum; health is defined as a positive state of physical, emotional, and mental vitality. As Americans seek to avoid the increasingly expensive costs of hospitalization, the alternative medical model's approach to health as a process, rather than a static state, may help them lead healthier lives (Box 1-4).

Diagnostic techniques and treatment were the sole domain of physicians until recently. Pharmaceutical books and disease descriptions were contained in their pocket manuals and were kept to themselves. This state of affairs has changed astonishingly—not by the choice of medical practitioners but by the public, who insist on knowing more about their bodies, what is wrong with them, and how to take care of themselves. Anyone is challenged to visit an ordinary pharmacy without finding published materials available for purchase by the public. One small pharmacy carries *Doctors' Book of Home Remedies,* edited by *Prevention Magazine, Vitamin Bible,* and books on diabetes, arthritis, diet, and similar subjects.

On another visit to a local bookstore in a shopping mall, numerous shelves of health-related books were found. One section was totally dedicated to books on diet and exercise, with many titles that implied self-help for loss of muscle tone, obesity, diet, and illness and disease prevention—particularly heart disease and cancer. Another section was predominantly filled with books on stress reduction, yoga, oriental approaches to pain control, and related materials. A further section included books such as *The Natural Remedy Bible,*[51] a pocketbook containing discussion and presentation of natural remedies for common ailments. The use of old-fashioned mustard plasters were included for specific symptoms. There were logical treatments for dandruff, bursitis, and fungal infections such as "jock itch." Hydrotherapy and Sitz bath treatments for hemorrhoids and treatments for certain female symptoms were described.

Above these were more sophisticated handbooks and textbooks, most of which were not available to the general public even 20 years ago. *Diseases and Disorders: The American Medical Association Family Medical Guide* and *Consumer Reports Books Complete Drug Reference* (produced by the United States Pharmacopeial Convention, Inc.) are examples that seemed to be comprehensive and well-written for the

*Homeopathy: a school of medicine that assumes that an effective medicine will cause effects in the healthy person similar to symptoms of illness. The inducement of these effects by administration of small doses of homeopathic drugs is believed to augment the body's inherent defensive response.[84]

Box 1-4 Comparing Assumptions: Conventional versus Alternative Models

	Conventional Medical Model	Alternative Medical Model
Definition of health	The absence of symptoms: a person is either healthy or not healthy	A positive state of physical, emotional, and mental vitality: health and disease are a continuum (we are always, to some degree, sick)
View of the body	Works mechanistically as a biochemical, physiologic entity	Not only a biochemical, physiologic entity; also surrounded by and suffused with energy fields (*chi, ki,* vital force, bioenergy)
View of symptoms	Evidence of breakdown	Evidence of the body's defenses
View of disease	An entity	A process
Source of knowledge	Derives initially from laboratories	Derives initially and primarily from clinical practice
Diagnostics	Practitioner relies on rational analysis of objective data and reductionistic interpretation of data. Diagnosis is based on the symptoms that fit a specific disease category. For example, a person with indigestion is examined by a medical doctor, who orders various tests, diagnoses a peptic ulcer, and prescribes drug treatment for the ulcer	Practitioner relies on subjective empirical findings and holistic assessment. Diagnosis is based on the idiosyncratic symptoms that fit a special body-mind pattern. For example, a person with indigestion is examined by a homeopath or an acupuncturist, who asks the person to describe all (not just digestive) physical and psychologic symptoms, makes various objective observations, provides an individualized treatment based on the totality of symptoms, and, if appropriate, refers the person to an internist for a conventional workup
Treatment	Seeks to excise disease tissue infecting organisms, and inhibit, manage, or control symptoms	Seeks to augment the person's own immune and defense processes
Role of practitioner	The authority	A partner

From Ullman D: The mainstreaming of alternative medicine, *Healthcare Forum Journal* November/December 1993.

average intelligent American citizen. At the very top of the display was the *Physicians' Desk Reference,* among other more sophisticated resources. This strongly points to a future in which self-help treatment, prevention, and individual responsibility will be standard.

Population Trends

Between 1900 and 1952 the nation's population doubled. After World War II impetus was given to the family-planning movement. Because of new awareness, readily available contraceptive methods, and society's desire to limit the rate of population growth, U.S. population growth was reduced to zero in 1973. This reversal of the population explosion, partly a result of the continued emancipation of women, resulted in closure of elementary and secondary schools. The population changes created a shift in focus to clinical facilities to care for the older age group, and caused difficulty for nursing students trying to obtain obstetric and pediatric clinical experiences.

Increased longevity has changed the health care delivery system. Statistics indicate that the number of persons 65 years of age or more increased from 3 million to 11.5 million between 1900 and 1952; by 1960 it reached 15.5 million. By 1990 the number had risen to over 31 million. This rise in the number of older Americans is only partly offset by the overall population growth in the United States. In 1940 Americans over age 65 constituted only 7% of the population; in 1997 they make up 13%.* That means that 34,044,000 persons of the total U.S. population of 267,368,000 are over the age of 65. The oldest age group, those over the age of 85 years, is a rapidly growing group. In 1900, 122,000 people were 85 years old or older. Their number had increased to 3 million by 1990; this is comparable to the 3 million persons over the age of 65 in 1900. In 1994, 10% of the nation's elderly (over 65 years of age) were 85 or over. This means that in 1994 only 1% of the American population was over 85. However, the projections are that this number will increase to 18.9 million (almost 20%) by the year 2050. One can only make conjectures about the impact that this trend will have on the nation's health and social service systems.* In 1991 the overall life expectancy was 75.5 years, in spite of an increase in HIV transmission and homicide.[24]

Two thirds of deaths in 1991 were caused by the three leading causes of death in America: heart disease, cancer, and stroke. Cancer deaths decreased only by a slender 3% between 1991 and 1995. Drugs to control cholesterol are effective but expensive, so in this cost-cutting time the impact that these drugs will have on heart disease and stroke remains uncertain. Deaths from HIV infection, crime and legal intervention, and chronic obstructive pulmonary disease and allied conditions are increasing. (They increased 15.3%, 6.9%, and 2%, respectively, from 1990 to 1991.) Causes of death vary according to ethnic group. For example, the leading cause of death among the black community is crime; this is not the case in other

---

*U.S. Bureau of the Census, Decennial Censuses for specified years and Population Projections of the United States by Age, Sex, Race, and Hispanic Origin: 1993 to 2050, Current Population Reports, P25-1104, U.S. Government Printing Office, Washington, DC, 1993. Data for 1990 from, 1990 Census of Population and Housing, CPH-L-74, Modified and Actual Age, Sex, Race, and Hispanic Origin Data.

groups. Indications are that alcohol-related deaths and injuries decreased since 1990, although roughly 40% of persons will be involved in an alcohol-related traffic accident during their lifetime.

There is increasing concern about HIV subtypes. Researchers have spent billions of dollars trying to develop vaccines based on HIV envelope proteins. For the first time in 15 years, researchers realized remission in AIDS in 1996. Treatment with triple-drug regimens combining new protease inhibitors with first-generation drugs can now suppress the virus to a level at which it is hardly detectable. This gives some AIDS patients a new lease on life, but 90% of the world's AIDS sufferers will be excluded from this treatment because of its cost. Researchers continue to learn more about the deadly virus and its subtypes, more questions are raised, and hope continues that an inexpensive treatment will be found as the disease continues to ravage large populations, including women, children, and the unborn. Organ transplants have also had a setback as a result of complications presented by HIV. It seems that when people sense a ray of hope from intense research efforts in one area, new problems loom, and progress is thwarted in another area of health.[24]

Changes in morbidity and mortality patterns indicate that today's nurse needs a different type of preparation from nurses of 50, 25, or even 10 years ago. Heart disease and cancer are still the leading causes of death, despite an increase in HIV and related diseases, such as tuberculosis. This era may go down in history as the war on drugs. Significant progress has not been made in that war. President Clinton's Republican opponent charged him with having "surrendered" in the drug war, leaving the world more awash in illegal drugs than ever.* AIDS and deaths related to narcotic and drug abuse are relatively new to the health scene.

Chronic problems associated with the increased incidence of degenerative diseases are more frequent. Alzheimer's disease and mental decline are becoming of great concern to Americans and others. As longevity increases so does the risk of living out the "golden years" with degenerative brain dysfunction. Throughout history people have sought the fountain of youth, and so it continues today. In 1975 researchers found that aspirin in low dosages helped avert heart attacks in people with heart disease. As evidence continues to support the positive effects of the drug aspirin to fend off such diseases as heart attacks and strokes, the quest for more evidence is sought regarding its possible impact on warding off cognitive disorders such as Alzheimer's. After all, physical well-being is as important as optimal mental functioning.† Alcoholism and other addictions, mental illness, and child and elder abuse are just some of contemporary society's other problems that nurses help prevent and treat.

Prevention and better treatment are replacing custodial care of the mentally ill. However, lack of finances, well-prepared personnel, and adequate facilities are making this change a slow process. Previously reduced maternal and infant mortality is on the rise, related to teenage pregnancy, lack of prenatal care, and use

---

*Gordon Witkin, "Why this country is losing the drug war," *U.S. News and World Report,* Sept. 16, 1996, p. 60.

†"Can Aspirin Help Block Alzheimer's? Maybe," Culture and Ideas, *U.S. News and World Report,* Sept. 16, 1996, p. 18.

of drugs and alcohol before and during pregnancy. Chemotherapy has revolutionized the treatment of many severe illnesses but has stimulated new strains of viruses and new diseases such as methicillin-resistant *staphylococcus aureus* (MRSA) infection. A common bacterium, *Escherichia coli* (0157-H7), has become a new threat. This bacterium, a normal inhabitant of the digestive systems of humans and animals, has now become the fourth leading cause of diarrhea. The reasons for this development must be reckoned with.[49] All of this demonstrates the dynamic state of health care and the internal and external pressures on nursing and other health services.

Growth of Junior and Community Colleges

The tremendous growth of junior and community colleges resulted from a population explosion after World War II and the increased demand for more institutions of higher learning. With the closure of 3-year diploma and 9 to 12-month licensed practical nurse (L.P.N.) hospital-based schools of nursing along with increased demand for nurses, junior and community college nursing programs came into their own. By 1970 nursing programs of this type increased 445%. Some are only state approved, whereas others are also NLN accredited. Junior and community colleges train various other auxiliary health personnel or provide portions of the preprofessional course of study. These institutions usually cost less, so it is financially more feasible for many students to obtain their education this way. These institutions are currently supported and used by health care facilities, especially large medical centers, as an inexpensive means of rapidly manufacturing nursing staff, regardless of quality. Graduates can earn prerequisites necessary to take the basic R.N. or L.P.N. license examination. Facilities can thereby satisfy minimum requirements in terms of hospital accreditation standards and federal and state criteria for funding and physically staff various units of the facility. Again the nurse is being manipulated; although on the positive side, this process may be a stepping-stone to a better education, independence, and an improved career.

Change takes place slowly and in cycles. This has been true throughout the history of nursing. The negative implications of the above-mentioned trend—lack of good education and conditions on the job—are documented. The task ahead includes better professional preparation, better formal education, and equal standing with other truly professional health care workers. The basic team from the beginning was and remains medicine and nursing. The formation of a true partnership between the two fields is addressed in the text that follows.

Continued Emancipation of Women

Not only are more women entering the labor force, but opportunities for employment in service occupations are also increasing. The predominately female occupation of nursing no longer has first claim on young women. Fewer women are entering this field now than in the 1950s and 1960s. Meanwhile the small fraction of male students in nursing seems to be increasing; however, the upward mobility of men in this profession still remains greater than that of women.

Medical schools still lag behind other programs in achieving true gender equality because of the traditional patriarchal system and the rigors that it perpetuates. With the issues of women's rights and sex discrimination coming to the fore, certain admission and progression criteria were bent, but not always in favor of those admitted nor the clients for whom they were responsible for caring. Now, as with the law profession and the sciences, the gender ratio has approached 50-50. Since this is a relatively new development in medicine, it will be interesting to learn how the nursing profession will be affected when the percentage of female physicians increases during the next decade and beyond. Will female physicians take a new view of nurses, or will they continue to demand the most money and power, as their male colleagues have for so long? Will female physicians be prevented from occupying positions of power so their voices will not be heard one way or the other? At this time, all remains open to speculation.

Women in any field are targets of sexual harassment. It is unfortunate that most female nurses will be harassed at some point in their career. The typical harassment scenario is still that of a power play by a person in authority (usually male), such as a physician, over a subordinate (usually female). This will gradually change as a result of current medical school admissions, which are increasingly more balanced between the sexes. Harassment can also be expected from clients, especially when they are male. Most female nurses and physicians who are sexually harassed by clients will tend to downplay the significance of any incident, fearing that complaining casts them as victims—as women first and professionals second. Since client harassers are often drunk or senile, targeted nurses or physicians assume that physical or vocal advances are unintentional. Yet men who are losing their physical or mental faculties often expose themselves to female nurses and physicians as a way of expressing their "ultimate male superiority." Some people still insist that a person's sexuality is more important than diplomas and credentials.

Perhaps the early emancipators of women visualized a world in which women and men would be equal in all respects of society. In fact, women have greater equality today than ever before. This has come about as a result of decades of work by activists, as well as related societal changes that have led to a continuing redefinition of "family" that incorporates greater equality between the members. As women carry more of the financial burden of running a family, anything that occurs in the overall job market affects them, especially downsizing. Downsizing on the one hand has caused unemployment and on the other hand has created opportunities for part-time employment that is often necessary to supplement family incomes. Employers have learned that workers often have to carry a second job to support themselves and their families. Part-time jobs at lesser wages are assumed by many nurses; such jobs are plentiful because they usually do not offer benefits and are consequently less costly to employers.

Adults living during the 1990s have been labeled "the Sandwich Generation." They are referred to in that way because they are taking care of both their children who are under the age of 18 and at least one parent or parent-in-law in their home. At the same time the concern over future responsibilities seems to be driving young people who are the potential parents of tomorrow to lower the anticipated number of children they plan to have. Increasingly more persons between the ages of 18 and 29 say they are not sure if they will have any or more children. This category of uncertain adults has doubled since 1989.*

*"Lifestyle Patterns," "Sandwich Generation" Isn't So Squeezed, *The Wall Street Journal,* Apr. 7, 1995, p. B1.

With a society on the move such as ours, children and relatives of the elderly are often far away from them. They are challenged to become long-distance caregivers. Maintenance of a successful support system that is able to keep up with the relative's physical and emotional state, as well as with his or her immediate living conditions, is required. Phoning, visiting, and running errands are some of the ways that long-distance care of the elderly is accomplished. In summary, long-distance caregivers often feel they are not doing enough, and telephone assurances from the elderly person saying, "Don't worry about me; I'm just fine" are not the most positive ends.

Many nurses in the workforce today are not only grandparents, but also become second-time parents. Three and a half million children live in such households.

■ HEALTH CARE REFORM

The average nationwide cost per day for a hospital stay is now $2400 for basic care. In 1994 the amount spent on health care per working American was already over $7000.[61] The costs have continued to rise so that in the past 5 years hospital costs alone have risen over 44.4%.[3] When health care costs rise, insurance premiums increase to pay the higher costs. This in turn has begun to exceed the ability of many citizens to pay for health insurance. The incredible, needless increases in health care costs are the root problem that has prompted the current efforts to reform the health care system.

Registered nurses and advanced practitioners can perform as much as 80% of health care for much less money than physicians charge. (See Chapter 16 for more discussion of this.) The high cost of care by physicians is partly a result of medical students' choice to specialize because of the much higher salaries specialists can command compared with general practitioners. Medical schools are now attempting to change this by promoting general practice. Physicians have traditionally had a much stronger lobby than nurses (or clients) in government, so sheer weight of power will continue to win over reason if the influence of physicians is not challenged.

Some nurses are publicly speaking out for extensive health insurance for all Americans—advocating the most care for everyone. As a society, Americans are giving, and giving more when not everyone is satisfied. However, there is the other side of reality: there really is no Santa Claus, and someone has to pay. After years of indoctrination, the U.S. citizenry had at least partially believed that the health care system, and more particularly physicians, had all the answers. Now, with the health care reform proposals in the 1990s, this attitude is shifting to emphasize personal responsibility for one's own health. Individuals, by their own behaviors and lifestyles, have a significant effect on their own health. Now they are expected to take responsibility for the way they live. Individuals must learn associations between risks and consequences, and what they are expected to know must be reasonable.

One snag in all this is that to place cause-and-effect responsibility on the client, the future health care system must be relatively certain that clients have caused the altered health status by their own voluntary behavior and are not to be blamed for uncontrollable variables such as hereditary predispositions. Nursing has been supporting consumer involvement in health care. Now it is coming. Nurses must become even more cautious because their responsibility for consumer advocacy remains with the focus shifted to one of protecting people so that the reformed system is not used to justify unintended and harmful consequences.[70]

Official nursing organizations such as the ANA have made public their statements regarding the position of nurses. However, as one interacts with nurses in various settings, it becomes clear that many nurses agree neither with the health reform package proposed by President Clinton nor with the official position of the ANA and other organizations. Many agree that the system, as it exists now, perpetuates escalating costs and that a major reform is necessary. However, the change is becoming only a new form of the old system to appease ANA, AHA, and the established system. The real issue is being lost because the focus is on ways to ensure powerful voters' support in the next election. Nurse speakers may find it expeditious to support the official position or join voices with the masses of Americans concerned that what is currently happening seems to resemble the negative experiences of other countries with national health coverage.

One position is that by abating abuse of the present system and ensuring that all people have access to preventive care, the savings can cover needs of others. Many anticipate that such reform will pay for itself. However, to realize such savings an expanded federal system must be created to ensure compliance. Such a system then requires a new bureaucracy to manage it. The danger is that present inefficiencies will be replaced by new inefficiencies. The main difference is that people would be paying for their health care with new higher taxes instead of insurance policy premiums. The intent of such social programs may be good but distant from people, and when its actual recipients finally receive the benefits those benefits may scarcely be recognizable as compared with the original intent. For example, the AMA states that the elderly are not helped much by dialysis treatment. Statistics indicate that 9 of 10 individuals 55 years of age and older die within 5 years of beginning dialysis treatment. The quality of life is also not significantly improved as measured by their outside activity. A study at the State University of New York Health Science Center in Brooklyn reported only one third of elderly persons receiving dialysis were active outside their treatment, compared to 78% who were active 2 years before they began treatment. Based on such data, cutting health care costs will require asking some hard questions such as who should receive dialysis as well as all other life-saving care.[65]

Some such hard questions must be addressed. Perhaps nothing is wrong with a utilitarian approach to the present health care crisis. It is not less human to pay for costly care for persons meeting certain criteria and lessen the interventions to those elderly who really do not want to extend their suffering. By early next century it may be that Dr. Kevorkian's campaign for the right to die and to be assisted by a health care practitioner in bringing a terminal illness to an early conclusion will be seen as a civilized idea promoted by someone ahead of his time. Regardless of how far one speculates, vast changes will most certainly take place. The changes have the capacity to make the United States a great nation in which to live and work, or a disgrace to the world. It is at a crossroads.

Konner [48] says that the very best care money can buy is often the cheapest. Specialists and their procedures, including hospitalization itself, are dangerous and should be used only when absolutely necessary. The primary care physician who knows the client can more frequently use less drastic interventions successfully. This level of care does not require an M.D. degree. Depending on each individual state's laws, specially trained nurses such as nurse practitioners can do this job well, and that is when the primary care physician's and nurse's roles overlap. Nurses can play a much larger role in family practice, internal medicine, pediatrics, obstetrics, and gynecology. Collaboration between physicians and nurses in these areas is the optimal solution. This directly addresses the bias that has existed in medicine against primary care in favor of specialty areas—balance is needed. There is a great need for client and family involvement as opposed to the authoritarianism of the medical model. Above all, emphasis needs to be on prevention, and everyone needs to develop a sense of responsibility for his or her own care.

Nursing Informatics and New Technologies

One of the latest developments in the nursing profession occurred in January 1992 when the ANA Congress of Nursing Practice established nursing informatics as a district area of nursing practice. The aim of nursing informatics is to coordinate data and information by integrating nursing science, information science, and computer science. According to the ANA, "The purpose of Nursing Informatics is to analyze information requirements; design, implement, and evaluate information systems and data structures that support nursing; and identify and apply computer technologies for nursing. Nursing Informatics is concerned with legitimate access to and use of data, information, and knowledge to: standardize documentation, improve communication, support the decision-making process, develop and disseminate new knowledge, enhance the quality, effectiveness, and efficiency of health care, empower clients to make health care choices, and advance the science of nursing."[5] This will surely benefit nursing practice, administration, research, and education, as well as help augment nursing knowledge. A certification examination became available in 1995 from the American Nurses Association Credentialing Center.

New technologies are being used in a variety of ways to improve accessibility to health care and control costs. Leading medical centers are experimenting with methods of using technology to monitor and diagnose patients in remote locations by using equipment such as two-way television, electronic stethoscopes, and long-distance x-ray transmission. Use of such "telemedicine" is transforming the way medical centers treat remote patients. More personal medical history data is becoming increasingly accessible on computer databases. This allows health care professionals working in remote places to have access to all necessary client history data. Growing numbers of procedures are being done by this method of long-distance medicine. Performing blood chemistry tests and administering fetal sonograms are only examples of the procedures that are now being conducted using telemedicine. Additionally, telephone triage is becoming increasingly common as a way to save money by eliminating unnecessary visits to emergency rooms.*

However, such new approaches to health care raise several issues. Greater accessibility of such personal information raises issues of privacy and confidential-

* *Wall Street Journal,* "Telephone Triage: How Nurses Take Calls and Control the Care of Patients From Afar," Vol. IC, No. 24, Tuesday, Feb. 4, 1997, pp. A1, A6.

ity. The quality of medical care clients would receive through telemedicine and telephone triage may not be as good as if the M.D. or nurse were in the same room. This remote health care may also change the physician-client or nurse-client rapport and relationship.

As technology puts an end to old problems and traditional caregiving roles, caregivers must find a new "twist" to their calling in order to earn a living. One example is the dental industry. As fluoride, early dental prophylaxis, and orthodontic care eliminated the major cause for dental expenses, the dental schools and profession turned to new ways to reap a significant annual income. One of the latest developments is the encouragement of braces for grown-up mouths; it is not uncommon to see middle-age persons smiling through a high-cost, full set of dental wires and braces. Nurses have gone through similar changes, although the economic rewards were not as significant to the individual practitioner because they were often instruments of a larger system that paid survival wages for long hours of hard work.

SUMMARY

The American nursing profession has been built on the work of people who held firm to their values. As the world enters the new information age, nurses who are knowledgeable and professional will command increasing ability to apply these values—possibly with increased pay. With an awareness of the past, nurses—male and female—can confidently help shape the future for themselves and the profession.

Nurses approaching the next century do not have to jump into any situation where they are needed. They are individuals with their own needs and aspirations. Nurses today sometimes find themselves frustrated and eager to plan their futures. The need for nurses is as great as it has ever been, but roles and responsibilities continue to change. It is hoped that the rewards of the career you plan be commensurate with the need. Choose carefully where you go, but never coldly turn your back on people who must have nursing care.

CRITICAL THINKING *Activities*

1. **During which period in history do you think nursing made its biggest strides toward professionalization? Where does it stand now?**
2. **What do you think have been major obstacles in the emancipation of women and the ancillary progress in the field of nursing? (Students might compare pursuit of women's rights to other groups that have sought recognition in the past, such as the 1960s civil rights movement.)**
3. **Discuss the present status of women in our society, and how that compares with nurses and nursing today. What major changes, if any, do you think will take place by the turn of the century? What could nurses do to enhance their position?**
4. **How does Dr. Abraham Flexner's 1915 definition of a profession compare with the state of nursing today? (See Early Nursing Schools section.)**

Some Significant Events Influencing the Development of Professional Nursing (some dates are approximations)	
1765	First school of medicine (Philadelphia)
1798	Marine Hospital Service (became USPHS in 1912) and U.S. Treasury Department established an Act for the Relief of Sick and Disabled Seamen, imposing a 20-cent tax on seamen's wages to provide funds for their health care
1813	Act to Encourage Vaccination
1839	First dental school (Baltimore)
1848	Imports Drug Act became the first federal statute to ensure the quality of drugs
1851	Florence Nightingale (1820–1910) went to Kaiserswerth
1859	First District Nursing Association, Liverpool (William Rathbone and Mrs. Mary Robinson)
1860	Nightingale Training School established in London; she described nursing and the environment
1861–1865	Civil War
1864	International Red Cross established by Henri Durant
1869	Massachusetts State Department of Health established
1872	First schools of nursing in United States (New England Hospital for Women and Children, in Boston, and Women's Hospital, in Philadelphia); American Public Health Association founded by Stephen Smith
1873	Linda Richards was the first nurse to graduate in the United States; she devised a system of written records and orders
1878	Act to Enforce Quarantine on Vessels and Vehicles
1877	Trained nurses sent into homes of sick poor by New York City Mission
1879	Act to Establish a National Board of Health to cooperate with states on matters of public health (4-year trial period)
1880	National Death Registration established by U.S. Bureau of the Census
1882	American Red Cross established by Clara Barton
1882–1884	Discovery of bacteria causing tuberculosis, diphtheria, and typhoid
1885	District Nursing Association in Buffalo, New York
1886	Visiting Nurse Association (VNA) started in Philadelphia
1889	Chicago Visiting Nurse Association
1890–1910	Much study of bacteria as cause of disease
1890	Pasteurization of milk developed; Act to Prevent Interstate Spread of Disease passed
1892	School of nursing established in London by Amy Hughes
1893	Henry Street Visiting Nurse Service, New York, established by Lillian D. Wald and Mary Brewster; American Society of Superintendents of Training Schools for Nurses (became National League for Nursing Education in 1912)
1895	Industrial Nursing started in the Vermont Marble Works by Ada Mayo Stewart
1897	Nurses' Associated Alumnae of United States and Canada (became American Nurses' Association in 1911); University of Michigan granted Master of Science degree in Hygiene and Public Health
1898	Los Angeles Health Department paid public health nurses; Detroit Visiting Nurse Association started; course in social work, New York Charity Organization Society
1899	International Council of Nurses; university education for nurses, Teachers College, Columbia University (course in hospital economics); Association of Superintendents became American Hospital Association in 1907)

Some Significant Events Influencing the Development of Professional Nursing (some dates are approximations)—cont'd

1900	*American Journal of Nursing* first published
1901	Fifty-eight public health nursing associations; 130 public health nurses in United States
1902	School nursing established in New York City by Linda Rogers
1903	Tuberculosis nursing, Baltimore; first Nurse Practice Acts; North Carolina was the first state to implement registration of nurses
1904	National Organization for the Study and Prevention of Tuberculosis (became National Tuberculosis Association)
1906	Food and Drug Act passed
1907	Alabama law permitting employment of public health nurses
1908	Detroit Health Department employed public health nurses
1909	University of Minnesota School of Nursing founded; Metropolitan Life Insurance Company contracted for visiting nursing service; first White House Conference; American Association for the Study and Prevention of Infant Mortality
1910	Public health nursing program, Teachers College, Columbia University; *Medical Education in the United States and Canada* by Abraham Flexner
1911	Boston Instructive Visiting Nurse Association added nutritional service
1912	USPHS established; National League for Nursing established
1913	Division of Public Health Nursing, New York State Department of Health; Harvard School of Public Health
1914	NOPHN suggested 4-month course in a visiting nurse association as essential preparation for public health nursing; Harrison Narcotics Act established federal controls over narcotics
1916	Cincinnati School of Nursing established a 5-year program leading to a bachelor's degree
1917–1918	U.S. involvement in World War I
1917	American Dietetic Association; Massachusetts and New York employed public health nutritionists
1918	USPHS organized a division of public health nursing to work in extra cantonment zones
1918	Compulsory education in all states; American Association of Medical Social Workers; Maternity Center Association established in New York
1919	*Public Health Nursing* by Mary S. Gardner; public health nursing program, University of Michigan; increase in public health nurses and public health nursing education
1919–1929	Demonstrations of child health and public health services
1920	NOPHN-approved university programs in public health nursing
1921	Industrial and school nursing sections of NOPHN; NOPHN set one academic year as minimum for public health nursing certificate; first university program in public health education, Massachusetts Institute of Technology, Harvard; National Health Council; American Association of Social Workers
1921–1929	Shepherd-Tower Act—federal aid for maternal and child health
1922	11,548 nurses in the United States; Sigma Theta Tau founded (became the International Honor Society in 1985)
1922–1935	American Child Health Association

Continued

Some Significant Events Influencing the Development of Professional Nursing (some dates are approximations)—cont'd

1923	Public health nursing section, APHA; Nursing and Nursing Education in the United States ("The Winslow-Goldmark Report"); Yale and Western Reserve Universities established collegiate schools of nursing
1924	U.S. Indian Bureau Nursing Service founded by Eleanor Gregg; Oil Pollution Act prohibited the dumping of oil in navigable waters
1925	Frontier Nursing Service founded by Mary Breckenridge; first NOPHN statement of qualifications for public health nurses; John Hancock Mutual Life Insurance Company Visiting Nurse Service
1925–1926	Chicago Infant Welfare Society and Boston and East Harlem public health nursing agencies employed psychiatric social workers
1926	Committee on Grading of Nursing Schools began studies; Goldmark Report criticized inadequacies of hospital nursing schools and recommended increased educational standards
1927–1931	Research by Committee on the Cost of Medical Care
1929	Beginning of the Depression
1930	Unemployment of nurses; study of maternal mortality in New York City; Act to Establish a National Institute of Health
1931	15,865 nurses in the United States
1932	Final report of Commission on Medical Education; Association of Collegiate Schools of Nursing; Lobenstine Midwifery Clinic and School (Maternity Center became responsible for the school in 1934); 7% of nurses employed in public health nursing had completed a 1-year program
1933	Pearl McIver appointed to USPHS as a public health nursing analyst; U.S. Birth and Death Registration Areas completed
1934	*Survey of Public Health Nursing* published by NOPHN
1935	*Facts about Nursing,* American Nursing Association; Social Security Act (designed to provide for the general welfare by establishing a system of federal old-age benefits and by enabling the states to make provision for aged persons, blind individuals, dependent and crippled children, maternal and child welfare, and the unemployed)
1935–1936	National Health Survey
1937–1947	Beginning of federal appropriations for cancer, venereal diseases, tuberculosis, mental health, heart disease, and so on
1938	Federal Food, Drug, and Cosmetic Act
1939	Reorganization of federal agencies; USPHS transferred from Treasury Department to Federal Security Agency
1939–1945	World War II
1941	Nurse Training Act
1942	American Association of Industrial Nurses
1943	Bolton-Bailey Act for nursing education and Cadet Nurse Program
1943–1947	Emergency Maternity and Infant Care Program
1944	Division of Nursing formed by USPHS with Lucile Petry (Leone) as director; commissioned rank for nurses; NOPHN accredited only public health nursing programs with professional content of at least 1 year, which is part of program leading to a degree; Skidmore College basic nursing program approved for preparation of public health nurses; Public Health Service Act consolidated all existing public health legislation into a single statute

Some Significant Events Influencing the Development of Professional Nursing (some dates are approximations)—cont'd

1945	End of World War II; educational privileges provided for nurse veterans by G.I. Bill of Rights; publication of *Local Health Units for the Nation;* APHA accreditation of schools of public health
1946	Nurses classified as professional by U.S. Civil Service Commission; Hospital Survey and Construction Act (Hill-Burton)
1947	Women's Medical Specialist Corps established a permanent nursing corps in the army and navy
1948	*Nurses for the Future* by Esther Lucile Brown recommended nursing education be moved from hospitals to universities; World Health Organization permanently established and meeting of World Health Assembly; National Heart Act authorized aid for research and training and established the National Heart Institute at NIH; National Dental Research Act established the National Institute of Dental Research in NIH; Water Pollution Control Act to help ensure clean water in the U.S.
1949	National Federation of Licensed Practical Nurses; national nursing organizations supported legislation for federal financial aid for practical nursing education
1950	Research Institutes Act expanded NIH to include research and training related to arthritis, rheumatism, multiple sclerosis, cerebral palsy, blindness, and leprosy
1951	National League for Nursing recommendation that collegiate basic nursing education programs include preparation for public health nursing; National Association of Colored Graduate Nurses integrated with ANA
1952	Hildegard Peplau developed the theory that nursing is an interpersonal process that must deal with the client's felt needs; reorganization of national nursing organizations, major functions transferred to American Nurses' Association and National League for Nursing
1952–1953	American Red Cross, Metropolitan Life Insurance Company, and John Hancock Mutual Life Insurance Company discontinued public health nursing services; last issue of *Public Health Nursing* printed in Dec. 1952
1953	*Nursing Outlook* published in January; Department of Health, Education, and Welfare established with Cabinet status
1955	National Association of Social Workers (seven associations combined); Air Pollution Control Act; Mental Health Study Act; Polio Vaccination Assistance Act
1956	National Health Survey Act provided for a continuing survey and special studies of sickness and disability in the United States
1959	NLN voted that no new specialized baccalaureate program be accredited and that after 1963 only baccalaureate programs that include public health nursing be accredited
1960	*NLN Criteria for the Evaluation of Educational Programs in Nursing That Lead to Baccalaureate and Master's Degrees;* International Health Research Act and Federal Hazardous Substance Labeling Act
1961	Eleven accredited schools of public health in United States, two in Canada; National Institute of Child Health and Human Development established; Vaccination Assistance Act aided programs to combat polio, diphtheria, whooping cough, and tetanus

Continued

Some Significant Events Influencing the Development of Professional Nursing (some dates are approximations)—cont'd

1963	Report of Surgeon General's Consultant Group on Nursing; Health Professional Educational Assistance Act and Clean Air Act
1964	*NLN Statement of Beliefs and Recommendations Regarding Baccalaureate Programs Admitting Registered Nurse Students;* Economic Opportunity Act of 1964 enacted to mobilize the human and financial resources of the nation to combat poverty (it established the Office of Economic Opportunity, authorized Volunteers in Service to America [VISTA], Upward Bound, the Job Corps, Neighborhood Youth Corps, Head Start, neighborhood health centers, community action programs; assisted small businesses; and was a stimulus to antipoverty programs); Civil Rights Act of 1964 forbade discrimination based on race or sex in public accommodations, facilities, and educational settings; Food Stamp Act
1964	Nurse Training Act
1965	Social Security Amendment of 1965 established Medicare and Medicaid; Federal Cigarette Labeling and Advertising Act, intended to inform the public of the hazards of cigarette smoking; Regional Medical Program established; Heart Disease, Cancer, and Stroke Amendments
1966	Child Nutrition Act establishing a federal program of research and support for child nutrition; Comprehensive Health Planning and Public Health Service Amendments; Social Security Amendments: Title XVIII (Medicare) and Title XIX (Medicaid)
1967	Air Quality Act
1968	Health Manpower Act extended Nurse Training Act of 1964
1969	Federal Coal Mine Health and Safety Act; National Environmental Policy Act; First Nursing Theory Conference held in Kansas City (the Nature of Science in Nursing was the theme)
1970	National Commission on Nursing and Nursing Education—Abstract for Action published; Family Planning Services and Population Research Act; Occupational Safety and Health Act; Comprehensive Alcohol Abuse and Alcoholism Prevention Treatment and Rehabilitation Act; Environmental Education Act; Comprehensive Drug Abuse Prevention and Control Act; Resource Recovery Act; Health Training Improvement Act; Emergency Health Personnel Act; Public Health Cigarette Smoking Act
1971	"Extending the Scope of Nursing Practice" report published; Comprehensive Health Manpower Training Act; National Cancer Act; Lead-Based Poisoning Prevention Act; Nurse Training Act of 1971 expanded and continued nurse training provisions of the 1964 and 1968 acts
1972	National Sickle Cell Anemia Control Act; National Cooley's Anemia Control Act; Federal Environmental Pesticide Control Act; National Heart, Blood Vessel, Lung, and Blood Act; National School Lunch and Child Nutrition Amendments; Federal Environmental Pesticide Control Act; Consumer Product Safety Act; Noise Control Act
1973	NLN required conceptual frameworks in nursing education; Health Maintenance Organization (HMO) Act; Endangered Species Act
1974	First National Transcultural Nursing Conference held at the University of Utah College of Nursing; formation of Nurses Coalition for Action in Politics (N-CAP); first certification examinations by the ANA for excellence in practice; Child Abuse Prevention and Treatment Act; Sudden Infant Death Syndrome Act; Narcotic Addict Treatment Act; Research on Aging Act; National Research Act; National Diabetes Mellitus Research and Education Act; Safe Drinking Water Act; National Arthritis Act

Some Significant Events Influencing the Development of Professional Nursing (some dates are approximations)—cont'd

1975	American Hospital Association published "Patients' Bill of Rights"; National Health Planning and Resources Development Act; Disabled Assistance and Bill of Rights Act; Health Services, Health Revenue, and Nurse Training Act
1976	Costs for health care in the United States rose 14% over 1975; Toxic Substances Control Act
1977–1978	Designated "Year of the Nurse" by the ANA to help the public better understand nursing; Rural Health Clinic Services bill passed in 1977
1977	Generic and brand names for drug legislation
1978	ANA Code for Nurses; Massachusetts became the seventh state to mandate continuing education as a requirement for relicensure of both registered and practical nurses; President Carter vetoes the Nursing Training Act; Robert Wood Johnson Foundation finances $5 million program to train nurses as school nurse practitioners and place them in areas where children receive inadequate care
1979	ANA board determined that future ANA conventions and conferences will be held only in states that have ratified the Equal Rights Amendment; President Carter's fiscal 1980 budget cut nursing education funds to $15 million, in contrast to previous levels of $122 million (only nurse practitioners came out well)
1980	Civil Rights of Institutionalized Persons Act; Colorado passed a new nurse practice act that enabled nurses to practice independently in private settings; the Supreme Court declined to review the discrimination suit brought by Nurses Under-Represented in Social Equality, which charged that the city of Denver paid women less than men for equal work; Maryland was the first state to pass a law that mandates that licensed health care providers, including nurses, be able to receive third-party reimbursement
1980s	Nursing diagnosis evolved as a separate component of nursing process; enrollments in higher education, including nursing, declined; decline in numbers of nursing students led to nursing shortages in most areas of the country (hospitals began to entice nurses with higher wages and more benefits, also produced more L.P.N.s and other less skilled help)
1981	The Robert Wood Johnson Foundation joined with the ANA to develop "teaching nursing homes" to improve long-term care; Ronald Reagan was elected President and began to pull back numerous health and social programs; Carolyn Davis became the first nurse to head the Health Care Financing Administration (HCFA); California legislature passed a vote mandating that women in female-dominated jobs be paid wages commensurate with those of males producing the same level or quality of work
1982	The Tax Equity and Fiscal Responsibility Act (TEFRA); to be licensed as R.N.s, students of nursing began taking a new comprehensive test developed by the National Council of State Boards of Nursing; North Carolina became the first state where R.N.s and L.P.N.s nominated and voted for members of their own board of nursing; federal support for nursing education was severely cut, and hundreds of nurses and nursing students protested in Washington, D.C.

Continued

Some Significant Events Influencing the Development of Professional Nursing (some dates are approximations)—cont'd

1983	Dr. Barney Clark became the first recipient of an artificial heart; Social Security Amendment
1984	National Organ Procurement Act; the University of Minnesota School of Nursing celebrated its 75th anniversary as the first school of nursing in the world to be located on a university campus where faculty held university appointments
1985	Consolidated Omnibus Budget Reconciliation Act
1986	North Dakota became the first state to require the B.S.N. for R.N. licensure and the A.D.N. for L.P.N. licensure; NLN changed its position and endorsed two levels of nursing practice—professional and associate; certified nurse midwives formed an independent mutual insurance firm to solve the malpractice insurance dilemma that threatened to shut down the profession
1987	UCLA found a sharp drop in the number of nursing students across the country; the Pennsylvania Nurses' Association won from the state the largest pay equity award in the history of nursing; candidates for nursing licensure took the first pass/fail test as a replacement for numerical scores; William Stern, as biologic father, won custody of "Baby M" and terminated parental rights for Mary Beth Whitehead, who had contracted to bear Stern's child for $10,000
1988	Medicare Catastrophic Coverage Act; the training of "registered nurse technologists" approved by the AMA to assume a new, technically oriented role at the bedside and carry out medical protocols
1989	A draft of *Promoting Health/Preventing Disease: Year 2000 Objectives for the Nation* was distributed for public review; 1900 nurses were named in liability and malpractice suits, 50% of those claims were upheld, the average claim against a nurse that resulted in payment was $145,397; RU 486, a controversial abortion pill, was increasingly popular in France
1990	Americans with Disabilities Act (ADA) enacted into law. The ADA became effective in 1992 and 1994 on a phase-in basis
1992	ANA Congress of Nursing Practice established nursing information as a distinct area of nursing practice
1993	Health Security Act proposed; Child Immunization Program; the NLN celebrated its 100th anniversary
1994	The Food and Drug Administration began enforcing nutritional labeling requirements for food
1995	The Social Security Administration is established as an independent agency
1996	The first Rural Health School was opened at the University of Minnesota. A federal jury verdict held a tobacco company responsible for the health effects of its product

References

1. A *century of nursing: Reprints of four historic documents, including Miss Nightingale's 1. Letter of September 18, 1872, to the Bellevue School,* Foreword by Elizabeth M. Stewart and Agnes Galinas for the National League of Nursing Education, New York: G. P. Putnam's Sons, 1950.
2. American Hospital Association: *Economic trends,* Winter 1992.
3. American Hospital Association: *Hospital Statistics,* 1992.
4. American National Red Cross: *The American Red Cross: a brief story,* Washington, D.C., 1951, American National Red Cross.
5. American Nurses Association Congress of Nursing Practice: *Report on the designation of nursing informatics as a nursing specialty from the Council on Computer Applications in Nursing,* Jan. 1992.
6. Andrews MR: *A lost commander: Florence Nightingale,* New York, 1938, Doubleday.
7. Austin AL, Steward IM: *History of nursing,* ed, New York, 1962, Putnam.
8. Banworth CA: Living memorial to Florence Nightingale, *Am J Nurs* 40:491–497, 1940.
9. Barton WE: *The life of Clara Barton—founder of the American Red Cross,* 2 vols, Boston, 1922, Houghton Mifflin.
10. Blackwell E: *Pioneer work for women,* New York, 1914, Dutton.
11. Blanchfield FA, Standlee MW: Organized nursing and the army in three wars, Manuscript on file, Historical Division, Office of the Surgeon General of the Army, Washington, D.C.
12. Bogdanich W: *Great white lie: dishonesty, waste and incompetence in the medical community,* New York, 1992, Simon & Schuster.
13. Brockett LP, Vaughan MC: *Woman's work in the Civil War: a record of heroism, patriotism and patience,* Rochester, N.Y., 1867.
14. Chayer ME: *School nursing,* New York, 1937, Putnam.
15. Christy TE: Portrait of a leader: Lavinia Lloyd Dock, *Nurs Outlook* 17:72, June, 1969.
16. Christy TE: Portrait of a leader: Adelaide Nutting, *Nurs Outlook* 17:20, Jan 1969.
17. Christy TE: Portrait of a leader: Isabel Hampton Robb, *Nurs Outlook* 17:26, March 1969.
18. Christy TE: Portrait of a leader: Isabel M. Stewart, *Nurs Outlook* 17:44, Oct 1969.
19. Clinton HR: Nurses in the front lines, *Nurs Health Care* 14:6(286), June 1993.
20. Cook Sir Edward: *The life of Florence Nightingale,* 2 vols, New York, 1942, Macmillan.
21. DeBarberey H: *Elizabeth Seton,* New York, 1931, Macmillan.
22. Dock L and others: *History of American Red Cross nursing,* New York, 1922, Macmillan.
23. Deutsch A: Dorothea Lynde Dix: apostle of the insane, *Am J Nurs* 36:987, Oct 1936.
24. Dodell D, ed: *The health Info-Com network newsletter,* Scottsdale, Arizona. Internet address: "david@stat.com." To subscribe, send "subscribe mednews *your full name*" message to "listserve@asuacad" (non-Bitnet users send mail "listserv%asuacad.bitnet@cuny vm. cuny.edu")
25. Doyle A: Nursing by religious orders in the United States, Part I, 1809–1840; Part II, 1841–1870; Part III, 1871–1928; Part IV, Lutheran deaconesses, 1849–1928; Part VI, Episcopal sisterhoods, 1845–1928, *Am J Nurs* 29:775, 959, 1085, 1197, 1466.

26. Dubos RJ: *Louis Pasteur: free lance of science,* Boston, 1950, Little, Brown.
27. Dulles FR: *The American Red Cross: a history,* New York, 1950, Harper.
28. Editorial—Dedication of the American Nurses' Memorial, Florence Nightingale School, Bordeaux, France, *Am J Nurs* 22:799, July 1922.
29. Editorial—The dedication of the Bordeaux School Building, *Am J Nurs* 36:491, May 1936.
30. Eisenberg DM and others. Unconventional medicine in the United States—prevalence, costs, and patterns of use, *N Engl J Med* 328(4):246, 1993.
31. Emanuelsson A: Pioneers in white, Doctoral thesis, 1990, Swedish Nurses' Union.
32. Extracts from letters from the Crimea, *Am J Nurs* 32:537.
33. Epler PH: *The life of Clara Barton,* New York, 1919, Macmillan.
34. Engleman RC, Joy RJT: *Two hundred years of military medicine,* Fort Detrick, MD, 1975, The Historical Unit, U.S. Army Medical Department.
35. Ferguson ED: The evolution of the trained nurses, *Am J Nurs* 1:463, April 1901; 1:535, May 1901; 1:620, June 1901.
36. Fishbein M: *History of the American Medical Association,* Philadelphia, 1947, Saunders.
37. Flexner A: Is social work a profession? In *Proceedings of the National Conference of Charities and Correction,* 1915, 578.
38. Florence Nightingale is placed among mankind's benefactors, *Am J Nurs* 50–265.
39. Frank CM: *Foundations of nursing,* ed 2, Philadelphia, 1959, Saunders.
40. Gaaserud MK: The invisible nursing, Doctoral thesis, Swedish Nurses' Union, 1990.
41. Gallison M: *The ministry of women: one hundred years of women's work at Kaiserswerth, 1836–1936,* London, 1954, Butterworth.
42. Hamilton SW: *The history of American mental hospitals: one hundred years of American psychiatry,* New York, 1944, Columbia University Press.
43. Hume EE: *Medical work of the Knights Hospitalers of Saint John of Jerusalem,* Baltimore, 1940, Johns Hopkins Press.
44. Improved knowledge base would be helpful in reaching policy decisions on providing long-term in home services for the elderly, Report to the Hon. Pete V. Domenici, U.S. Senate, Washington, D.C., 1981, GAO.
45. Jensen DM: *History and trends of professional nursing,* St. Louis, 1959, Mosby.
46. Jones MC: *The training of a nurse,* New York, 1980, Scribner's.
47. Kernodle PB: *The Red Cross nurse in action, 1882–1948,* New York, 1949, Harper Brothers.
48. Konner M: *Medicine at the crossroads: the crisis in health care,* New York, 1993, Pantheon.
49. *La Crosse Tribune:* Bacteria with four numbers has become U.S. menace, Jan 9, 1994, A3.
50. Lee E: A Florence Nightingale collection, *Am J Nurs* 38:555, May 1938.
51. Livermore MA: *My story of the war, a woman's narrative of the four years' experience as a nurse in the Union Army,* Hartford, CT, 1888, Worthington.
52. Loeb S, ed: *Diseases,* Springhouse, PA, 1993, Springhouse.
53. Lust J, Tierra M: *The natural remedy bible,* New York, 1990, Simon & Schuster.
54. Marshall HE: *Dorothea Dix,* Chapel Hill, 1937, University of North Carolina Press.

55. McGinley P: *Saint-watching,* New York, 1969, Viking.
56. Morganthau T: The Clinton solution, *Newsweek,* Sept. 20, 1993, 30.
57. Noyes CD: American nurses complete fund for Memorial School in France, *Am J Nurs* 29:1189, Oct 1929.
58. Nightingaliana, *Am J Nurs* 288, May 1949.
59. Nursing and the League of Nations, *Am J Nurs* 31:1283, Nov 1931.
60. Nutting MA (in collaboration with Dock LL): *History of nursing,* vols. 1 through 4, New York and London, 1907, 1912.
61. Office of the Press Secretary, White House, The Health Security Act of 1993: Health care that's always there, Sept. 22, 1993.
62. Payne JF: *Thomas Sydenham,* New York, 1900, Longmans, Green & Co.
63. Pavey AE: *The story of the growth of nursing,* London, 1938, Faber & Faber.
64. Pickett SE: *The American National Red Cross,* New York, 1924, Century.
65. Post-Bulletin: Studies: elderly are not helped much by dialysis, *Seattle Post-Intelligencer,* Rochester, MN, Jan 5, 1994, 5A.
66. Prevention Magazine: *Doctors book of home remedies,* Emmaus, PN, 1991, Rodale Press.
67. Robb IH: *Educational standards for nurses,* Cleveland, OH, 1907, E. D. Koechart.
68. Roberts MM: Florence Nightingale as a nurse educator, *Am J Nurs* 37:773, July 1937.
69. Roberts MM: *American nursing: history and interpretation,* New York, 1954, Macmillan.
70. Salsberry P: Assuming responsibility for one's health, *Nurs Outlook* 41:5, 212, 1993.
71. Scovil ER: Florence Nightingale's notes on nursing, *Am J Nurs* 27:355, 1927.
72. Seymer L: St. Thomas' Hospital and the Nightingale Training School, *Int Nurs Rev* 11:340, 1937.
73. Sharp EE: Nursing during the pre-Christian era, *Am J Nurs* 19:675, 1919.
74. Stephen B: Florence Nightingale's home, *Int Nurs Rev* 11:331, 1937.
75. Stevens R: *In sickness and in wealth: American hospitals in the twentieth century,* New York, 1990, Basic Books.
76. Strachey L: *Eminent Victorians,* New York, 1963, Putnam.
77. The American National Red Cross: *Jane A. Delano: a biography,* ARC 781, Washington D.C., 1952.
78. *The A.N.A. and you,* New York, 1941, American Nurses Association.
79. Tiffany F: *Life of Dorothea Lynde Dix,* Boston, 1890, Houghton Mifflin.
80. Toffler A: *Powershift: knowledge, wealth, and violence at the edge of the 21st century,* New York, 1990, Bantam Books.
81. *Transactions of the American Hospital Association,* 1913, pg. 91.
82. Trevelyan GM: *History of England,* London, 1928, Longmans, Green & Co.
83. Tyson LD: Chair of Council of Economic Advisers: The costs of failing to reform health care, press release from the office of the Press Secretary, The White House, October 6, 1993.
84. Ullman D: The mainstreaming of alternative medicine, *Health Forum J* 24, 1993.
85. Whittaker EW, Olesen VL: Why Florence Nightingale? *Am J Nurs* 67:2338, 1967.
86. Williams BC: *Clara Barton: daughter of destiny,* Philadelphia, 1941, Lippincott.

87. Vreeland EM: Fifty years of nursing in the federal government nursing services, *Am J Nurs* 50:626, 1950.

88. Wald LD: *Windows on Henry Street,* Boston, 1934, Little, Brown.

89. Woodham-Smith C: *Florence Nightingale,* New York, 1951, McGraw-Hill.

Suggested Readings

American Association for the History of Nursing: *Nursing History Review: Official Journal of the AAHN,* University of Pennsylvania Press, Baltimore, MD.

Boston C, Estes C, eds: *Health policy and nursing: crisis and reform in the U.S. health care system,* Boston, 1994, Jones & Bartlett.

Debella S, Martin L, Siddall S: *Nurse's role in health care planning,* Norwalk, CT, 1986, Appleton-Century-Crofts.

Ginsberg E: *Medical triangle: physicians, politicians and the public,* Cambridge, MA, 1992, Harvard University Press.

Hicks L, Stallmeyer JM, Coleman J: *Role of the nurse in managed care,* Washington, D.C., 1993, American Nurses Publishing.

Jonas S: *An introduction to the U.S. health care system,* New York, 1993, Springer.

Konner M: *Medicine at the crossroads: the crisis in health care,* New York, 1993, Pantheon Books.

Mason DJ and others, eds: *Policy and politics for nurses: action and change in the workplace, government, organizations and community,* Philadelphia, 1993, Saunders.

Payer L: *Disease-mongers: how doctors, drug companies, and insurers are making you feel sick,* New York, 1992, Wiley.

Toffler A: *The third wave,* New York, 1980, Morrow.

Toffler A: *Powershift: knowledge, wealth, and violence at the edge of the 21st century,* New York, 1990, Bantam.

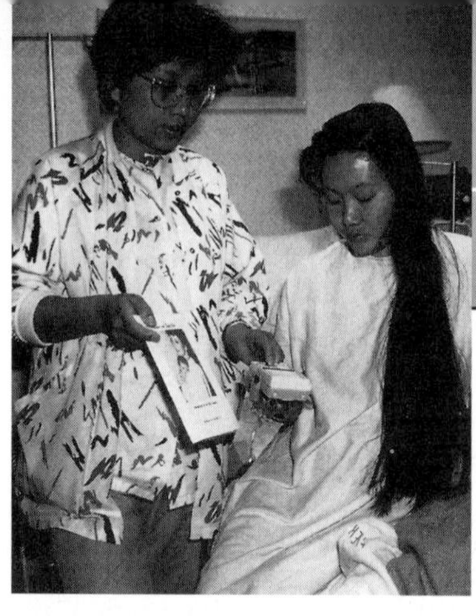

CHAPTER 2

The Evolution of Nursing Science and Practice

*M. Patricia Donahue**

OBJECTIVES

After completing this chapter the reader should be able to:

- **Discuss what is meant by *nursing art* and *nursing science***
- **Examine changes in nursing practice over the last 50 years**
- **Analyze historic events, reports, and studies that have had an impact on nursing education and practice**
- **Discuss the nursing process model with its currently accepted components**
- **Describe the interdependence of nursing practice, theory, and research**
- **Differentiate between a nursing model and a nursing theory**
- **Compare three contemporary nursing theorists who have made a contribution to the scientific body of nursing knowledge**
- **Examine the nursing profession's movement toward standardized language and classification systems**

During the past five decades the nursing profession made significant progress toward developing a body of scientific knowledge and establishing the credibility of nursing science. Nursing science encompasses knowledge of the field of nursing based on research and practice. Changing trends in many areas, including medical science and technology, the health care system, consumers' demands, professional nursing education and organizations, and other humanistic disciplines influence the evolution of nursing science. Nursing's body of knowledge grows as nurses are educated to critically study nursing practice, develop nursing theories and conceptual models, conduct nursing research, and test nursing theories. Concurrently, nursing practice changes in response to consumer demands for accessibility and involvement in decision making, new technology, changes in health care delivery systems, health care reimbursement plans, and public policy.

*The majority of the content for this chapter was originally written by Janet W. Kenney.

These changes in response to societal needs lend credence to the fact that nursing is a *reflection of social reality.* Nursing changes, grows, and advances continually in response to perceived social needs. Nursing also changes in response to advances in medical science, knowledge, and technology. Thus nursing roles, functions, and responsibilities are in almost constant flux, ever-responsive to necessary changes to effect quality care. As health care systems worldwide are caught in a web of social problems, financial crises, and scarce resources, nursing practice continues to adapt to these shifting realities while taking into account the need for internal change to meet new opportunities created by such upheaval.

Nursing is more than just a technique or a highly skilled trade—it is a dynamic process. It includes all those elements that have contributed to its foundation: the elements of soul, mind, and imagination. Its very essence lies in the sensitive spirit, the intelligent understanding, and the creative inspiration that underlie the basic structure for effective nursing practice. It embodies those traditional attributes of compassion, humanity, advocacy, commitment, and caring that make nursing unique in the "care of strangers." Nursing is both simple and complex; it is concrete in result, yet abstract in practice. Nursing is truly an art and a science.

This chapter describes the evolution of nursing as a science and a practice discipline. It begins with a discussion of the development of knowledge and the interdependence of nursing practice, theory, and research. The development of nursing science reflects the ongoing struggle with various philosophic and methodologic issues. These are presented as historical background, followed by a summary of major societal changes that affect nursing practice and nursing theory development. The evolution of the nursing process and theory development is described through historical events, publications, and contributions of nursing leaders. Nurse scholars and leaders who have shaped the nursing profession are acknowledged and their contributions emphasized. Current views of nurse leaders and their projections of the future of nursing practice, theory, and research are presented. The chapter concludes with suggestions for the future of professional nursing.

■ EVOLUTION OF NURSING KNOWLEDGE

Each discipline is distinguished by a specific field of inquiry that is agreed upon by its members and by its unique body of knowledge in that field.[69] The discipline's field is identified by how specific concepts are defined and interrelated. The nursing discipline has reached consensus on four concepts that are central to its focus: human being or person, environment, health, and nursing.[24] As a practice discipline, nursing develops knowledge for application by designing conceptual models and theories that may be applied and tested in practice.

Over the past 50 years nursing has been defined as a series of tasks: a caring, comprehensive service; a process involving cognitive, psychomotor, and interpersonal skills; and as an art and science of human health.[28] As nurse leaders and scholars have sought to elevate nursing to a scientific discipline with its own body of knowledge, they have addressed the following questions:

- What is nursing science?
- What is the purpose of nursing science?
- How can we develop a science of nursing?

What Is Nursing Science?

As early as 1959 D. E. Johnson[38] wrote about the science of nursing, citing several definitions. Johnson noted that professional disciplines usually represent applied sciences rather than basic sciences. Their goals are to use knowledge in practice. Johnson believes that nursing should be a body of knowledge with the following goals:

1. Preventing illness
2. Promoting and maintaining health
3. Providing comprehensive care

In 1969 Abdellah[1] described nursing science as "a body of cumulative scientific knowledge, drawn from the physical, biological, and behavioral sciences, that is uniquely nursing." She explained the need for nursing to develop a highly organized and specialized field of knowledge and listed steps to achieve a nursing science. Abdellah emphasized the need for concept identification and nursing research to clarify nursing theory.

The question "What is science?" was addressed by Jacox[33] in 1974. She described science as a *process* (research and inquiry) and a *product* (body of knowledge). She (1) emphasized the importance of empirical knowledge, which can be perceived and verified through the senses by others, and (2) described how knowledge accumulates through examination of phenomena, concept identification, model building, and theory testing. Jacobs and Huether[32] support the viewpoint that "science is a product created by a process" that is directly related. They assert that the major aim of nursing science is to develop theories to explain, predict, and control nursing practice. In other words, they believe that the purpose of nursing science is to develop knowledge for direct application in practice rather than developing knowledge simply for the sake of knowledge. J. L. Johnson[36] wrote that each science emerged from the study of different phenomena or from a unique perspective of observation and interpretation of a specific field. Silva[87] described the development of a science as originating in the need to categorize and structure different fields of knowledge. She listed the following six principles of science that are still relevant today:

1. Science must show a certain coherence
2. Science is concerned with definite fields of knowledge
3. Science is preferably expressed in universal statements
4. The statements of science must be true or probably true
5. The statements of science must be logically ordered
6. Science must explain its investigations and arguments

These six principles must be applied for science to be a body of knowledge (product) and a research methodology (process). Nursing, as a profession, is striving to meet these principles today.

Meleis[57] wrote that nursing science consists of knowledge based on its evolving philosophy and former practice, as well as on emerging ideas, theory, and research. She concluded that the nursing domain consists of the following four major elements:

1. Major concepts and problems of nursing
2. Process for assessment, diagnosis, and intervention
3. Tools to assess, diagnose, and intervene
4. Research designs and methods congruent with nursing knowledge

If an emerging discipline establishes its major concepts and identifies the problems to be addressed, the other three elements will gradually evolve. Nursing continues to make dramatic progress in each of these areas.

What Is the Purpose of Nursing Science?

The nature, purpose, and direction of nursing science has been a subject of debate among nursing scholars for over 35 years and continues to be so today.[36,59,78] Early debate focused on whether nursing is a basic or applied science. Many nurse scholars agree with Kerlinger,[41] a noted authority, who believes that the purpose of science is to describe, explain, predict, and ultimately control natural events. "Traditional," or empirical, science, which evolved from the natural sciences, relies on theory-neutral facts, objective and quantitative data, and the search for universal laws of cause and effect to predict and control events, as shown in Table 2-1.

During its evolution nursing sought professional status by conducting empirical research to establish a scientific base for its practice and by developing conceptual models of nursing. Thus this strong desire for professional status was probably the primary motivation for the development of a theoretic basis for nursing practice. The search for empirical knowledge became predominant and was based on

TABLE 2-1

Nursing Science's Shifting Perspectives (world views)

Characteristics	Traditional Natural Science	Biopsychosocial Integrative Science	Humanistic-Phenomenologic
Types of knowledge	Reductionistic Mechanistic Objective	Multidimensional Organismic Subjective and Objective	Holistic Contextual Relative Interactional
Research controls	Measurable Observable Verifiable	Desires objectivity, controlability, and predictability	Participant validation
Searches for	Laws and principles Linear causal relationships to predict and control	Probabilistic relationships and influential factors	Understanding of patterns and relationships
Change attributed to	Linear cause and effect	Multifactorial Probabilistic	Unidirectional, unpredictable, interactive processes
Views knowledge as	Verifiable facts, laws, and principles—a product	Contextual, relative, multifaceted, and interrelated	Personal interpretation of patterns, meanings Context of lived experience—a process of discovery

observable, objective, logical data and rational thought. Other forms of knowledge were considered less acceptable. However, empirical knowledge alone provided an incomplete view to understand humans and their environments, nursing, and health.

As early as 1929, Isabel Stewart[91] recognized a weakness in such a method that endorsed virtue in an accumulation of a fund of scientific knowledge derived strictly from observation. Her method of science included not only observation-getting but also a way of doing things that had direction and kept thought moving with experience. Stewart cautioned that science must focus on the scientific methods of thinking rather than purely on the "empirical," since naive empiricism held that sensation, or sense-perceptual experiences, was the only medium through which knowledge was gained. To her, sense perception was neither passive nor purely receptive. Experience was part of the objective world, joining with the actions of humans, and capable of being modified through human response. According to Stewart[90] it was imperative that nurses be educated in the methods of scientific inquiry, since the power of scientific knowledge was a valuable educational product. She stressed, however, that emphasis not be on general observation but on observation that was direct, exact, rational, and selective.

In 1978 Carper[10] described four basic patterns of knowledge that are used in nursing and many other disciplines. Each pattern is an equally necessary component of nursing and has its own method for determining credibility of knowledge in each field. The four patterns of knowledge are described as follows:

1. *Empirical knowledge:* is based on objective evidence obtained by the senses and requires validation and verification by others
2. *Ethical knowledge:* examines the philosophic premises of justice and seeks credibility through logical justification
3. *Esthetics:* judges creativity, form, structure, and beauty through criticism of the meaning of the creative process and product
4. *Personal knowledge:* integrates and analyzes the current interpersonal situation with past experience and knowledge

A discipline's body of knowledge would be incomplete if it relied exclusively on one form of knowledge. Most disciplines, including nursing, integrate all four patterns of knowing to form a more complete picture of reality.

Nurses are beginning to recognize the value and validity of different ways of knowing and to realize that no single form of knowledge is superior. Peggy Chinn[11] wrote extensively in support of Carper's patterns of knowing. She refuted the superiority of empirical knowledge as the only relevant model of science. With assistance from members of the Nursing Theory Think Tank, Chinn and Kramer[12] developed a process for determining the credibility of knowledge and clarified the patterns of knowing as follows:

1. *Empirics:* scientific theory, models, and linguistic descriptions of observable reality
2. *Ethics:* standards, codes, and normative theory
3. *Esthetics:* expressed in an art or act
4. *Personal knowing:* expressed in the authentic self

Contemporary nurse scholars and theorists have shifted the focus away from the rationality of searching for principles of cause and effect to view science as examining "real" changing life patterns and experiences as lived by humans. Table 2-1 compares traditional views of science with the changing and emerging views in nursing science.

Development of the Science of Nursing

As recognition of the four patterns of knowledge emerged and nurses agreed that the interrelationship of the four major concepts of person, environment, health, and nursing were the focus of the discipline, there was a move away from belief in the superiority and infallibility of traditional empirical science.[11,68,99] Several nurse scholars suggested that nursing consisted of more than just verifiable, quantitative data as knowledge and the search for universal laws. Their arguments suggested that empirical science alone was not congruent with contemporary nursing science and that alternative research methods for developing nursing science were warranted.[86] Critical social theory and feminist philosophies also influenced changes in nursing and the movement toward development of a human science in nursing.

Nursing science consistently undergoes change as new views emerge that challenge the traditional methods of natural science and biomedical nursing. Development of knowledge in a discipline may be based on different philosophies and perspectives (world views).[69] Several alternative perspectives for developing nursing models, theories, and science have been suggested.[36,69] According to Mitchell and Coldy, Wilhelm Dilthey believed that we must understand life as a process that is humanly lived—a living knowledge of "reflective" life that manifests itself in the dynamic unity of experience. Based on Dilthey's work, nursing began to develop as a human science paradigm.[59] This perspective views human beings as valued, intentional, and free-willed persons who are engaged in dynamic interaction with others and their environment. The individual's life experience is the focus of both practice and research. Practitioners and researchers are regarded as coparticipants; they both value the lived experiences and must work together to understand life's complex interactions, meanings, and values in their lives.

As nurses embrace the human science paradigm, nursing practice, theory development, and research change to reflect this new perspective. Four nursing theories have abandoned the natural science approach and developed new and different frameworks congruent with the human science paradigm.[68] These theories are Paterson and Zderad's[78] humanistic nursing, Newman's[66] model of health as expanding consciousness, Parse's[77] theory of human becoming (formerly called man-living-health), and Watson's[6,99] human science and human care.

Nurse scholars are redefining the meaning of nursing and health, thereby expanding nursing knowledge. As nursing science evolves and new conceptual models and theories are developed, new implications for nursing practice will arise.

■ INTERDEPENDENCE OF NURSING PRACTICE, THEORY, AND RESEARCH

Historically, nursing practice was based on apprenticeship and the performance of technical skills, with little consideration for a knowledge base. As nursing education shifted from hospital programs to academic institutions, there was a gradual increase in emphasis on developing a body of nursing knowledge that could be applied in practice.

Although the movement of nursing education from hospitals to academic institutions was a positive move, it created several problems. Nurse educators and scholars were isolated from practice and had difficulty identifying appropriate questions, developing relevant nursing practice models and theories, and applying nursing theory and new knowledge to nursing practice. They were frequently regarded by practicing nurses as being uninformed or oblivious to the "real world" of nursing. This created a division between nursing education and nursing practice that often hindered effective communication and exchange of information, potential collaborative research efforts, and movement toward the integration of theory in practice.

Ideally, nursing theory, research, and practice are interrelated. From observations in nursing practice, questions arise and conceptual models are formulated. This may lead to theory development and testing through research. Although theory is used primarily to guide research, it also interacts with and guides nursing practice. Research validates and modifies theory, which then changes nursing practice. Interestingly enough, this particular question of theory and practice has long been a bone of contention among various factions of nurses. In the past the prevailing notion of a nurse's work was that of being a matter of skill of hand and technical efficiency. The intellectual and social element and the need of knowledge, judgment, and social insight for nurses was not well recognized nor accepted. Yet to some nurses the welding or fusing of theory and practice was a crucial issue. Practice tested theory and made it more intelligible. Theory explained practice, made it more interesting and vital. In other words, a symbiotic relationship existed between the two, as demonstrated by Stewart[90]: "It is now beginning to be seen that all theory exists for the sake of practice, without which it is empty, and that practice without theory is relatively blind and untrustworthy."

Nursing models and theories serve many purposes in practice. Conceptual models provide a frame of reference to guide the nurse's situation.* Models assist nurses to organize information about the client, decide on appropriate nursing diagnoses, and plan nursing interventions that can effectively achieve the desired outcomes.[13] Several well-developed conceptual models of nursing have been adopted by nurses in health care institutions.[13,32,39] Nursing practice provides the necessary observations and experiences for nurses to develop and test theory. As theories are applied, nurses gain greater control over practice because the rationale for their actions is based on tested theories.

The application of nursing models and theories in practice is difficult and requires advanced education, critical analysis, and creativity. Several major problems have hindered progress in this area. Many nursing programs did not include knowledge and application of nursing theories or models in their curriculum, and therefore graduates were not prepared to use them in practice. However, the trend toward incorporating such content in nursing programs has steadily continued, particularly in graduate programs. Some nurse leaders contended that nursing models and theory were not sufficiently developed to apply in practice.[32,104] Since 1980 several textbooks have been written that explain how to apply nursing models in the nursing process.[13,81] In addition, nursing models and theories continue to be

---

*References 13, 23, 25, 30, 32, 33.

refined and explicated, with testing of either components of theories or the theories themselves occurring.[51,72] The application of theory in clinical practice is thus evolving as emphasis is placed on theoretic content in curricula, the acquisition of advanced degrees, and the collaborative efforts of nursing education and nursing practice in research endeavors.

Walker[93] believes that to apply abstract nursing models to practice the nurse must have the following:

1. A solid understanding of relevant theories
2. Knowledge of contextual factors affecting the client
3. Creativity to synthesize theory within the situational constraints
4. The ability to apply theory to a unique client situation

That is, the nurse must consider and synthesize the major concepts of a theory, the client's health/illness variables and uniqueness, and the constraints and variables of the employing agency. The ability to synthesize all of these variables in practice requires previous learning and practice in critically analyzing each individual factor. Nurse educators who know and value nursing models and theories can teach students to apply these models appropriately by considering all the variables. In practice settings, the incorporation of theory and research is an evolutionary process that has gained increasing momentum. It requires a nursing staff that asks questions, seeks answers, and looks for new ways to handle old problems. It requires nursing and hospital administrators who value and encourage research and render support in every possible way.

The link between nursing practice and research has been under scrutiny and discussion for years. With the growing cadre of nurse researchers and the increasing number of nurses who understand research and can translate findings into practice, there is a stronger link between research and practice. Increasingly more nurses, in both practice and academic settings, are involved in nursing research. Findings from their studies are reported in nursing journals and presented at various national and international conferences. Presentations of nursing research at conferences sponsored by other disciplines are also intensifying. As knowledge from studies is disseminated, many practitioners welcome the opportunity to creatively implement it in practice to test the findings. Reports of the effectiveness on client outcomes in practice settings support the theorist's and researcher's work. Reports of ineffectiveness or negative results lead to modification of their theories and research.

The following major factors have facilitated the integration of research in nursing practice:

1. More nurses are knowledgeable about the research process and recognize the value of applying research in practice
2. More nurses are conducting research
3. Information about research studies and implications for findings in practice are being disseminated through nursing publications and conferences
4. Nurses are attending both in-service education programs and conferences to improve and update their knowledge based on research
5. Increasing numbers of nursing administrators are encouraging and supporting research by clinicians and practitioners in health delivery settings
6. Nursing educators, nursing administrators, and nurses in practice are collaborating in research efforts

7. Departments or centers for nursing research are being established in health care agencies and colleges of nursing
8. Nurses are participating in interdisciplinary research

The establishment of the National Center for Nursing Research (NCNR) in 1986 was another milestone in the evolving success of nursing research and the development of nursing science. The center became a reality through an intensive effort by nurses across the country and organized national, state, and specialty nursing associations. However, it took a congressional override of a presidential veto to enact legislation to establish the center at the National Institutes of Health (NIH) in Washington, D.C. Its threefold purpose was to provide a focal point for promoting the growth and quality of research related to nursing and client care, to provide leadership to expand the pool of experienced nurse researchers, and to promote closer interaction with other bases of health care research.[61,92] The National Institutes of Health Revitalization Act of 1993 elevated the center to the status of an institute. It confirms nursing's accountability for developing new knowledge for its practice and nursing's commitment to society to use that knowledge to improve practice.

In nursing education fundamental research questions may also arise about student learning and faculty teaching. These questions lead to fundamental research in practice or education. Specific research in specialized areas of nursing practice, delivery of nursing care, and nursing education follow. Research tests nursing models and theories and generates nursing theory, which forms the base for the growing body of knowledge essential to nursing science. With continued testing and replication of studies and clinical trials theories are modified, refined, and disseminated through the literature and at conferences. New knowledge of supported theories and models can then be applied in practice and education.

In the development of nursing science, nursing practice, theory, and research are inseparable.[23,30,53,104] Both basic and applied (practice) research is necessary to identify effective nursing interventions for application in practice. Sometimes the importance of applying theory *to practice* is overemphasized, while the value and usefulness of developing theory *from practice* is underestimated. To paraphrase Firlet,[25] nursing theory is generated from practice, tested in research. Findings are then used to explain or direct nursing practice, where it may be refined or expanded. Most nurse scholars agree that the basic goal underlying the development of nursing models and theories is to generate knowledge for the improvement of nursing practice.

Although current nursing theories and models need further development, nurses are applying theoretic concepts to practice and validating theories through testing and research. As theories acquire continued support, the body of knowledge in nursing science grows.

■ EVOLUTION OF THE NURSING PROCESS

Early Nursing Practice: 1920 to 1950

During the first half of the nineteenth century, the status of nursing in the United States was similar to that in England before Nightingale's influence. Before the Civil War there were few trained nurses and no formal training programs. Large numbers of lay men and women volunteered as nurses during this war; many emerged as leaders and strong contributors to the nursing cause. The experiences of the Civil War emphasized the need for skilled nurses, which aroused the interest of government agencies and precipitated the first major nursing reforms in the United States. The time was ripe for the organization of schools of nursing. In the latter part of the century nurses' training and improved nursing practice occurred, facilitated by the improved status of women, increasing public interest in nursing, greater social commitment for health, and the establishment and success of the Nightingale school.

Early in the 1900s nurses' training was accomplished through hospital apprenticeship. The emphasis was on experience, with little concern for education. Donahue[21] expands on this concept with the following description:

> The earliest schools were created independent of hospitals by committees or boards that had the power to develop the schools. They were soon absorbed, however, into the hospitals to which they were attached because of a lack of endowment. This factor proved to be the greatest weakness in the system, since many hospitals soon discovered that schools could be created to serve their needs and a valuable source of almost free labor could be obtained. Nursing care became the major product dispensed by hospitals. The real function of the school of nursing became *not education,* but *service.* In addition, no policy for control of the numbers of nursing schools or the standards for admission and graduation was established or accepted. Consequently a proliferation of nursing schools occurred. The first decade of the twentieth century demonstrated a period of phenomenal growth, with the establishment of close to seven hundred schools. All school functions were ultimately placed under the control and general direction of hospital authorities.

The educational needs of nursing students were consistently sacrificed to meet hospital demands for service. The primary emphasis was on technical mastery and number of clinical hours worked. A school of nursing became almost indispensable to the running of a hospital.

Efforts to upgrade nursing education soon became a priority. Nursing leaders banded together to support educational standards and prevent the spread of inferior schools and unlimited expansion through legal control. By the 1930s many of the smaller and weaker schools had disappeared, the number of hours of service had been decreased, and the theory hours had been increased. Emphasis, however, still remained on technical proficiency.

Numerous studies were conducted between 1920 and 1950. In addition to the profession, other groups such as government agencies, sociologists, allied health organizations, and private foundations became involved in investigating nurses and nursing. Each of the studies provided varying levels of significance in terms of effect on nursing education and/or practice. Fitzpatrick[26] referred to those that affected the profession and contributed to its progress as *landmark studies.* The following studies are those that exerted a profound influence on the development of nursing:

- 1923—*Nursing and Nursing Education in the United States* (The Goldmark Report)[14]
Financed by the Rockefeller Foundation, this study was originally intended to consider the status of public health nursing in the United States. It soon became evident that its scope was too narrow; work was expanded to encompass the study of nursing and nursing education as a whole. The study clearly demonstrated that the traditional apprenticeship system of diploma education was not adequate for preparing nurses for professional practice and strongly urged school reorganization and improved methods of training. The conclusions indicated that adequate public financing was needed to support nursing education independently of hospitals, that more nursing schools needed to be established as independent units in universities, and that educational standards and admission requirements should be increased.
- 1928—*Nurses, Patients, and Pocketbooks*[15]
This study focused on the supply and demand of nursing service. Specific findings included the following: educational entrance requirements for nursing schools were minimal, most nursing schools were of poor educational quality, nursing schools existed to service hospitals, a serious overproduction of graduate nurses had led to chronic unemployment, and salaries and working conditions were extremely poor. In general, the conclusions of this committee agreed with those of the Committee on Nursing and Nursing Education in the United States.
- 1934—*Nursing Schools Today and Tomorrow*[16]
This final report outlined the essentials for a professional program of education for nurses. It contained facts necessary for nursing school reform, clear descriptions of weaknesses in nursing education, and the lack of adequate financial support as the greatest problem in positioning nursing education at a higher level. Professional standards that were emphasized and stressed included a collegiate level of education, an enriched curriculum with more and better theory and better practice, and faculty comparable with those in other professional schools.
- 1934—*An Activity Analysis of Nursing*[34]
Two primary questions were addressed in this study: What is good nursing? and How can it be taught? An attempt was made to document the exact functions of nurses in different occupational categories: hospital bedside nursing, private duty nursing in the home, and nursing in the public health field. A list of personal activities that should be practiced by the professional nurse were also described. Finally, the report included a clear and concise description of what the client, the physician, the hospital, and the general public expected of nursing. Once again it was clear that reform in nursing education was necessary. Four basic goals with accompanying strategies were also identified: to reduce and improve the supply of nurses, to replace students with graduates as the primary workforce in hospitals, to help hospitals meet costs of graduate services, and to get public support for nursing education.

Three important studies emerged from the Curriculum Committee of the National League of Nursing Education (NLNE). The first was the 1917 *Standard*

Curriculum for Schools of Nursing,[63] the second was the 1927 *Curriculum for Schools of Nursing,*[64] and the third was the 1937 *A Curriculum Guide for Schools of Nursing.*[65] The last, *A Curriculum Guide,* proved to be the one of the most far-reaching and ambitious efforts undertaken in the area of nursing education. It was essentially a cooperative research project lead by Isabel Stewart and the NLNE that involved the participation of representatives of all the professional organizations, allied professions, and the community. The study called for a review and reevaluation of existing curricula as well as the traditional philosophies underlying them. Its main purpose was to produce a curriculum guide that would be beneficial in the critical years ahead. It is considered by some to be one of the first major mass studies in nursing. Nursing schools were motivated to improve their educational standards as a result of these three curriculum projects.

Two additional studies that continued the dialogue on nursing education were completed before 1950:

- 1948—*Nursing for the Future*[6]

  This study was initiated in connection with the postwar planning of the National Nursing Council. Esther Lucile Brown, a social anthropologist and director of the Department of Studies in the Professions at the Russell Sage Foundation, conducted this study to determine the "needs of society" for nursing; nursing education and nursing service would be viewed from the aspect of what was best for society. Brown's twenty-eight recommendations called for a total reorganization of nursing education and service and that nursing be divided into two categories of personnel—professional and practical levels. One of the strongest proposals was "that effort be directed to building basic schools of nursing in universities and colleges, comparable in number to existing medical schools, that are sound in organizational and financial structure, adequate in facilities and faculty, and well-distributed to serve the needs of the entire country."

- 1950—*Nursing Schools at the Mid-Century*[101]

  A Joint Committee on Implementing the Brown Report was established by the NLNE in 1948 (renamed the National Committee for the Improvement of Nursing Services in 1949). Its purpose was to establish programs to strengthen nursing schools as a response to the need for increased and better prepared nurses. The early work of the committee involved data collection of factual information about nursing school programs and the interim classification of schools. This was to be a precursor to the development of a more comprehensive accreditation system and program. Schools were classified according to a total score obtained by the weighting of various criteria. The "Interim Classification of Schools of Nursing Offering Basic Programs" was published in the *American Journal of Nursing* in 1949. The overall findings of the study were published in 1950 as *Nursing Schools at the Mid-Century,* which provided a method for schools of nursing to evaluate their programs.

The studies were indeed significant. Eventually inferior hospital schools were closed. Yet nursing has experienced considerable difficulty in implementing the recommendations that were put forth on the education and practice of nursing.

Impact of the Scientific Era: 1950 to 1970

After World War II the United States and Russia competed for technologic and nuclear supremacy. The competition for world power spearheaded the emphasis on scientific advancement in all major fields, including medicine and nursing.

In their initial quest to develop a scientific body of knowledge, nurses used traditional empirical methods from the medical sciences. This research perspective, known as *logical positivism,* emphasized obtaining objective, observable, measurable data that could be verified and controlled.[28] It also focused on examining separate parts of systems to identify linear causal relationships, thus enabling prediction and control of these relationships, as shown in Table 2-1. Since an investigator is supposed to be objective, empirical research was assumed to be superior and infallible. However, nurse scholars began to question the value and usefulness of sterile facts and principles in the real world of contextual relationships.* Yet logical positivism is still prevalent in nursing today and represents one major world view of science.

In response to the growing scientific perspective, nursing recognized the need for new knowledge, skills, and techniques. In an effort to define nursing, Peplau[79] described nursing as an *interpersonal process* between the client and the nurse. Peplau's classic work was deemed one of the first models in nursing. Yura and Walsh[102] credit Lydia Hall with first naming nursing a "process" in 1955. The term *nursing process* also appeared in Orlando's text, *The Dynamic Nurse-Patient Relationship.*[76] Orlando described the nursing process as the interaction between the client's behavior, the nurse's action, and the nurse's reaction. She emphasized that nurses must deliberate and validate client needs rather than respond intuitively.

It is also important to remember that the concept of what is now labeled the "nursing process" was being considered in the late 1940s and early 1950s by early nurse theorists. Note that the nursing process is not unique to nursing. Systematic approaches have long been used in other fields to answer questions and solve problems. The most familiar of these approaches are labeled the *problem-solving method* and the *scientific method.* The steps of the nursing process are identical to the steps in the problem-solving method. What is different, however, is the terminology used to identify the steps. The focus of the nursing process is client care; problem solving is used daily in all facets of life.

In the early 1960s nurse leaders suggested that nursing was a dynamic process that changed as the client's health changed. Nurses were encouraged to collect information about the client. Kelly[40] described the data available for nursing assessment as the client's physical signs and symptoms, medical history and diagnosis, social history and cultural background, and environmental factors. Knowles[44] identified the importance of discovery, delving, deciding, doing, and discriminating in nursing, thus linking nursing with the scientific process. Systematically collecting data and rigorously analyzing them was stressed by Johnson.[35] Nursing diagnosis was defined at that time as *determining the etiology of a symptom.* Also in 1967, Yura and Walsh[103] published the first comprehensive book describing

---

*References 11, 12, 36, 59, 68, 86.

the nursing process as four components: assessing, planning, implementing, and evaluating. These authors emphasized the intellectual, interpersonal, and technical skills of nursing practice.

Defining the Nursing Process: 1970s to the Present

Nurse educators originally developed the nursing process as a teaching tool to guide students in learning the scientific approach to nursing practice. In 1973 the ANA adopted, and thereby legitimized, the components of the nursing process in the ANA Standards of Nursing Practice. The ANA Standards consisted of eight specific nursing activities that described the nursing process. However, most nurse educators taught the nursing process as the four-step method during the 1970s.

The trends in the development of nursing knowledge and science also shaped the movement toward greater control over nursing education and practice. As developments occurred, changes in Nurse Practice Acts were sought. Bullough's[8] three phases of nursing licensure describe this progression:

Phase 1: 1900–1923	Nurse practice acts concerned solely with registration of nurses
Phase 2: 1938–1955	Goals determined to define the scope of nursing functions of registered nurses and practical nurses, condense educational standards, and prevent unlicensed individuals from practicing nursing
Phase 3: 1971–present	Amendments promoted to permit diagnosis, prescription, and treatment for the expanded role of nurses in delivering health care

It was during this third and current phase that most states revised or amended their Nurse Practice Acts to reflect changes in nursing practice, including use of the nursing process.

Nursing licensure was also affected by progression in the development of the nursing process, nursing knowledge, and nursing science. The single, uniform examination for nurses (originally known as the State Board Examination) to be used by all state boards of nursing was implemented in 1950. It was revised in 1982 and renamed the National Council Licensure Examination (NCLEX) in 1987. The computerized version of the examination was implemented in 1994 and named the National Council Licensure Examination—Computerized Adaptive Testing, for Registered Nurses (NCLEX-CAT, RN). It measures nursing knowledge covering a broad scope of material and encompasses three primary components: nursing process, client health needs, and levels of cognitive ability. It currently tests knowledge of the five phases (steps) of the nursing process: assessment, analysis, planning, implementation, and evaluation. Nursing process questions are equally divided for each phase.

The components in the nursing process often developed independently as different nurse scholars focused on a specific step. Many nurses described relevant aspects and important factors to consider in nursing *assessment.* Numerous tools to assess the client, family, and community appeared in the nursing literature in the 1980s. The amount of assessment data available expanded considerably. Currently the application of nursing models and theories in assessment has been emphasized.[13,30,81]

In the mid-1970s several nurses described nursing diagnosis as separate from the assessment or planning steps.[4,60] Other writers combined data collection, analysis, and diagnosis with nursing assessment.[9,50] The First National Conference for the Classification of Nursing Diagnoses was held in 1973 in St. Louis. The conference was invitational, with its participants placed into working groups to generate diagnoses related to a specific functional system. Thirty-seven nursing diagnosis labels were approved at the second conference; additional diagnoses were approved at subsequent conferences. In 1982 the conferences were opened to the nursing community and the name of the organization was changed to the North American Nursing Diagnosis Association (NANDA). Eleven conferences have been held thus far, with the last, the twelfth, being held in 1996. The current and approved list of 137 nursing diagnoses describes the phenomena that nurses treat, provides a common language to assist nursing practice, differentiates nursing from medicine, and serves as a framework for future nursing research. It is the first developed taxonomy in nursing that provides a conceptual basis for the organization and advancement of nursing knowledge and for furthering progress in nursing theory.[74] Currently the task of extending and refining nursing diagnoses has been undertaken through a collaborative effort of NANDA and the Nursing Diagnosis Extension and Classification (NDEC) team of researchers at The University of Iowa College of Nursing.[17]

Contrary to what many nurses believe, the concept of nursing diagnosis had been discussed before the 1950s by Lesnik and Anderson in *Legal Aspects of Nursing.*[48] In 1947 they described diagnosis as the "art or act of recognizing disease from its symptoms; also, the decision reached." In a long commentary similar to an anecdotal footnote, they emphasized that although diagnosis had long been the province of physicians, clarification was warranted regarding nursing activities. They argued that not every aspect of the "art of diagnosis" is the exclusive right of the physician:

> Approached basically, diagnosis involves the utilization of intelligence in interpreting known facts. The decision is the result of interpretation. Certainly the utilization of intelligence is not the exclusive province of the physician, insofar as this inseparable aspect of the science of diagnosis is concerned. A definition of nursing which embraces the functions of supervision of symptoms and reactions assumes that aspect of diagnosis which requires the exercise of intelligence.

Lesnik and Anderson in their 1955 second edition, now titled *Nursing Practice and the Law,*[49] again discussed the nurse's responsibility for diagnosis in even greater detail. The content was no longer relegated to fine print and was even stronger in tone and importance. According to these authors, "There can be no question that a nurse is required to interpret known facts and make a decision based upon them. Although the action that she may be permitted to adopt differs from that of the physician, nevertheless there are courses that are not only available but obligatory."[49] They thus proposed an area with which the nurse is charged and that might well be called "nursing diagnosis."

Nursing diagnosis gradually evolved into a separate component of the nursing process in the early 1980s.[13] In current nursing literature it is referred to as either

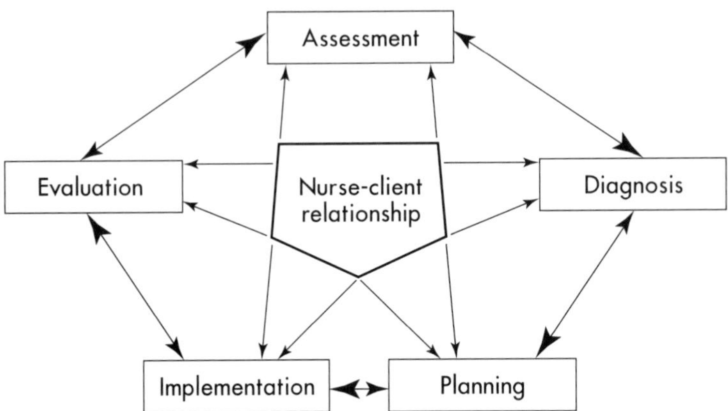

FIG. 2-1 Nursing process: feedback system. (Redrawn from Christensen PJ, Kenney J: *Nursing process: application of theories, frameworks, and models,* ed 4, St. Louis, 1994, Mosby).

the *diagnosis* or *analysis* step. In 1980 the ANA refined its definition of nursing to read, "Nursing is the diagnosis and treatment of human responses to actual or potential health problems."[2]

The *planning* component of the nursing process evolved over the years through the contributions of many nurses.[9,54] Planning divides into several sequences: prioritizing nursing diagnoses, establishing goals and objectives, developing strategies, and writing nursing orders.[13]

Evaluation in the nursing process was addressed by other nurses and includes establishing criteria and describing the differences between structure, process, and outcome evaluation.[80,95] Quality assurance mechanisms were occasionally integrated in the evaluation component. The nursing process components were originally depicted as logical sequential steps, beginning with assessment and ending with evaluation. Currently the five components are usually viewed as an open system, with an interacting network of smaller units.[77] The feedback model developed by Christensen[13] illustrates the interaction of each component with all the other components to varying degrees. This model is illustrated in Figure 2-1.

Currently Accepted Components of the Nursing Process

The nursing process is a systematic approach to nursing practice that leads to sound judgments and actions. Nurses use a comprehensive knowledge base to assess the client's health status; make judicious decisions and diagnoses; and plan, implement, and evaluate appropriate nursing actions. As the core of nursing practice, the nursing process provides the structure for nursing care. Five interacting (not linear) components, with various steps, make up the nursing process (Figure 2-1 and Table 2-2).

The nursing process model, Figure 2-1, depicts the usual flow of information by the dark lines and heavy arrows clockwise from assessment to diagnosis, planning, implementation, evaluation, and back to assessment. The small arrows in the opposite direction show that information from the succeeding components affects the previous ones by providing feedback. The lighter lines intersecting with the nurse-

TABLE 2-2

Components, Definitions, and Activities in the Nursing Process

Components	Definitions	Activities
Assessment	Ongoing process of data collection to determine client strengths and health concerns	Data collection Interview History Examination Review records
Diagnosis	Analysis/synthesis of data to identify patterns and compare with norms and models	Data analysis and synthesis Identify gaps Categorize Recognize patterns Compare to norms and models
	Clear, concise statement of client health status and concerns appropriate for nursing intervention	Diagnostic statements Actual concerns Potential concerns Etiology
Planning	Determining how to assist client in resolving concerns related to restoration, maintenance, or promotion of health	Establish priorities Set goals/objectives Select strategies Write nursing orders Describe rationale
Implementation	Client and nurse carry out the plan of care	Perform interventions Collaborate Ongoing assessment Update/revise plan Document responses
Evaluation	Systematic, continuous process of comparing client response with written goals/objectives	Compare responses to objectives/goals Determine progress Revise plan of care

From Christensen P, Kenney J, eds: *Nursing process: application of theories, frameworks and models,* ed 4, St. Louis, 1994, Mosby.

client relationship show that this relationship affects each component of the nursing process and that each component is interdependent with all other components.

The purpose of the nursing process is to provide a systematic framework for nursing practice. As such, it unifies, standardizes, and directs nursing practice. The nursing process defines nurses' roles and functions and enhances communication, collaboration, and synchronization of health team members. Equal emphasis is given to health prevention, maintenance, restoration, and/or a peaceful and dignified death.

The nursing process includes the following seven major characteristics:

1. Goal-directed, to provide quality client-centered health care
2. Systematic, providing organized logical approach to nursing care
3. Dynamic, because it involves an ongoing process focused on the changing responses of the client
4. Applicable to individuals, families, and community groups at any point on the health-illness continuum

5. Adaptable to any practice setting or specialization; components may be used sequentially or concurrently
6. Interpersonal, based on nurse-client relationship
7. Useful with any type of model, especially nursing[13]

Future Trends in the Nursing Process

The nursing process is now an integral and essential part of the curriculum in nursing education. It is the basis for learning nursing practice and for making decisions about nursing care. However, as nurses acquire advanced knowledge and experience, they internalize this thinking process and develop an intuitive grasp of the client's situation.[5] From her study of different ways practicing nurses think, Benner[5] identified five levels of nursing proficiency. The first level (novice, or student) relies on a set of rules or guidelines such as the nursing process. With increasing experience, nurses attain a proficient, or expert, level of practice in which they perceive the client situation as a gestalt and initiate actions without separately analyzing each factor. Benner's research suggests that as nurses develop proficiency they use a more holistic approach and can visualize future possibilities for their clients. Reliance on the structured nursing process by proficient nurses may reduce their creative approaches to nursing practice.

Increasingly, baccalaureate nursing programs introduce the application and integration of nursing models into the nursing process. These models provide a framework that defines the nurse's role, the client, and the meaning of health. Nurses use several models to guide their practice, some of which include Maslow's[52] hierarchy of needs, Erikson's[22] stages of man's development, Orem's[75] self-care model, and Roy's[84] adaptation model. Nursing models can direct each component of nursing practice and assist nurses to:

- Collect, organize, and classify data
- Understand, analyze, and interpret the client's health situation
- Plan, implement, and evaluate nursing care
- Explain nursing actions

As more nurses learn about nursing models and theories and their application in practice, the commitment in the nursing profession to theory-based nursing practice will grow.

In the future the five components of the nursing process will be further refined. Standardized nursing assessment data sets will be used to collect client data either on the computer record or on a standardized form for the chart. These client data sets will be based on nursing models instead of the medical systems model. Nursing diagnostic classifications will be expanded through efforts such as that of the NDEC research team. As clients' total charts are entered into computers, data from nursing diagnoses, interventions, and outcomes evaluation will be used in research studies to analyze the efficacy and cost-effectiveness of various interventions. Nursing interventions may also be changed after replicative research studies are based on client data. Finally, the use of client computerized records will mandate the development of new evaluation tools and research methods.

With the advent of managed care and case management, tools such as standardized care plans, critical pathways, or care maps have been evolving. These provide options for innovative and creative nursing interventions in specialized areas such as obstetrics, oncology, or cardiology. They briefly and concisely define the

TABLE 2-3

Theory Development System

Process	Activities	Product
Identify values, beliefs, and assumptions	What do nurses do (actions, skills), for whom (individuals, families, community) When (under what conditions) Where (in what settings) How (roles, i.e., practitioner, researcher)	Philosophy of nursing
Concept analysis	Define and describe major concepts Nursing (action, interactions, process) Clients (individual, family, community) Health (maintenance, prevention, restoration) Environment (hospital, community, clinic)	Concept identification
Construct relationships	Descriptive theory Describes relationships between concepts, but the relationship between *all* concepts is not clearly defined	Conceptual model
Test relationships	Explanatory theory Explains the interrelationship between major concepts; however, logical and empirical adequacy of relationships requires further explication	Theoretical framework
Validate relationships in practice	Predictive and prescriptive theory Provides a set of interrelated concepts and relational statements that are logical and amenable to empirical testing and explain or predict phenomena	Theory

sequence and timing of key tasks and technical aspects of the treatment plan and provide the framework for planning client care. Daily events, tasks, and interventions that caregivers must provide for the "usual" client with a specific condition are spelled out. Since hospital stays are being reduced, the focus will of necessity be on monitoring the clients' physiologic responses with the teaching of self-care responsibilities delegated to community case managers for follow-up.

In summary, the nursing process as it is known today evolved over a 50-year span as the result of the nursing profession's response to societal needs. Many nurse leaders contributed to its development and refinement. As consensus was reached by the profession, the ANA formulated the Standards of Nursing Practice, and clinical specialty groups adopted modified versions. State Board Examinations were changed to reflect the five components of the nursing process and most state nurse practice acts were revised to reflect the current scope of nursing practice and the use of the nursing process and nursing diagnoses.

Theory Development in Nursing

Theory development is considered both a process and a product.[33] The process includes many cognitive activities, such as analyzing, synthesizing, testing, and refining. This process is not linear: the theorist may move back and forth in the various phases. The product of these activities is expressed as a philosophy of nursing, a conceptual model or a theory, as shown in Table 2-3.

There are several views on how nursing theory develops. Initially most nurse theorists began by identifying their beliefs, values, and assumptions about human beings, how people's health is affected by their interactions with the environment, and how nurses can assist them to maintain or regain health. The theorists' views of these concepts reflect their philosophies. Major concepts are then identified, analyzed, and defined. Walker and Avant[94] proposed that theory development begins with *concept analysis,* whereby the theorist defines all concepts relevant to a proposed theory. Next, the concepts are linked in *relational statements,* and the statements are analyzed for their internal logic and consistency with other validated theories, laws, and principles. Next, the concepts, statements and theory are tested and further refined as necessary. According to Stevens,[89] once a theorist identifies the relationship between some concepts, this is considered *descriptive theory,* with a conceptual model being the product. When the relational statements of all the concepts are explicit, the work may be considered at the level of *explanatory theory* and is called a *theoretical framework.* A theorist's work may be considered a *theory* when it provides a set of interrelated defined concepts and logical statements relating all the concepts, and the statements are amenable to testing. However, the relationship must be tested and validated in a variety of practice settings to be supported and accepted by the discipline as a theory.

Chinn and Kramer[12] recommend a similar process that includes creating conceptual meaning, structuring and contextualizing theory, generating and testing theoretic relationships, and, finally, deliberately applying theory to practice. A model of the process of theory development is illustrated in Figure 2-2 and described as follows:

1. Philosophy—a theorist's viewpoint; in other words, what the theorist assumes, believes, or holds to be true. The theorist examines: What is nursing? What does the nurse do? How? For whom? Each of the well-known nursing theorists has unique views about the nature of nursing, health, and clients, which will be discussed later.
2. Concept—an abstract word that conveys a mental image. Concepts are names, labels, or categories for objects, persons, or events. Each individual interprets a concept based on past experiences and perception of its present use. Concepts must be specifically defined within a contextual statement if they are to have meaning. Alone, concepts are useless. For example, the concept *nurse* has different meanings for everyone. Concepts can be variable or nonvariable. With simple labeling of an item such as a dish, the concept is nonvariable. With more than one form, a concept is variable, such as with *excited,* which can be designated as less to more. In theory development the theorist identifies the major concepts, then analyzes and describes what each concept means.
3. Conceptual model—a group of related concepts whose relationship is not explicit.[19] In nursing the difference between conceptual model, theoretic framework, and theory continues to be debated. What one writer considers a conceptual model, another writer calls a theory. Conceptual models attempt to represent the real world, but they are not reality. The concepts symbolize meanings, but the relationships between the concepts are obscure and subject to many different interpretations.

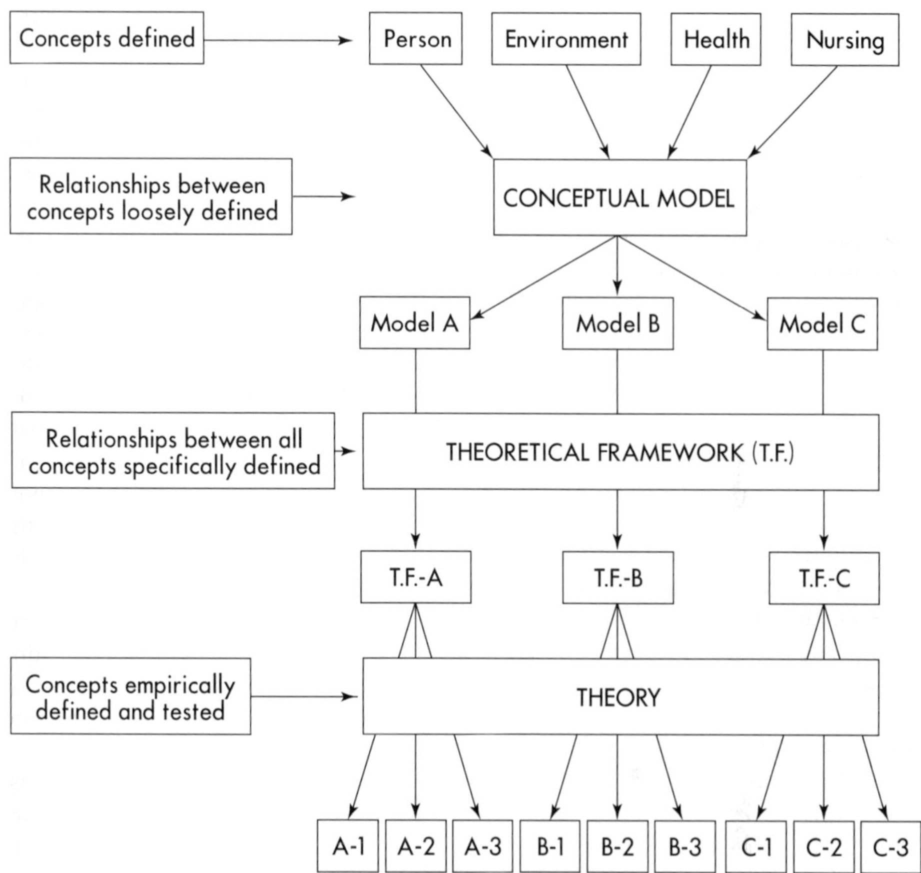

FIG. 2-2 Model of nursing theory development process.

4. Theoretic frameworks—a set of defined concepts and some relational statements linking them. A relational statement is a proposition stating how the concepts interact: their positive or negative association, or cause-effect relationship. A theoretic framework is less tentative than a conceptual model and requires explication of the specific relationships between *all* major concepts before it may be considered an "acceptable" theory. The relationships that are clearly specified may be tested for empirical adequacy.
5. Theory—a set of explicitly defined concepts and relational statements that explain a phenomenon and project a tentative, purposeful, and systematic view. The term *theory* is very complex, with many arbitrary meanings and little agreement among the disciplines. For some, theory includes ideas or hunches. Others argue that a theory must be rigorously tested and can be accepted only on consensual agreement within a discipline. A theory symbolically represents reality. It is abstract and tentative. The level of abstraction varies with the types of concepts and relational statements in the theory. Theory is considered tentative until it is repeatedly tested and validated in practice.

■ EVOLUTION OF NURSING THEORY: CHRONOLOGY OF DEVELOPMENT

Many nurse scholars cite Florence Nightingale as the first nurse theorist. Nightingale had sets of principles related to cleanliness, fresh air, good food, rest, sleep, and exercise; good health care seemed synonymous with good health habits and a healthy environment. The emphasis was on nursing as health oriented, to put the client in the best condition for nature to restore or preserve health and to prevent or cure disease or injury. This philosophy was consistent with the fact that Nightingale accepted the theory of *miasma* (a form of bad air, or bad odor, that permeated places where rotting organic material was located) as the cause of illness. She did not accept the germ theory as an explanation for the cause of disease. One cannot dispute that Nightingale had significant thoughts, ideas, and principles that, at times, were even disjointed. These must, however, be systematically analyzed according to defined criteria to establish her credibility as a theorist. Some believe her to be the first nurse theorist; others do not. In her *Notes on Nursing, What It Is and What It Is Not,* Nightingale[73] described her philosophy of nursing and her view of the nature of nursing practice. Undoubtedly the book was an inspiration not only for nursing theorists but also for all nurses.

With the exception of Nightingale's work, nursing theory development had its initial beginnings in the 1950s as nurses began to formulate definitions and descriptions of nursing. In 1952 Peplau[79] published *Interpersonal Relations in Nursing.* Nursing was represented as an interpersonal process between nurse and client; four phases of the nurse-client relationship were described. This work led to numerous studies in the communication area and brought interpersonal theories from psychiatry into nursing. Virginia Henderson's[29] first definition of nursing was published in 1955 and revised in 1966:

> The unique function of the nurse is to assist the individual, sick or well, in the performance of those activities contributing to health or its recovery (or to a peaceful death) that he could perform unaided if he had the necessary strength, will or knowledge. And to do this in such a way as to help him gain independence as rapidly as possible.

In this same decade the federal government initiated numerous programs to assist nurses with graduate education and for various research projects and grants. In 1955 the U.S. Public Health Services National Institute of Health (NIH) offered special predoctoral research fellowships. These were awarded directly to students to finance doctoral study. In addition, the Nurse Scientist Training programs offered grants to schools of nursing to support doctoral education of faculty. Many nurses were assisted by these grants and the development of doctoral programs in nursing was facilitated. Through these efforts nursing theory and science were catalyzed. Many nurses seeking doctoral education studied behavioral sciences such as sociology, psychology, and education until well into the 1980s. Lack of access to doctoral programs in nursing still leads nurses to seek the doctoral degree in these fields in the 1990s. Having been grounded in these disciplines, nurses eventually developed theories derived from the social sciences.[85] By the 1960s four universities offered doctoral programs in nursing: Teachers College, Columbia University with doctorates in nursing education (Ed.D.); New York University, with doctorates in philosophy (Ph.D.); the University of Pittsburg, with a doctoral program in maternal-child health nursing; and Boston University, with the first doctorate in nursing science (D.N.S.) in psychiatric nursing. These programs were small, and the few students attending were challenged to identify what made nursing unique from other disciplines.

With the emergence of the scientific era in the 1960s, nurse scholars criticized uneducated intuitive nursing practice. The nature of practice was debated during this decade as nursing leaders recognized the need to define nursing practice, develop nursing theory, and create a substantive body of knowledge. Several nurse leaders, including Abdellah, Orlando, Weidenbach, Hall, Henderson, and Levine, developed and published descriptions of nursing. Their work evolved from personal, professional, and educational experiences, and reflected their perception of "ideal" nursing practice.

Table 2-4 lists the nursing leaders who made scholarly contributions to the development of nursing theory. These theorists described nursing as an interpersonal process, meeting clients' needs, and/or providing care. A brief overview of their work follows:

- 1960: Fay Abdellah published the first of her three textbooks on client-centered approaches. She advised nurses to use a problem-solving approach in resolving 21 nursing problems related to individual health needs.
- 1961: Ida Jean Orlando described nursing as a dynamic interaction between nurse and client. She described the nursing process as the nurse's perception of the client's thoughts, feelings, and actions and the nurse's actions to meet the needs of ill clients.
- 1964: Lydia Hall described nursing practice at the Loeb Center for Nursing at Montefiore Hospital. She viewed nursing as three intersecting circles: the core, the care, and the cure. The *core* represents application of the biologic sciences and therapeutic use of self by the nurse; the *care* reflects intimate bodily care and nurturing; and the *cure* is based on understanding and implementing the physician's orders.
- 1964: Ernestine Wiedenbach delineated four components of nursing: philosophy, purpose, practice, and art. She defined nursing as helping clients through identification, ministration, validation, and coordination.
- 1966: Virginia Henderson's major contribution was a concise definition of nursing. She described nursing as assisting individuals, sick or well, to regain independence. She listed 13 components of basic nursing care.
- 1967: Myra Levine defined nursing as supportive and therapeutic interventions based on scientific or therapeutic knowledge. She believed that all nursing actions are based on four principles: conservation of energy, structural integrity, personal integrity, and social integrity.

The work of nurse theorists from Peplau through the 1960s focused on defining the nurse's role and nursing actions to assist clients toward healthy outcomes. After the 1960s several nurse theorists expanded the earlier models in different directions.

In the 1960s Lucille Notter became editor of the journal *Nursing Research.* Under her guidance the articles published and the topics they addressed encouraged open discussion of the nature of nursing and theory development. Another important influence on nursing theory development was the federal financial

TABLE 2-4

History of Nursing Theory Development

Events	Year	Nurse Theorist
	1860	Florence Nightingale Described nursing and environment
	1952	Hildegard E. Peplau Nursing as an interpersonal process Patients with felt needs
Scientific era: nurses questioned purpose of nursing	1960	Faye Abdellah (also 1965, 1973) Patient-centered approaches
	1961	Ida Jean Orlando Nurse-patient relationship Deliberate nursing approach
Process of theory development discussed among professional nurses	1964	Ernestine Wiedenbach (also 1970, 1977) Nursing: philosophy, purpose, practice, and art Patient with needs
	1966	Lydia E. Hall Core (patient), care (body), cure (disease)
	1966	Virginia Henderson (also 1972, 1978) Nursing assists patients with fourteen essential functions toward independence
Symposium: theory development in nursing	1967	Myra Estrin Levine (also 1973) Four conservation principles of nursing
Symposium: nature of science and nursing Dickoff, James, and Wiedenbach wrote "Theory in a Practice Discipline" in *Nursing Research* Symposium: theory development in nursing	1968	
First nursing theory conference: the nature of science in nursing	1969	
Second nursing theory conference	1970	Martha E. Rogers (also 1980) Science of unitary man: energy fields, openness, pattern, and organization
Consensus on nursing concepts: nurse/nursing, health, client/patient/individual, society/environment	1971	Dorthea E. Orem (also 1980, 1985) Nursing facilitates patient self-care

TABLE 2-4

History of Nursing Theory Development—cont'd

Events	Year	Nurse Theorist
Discussion on what is theory, its elements, criteria, types and levels, and its relation to research	1971	Imogene King (also 1975, 1981) Theory of goal attainment through nurse-client transactions
NLN required conceptual frameworks in nursing education	1973	
Borrowed theories from other disciplines Expanded theories from other disciplines	1974	Sister Callista Roy (also 1976, 1980, 1984) Roy's adaptation model nurse adjusts patient's stimuli (focal, contextual, or residual)
Recognized problems in practice and developed theories to test and use in practice	1976	Josephine Paterson and L. Zderad Humanistic nursing
Nurse educator conference on nursing theory	1977	Madeline Leininger (also 1980, 1981) Transcultural nursing Caring nursing
Articles on theory development appeared in *ANS, Nursing Research,* and *Image*	1978	
	1979	Jean Watson (also 1985) Philosophy and science of caring Humanistic nursing
Books were written for nurses on how to critique theory and how to develop theory, and described application of nursing theories	1980	Dorothy E. Johnson Behavioral system model for nursing
Graduate schools of nursing developed courses in how to analyze and apply nursing theories		Betty Neuman Health-care systems model: a total person approach
Research studies in nursing identified nursing theories as framework for study	1981	Rosemarie Rizzo Parse (also 1987) Man-living-health: a theory of nursing
	1982-present	Numerous books published on analysis, application, evaluation, and/or development of nursing theories

From Christensen PJ, Kenney JW: *Nursing process: application of conceptual models,* ed 4, St. Louis, 1994, Mosby.

support given to nursing schools to sponsor conferences on the nature and development of nursing science. Three landmark conferences were held in the late 1960s. These conferences were:

- Theory Development in Nursing at Case Western Reserve, 1967
- The Nature of Science and Nursing at the University of Colorado, 1968
- The Nature of Science in Nursing at the University of Colorado, 1969

The proceedings of the conferences were published in *Nursing Research.*

The purpose of these conferences was to gather nurse scientists together to discuss the nature of nursing, the development of basic and applied research, and ways to develop a nursing science. These conferences provided a forum for discussing and synthesizing knowledge from a variety of disciplines. Nurses developed a commitment to regular conferences for nursing research, theory, and practice.

Dickoff and James[19] presented their position paper, "A Theory of Theories," at the first conference. They introduced the idea that significant nursing theory must be "situation producing"; in other words, nursing must develop theories that prescribe nursing actions for predictable client outcomes. Their controversial position has been debated for many years.

In 1969 the First Nursing Theory Conference was held in Kansas City, with the second conference the following year. These conferences brought nurse theorists and scholars together to debate the issues of the purpose of nursing theory and science, how theory can be developed, and what types of theory are needed in nursing.

By the 1970s there were numerous publications on the development of nursing theory and nursing science. However, the 1970 report by the Joint Commission on Nursing Theory and Nursing Education noted the absence of nursing theory and research in practice. The report indicated that the commission believed this omission hindered the development of nursing. As more nurses received doctoral education in nursing and other disciplines, they recognized the value of theory in explaining nursing actions and in developing a science of nursing. Nurses also became aware that theories developed in other disciplines were insufficient to describe nursing. They concluded that nurses needed to develop their own theories. Dickoff and Wiedenbach[20] stimulated this trend by describing how theory is developed for a practice discipline. Although their approach to theory development was debated, it sparked a growing commitment by nurses to develop their own models and theories.

In 1972 Newman[67] described the following three approaches that nurses used to develop nursing models:

1. Theories were borrowed from related disciplines and integrated into a science of nursing
2. Nursing practice situations were analyzed to identify theoretic underpinnings
3. Conceptual models of nursing were created from which theories could be derived

Newman's classification of the evolution of nursing theory provided one view. In reality many nurse theorists combined several approaches in developing nursing models. New models in the 1970s often expanded the work of earlier theorists. One theorist would pick up where another left off, adding insight to a missing piece. The nursing models that evolved in the 1970s were a product of accretion rather than accumulation.[71]

■ CURRENT NURSING MODELS: CONTEMPORARY THEORISTS

The work of early nurse theorists contributed to the development of the central concepts in nursing. In the 1970s a consensus among nursing leaders included the following major concepts:[23]

1. Nursing—roles and actions of nurses
2. Client—recipient of nursing care
3. Health—client's place on the health-illness continuum
4. Environment—context for nurse-client interactions

These four concepts and their interrelationships were accepted as the bases for nursing models and theories, which would become a science of nursing. For several years nurse leaders debated whether there would be one model or theory to describe nursing or several models to describe the relationships between the four concepts. Since 1970, 10 nurse theorists have published books describing their models. Each nursing model or theory represents the theorist's unique view of each of the four major concepts. In addition to describing the major concepts, each theorist developed several subconcepts that describe the interaction between the nurse and client or further clarify the activities or role of the nurse.

The essence of the work of these 10 contemporary nurse theorists is presented in chronologic order (Box 2-1). For a thorough understanding of each theorist's viewpoint, the literature includes numerous primary and secondary sources.

Categories of Nursing Models

Nursing models may be categorized in the following ways:

1. Underlying theoretic base
2. Level of theory development
3. Level of abstraction

These categorizations provide different ways of looking at the theorist's work. The three categorizations are explained below.

Underlying theoretic base. Although each nursing theorist's model is unique, some similarities between models exist. Each model is based on one or two theoretic premises that ultimately influence the overall work. Three theoretic themes evolved in nursing since the 1970s. The first predominant theme was introduced in the early "interactional" models of Peplau, Orlando, and King, and focused on the interpersonal nurse-client process. Peplau[79] integrated theories from psychiatry to help nurses analyze nurse-client interactions. Orlando[76] used psychiatric and communications theory to describe the nurse's deliberative approach of analyzing the client's behavior, actions, and reactions. Building on these theories, King[42,43] described the transactional process of goal attainment in the nurse-client relationship. She added systems theory, which incorporated the family and community social systems, thereby broadening the client's environment.

Subsequent theoretic approaches that emerged in nursing include the following:

1. Systems theory—serves as the basis for the models developed by King, Johnson, and Neuman. Neuman's model was an outgrowth of systems theory used in organizational behavior theory.[18] The client is viewed as a system interacting with and adjusting to other systems, such as the family, community, or environment.

Box 2-1 Contemporary Nurse Theorists

ROGERS' SCIENCE OF UNITARY HUMAN BEINGS (1970)

Nursing: A science and art to facilitate and promote symphonic interaction between human beings and their environment

Client: Any human being or individual and personal environment

Health: An expression of the life process characterized by behaviors emerging from mutual simultaneous interaction between human beings and their environment; a continuum based on value judgments

Environment: A four-dimensional negentropic energy field identified by pattern and organization, and encompassing all that is outside any given human field; any setting worldwide where nurse and client meet

OREM'S SELF-CARE MODEL (1971)

Nursing: A service of deliberately selected and performed actions to assist individuals or groups to maintain self-care, including structural integrity, functioning, and development

Client: An individual who is unable to continuously maintain self-care in sustaining life and health, in recovering from disease or injury, or in coping with their effects

Health: An individual's ability to meet self-care demands that contributes to the maintenance and promotion of structural integrity, functioning, and development

Environment: Any setting in which a client has unmet self-care needs and a nurse is present

KING'S MODEL—A THEORY OF GOAL ATTAINMENT (1971)

Nursing: An interaction process between client and nurse in which transactions occur and goals are achieved as a result of perceiving a need, setting goals, and acting on them

Client: An individual (personal system) or group (interpersonal system) who is unable to cope with an event or a health problem while interacting with the environment

Health: An ability to perform the activities of daily living in one's usual social roles. A dynamic life experience of continuous adjustment to environmental stressors through optimum use of resources

Environment: Any *social system* in society; social systems are dynamic forces that influence social interaction, perception, and health, and include hospitals, clinics, community agencies, schools, and industry

ROY'S ADAPTATION MODEL (1974)

Nursing: Uses the nursing process to promote client adaptation in the four modes to enhance health

Client: A person, family, group, or community with unusual stresses or ineffective coping mechanisms

Health: A state and process of being and becoming an integrated and whole person

Environment: All conditions, circumstances, and influences surrounding and affecting the development and behavior of persons or groups: any health-related situation is implied as the setting

PATERSON AND ZDERAD'S HUMANISTIC NURSING (1976)

Nursing: An existential experience of being and doing with another person to respond to their fundamental needs

Client: A unique individual who is struggling to know about self and others

Health: A state in which basic needs are addressed by another to assist growth of awareness and make responsible choices

Environment: Any situation whereby nurse and client seek awareness of the experience by responding to the client's needs

Box 2-1 Contemporary Nurse Theorists—cont'd

LEININGER'S TRANSCULTURAL NURSING MODEL (1978)

Nursing: A humanistic and scientific mode of helping a client, through specific cultural *caring* processes (cultural values, beliefs, and practices), to improve or maintain a health condition for life or death

Client: An individual, family, group, society, or community with possible physical, psychologic, or social needs within the context of their culture

Health: Defined by the specific culture; technology-dependent cultures view health and health care differently than non–technology-dependent societies do

Environment: Any culture or society in which ethnocaring is practiced by nurses assisting clients

PARSE'S MAN-LIVING-HEALTH MODEL (1981)

Nursing: Guiding of individuals and families to share and uncover personal meaning of their living health situation

Client: Person or family concerned with their quality of life situation; man is viewed as an open, whole being, influenced by past and present lived experiences, who interchanges with the environment through choices and responsibility for those choices

Health: A process of unfolding, continuously changing, lived experiences, including a synthesis of values and a way of living

Environment: Setting is undefined but implied to be any health-related setting

D.E. JOHNSON'S BEHAVIORAL SYSTEM MODEL (1980)

Nursing: Regulates external forces to stabilize client's behavioral system and restore, maintain, or attain balance

Client: A behavioral system (person) threatened or potentially threatened by illness (imbalance) and/or hospitalization

Health: An efficient and effectively functioning behavioral system (person) that is in balance/stable as a result of adapting/adjusting to outside forces

Environment: No specific setting identified

NEUMAN'S HEALTH-CARE SYSTEMS MODEL (1980)

Nursing: Assists clients to reduce stress factors and adverse conditions that affect optimal functioning

Client: Individual, family, or group with an identified or suspected stressor that may disrupt harmony and balance

Health: A level of wellness in which all needs are met and more energy is built and stored than is expended

Environment: Includes internal and external forces surrounding the client; nurse-client settings are not described

WATSON'S MODEL OF HUMAN CARING (1985)

Nursing: A transpersonal process of caring that enables the client to find meaning in wellness, gain self-knowledge and control, and restore inner harmony for self-healing

Client: Any individual who enters into a transpersonal caring process with a nurse

Health: Unity and harmony within the mind, body, and soul, which is associated with the degree of congruence between the self as perceived and the self as experienced

Environment: The setting is undefined but is implied to be any situation in which the nurse interacts with a client

2. Stress-adaptation theory—used in the models developed by Roy, Johnson, and Neuman. These theorists believe the client experiences stress, which leads to disequilibrium. The nurse's role is to restore equilibrium and facilitate adaptation.
3. Humanistic health experience—the theoretic basis for the work of Rogers,[83] Paterson and Zderad,[78] Leininger,[46,47] Neuman,[66] Parse,[77] and Watson.[9]

These theorists emphasize the humanistic transactional relationship in nursing that transcends the body and mind and includes the spiritual and higher levels of consciousness.[68] Models based on this perspective are often described within the "human science of caring."[59,70] Humans are viewed as unitary wholes who are free-willed, intentional beings and who actively participate in continuous interactions within their dynamic social, cultural, and historical world. The human's lived experience is the fundamental, preeminent reality of concern to nursing and includes what the person thinks and feels, along with their complex past, present, and future as perceived and experienced in relation to the here and now. This emerging perspective of nursing is a major shift from the biologic model, as shown in Table 2-1, and is gaining tremendous support among nurse scholars.

From the mid-1960s professional nursing attempted to define nursing and differentiate nursing practice from medical care. Henderson's[29] definition of nursing as "do for the patient what he cannot do for himself to promote independence" was widely accepted. In a similar theme, Orem[75] proposed a model delineating three roles for nurses to promote the client's self-care. Johnson's[39] behavioral systems model describes nursing as assisting patients to regain stability or equilibrium. Roy's[84] adaptation model describes nursing as reducing the client's stimuli and promoting adaptation. These theorists viewed clients as somewhat incapacitated within the health-illness continuum. The nurse's role was to help the client regain independence and equilibrium or perform self-care activities.[68] The various philosophical schools of thought are discussed in Chapter 7.

The shift from the traditional world view of science to the humanistic transactional view of health and caring in nursing began with the late Martha Rogers[82] at New York University. Based on her knowledge of physics and laws of thermodynamics, she described unitary human beings as open systems, inseparable from and in constant interaction with their environment. Human beings are all different in the way they interact with their environment, but their behaviors can be distinguished and create patterns that can be identified and labeled. According to Rogers, the purpose of nursing is to recognize these patterns and promote symphonic interaction between humans and their environment.[83] Roger's new view of humans, their interaction with the environment, and the purpose of nursing directly influenced models proposed by Newman, Parse, and Watson, although each of these theorists proceeded in slightly different directions.[70] The shift from nurses' empirical view of nursing science to a more humanistic, experiential view is illustrated in Table 2-1.

Level of theory development. Classification of nursing models according to the level of theory development was first described by Stevens.[89] She classified nursing theory as descriptive, explanatory, or predictive, as shown in Table 2-3. *Descriptive theory* is the first level of development. Major concepts such as *client, nursing,* and *health* are identified and described by the theorist. The relationship between concepts, however, is not described. *Explanatory theory* attempts to describe how or why the major concepts are related. The theorist explains the relationship between some concepts. However, further clarification of the logical and empirical adequacy of the relationships is needed for testing. *Predictive theory* is achieved when the conditions under which concepts are related are stated and the relational statements consistently describe future outcomes. This highest level of theory development permits repeated testing of the theory for validation. In nursing and the social sciences it is generally accepted that predictive theories are actively being pursued but presently do not exist.

Level of abstraction. Walker and Avant[94] classified nursing theory according to the level of abstraction. They identified the following four levels:

1. Meta-theory—highest level of abstraction; focuses on broad philosophic and methodologic issues related to theory development; at this level, nurse scholars analyze the purpose and type of theory nursing needs, propose sources for theory development, and examine criteria for evaluating theory in nursing
2. Grand nursing theories—provide global conceptual frameworks for nursing practice and education; broad abstract descriptions of the nurse's actions or roles
3. Middle-range theories—more limited in the scope of nursing practice than grand theories; also provide more direction for practice and research
4. Practice theory—first described by Dickoff and James;[19] specifies the goal and the nursing actions necessary to achieve the goal; can be tested in practice; nursing is moving in this direction

Acceptance of Nursing Models

The publication of nurse theorists' work in journals and textbooks has sparked a growing interest among nurses to understand, analyze, apply, test, and evaluate their models. As nurse educators first became familiar with the theorists' models, a few were taught in some nursing programs, notably Roy's stress-adaptation model and Orem's self-care model. In the mid-1970s several nurse theorists expanded and revised their earlier work in attempts to describe their theories within the framework of logical empiricism. Orem, King, Roy, and Rogers published more explicit definitions of their concepts and relational statements and tried to show the logical adequacy of their theories. Some nurse scholars describe the application of selected models in practice, and others describe research studies based on a nurse theorist's framework. This growing body of literature contributes to the gradual acceptance of several theorists' models. In addition, the theorists presented their models at national conferences where nurse educators sought an understanding of how to apply the models in practice.

Acceptance of a theorist's model by the nursing profession is contingent on numerous factors. The theorist's work must be a substantial publication, well disseminated and widely read. The model must be sufficiently described and clearly explained for nurses to grasp the ideas and comprehend their application in nursing. There must also be a cadre of educated nurses who thoroughly understand the theorist's work, can teach it to others, apply it in practice, and test it in research. Martha Rogers taught her theory at New York University in the master and doctoral programs in the 1970s. Many of her graduate students wrote their dissertations based on her theoretic work, and some have continued to conduct research based on her work. Rogers' protégés include Margaret Newman, Jacqueline Fawcett, and Rosemarie Parse. The work of Rogers, and those of her followers, continues to strongly influence nursing practice, theory, and research. The nursing diagnostic conference group is well represented by Rogers' protégés, who have influenced the list of accepted diagnostic categories. The nursing models by Newman,[66] Parse,[77] and Watson[97] reflect the strong influence of Rogers' work.

By the 1980s most graduate nursing programs included a core course in theory development that provided an overview of nursing theorists' work. Concurrently, various nurse scholars continued to debate how theory is constructed and what evaluation criteria must be achieved for a theorist's work to be called a theory. During the 1970s most nurse scholars believed that the purpose of theory was the description, explanation, and prediction of phenomena. A strong commitment to logical empiricism is reflected in the writings of Fawcett[24] and Walker and Avant.[93,94] It was believed that rigorous and logically structured theory, with operational definitions of the concepts, was necessary for theory testing and validation—the ultimate criteria of a theory. In the late 1970s nurse scholars recognized the limits of logical empiricism and quantitative research in dealing with nursing phenomena. As nursing began to emphasize humanism and holism, scholars sought more meaningful and creative ways to describe nursing theory and research.[88] By the mid-1980s there was a gradual shift from acceptance of empirical scientific knowledge as the sole way of knowing to a broader view of knowledge based on the inclusion of ethical, aesthetic, and personal knowledge. This shifting viewpoint reflects a synthesis of the influences of Rogers (1970), Carper,[10] Parse,[77] Benner,[5] Chinn and Kramer,[12] and Watson.[98]

Future Trends in Theory Development

Nursing, like any scientific discipline, will continue to experience shifts and new trends in its evolution. Nursing theory will continue to respond to the dynamic changes in society and science. As the body of nursing science grows, older models and theories will be replaced by newer ones that more completely explain nursing. Nurse practitioners and researchers will continue to apply and test nursing models in practice settings. Nurse theorists will continue to develop, refine, and test their models and theories. Practice theories may be constructed and tested in specific clinical situations.

The nurse scholars in education will establish closer working relationships with practitioners, researchers, and theorists to keep abreast of changes in society and in nursing practice. Collaboration in theory construction among these professionals, and cooperation in testing theory through conducting research in practice settings and disseminating findings, will advance the science of nursing.

The establishment of nursing research centers in state and national institutions and academic settings will continue as the integration of research, theory, and practice continues to escalate. Interdisciplinary and international research will increase, creative strategies will be developed to attract research funding, and research application in nursing practice will be demonstrated. Nursing organizations will increase their efforts to enhance scholarship so that knowledge and theory development will continue their momentum toward the goal of nursing science. Finally, the world will become even smaller as emphasis is placed on global health concerns and the research needed to resolve them.

■ PROFESSIONAL NURSING'S RESPONSE TO SOCIAL CHANGE

Professional nursing continually changes and evolves in response to major trends in the medical and human sciences and technology, in consumers' health care problems and needs, and in the health care systems. These major trends, which are depicted in Figure 2-3 and Table 2-5, continue to influence nursing today. Trends in medical science (such as the diagnosis and treatment of HIV and AIDS) along with advanced technology (such as computer imaging of the brain or laser surgery) have a direct effect on nursing. Changes in health care insurance carriers and coverage influence health care services provided to consumers. Nursing education, licensure, and trends for certification in advanced practice specialties also influence nursing and the types of health care provided. Within each of these areas, many complex issues involving economic, social, political, cultural, and ethical considerations provide an important contextual background for understanding their impact on nursing. Some of these major trends are described in the next sections, whereas others are presented in greater depth in subsequent chapters.

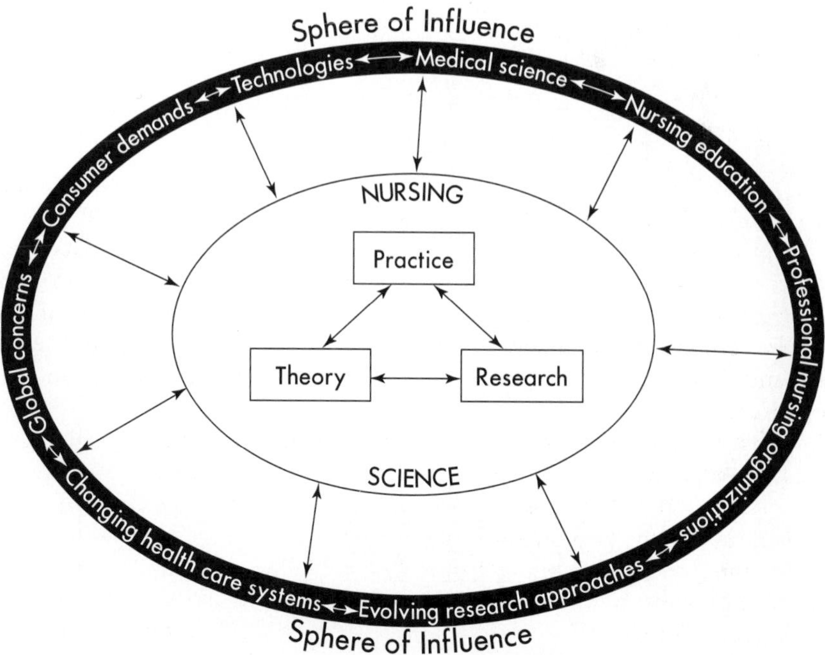

FIG. 2-3 Model showing the relationship of trends in the sphere of influence on nursing. (Redrawn from original design by Steven Warner, The University of Iowa—College of Nursing.)

TABLE 2-5

Trends Influencing Nursing

Medical Science	Nursing Education	Professional Nursing Organizations	Evolving Research Approaches	Health Care Systems	Global Concerns	Consumer Demands	Technologies
Diagnostic tests	Undergraduate programs	Standards of practice	Phenomenology	Case management	Epidemiology	Accessibility	Drugs
Monitoring devices	Graduate programs	Specialty certification	Heuristics	Total quality management	Worldwide disease transference	Affordability	Devices
Treatment regimens	Faculty research programs	Code of ethics	Critical social theory	Cost containment	Population growth	Quality of life	Procedures: biomedical
	Faculty practice	Levels of practice	Large databases	JCAHO outcomes focus	WHO strategies for healthy populations	Rural clinics	Behavioral/ interpersonal relationships
	Advanced practice		Interdisciplinary	Computerized patient records	Ethics	Comprehensive health insurance	Administrative/ organizational arrangements
			Informatics	Managed care		Minority health care	Health services delivery model
			Large teams	Integrated delivery systems		Self-care	
				Population-based case management		Treatment options	
						Health promotion	
						Women's health issues	
						Viable information	
						Education	

The Scientific Era

In the 1950s a second scientific explosion marked the age of Sputnik, television, computers, and future spaceships. Science was a way of discovering, organizing, and controlling the world. It was thought that knowledge discovered by logical, systematic, empirical research would pave the way to the control of nature and destiny. Research, considered the most extensive investigative process of science, would lead scientists to discover new facts, theories, or applications and revise old ones. Science would provide new technology and the power to conquer new worlds and disease. In this era medical scientists made significant discoveries that have controlled many diseases and dramatically extended life.

With the scientific explosion and rapid advancement of knowledge in every field, it is estimated that cumulative knowledge doubles every 2 years. Today's discoveries make yesterday's knowledge obsolete. Major scientific revelations are rapidly disseminated to the public with the assistance of high-technology communication. Present society religiously seeks the "best scientific evidence" and welcomes each new major development with new questions raised about its effect on humans. Each new development must be considered for its risks, benefits, consequences, and impact on the environment and society.

Nursing responded to the scientific era by developing ways to incorporate the scientific process into nursing. This integration began in the 1950s as nurse leaders encouraged practitioners to search for objective data and to diagnose human responses. In 1973 the American Nurses Association (ANA) wrote the *Standards of Nursing Practice*,[3] which incorporated the scientific method into the nursing process and were soon adopted by the profession. The standards remain the major guidelines for general practice today and have been modified and accepted by most clinical specialties.

In this age of scientific advancement nurses seek advanced education in various disciplines that rely on research and empirical methods. Although initial experiences in research are usually limited to the execution of theses and dissertations and/or performance as research assistants, nurses recognize the value of nursing research in establishing the credibility of nursing as a profession. Nursing research assists the profession to develop nursing theories and to describe, explain, and predict nursing actions. As research and theories evolve, nursing accumulates a unique body of knowledge and moves toward becoming a science. In the past 3 decades the number of nursing research studies in clinical practice, administration, education, and theory increased substantially. The quality of these studies has improved tremendously as a result of competition for federal and state grants to support the research. Numerous research conferences are held annually throughout the United States to disseminate the results of nursing research studies. The science of nursing is gradually evolving as nursing theories are generated and tested and as knowledge unique to nursing grows.

Technology and use of computers. Scientific discoveries in the medical disciplines have influenced nursing practice, education, and research. Advanced medical technology includes new high-tech devices such as cardiac, respiratory, and oxygen monitors; pulmonary artery and central venous pressure catheters; fetal monitors; and mechanical ventilators. Advanced technology requires highly skilled nurses. Hospitals employ over 70% of the practicing nurses, and acute-care clients occupy the majority of hospital beds. Consequently, because nursing has changed to provide expert care to acutely ill clients, this care often involves the use of high-tech equipment. Nurses receive specialized education to operate, monitor, and use these devices. Life-and-death decisions are based on the nurses' interpretation of the information provided by high-tech equipment. Unfortunately, the cost of scientific advances surpasses economic resources, and the application of advanced technology may not be available to everyone.

As new technologic equipment is developed and used, nurses are forced to address difficult ethical, economic, and values questions, such as the following:

- What criteria will be used by different health care systems (such as government programs or insurance groups) to decide who is worthy to receive costly diagnostic tests, operations, and treatments, given our limited resources?
- Who has the right to decide which expensive tests, operations, or treatments will be used—the client, the parents, the physician, an institutional review board, the insurer, or all parties with a vested interest?
- Who deserves and who might benefit from the use of expensive technology? Would a young prisoner be considered as qualified for a heart transplant as an 80-year-old person?
- What are the risks and chances for an acceptable quality of life based on use of new technologies?
- Who pays for the use of expensive high-tech diagnostic and treatment equipment—the insurance company, the client/family, or society (Medicare/Medicaid)?
- What are the chances that a diagnostic test may be harmful (such as placenta sampling to detect genetic anomalies, which also may cause a fetal defect)?
- What constitutes extraordinary versus ordinary diagnostic workup and treatment?
- Is selective nontreatment an option when there is uncertainty in the efficacy of the treatment or the client refuses treatment?
- If a treatment is experimental, who will evaluate the potential value and risks, and who will decide whether they are worthwhile?
- How can society balance the costs of prevention of illness with the costs of treating diseases?

Nursing roles change with the growth in the number and types of technologic equipment to diagnose, monitor, and treat patients. Some nurses are skilled technicians in acute intensive care settings. Others study the impact of these new devices on the client's needs and the evolving role of the nurse. They are also examining the effect on nurses who use high-tech devices and work in intensive care units. Nurse educators are exploring effective and efficient methods to teach students about new technology and nurses' roles. One outcome is that since May 1994 graduates take computerized state board examinations, called NCLEX-CAT, upon graduation from state-approved nursing programs. This computerized test provides for a quick turnaround of results, which are received 7 to 10 days after completion of the examination.

Computer technology rapidly developed concurrently with medical technology. The silicon chip boosted the computer's capacity for seemingly infinite scientific discoveries and technologic innovations. Computers automate and consolidate information and increase the speed and efficiency of data processing, thus improving control over client data, including costs, diagnoses, orders, plans, and outcomes. Increased numbers of nursing schools offer informatics and computer courses that soon may be required as a "second language." Most health care institutions and agencies use computers; some hospitals have a computer at every client's bedside. At other hospitals nurses use computers to enter client data, check nursing or medical orders, and order services from other hospital departments. New computer programs have tremendous flexibility, with integration of word processing, data processing, spreadsheets, and graphics. In this scientific era, characterized by a rapid knowledge explosion, nurses' roles are changing. They now include rapid processing of multicomplex data, which affects the client, the nurse, and the health care delivery system.

Standardized language and classification systems.* Now as never before has it become necessary for nurses to develop a standardized language of nursing. Concerns for the cost of health care and computerization will continue to force the nursing community to identify the structure and components of nursing practice. The clinical, theoretic, and research dimensions of nursing must be brought together in a unified whole with recognition of the influence of the political, economic, and ethical domains. It is believed that professional advancement of the discipline can be achieved only when a consistent language representing all settings and all levels can be used to communicate nursing activities. Nursing individuals, groups, and organizations have steadily moved toward that end with the development of classification systems that have been appearing in the nursing literature since the early 1970s.

Classification systems are often called *taxonomies* or *taxonomic approaches.* They are developed with particular goals or purposes in mind. The usefulness of classification systems cannot be denied: enhanced communication, generation of research hypotheses, projections of future trends, and other benefits can be realized. The classification system movement in nursing has led to the generation of various types. It would be well to remember, however, that nursing classification systems actually began in the late 1950s as client classifications for nurse staffing.

The initial work toward the development of the Nursing Minimum Data Set (NMDS) began in the 1970s. Based on the concept of the Uniform Minimum Health Data Sets, the NMDS is an initial attempt to establish uniform standards for the collection of comparable, minimum, essential nursing data. According to Werley and others,[100] it is "a standardized approach that facilitates the abstraction of essential, core minimum data to describe nursing practice. It is intended for use in any and all settings where nursing care is provided. The NMDS is unique in that it is the only data set whereby the practice of nursing can be described, resulting in a nursing database." Following the earlier work, the NMDS was developed in 1985 through the efforts of a national group of 64 experts. Three broad categories of elements were identified: nursing care (four elements), patient or client demographics (five elements), and service (seven elements). These 16 elements include nursing diagnosis, intervention, outcome, and intensity of nursing care. As the title

*This section was published in *Nursing: The Finest Art, An Illustrated History,* St. Louis, 1996, Mosby.

itself implies, the NMDS consists of a minimum set of items that have both uniform definitions and categories concerning nursing practice. Thus through the use of this system two primary aspects can potentially be achieved: the description of the essence of nursing and the development of a database.

Although individual nurses were involved in nursing diagnosis activities before the 1970s, NANDA is considered the forerunner in this activity. Since 1973 its members have diligently endeavored to develop nursing diagnoses and, more recently, a taxonomy for their classification. The NANDA Nursing Diagnosis Taxonomy[74] has had great significance for both the discipline of nursing and for the organization of its knowledge. This taxonomy is currently the best known and most widely used classification system in nursing. It is also, perhaps, one of the most controversial for a variety of reasons. Each NANDA-approved nursing diagnosis includes a definition of the diagnosis, defining characteristics, and related factors. A great number of nursing diagnoses have been approved for clinical testing. NANDA's Taxonomy I has been translated into the format used by the World Health Organization (WHO), the organization that revises and publishes the International Classification of Disease (ICD). This format provides for an organized international database for health care; the inclusion of nursing diagnoses assists the development of an international nursing database within the ICD framework.[96] Ongoing work on the taxonomy involves the refinement and clinical testing of the existing nursing diagnoses, as well as the identification, development, and testing of new diagnoses. Movement toward a Taxonomy II is proceeding.

The Nursing Interventions Classification (NIC) was developed by a large research team and is continuing at the University of Iowa College of Nursing. The work of the team was begun in the late 1980s and has been facilitated by the help of nurse experts from many specialties. The primary usefulness of the classification of treatments that nurses perform is in the planning and documenting of nursing care, the communication of the nature of nursing, and the development of large databases for research related to the effectiveness of nursing care. In May 1992 the *Nursing Interventions Classification*[55] was published with a standardized list of 336 direct-care nursing interventions. Each of these is elucidated by a definition, nursing activities necessary to carry out the intervention, and background reading. "NIC includes all direct care interventions that nurses do on behalf of patients, including both independent and collaborative interventions. The classification applies to nurses in all specialties and in all settings. While an individual nurse will have expertise in only a limited number of intervention, the entire classification is meant to capture the expertise of all nurses."[55] The second edition of the book was published in 1996 and contains 433 interventions. It includes the revised NIC taxonomy and a list of linkages with NANDA diagnoses.[56]

The evaluation of health care effectiveness is one of the great challenges of the 1990s. Emphasis has thus been placed on the use of client outcomes, which have been studied primarily in relation to specific diagnoses, whether medical or nursing, and specific interventions. The outcome models that have been generated, however, did not embrace the multivariate influences on client outcomes. Going one step further, the models do not necessarily reflect nursing practice. The landmark research of Horn and Swain was a grand effort to organize nursing-sensitive client outcomes. Their research was conducted to identify client outcomes influenced by nursing care. Other research efforts have focused on the identification and categorization of those outcomes used to measure the effects of nursing care. Currently a large research team at the University of Iowa College of Nursing is studying nursing-sensitive client outcomes. The overall purpose is to identify, label, define, and classify these outcomes and ultimately develop valid and reliable outcome measures. Although the project is painstaking and laborious, considerable work has been done. *Nursing-Sensitive Outcomes Classification (NOC)*, 1997, was recently published.[31]

The description of nursing practice remains at the forefront of nursing thought. A standardized language is believed to be the answer to facilitating that description and making it operational and measurable. The preceding examples of classification system and possible others that exist may provide the mechanism for achieving this goal as linkages between diagnoses, intervention, and outcomes are identified in the developmental processes. Perhaps most beneficial, standardized languages can be computerized. This is particularly significant since information system activities and the drive toward computer-based client records are influencing, and will continue to influence, the day-to-day practice of nurses. The Institute of Medicine has set the year 2000 as the date for the actual achievement of a computer-based client record.

Changes in Consumers' Health Care Needs

Although America offers the best in health care, almost 50% of Americans cannot afford it. The recent economic depression and subsequent unemployment, along with the escalating costs of health insurance, have contributed to the growing number of uninsured or underinsured Americans. In 1991 about 60 million Americans had inadequate or no health care insurance.[58] In 1993 an estimated 25% of Americans (the working poor) had no health insurance but did not qualify for government health coverage, and another 25% or more were covered by government health care programs. More than half of blacks and Hispanics (53%) could not pay for health services in 1992, and physicians refused to treat 22% of those insured by government programs. Minority groups have also had inadequate access to preventive health care; thus when disease occurs it is usually more advanced and requires more costly interventions. Americans are living longer, so the number of older people is increasing. Older persons tend to have more health problems but have fewer resources to pay for them, which increases the burden on society. Thousands of Americans suffer from chronic diseases that require ongoing health care, and the number of Americans diagnosed as being HIV-positive and having AIDS is rapidly growing. These people require lengthy care and treatment, which contributes greatly to health care costs.

Currently the health care system focuses on diagnosis and treatment of disease, provided by health maintenance organizations, outpatient clinics, and hospitals. Consumers are expected to assume more and more responsibility for their health with less and less assistance from health care professionals. Following surgery and major acute illnesses, clients are discharged from hospitals "quicker and sicker." Minimal attention is given to follow-up of chronic health problems. But clients require more assistance after surgery, childbirth, or acute illness, especially when placed on home electrical monitors or when their treatments require special monitoring or regulation. Their lifestyles and living patterns must be considered in planning their care and in managing their illnesses.

In the 1970s the women's movement and other activist groups began to assert their rights in health care. One result was that several versions of a "Patient's Bill of Rights" appeared. In response to consumer demands for greater participation in determining health policies at the state and local level, consumer health care advocates were frequently appointed to serve on various advisory boards.

In recent years some consumers have become more knowledgeable and involved in their own health care decisions and have learned ways to improve their health and treatment options. Some have become informed about "alternative treatment modalities" and are using these, either alone or in conjunction with traditional, medically accepted treatments. In addition, consumers have been encouraged to discuss and document their treatment and care wishes (e.g., life-sustaining treatment) in advance. According to the Patient Self-Determination Act, a federal law enacted in 1990, all federally funded institutions must inform clients of their right to prepare these advance directives. With the increasing emphasis on consumer responsibility, it is hoped that the media will also become more responsible for promoting and encouraging healthy lifestyle behaviors.

Changes in the Health Care System

The crisis in today's health care system is the result of high costs for health care and insurance, limited access of impoverished people and minority groups, the emphasis on treatment of disease rather than prevention, and concerns about the quality of care. Each of these contributing factors will lead to changes that will affect nursing practice and research.

New technologies are a double-edged sword. They may assist in refining our knowledge of disease and improve treatment, but at the same time the financial costs may be prohibitive for those without private health insurance. The increased use of high-tech equipment has also contributed to depersonalization of health care, although consumers are demanding these new diagnostic techniques and treatments, such as ultrasound, CAT scans, kidney dialysis machines, and organ transplantation. Poor quality of health care, along with a fragmented, depersonalized health care system, has angered many consumers.

Along with the increasing costs of equipment, laboratory tests, and health care personnel, other factors have contributed to the changes in health care. The use of diagnostic related groups (DRGs), which determine hospital reimbursements in the prospective payment system, along with utilization review of cases to minimize expenses, has led to many changes in the provision of health care. As a result, more consumers are increasingly treated in outpatient surgery, discharged to nursing homes or rehabilitation units, or sent home sooner.

In the early 1900s the movement toward managed care as a method to solve the issue of high health care costs began, although it was actually pioneered in the 1930s. It was seen as a system of organizing care and providing comprehensive coverage. The effect of this efficiently run system, which would incorporate a full range of services, continuity of care, emphasis on prevention, and early intervention, would potentially save costs. A variety of models of managed care thus had a rapid influence on both the private insurance market and government insurance programs within the United States. Many areas of the country are now dominated by managed care, while other areas are attempting to follow suit.

Managed care has provided the impetus to the increased use of case management as a mechanism for the coordination and sequencing of care and the development of critical paths. This shift toward managed care has also had a major effect on nursing. Frequently it is being advanced as the rationale for the use of fewer nurses for client care, layoffs, and job losses. Nurses fear that erosion of care will occur in health care institutions.

Nurses' Response to Societal Changes

Professional nursing organizations and health care agencies have responded to some changing trends in various ways. Total quality management (TQM) programs have been initiated in many hospitals and agencies to improve the efficacy and response to consumer and provider needs. Self-governance has been implemented in some hospital systems to strengthen nurses' involvement in decision-making areas and to increase their autonomy and accountability. Some health care institutions have introduced case management programs so that nurses follow and relate to clients with chronic health problems in a variety of settings. Using the case management approach, nurses may coordinate an interdisciplinary health team to promote health and reduce the need for hospital admissions.

In response to the health care crisis the National League for Nursing, along with other nursing organizations, developed a plan called *Nursing's Agenda for Health Care Reform.* This agenda called for development of a health care system to:

- Provide universal access to basic health care
- Ensure the provision of quality, cost-effective, ethically responsible care
- Focus on health promotion and disease prevention within communities
- Support consumers as responsible partners in health care[62]

Several other critical elements in the *Agenda* to improve health care are to:

- Inform and empower consumers through education
- Provide clear choices among health care plans, including data on quality and costs
- Offer a comprehensive benefit package that incorporates mental health services and long-term care
- Give incentives for Associated Health Providers (AHPs) and new networks to assure access to services responsive to the culturally diverse populations in rural and inner city areas
- Provide opportunities for nurses to participate in decision making at all levels, from national board and state Health Insurance Purchasing Cooperatives (HIPCs) to clinical decisions as primary care providers in AHPs
- Offer incentives to reduce administrative costs, create uniform data systems, and keep costs of premiums linked to costs of services[62]

To accomplish these objectives, several legislative and administrative changes are necessary. According to ANA past president Virginia T. Betts, professional nurses in advanced practice roles can deliver primary health care as competently as physicians at a 40% savings.[58] Unnecessary restrictions in nurse practice acts, unnecessary limitations on prescriptive authority, and significant barriers to reimbursement of nurse practitioners must be removed. Nurses continue to lobby and advocate for these changes. If anticompetitive barriers for primary care are removed, nurses can deliver high-quality health care at lower costs and in multiple new sites.

Future of Professional Nursing Science and Practice

The nurses of tomorrow will blend the scientific, pragmatic, spiritual, and intuitive aspects of nursing to provide increased humanistic care. Research must be expanded in the physical science area, since the majority of nursing research to date has been social-science oriented. Less energy will be devoted to tasks that do not require a professional nurse. Already, in hospitals across the country, nurses are being replaced by less-trained personnel. This is causing an increasingly tight job market for nurses. Nurses need to direct their efforts toward prevention and cost effectiveness, because this combination is their forte and also seems to be the wave of the future. Some nurses will use high-tech procedures combined with the efficacy of the traditional arts of nursing, such as touch, massage, and listening for the meaning of unspoken words. Other nurses will assist clients to achieve synchrony between themselves and their environment through health maintenance and promoting the basics of adequate rest, suitable exercise, proper nutrition, and weight control. By emphasizing disease prevention and health promotion, nurses can reduce the need for costly health care while providing cost-effective, high-quality health care for all Americans.

In the future the needs of people living in each community, not the hospitals' or physicians' needs, will determine the types of health services offered. Since community-based settings are essential for providing universal access to health care, nursing care may shift from traditional hospitals to lower acuity alternative sites, such as ambulatory facilities, short-stay hospitals, day surgery centers, and hospice settings. In addition, more alternative health care services such as free clinics and primary care clinics will serve culturally diverse populations. Nurses in these diverse settings will fill roles such as primary care practitioners in acute care units, case managers and coordinators of services across settings, utilization review managers, and entrepreneurs who develop transitional services. In addition, nurses will collaborate with interdisciplinary and multidisciplinary health care teams. Collaboration, team building, health promotion, disease prevention, and health maintenance will be essential in the economics of health care delivery.

With the rapid expansion of new technologies, nurses are faced with conflicting paradigms as medical care relies on new technologies that require advanced technical skills. However, nurses may choose to provide holistic transactional human care in which the clients' lived experiences and their interrelationships are the focus of care. Thus future nurses must be skilled in both technical and humanistic knowledge so they may provide sensitive health care with an awareness of the effect of technology on the client and guide the client toward enlightened, empowered self-care, self-responsibility, and the ability to control his or her own destiny.

The professional nurse will want to be knowledgeable about current nursing research and to creatively apply valid findings in practice. To accomplish this task, practitioners must visualize possibilities beyond the common clinical constraints. They must recognize the effect and application of changing world views, scientific discoveries, and shifts in nursing models and theories.

Having internalized the nursing process, professional nurses will see the client's situation as a gestalt and creatively apply appropriate nursing models. With experience, professional nurses will identify common patterns in client situations and raise new questions. Some of these questions (such as "Would this nursing action or another action be more effective in assisting the client?") are worthy of further pursuit. The nurse may discuss these questions with peers, search the literature for answers, initiate a research study, or develop clinical impressions for publication. The professional nurse always looks for new meanings in nursing phenomena. The ability to see new relationships in human behaviors or new patterns of response leads to more questions about nursing actions. Rather than revert to lock-step thinking—where if X happens, then Y is the appropriate nursing action—the professional nurse critically analyzes multiple factors and examines all feasible possibilities.

Experience in practice, a broad knowledge base, and continuous updating of research on theory stimulates the professional nurse to raise new questions about practice and seek greater knowledge. It is in the practice arena that theories are generated and tested. New questions and problems lead to continual refinement of theory and development of new theories. Like other disciplines, nursing knowledge and science will never be static. As trends and shifts occur in technology, economics, education, politics, and cultures, the professional nurse seeks an understanding of these changes by raising questions and searches for answers in theory, research, and practice. The continuous search for answers to new questions is what stimulates the development of new knowledge and contributes to the growing body of nursing science.

Summary

Nursing science has made great strides in the last 50 years. During the 1950s and 1960s the emphasis on empirical knowledge stimulated the profession to develop and refine the nursing process. By the 1980s the five components of the nursing process were legitimized in the Standards of Nursing Practice and the National Council Licensure Examination.

Professional status was brought about in large part through the efforts of those nurses who sought doctoral degrees in other disciplines. Nurses then developed doctoral programs in nursing. Some nurses described their conceptual models for practice and initiated research studies to test their models and theories. The profession reached consensus on four major concepts in the nursing domain. Although a dichotomy continues to exist between nursing practice and nursing theorists and researchers, there is a growing commitment toward integration of theories, research, and practice. Nursing science and research are moving toward acceptance of other ways of knowing, such as ethical, aesthetic, and personal knowledge.

New approaches in practice, theory development, and research will be developed to expand nurses' understanding of humans and their health care needs. The future will bring stronger collaboration between practitioners, scholar-theorists, and researchers to improve nursing science. In this way, the nursing profession can best respond to the ever-changing social forces of our time and to the effect that these major social forces have on the health care needs of individuals, groups, and society.

CRITICAL THINKING *Activities*

1. How well do you feel that nursing as a profession is responding to the knowledge explosion and rising health care costs?
2. To what extent do you consider that nursing theory is influencing nursing practice?
3. Which of the various nursing models and theories do you personally find most adaptable to your nursing practice? Why?
4. To what extent do you believe that theories and models are important to the profession of nursing?
5. What effect do you believe technology and information systems are having on health care, nursing practice, and ethical issues?
6. Do you believe that theories should be tested?

References

1. Abdellah FG: The nature of nursing science, *Nurs Res* 18(5):393, 1969.
2. American Nurses Association: *Nursing: a social policy statement,* ANA Publication Code NP-63, 35M, December 1980.
3. American Nurses Association: *Standards of nursing practice,* Kansas City, MO, 1973, American Nurses Association.
4. Aspinal MJ: Nursing diagnosis: the weak link, *Nurs Outlook* 24(7):433, 1976.
5. Benner P: *From novice to expert,* Menlo Park, CA, 1984, Addison-Wesley.
6. Brown EL: *Nursing for the future,* New York, 1948, Russell Sage Foundation.
7. Brown MI: Research in the development of nursing theory: the importance of a theoretical framework in nursing research, *Nurs Res* 13(2):109, 1964.
8. Bullough B: The first two phases in nursing licensure. In Bullough B, ed: *The laws and the expanding nursing role,* New York, 1975, Appleton-Century-Crofts.
9. Carnevali D: *Nursing care planning: diagnosis and management,* ed 3, Philadelphia, 1983, Lippincott.
10. Carper B: Fundamental patterns of knowing in nursing, *ANS* 1(1):13, 1978.
11. Chinn P: Debunking myths in nursing theory and research, *Image* 17(2):45, 1985.
12. Chinn P, Kramer M: *Theory and nursing: a systematic approach,* ed 3, St. Louis, 1991, Mosby.
13. Christensen PJ, Kenney JW, eds: *Nursing process: application of theories, frameworks, and models,* ed 4, St. Louis, 1994, Mosby.
14. Committee for the Study of Nursing Education: *Nursing and nursing education in the United States,* New York, 1923, The Committee.
15. Committee on the Grading of Nursing Schools: *Nurses, patients, and pocketbooks,* New York, 1928, The Committee.
16. Committee on the Grading of Nursing Schools: *Nursing schools today and tomorrow,* New York, 1934, The Committee.
17. Craft-Rosenberg M: *Nursing diagnosis extension and classification (NDEC),* grant proposal submitted to National Institutes of Health, October 1, 1995.

18. Deloughery GL, and others: *Consultation and community organization in community mental health nursing,* Baltimore, 1971, Williams & Wilkins.
19. Dickoff J, James P: A theory of theories: a position paper, *Nurs Res* 17(3):197, 1968.
20. Dickoff J, and others. Theory in a practice discipline, part 1: practice-oriented theory, *Am J Nurs* 17(5):415, 1968.
21. Donahue MP: *Nursing: the finest art, an illustrated history,* ed 2, St. Louis, 1996, Mosby.
22. Erikson E: *Childhood and society,* ed 2, New York, 1963, Norton.
23. Fawcett J: Conceptual models and theory development, *JOGNN* 17(6):400, 1988.
24. Fawcett J: *Analysis and evaluation of conceptual models of nursing,* ed 2, Philadelphia, 1989, Davis.
25. Firlet SL: Nursing theory and nursing practice: separate or linked? In McCloskey JC, Grace HK, eds: *Current issues in nursing,* ed 2, Boston, 1985, Blackwell Scientific.
26. Fitzpatrick ML: *Prologue to professionalism,* Bowie, MD, 1983, Robert J. Brady.
27. Gortner SR: Nursing values and science: toward a science philosophy, *Image* 22(2):101, 1990.
28. Gortner SR: The history and philosophy of nursing science and research, *ANS* 5(2):1, 1983.
29. Henderson V: *The nature of nursing: a definition and its implications for practice, research, and education,* New York, 1966, Macmillan Company.
30. Huckabay L: The role of conceptual frameworks in nursing practice, administration, education, and research, *Nurs Admin Q* 15(3):17-28, 1991.
31. Iowa Outcomes Team; Johnson M, Maas M, eds: *Nursing-Sensitive Outcomes Classification (NOC),* St. Louis, 1997, Mosby.
32. Jacobs MK, Huether SE: Nursing science: the theory-practice linkage, *ANS* 1(1):63, 1978.
33. Jacox AK: Theory construction in nursing: an overview, *Nurs Res* 23(1):4, 1974.
34. Johns E, Pfefferkorn B: *An activity analysis of nursing,* New York, 1934. Committee on the Grading of Nursing Schools.
35. Johnson D: Professional practice in nursing. In *The shifting scene: directions for practice,* Pub. No. 15-1252, New York, 1967, National League for Nursing.
36. Johnson JL: Nursing science: Basic, applied, or practical? Implications for the art of nursing, *Adv Nurs Sci* 14(1):7-16, 1991.
37. Johnson DE: Development of theory: a requisite for nursing as a primary health profession, *Nurs Res* 23(5):372, 1974.
38. Johnson DE: The nature of a science of nursing, *Nurs Outlook* 7(5):291, 1959.
39. Johnson DE: The behavioral system for nursing. In Riehl JP, Roy Sister Callista, eds: *Conceptual models for nursing practice,* ed 2, New York, 1980, Appleton-Century-Crofts.
40. Kelly K: Clinical inference in nursing, *Nurs Res* 15(1):23, 1966.
41. Kerlinger F: *Foundations of behavioral research,* New York, 1973, Holt, Rinehart & Winston.
42. King I: *Toward a theory in nursing,* New York, 1971, Wiley.
43. King I: *A theory for nursing: systems, concepts, process,* New York, 1981, Wiley.
44. Knowles LN: Decision making in nursing: a necessity for doing. In *ANA clinical sessions 1966,* New York, 1967, Appleton-Century-Crofts.

45. Leininger M: *Transcultural nursing: concepts, theories and practices,* New York, 1978, Wiley.
46. Leininger M, ed: *Care: the essence of nursing and health,* Thorofare, NJ, 1984, Slack.
47. Leininger M, ed: *Cultural care diversity and universality: a theory of nursing,* New York, 1992, National League for Nursing.
48. Lesnik MJ, Anderson BE: *Legal aspects of nursing,* Philadelphia, 1947, Lippincott.
49. Lesnik MJ, Anderson BE: *Nursing practice and the law,* ed 2, Philadelphia, 1955, Lippincott.
50. Little DE, Carnevali DL: *Nursing care plans,* ed 2, Philadelphia, 1976, Lippincott.
51. Marriner-Tomey A: *Nursing theorists and their work,* ed 3, St. Louis, 1994, Mosby.
52. Maslow A: *Motivation and personality,* ed 2, New York, 1970, Harper & Row.
53. Mayberry A: Merging nursing theories, models, and nursing practice: more than an administrative challenge, *Nurs Admin Q* 15(3):44, 1991.
54. Mayers J: *A systematic approach to the nursing care plan,* ed 3, New York, 1983, Appleton-Century-Crofts.
55. McCloskey JC, Bulechek GM: *Nursing interventions classification (NIC),* St. Louis, 1992, Mosby.
56. McCloskey JC, Bulechek GM: *Nursing interventions classification (NIC),* ed 2, St. Louis, 1996, Mosby.
57. Meleis AI: *Theoretical nursing: development and process,* Philadelphia, 1985, Lippincott.
58. Mikulencak M: Reform discussions include ANA input, *The American Nurse* 25(5):3, 1993.
59. Mitchell GJ, Cody WK: Nursing knowledge and human science: ontological and epistemological considerations, *Nurs Sci Q* 5(2):54, 1992.
60. Mundinger MO, Jauron GD: Developing a nursing diagnosis, *Nurs Outlook* 23(2):94, 1975.
61. National League for Nursing: *Legislative update,* p. 1, December 5, 1985.
62. National League for Nursing: *Nursing's agenda for health care reform,* 1992, NLN.
63. National League of Nursing Education: *Standard curriculum for schools of nursing,* New York, 1917, The League.
64. National League of Nursing Education: *A curriculum for schools of nursing,* New York, 1927, The League.
65. National League of Nursing Education: *A curriculum guide for schools of nursing,* New York, 1937, The League.
66. Neuman B: *The Neuman systems model,* New York, 1982, Appleton-Century-Crofts.
67. Newman MA: Nursing's theoretical evolution, *Am J Nurs* 20(7):449, 1972.
68. Newman MA: Prevailing paradigms in nursing, *Nurs Outlook* 40(I):10, 1992.
69. Newman MA, Sime AM, Corcoran-Perry SA: The focus of the discipline of nursing, *Adv Nurs Sci* 14(1):1, 1991.
70. Newman MA: Shifting to higher consciousness. In Parker ME: *Nursing theories in practice,* New York, 1990, National League for Nursing.
71. Newman MA: The continuing revolution: a history of nursing science. In Chaska NL: *The nursing profession: a time to speak,* New York, 1983, McGraw-Hill.
72. Nicoll LH: *Perspectives on nursing theory,* ed 2, Philadelphia, 1992, Lippincott.

73. Nightingale F: *Notes on nursing, what it is and what it is not,* New York, 1860, Appleton.
74. North American Nursing Diagnosis Association: *NANDA nursing diagnosis: definitions and classification 1995-1996,* Philadelphia, North American Nursing Diagnosis Association.
75. Orem DE: *Nursing: concepts of practice,* ed 4, St. Louis, 1991, Mosby.
76. Orlando IJ: *The dynamic nurse-patient relationship,* New York, 1961, Putnam.
77. Parse RR: *Man-living-health: a theory of nursing,* Philadelphia, 1981, Wiley.
78. Paterson JG, Zderad LT: *Humanistic nursing,* Philadelphia, 1976, Wiley.
79. Peplau HE: *Interpersonal relations in nursing,* New York, 1952, Putnam.
80. Phaneuf M: *The nursing audit: profile for excellence,* New York, 1972, Appleton-Century-Crofts.
81. Pinnell NN, deMeneses M: *The nursing process: theory, application and related processes,* Norwalk, CT, 1986, Appleton-Century-Crofts.
82. Rogers ME: *An introduction to the theoretical basis of nursing,* Philadelphia, 1970, Davis.
83. Rogers ME: Space-age paradigm for new frontiers in nursing. In Parker ME: *Nursing theories in practice,* New York, 1990, National League for Nursing.
84. Roy C Sr: *Introduction to nursing: an adaptation model,* ed 2, Englewood Cliffs, NJ. 1984, Prentice-Hall.
85. Schmidt M: The current status of practice theories in nursing. In Woodridge PJ and others: *Behavioral science and nursing theory,* St. Louis, 1983, Mosby.
86. Schumacher KL, Gortner SR: (Mis)conceptions and reconceptions about traditional science, *Adv Nurs Sci* 14(4):1, 1992.
87. Silva MC: Philosophy, science, theory: interrelationships and implications for nursing research, *Image* 9(3):59, 1977.
88. Silva MC, Rothbart D: An analysis of changing trends in philosophies of science on nursing theory development and testing, *ANS* 6(2):1, 1984.
89. Stevens BJ: *Nursing theory: analysis, application, evaluation,* ed 2, Boston, 1984, Little, Brown.
90. Stewart IM: Problems of nursing education, *Teachers College Record* 11:7, 1910.
91. Stewart IM: The science and art in nursing, *Nursing Education Bulletin* 11:1, 1929.
92. *The American Nurse:* Congress overrides veto, nursing gets center for research, pp. 1, 24, January, 1986.
93. Walker LO: Theory and research in the development of nursing as a discipline: retrospect and prospect. In Chaska N, ed: *The nursing profession: a time to speak,* New York, 1983, McGraw-Hill.
94. Walker LO, Avant KC: *Strategies for theory construction in nursing,* ed 2, Norwalk, CT, 1988, Appleton-Century-Crofts.
95. Wandelt MA, Ager JW: *Quality patient care scale,* New York, 1974, Appleton-Century-Crofts.
96. Warren JJ: Nursing diagnosis taxonomy development: overview and issues. In McCloskey J, Grace HK, eds: *Current issues in nursing,* St. Louis, 1994, Mosby.
97. Watson J: *The philosophy and science of caring,* Boston, 1979, Little, Brown.
98. Watson J: *Nursing: human science and human care: a theory of nursing,* Norwalk, CT, 1985, Appleton-Century-Crofts.

99. Watson MJ: Transpersonal caring: a transcendent view of person, health, and healing. In Parker ME: *Nursing theories in practice,* New York, 1990, National League for Nursing.
100. Werley H, Ryan P, Zorn CR, Devine EC: Why the nursing minimum data set (NMDS)? In McCloskey J, Grace HK, eds: *Current issues in nursing,* ed 4, St. Louis, 1994, Mosby.
101. West M, Hawkins C: *Nursing schools at the mid-century,* New York, 1950, National Committee for the Improvement of Nursing Services.
102. Yura H, Walsh MB: *The nursing process: assessing, planning, implementing, evaluating,* ed 2, New York, 1973, Appleton-Century-Crofts.
103. Yura H, Walsh MB: *The nursing process: assessing, planning, implementing, evaluating,* New York, 1967, Appleton-Century-Crofts.
104. Zeluskas BA and others: Bridging the gap: theory to practice, research application, *Nurs Man* 19(9):50, 1988.

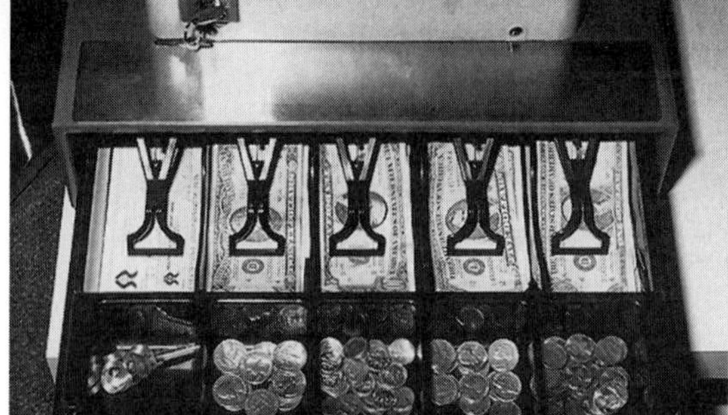

CHAPTER 3

Economics of Health Care

Philip Jacobs

OBJECTIVES After completing this chapter the reader should be able to:

- **Define *health status, health care,* and *health outcome,* and specify a relationship between these concepts**
- **Identify the main economic groups in the health care system and describe how money and services flow between these groups**
- **Specify what health insurance is and how it affects what consumers pay when they receive medical care**
- **Identify the difference between paying providers on a retrospective and on a prospective basis**
- **Identify what an HMO is and specify how they are paid**
- **Describe preferred provider organizations and managed care**
- **Define *cost* and identify how it can be measured in the health field**
- **Specify the effects of paying providers on a fee-for-service basis, on a retrospective basis, and on a capitation basis**
- **Specify the goals of health policy and identify how these goals have been pursued in different ways in the decades since the 1970s**

Economics is the discipline that deals with the analysis of behavior when scarcity exists. In the health care field scarcity has always existed, in the sense that the resources devoted to health care could have been used in other ways, although emphasis on this fact is now increasing. Since at least 1966, when the two large government health insurance programs, Medicare and Medicaid, were instituted, the proportion of the total final production of *all* goods and services that was devoted to medical care has been rising dramatically. As can be seen in Figure 3-1, national expenditures on medical care have risen from 6% of the nation's gross domestic product (that is, production of all final goods and services) in 1966 to

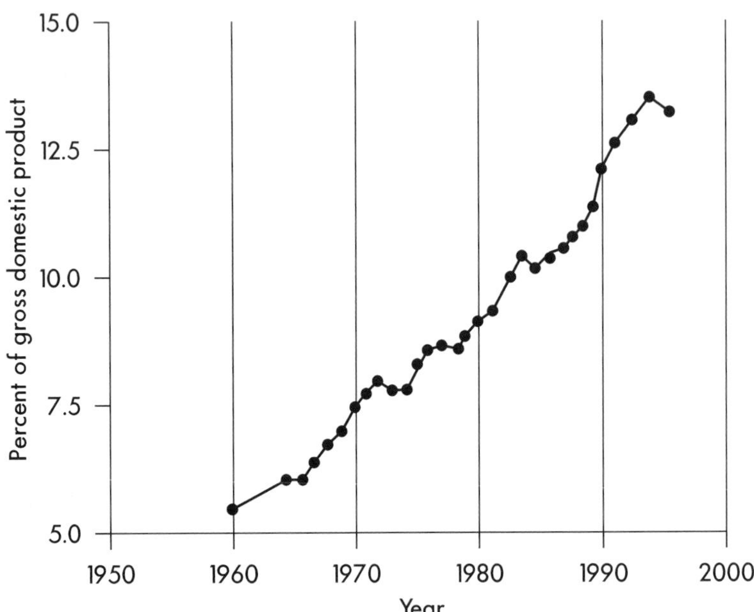

FIG. 3-1 National health expenditures as a percentage of gross domestic product.

13.7% in 1994. What is so striking about this statistic is that it represents a *share* of the total economic pie, not merely a dollar amount. But is this increasing share, dramatic as it is, bad, per se? In itself this increasing share would not *necessarily* constitute an economic problem if the benefits from these expenditures were readily apparent.

Central to the "economic problem" in health care is the belief that in many instances the benefits are *not* there. The hypothesis has been forwarded that medical care is subject to diminishing returns. This means that as we spend more and more on medical care, the effectiveness or impact on health of the additional expenditures is somewhat diminished. Such a relationship between health and medical care is very difficult to measure, and it certainly would not hold for all types of medical care under all circumstances. The essential question is whether it holds true *in general.* If it does, then this makes the case for a careful examination of medical care expenditures all the more compelling.

This *hypothesized* relationship between health and medical care has been presented pictorially with a famous curve, shown in Figure 3-2. This figure shows the population's health status on the vertical axis and the quantity of medical care on the horizontal axis. Notice how, at low amounts of medical care, the level of health rises quickly; at these levels of care, medical care is effective. However, additional amounts of medical care are, while still effective, not *as* effective as when the population had less care. And farther along the curve becomes almost flat, which is to say that, as we provide more medical care, there is very little net addition to health. At this position on the curve we are providing what has been termed "flat of the curve" medicine. Since we are paying for the additional care we are, in effect, paying without deriving much benefit. A growing number of commentators are suggesting that, in America, we have reached this level of medical care.

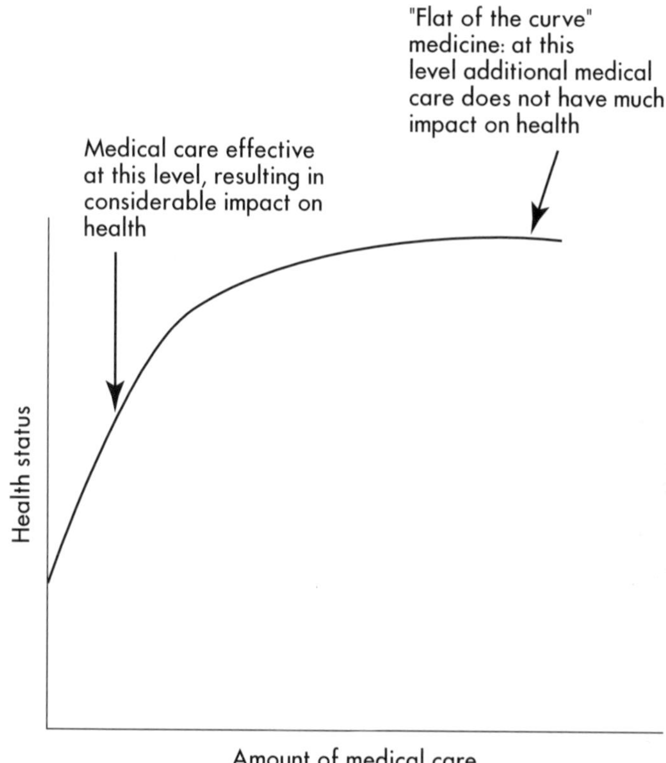

FIG. 3-2 Hypothesized relationship between medical care and health.

Numerous examples of waste, or potential waste, have been suggested to pinpoint areas that are contributing to this phenomenon. These include the expenditures on intensive care for clients who will never recover[7]; the excessive use of "little ticket" items such as lab tests and ultrasound[1]; and the use of cesarean sections as opposed to normal deliveries.[3] If "flat of the curve" medicine is a reality, substantial savings could be made by paying more attention to the economic aspects of health care delivery, and selected cutbacks could be initiated with little if any resulting loss of health.

It is here that the overall importance of health care economics lies. This chapter provides an introduction to the topic of health care economics. I will demonstrate a few of the important techniques in the field and show how they can be applied. You can go a long way towards understanding many economic policies and events with only a few very basic economic concepts. The basic economic topics that will be presented are the measure of the "output" of the health care system; the tracing out of economic flows in the system; the measurement of costs of various activities in the system; and the analysis of incentives in the system, how these incentives can be understood using cost analysis, and how they affect economic behavior. Finally, using these concepts, I will examine several of the different types of economic organizations.

■ HEALTH STATUS AND OUTCOMES

At the start it is important to focus on specific concepts that form the focal point of the study of the economics of health. Three important terms in this endeavor are

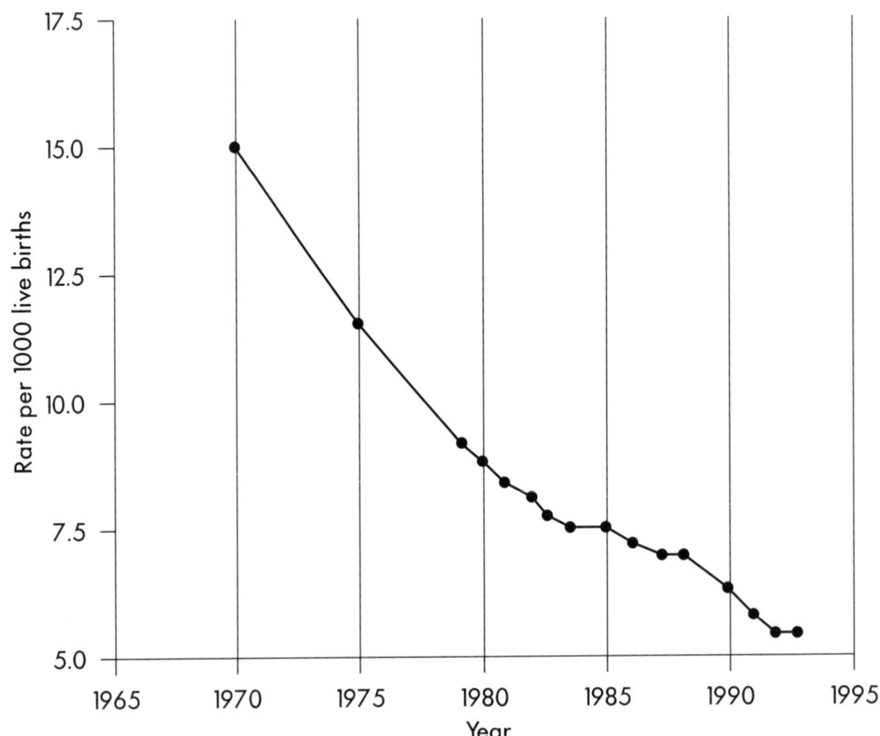

FIG. 3-3 Neonatal (age <28 days) mortality rate.

health care, health status, and health outcome. *Health (and medical) care* refers to the services actually delivered by a provider (a nurse, a physician, a hospital, and so on) to a client. A visit to a public health nurse for a vaccination is an example of an episode of health care. It is essential to note that measures of the numbers of services used, per se, tell us nothing of how "healthy" the population is that received these services; that is reserved for the next concept, health status.

Health status refers to the actual health state of an individual or a population. The simplest measures of health status are alive and dead; thus the number of individuals in a population who passed from one state (alive) to the other (dead) could be used as a very crude measure (called *mortality*) of the health status of the population. Figure 3-3 shows the neonatal mortality rate (deaths from birth to 28 days) per 1000 live births in the United States since 1970. This rate has been falling over this period. Using this measure, we conclude that health status has improved for the newborn population.

Further refinement of health status measures are needed to gauge the health status of individuals who are alive. Measures of the numbers of individuals who are "ill" (called *morbidity measures*) are used. One such measure is the percentage of a population that is hospitalized. Such measures really are *utilization* measures and do not say much about the health status itself of those who are not hospitalized, many of whom may need hospitalization or some other treatment; and, indeed, current research indicates that many who are hospitalized do not require it. Current work

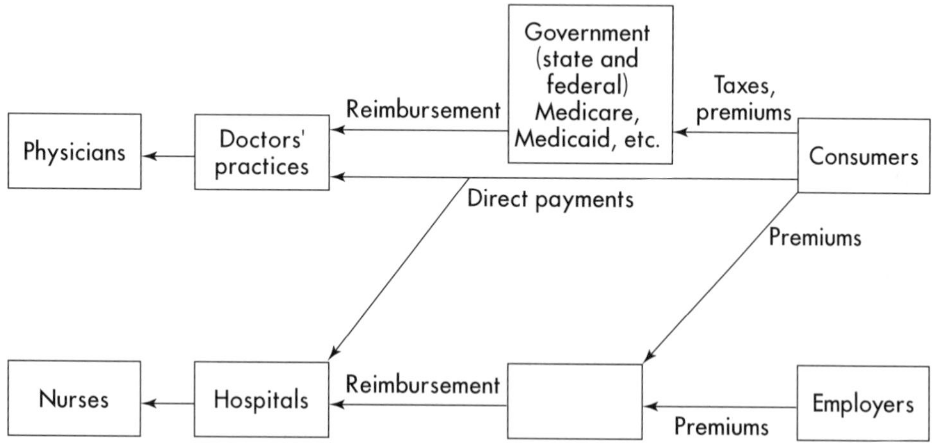

FIG. 3-4 Simplified presentation of financial flows in the health care system.

is ongoing to measure health status in a more direct fashion, such as examining the proportion of a population who have above-average hypertension levels.

The third, related measure is that of *health outcome*. This concept relates to the net impact of health care on health status. Health outcomes are not easy to measure, because to do so one must disentangle a host of other events that also affect health status, such as personal lifestyles and environmental factors. For example, the neonatal mortality rate previously discussed can be associated with the growth in neonatal intensive care units in hospitals. One might conclude that the spread of such units are responsible for this increase in health status of neonates. However, this reduction has also coincided with other factors, such as more thorough prenatal care and mothers' improved lifestyles, that have also changed over time. It would therefore be incorrect to attribute all of the change in health status to medical care. And although it would also be difficult to disentangle the impact of the other factors, if one wanted to determine health outcomes—the impact of medical care on health—this is what would have to be done.

■ ECONOMIC FLOWS IN THE HEALTH CARE SYSTEM

Economic flow analysis is a very simple tool that is of enormous usefulness in understanding economic systems. It involves identifying the various financing, spending, and consuming bodies within the system and tracing the flows of money and services between these groups. It should be stressed that this is simply a *descriptive* task. That is, one does not explain what caused the behavior to occur, but simply describes what happened. Though it is limited, this task is nevertheless one of considerable importance. One must get the flows straight in any economic system before understanding the economic relationships in the system.

As a partially simplified beginning, I present a picture of the flows in the traditional American health care system circa 1980. Many of these relationships still exist, although the scene has become more complicated since that date. Figure 3-4 shows the money flows from the ultimate payers for medical care through to two key groups of providers, physicians and hospitals. These flows are described with arrows; note that not all the participating groups in the systems have been included (for instance, nursing homes have been omitted), and I have not drawn all the flows possible; this is to keep the illustration simple.

Households: Consumers and Insurees

The example begins with the ultimate payers for medical care—consumers (households) and employers (business firms, and so on). Households pay for medical care in three major ways. First, they purchase insurance from health insurance companies. The payments for these purchases are called *premiums.* In return for premiums the insurance companies "insure" the households: that is, when some member of the household receives medical care, the insurance company pays part or all of the bill (depending on how complete the insurance coverage is). The second form of payments—extremely important ones—are called "out-of-pocket" payments. These are payments made directly by households to providers. These payments may be for the full amount charged by the provider (if the individual is not insured), or for the part of the bill that the insurance company does *not* cover. These noncovered portions of the total bill are also called *co-payments* or *deductibles.* The consumer is not reimbursed for these out-of-pocket expenses by anyone else. As an example, say Mrs. Smith was hospitalized and her total hospital bill was $4000. Mrs. Smith's husband has Blue Cross coverage for his family, which he purchased for $1200 a year. The nature of his coverage is such that he pays a deductible of $200 for each episode of hospitalization, and Blue Cross covers the rest. The Smith's premiums will be $1200. Their out-of-pocket cost of hospitalization was $200. The rest is paid for by the insurer. As an example of the size of a deductible, individuals who are covered for hospital insurance coverage under Medicare in 1995 had deductibles of $716 when they were hospitalized. The third form of payments consist of taxes paid by households to the government, which in turn reimburses providers when they provide services for certain individuals who are covered by government programs such as Medicare and Medicaid. These taxes can take many forms: they can be part of the general income tax, social security taxes, and so on.

To put these flows in perspective, in 1995 consumers paid out of pocket for 4% of their hospital bills and 18% of their physician bills. Of course, this is just an average figure for the nation as a whole, and hides the enormous distributions of payment between different classes of users. Medicare direct payments, for example, are considerable. The Medicare program was instituted on July 1, 1966 by the federal government to cover high medical expenses for people over 65 (its current coverage is somewhat broader and includes disabled individuals, as well as those with end-stage renal disease). Medicare is designed in two parts. Its compulsory component (with zero enrollment premiums for beneficiaries) is called hospitalization insurance (HI) and covers hospital expenses and some extended care benefits as well. Initially HI was designed with limited out-of-pocket payments by the beneficiaries, but because hospital expenses rose rapidly throughout the period since Medicare was instituted, direct user fees were raised annually. By 1995 the out-of-pocket deductible for HI was $716 in total for the first 60 days of hospitalization. In addition, if the individual required over 60 days of hospitalization during a year, there was a co-payment of $179 a day, up to 90 days. The individual had a lifetime reserve of 90 days in addition, and he could dip into this reserve if he went over the 90 days in a year; the co-payment for this was $358 per day. Beyond this, no coverage was provided. As an example, say that Mrs. Rubin was 66 years old and was hospitalized at City General Hospital for 10 days in 1987. Mrs. Rubin's total payment would be the deductible, or $716. If she were hospitalized five times in 1995, and in total she was in the hospital for 65 days, she would have to pay the deductible (just once), and additionally $179 for each of the five days above 60.

In addition to this compulsory component, Medicare has a *voluntary* component called Supplementary Medical Insurance (SMI) that the individual can join upon payment of a premium of $46.10 per month (in 1995). SMI covers physicians' fees and other outpatient benefits. In 1995 it had a deductible of $100 (that is, the first $100 of expenses incurred by the individual was paid out of pocket by the individual) and a co-payment of 20% of expenses beyond that. For example, Mr. Hall, 70 years old, purchased SMI in 1995 for $46.10 per month. He went to a physician and was treated on an outpatient basis for a stomach disorder. The treatment required 5 visits, and the physician's bill was $25 a visit, or $125 in total. Mr. Hall would have to pay the first $100 out of pocket, and then he would have to pay 20% of the remaining $25, or $5. Medicare would pay $20. If Mr. Hall needed additional physician care during the year, he would pay 20% of the bill.

As medical care costs have increased over the years, so have the out-of-pocket expenses of the Medicare beneficiaries. In 1962, before the institution of Medicare, the average elderly person spent about 8% of per capita household income on medical care. By 1985 this figure had risen to 15%.[10] The poor elderly spend even larger portions of their income on medical care.

Premium Payers: Businesses

Business firms are primarily involved as payers because the bulk of nongovernment health insurance in America is provided through employers. The internal revenue tax code currently exempts from employees' income tax the benefits received by workers in the form of health insurance premiums. This means that if a nurse in a hospital receives a salary of $20,000 yearly, she will pay a tax based on that salary. However, if the hospital additionally provides her with health insurance coverage by paying an insurance company a premium of $800, she will not be taxed on these benefits. This makes benefits such as health insurance coverage a very attractive form of compensation, because otherwise health insurance is quite costly. Many companies pay only part of the premium for health care, and the employee pays the rest. Businesses, of course, also pay taxes, some of which support government health care programs.

Intermediaries: Governments and Insurers

The next group involved in the flows of the health care system can be called intermediaries because they act as insurers *and* reimbursers. These intermediaries include Blue Cross (for hospitalization) and Blue Shield (for insurance of physicians' services), as well as the "commercials," a term covering all of the other health insurance companies including such well-known insurers as John Hancock, Aetna, and Prudential. The intermediaries receive premiums from individuals and employees and, when the insured individuals require medical care, they reimburse the providers on a specific contractual basis. Remember, they may or may not pay the *whole* bill, depending upon whether they require a co-payment on the consumer's part. As a simple example, Blue Cross may have 3000 subscribers whom it insures;

its premium *rate* might be $1000 annually for each subscriber. Blue Cross's total receipts, its premiums, are $3 million. Its payments are its reimbursements to hospitals (say, $2.5 million) and its other expenses, such as salaries (say $0.3 million). Blue Cross is left with a surplus of $0.2 million.

The other intermediary is the government. The government receives payment in taxes and sometimes premiums, and reimburses the providers for covered care. Two important government programs, already mentioned, are Medicare and Medicaid. Medicare's hospitalization insurance plan is operated through the Hospital Insurance (HI) Trust Fund. Government *receipts* for this fund come almost exclusively from a flat rate tax on taxable income, called an employment tax. In 1966 this tax amounted to about one third of 1% of taxable income from both the employee and employer (two thirds of 1% of taxable income in total.) By 1983 this had increased to 2.6%, and by 1995 it was 3.2% in total. This tax rate, like all tax rates, can be changed by law, but not without a good deal of opposition. It should be noted that government receipts from the tax depend on the tax rate and the number of employees.

The HI Trust Fund's expenses are primarily reimbursements to hospitals; in addition, the government wants to keep reserve in the fund. The expenditures of the fund are determined by the hospital expenses (reimbursements) per beneficiary and the number of beneficiaries hospitalized.

As the population has aged and hospital costs have increased, reimbursements to hospitals have increased considerably. In fact, the increase in expenditures paid out by the fund has grown much more rapidly than has the increase in receipts from the employment tax. Although in the mid-1980s the receipts from the tax were less than the expenses, conservative projections based on the growth of hospital expenditures and on the use of hospital services by the aged forecast a narrowing of the receipts-expenditures gap, and by the mid-1990s the projections indicated a deficit of the Trust Fund. This projected deficit caused a good deal of alarm in policy circles. Any search for a solution had to recognize that (1) further increases in taxation would be limited, and (2) the population would continue to age (and thus hospitalization would continue to grow). Any solution to this deficit problem had to control hospital expenditures per beneficiary, which meant containing the reimbursements per unit of hospitalization. This led to the dramatic policy shifts in hospital reimbursement, as will be discussed.

Medicare's voluntary program, the Supplementary Medical Insurance (SMI) program, has also experienced increased economic pressures. This program's revenues come from two sources: a premium for enrollees and receipts from government general tax revenues. The fact that nonpremium receipts come from general revenues means the SMI Trust Fund is not nearly as constrained in its revenue sources; projected deficits can be met by additional appropriations. The SMI program's expenditures are primarily for Medicare's share of reimbursement for physician care and outpatient services. It should be recalled that the co-payment and deductible under SMI (i.e., the beneficiary's share) is quite significant.

Providers: Recipients of Funds

The next stage of the flow system is the reimbursement of the providers by the payers (households, governments, and insurers). Hospital reimbursement has taken several different forms in recent years. Before 1983 Medicare and Medicaid reimbursed hospitals on the basis of the costs *that they had already incurred.* This basis of payment is called *retrospective reimbursement.* What this term means is that if the hospital spends $1200 for treating a Medicare client, then Medicare will base its reimbursement on that $1200. The reimbursement may not be exactly $1200 because the intermediary may make certain adjustments, like taking discounts. As we will see in the "incentives" section of this chapter, this form of reimbursement does not foster efficiency, in that hospitals are reimbursed more if they spend more.

Private insurers generally reimbursed hospitals on the basis of what they charged (i.e., their prices). Prices are usually greater than costs, because hospitals add a mark-up to their costs to set their rates. For example, if the mark-up is 20%, then the charges associated with the Medicare client just discussed would have been $1200 (the costs incurred) plus 20%, or $1440. The private insurers would have had to pay that amount for their insured clients.

In 1983 a virtual revolution occurred in hospital reimbursement. Induced by the projected deficits in the HI Trust Fund, Medicare began paying hospitals on the basis of diagnosis related groups (DRGs). This means that each Medicare client is assigned to a category based on his or her diagnosis, age, and procedure. There are a total of 495 DRG categories, and each category is supposed to contain clients with similar cost experiences. As a result, a prospective price is set for each category, and this is what the hospital is paid. The reimbursement rate for each client within a DRG category is based on two numbers: a relative weight for the particular DRG category and an overall rate applied to this weighted figure. For example, if the relative weight set by Medicare for DRG 159, hernia procedures for persons over 69 years of age, is .9297, and the DRG rate is $3000, then the hospital will receive $2789 (=. 9297 × $3000) for each case it treats in that group. There has been considerable controversy over the particular weights for specific DRGs as well as the setting of the overall rate. One objection relating to the weights is that they are not good reflections of economic costs; for example, it has been claimed that actual nursing costs vary considerably from DRG weights, and in setting the weights more attention should be paid to the nursing input.

Notice that this payment is *prospective:* that is, the price is set before the client is treated, and the hospital knows what this price is. As we will see later, this form of reimbursement dramatically changed the incentive system in hospital reimbursement; in this case, unlike the retrospective case, if the hospitals spent more they did *not* get any more reimbursement.

Physicians have traditionally been reimbursed on a fee-for-service basis. That is, for each service performed, a separate charge was made. For example, for each initial pediatric check-up, U.S. physicians received on average a payment of $120 in 1994. Under fee-for-service payment each visit to a physician can result in several procedures being performed and billed for. For example, a visit for a check-up can result in a complete examination ($120), a chest x-ray ($16), a blood test ($9.80), and an electrocardiogram ($8.60). The total billings for this are greater than that for a simple examination. In the past physicians set these fees themselves. Recent changes suggest a much greater involvement in the setting of fees by insurers, based on factors such as the average fee level for all physicians in an area. Medicare and some private insurers now base their physician fees on estimated costs of each procedure, a system called the Resource Based Relative Value System. As we will see, fee-for-service reimbursement has a built-in incentive for the doctor to perform more services, and for this reason an alternative form of reimbursement, called prepayment, has been promoted by payers. This important development will be covered later.

The providers, physicians and hospitals in this simplified example, must spend some of their receipts on expenses, such as nurses' salaries, supplies, drugs, and so on. The rest they retain in surpluses or profits for themselves. Thus if the Coosa Community Hospital receives $2 million in reimbursement from Blue Cross, $1 million from self-pay sources, and $4 million from Medicaid and Medicare, its total receipts are $7 million. Coosa's expenditures are $4 million for nurses' salaries, $1 million for supplies, and $1.5 million for other expenses. Its surplus, what it has left over, is half a million dollars.

Inputs

To complete the simplified picture of the flow of funds in the medical marketplace, we need to add those groups who produce the inputs (the physicians, the nurses, and so on). These input-producing groups include medical schools, nursing schools, drug companies, and so on. In the case of nursing schools, their revenues are students' fees and government funds, and they graduate nurses to work in the system.

I now have drawn a simplified picture of the flows in the health care system. It is designed to provide an understanding of who the prime actors are in the health care system and how money flows between them. Although not all the actors, or flows, have been identified in this presentation, this overview should give an idea of where things fit. This picture is really one of the traditional system, which was predominant around 1980. Since then a number of changes have been made. One in particular has been the emergence of several new types of actors on the scene: the health maintenance organization (HMO) and the preferred provider organization (PPO). Let us first look at the flows of the HMO.

Health Maintenance Organizations (HMOs)

Figure 3-5 presents a modified version of the flow diagram that incorporates the HMO. From a funds flow standpoint, the essential point about the HMO is that it is both an insurer and a provider. That is, the consumer, employer, or government pays annual premiums to the HMO; in return the HMO undertakes *directly* the responsibility of providing care—basic medical, hospital, and drugs, among others—when required. Notice the difference between this form of "prepaid" care and traditional care, as outlined above. Under traditional care the premiums are paid to the insurer who, in turn, separately reimburses the physicians and hospitals for each unit of care they provide to the insured client. Under prepayment, it is the HMO that undertakes the responsibility for the provision of care and must cover its costs out of its premiums. It does not receive any additional money if more care is provided to any single enrollee.

The HMO incorporates insurance functions as well as provider functions within its organization. Figure 3-5 shows this by incorporating the participating components of the HMO in a dotted line area. It is important to note, however, that an HMO need not have physicians, hospitals, and insurers all in the same institution. An HMO can take the form of a contractual arrangement, with insurers, hospitals, and physicians all independent of one another but each contracting to provide the agreed-upon service.

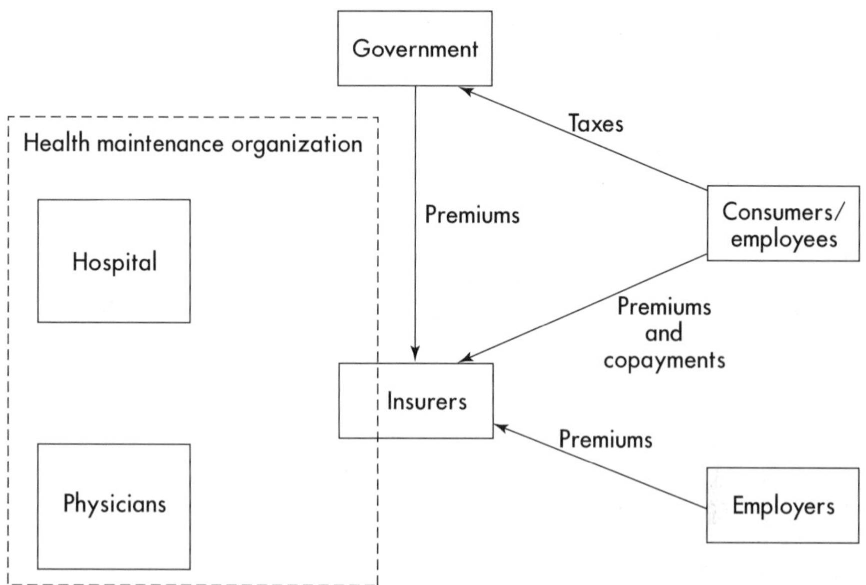

FIG. 3-5 Flow presentation of the health maintenance organization (HMO).

As an example, assume that the Broad River Textile Company has 1000 employees. It decides to provide them with HMO health insurance coverage as an employment benefit. It contracts with Blue Ridge HMO for $1000 an employee. For this fee Blue Ridge agrees to provide all physician, hospital, and drug care for the 1000 employees and their dependents. Now Blue Ridge has received $1 million in premiums. Since it has undertaken to provide medical care for the 1000 employees and their dependents, it must make some arrangements to do so. The alternative arrangements that Blue Ridge can make are numerous. It can purchase its own hospitals and hire its own (salaried) physicians and can actually be a provider; or it can contract out with doctors and hospitals to provide care for its members. In the latter case Blue Ridge becomes a reimburser of care; but what distinguishes it from a traditional insurer is the fact that it is responsible for *providing* the care (or seeing to it that care is provided) rather than merely paying for it. Under HMO membership the member must be treated by the HMO's own selected providers. Under traditional care the consumer is free to select her own providers. This gives the HMO a greater degree of control over the providers. It can select providers with conservative practice patterns and thus reduce the degree of hospitalization of its members. The traditional insurer has no such control over its insurees' providers.

Notice that the HMO premium is a fixed prepaid amount (e.g., $1000) per employee. The HMO as *insurer* receives this sum as its receipts. But the HMO is also a *provider,* or a contractee for providers, and as a provider it receives a fixed sum per member. Unlike a hospital or a physician under traditional care, the more care an HMO provides, the more it costs the HMO, but *it does not get reimbursed any additional amount for providing more care.* It still gets the same $1000. As we will see, the HMO operates under radically different incentives from the provider under traditional insurance. Membership in HMOs has been growing dramatically in

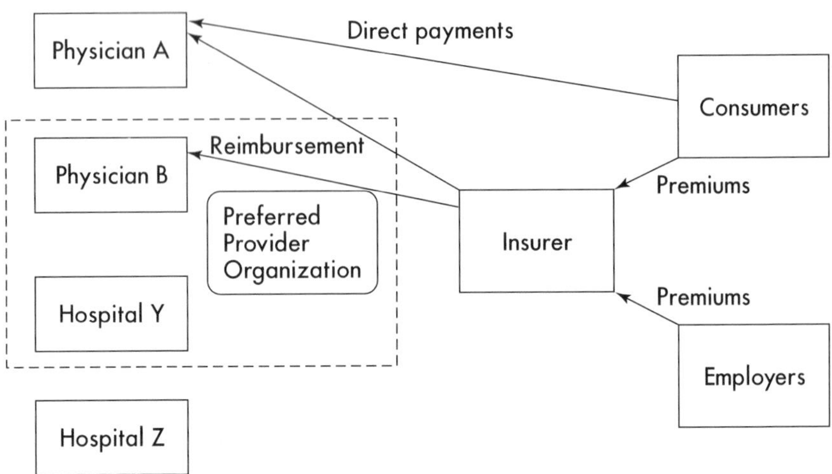

FIG. 3-6 Financial flows and the preferred provider organization (PPO).

recent years. In 1971 there were 3.6 million subscribers nationally. By 1994 this number had grown to 51 million, or 20% of the population.

Preferred Provider Organizations (PPOs)

The final addition to the scene that we will look at is the preferred provider organization (PPO). The PPO is not an insurer, nor is it a provider, although it may have links to both. It is a true "middleman," a creature of the competitive marketplace. To illustrate what a PPO does, I have again redrawn the flows diagram slightly in Figure 3-6. This figure shows two competing physicians and two competing hospitals (I could have included more, but the diagram would have been complicated). Now each physician and each hospital is vying for clients. The problem for them, in a competitive environment, is how to sign up clients. One possibility is to try to attract them with favorable prices.

Now the insurer is also part of this picture. The insurer wants to keep its premiums down so it can attract the business of employers, who will contract with it to insure its employees. The prime way that the insurer can keep its rates down is to contain its reimbursements to physicians and hospitals. If the insurer can contain the reimbursement rates that it pays to these providers, as well as the number of times the consumers are hospitalized, it can succeed in lowering its costs, and also its premiums. Enter the PPO.

The PPO is an intermediary that tries to develop favorable terms for physician and hospital care and sell it to insurers. First the PPO signs up physicians with conservative practice patterns and hospitals with low charges. It then develops a system of reviewing the usage of potential clients so that the utilization will be kept low. Because of the favorable utilization experience of consumers, as well as reasonable rates, the PPO will have a favorable package, which it in turn can promote at reasonable premium rates, *if the consumers use these "preferred" providers.* The problem is to induce them to do so.

Under PPO arrangements, as with traditional insurance, the consumers have free choice of providers. They can select doctors with nonconservative practice patterns (Doctor A in the diagram), and they can select high-cost hospitals (Hospital Z). The insurer builds an incentive into its package to induce consumers to use the conservative and low-cost providers (B and Y). They can do this in a number of ways. Most notably, they can write up insurance policies such that, when the consumers go to "preferred" providers B and Y, they make little or no direct payments. When they go to the nonmember providers A and Z, they have to make a direct payment. For example, the Green Hills Insurance Company can offer employers a preferred package consisting of a specified list of physicians, Smith and Jones, and a specified hospital, Gander County Memorial. The premium is $1200 a year per employee. If the employees seek treatment from these preferred providers, there is no additional payment (as per agreement with the insurers). If, however, they go to Dr. Brown, who is not on the preferred list, Green Hills will reimburse Dr. Brown only $20 for the visit. If Dr. Brown's bill is $50, those consumers who chose to go to Dr. Brown would pay the additional $30 directly. Thus there is a penalty to consumers for using nonpreferred providers. Note that unlike other HMO arrangements, under a PPO system the consumer can use nonmember providers. There is a penalty for doing so, however.

The PPO can be operated by providers, by insurers, by independent contractors, or by anyone else, for that manner. The essential ingredient in the PPO is that it contracts with providers and manages the care they provide. In performing this monitoring function the PPO can offer a group of services at reduced rates. The PPO is not directly an insurer or a provider; it does not collect or pay out funds. It performs a flow-through function, and tries to ensure that the funds flowing through are reduced. The PPO might, therefore, be reimbursed on a commission basis, and so it gains a portion of any savings it creates. In 1994 about 44 million Americans were covered under PPO-type plans, just slightly under the 51 million covered by HMOs, out of a total covered population of about 180 million persons.

Managed Care

Managed care is a term that is used to indicate a broad set of arrangements between insurers and providers. Under managed care the "manager" will have some degree of control over the provider's behavior. This could be because the manager (often also the insurer) either employs the provider directly or else owns the provider (hospital) outright. It could also be because of contractual arrangements that are set up between the insurer and the provider; under contractual arrangements the provider agrees to submit to some form of scrutiny of its provision practices as part of the reimbursement agreement. Managed care is most closely associated with HMOs, somewhat less with PPOs, and least of all with conventional fee-for-service insurance arrangements. Increasingly, however, conventional insurance arrangements between insurers and providers incorporate elements of managed care. Among the techniques that are frequently employed in managed care are the requirement that the insurer approve that a client needs hospitalization before the admission occurs, and a requirement that a person who has been recommended for surgery by a surgeon get a second opinion from another surgeon.

Nowadays insurers (including HMOs) exert considerable direct control over what care the provider gives the clients. Their payment to providers is based on specific contractual criteria, and in this sense the care is "managed."

■ COSTS

Cost is a fundamental economic concept that refers to the value of a resource commitment. One measures an activity by its cost, which refers to the quantity and value of resources that have gone into that activity. Often costs are associated with dollar expenditures; for example, let us say Mrs. White gets ill and needs $800 in treatment costs (measured by physicians' fees and drug costs.) In addition, Mrs. White loses 3 days from her part-time job as a ballpoint pen assembler in a factory; she gets $60 a day from this job. Mrs. White's husband has insurance coverage, with some deductibles, such that Mrs. White ends up paying $200 of the $800, with the insurance company paying $600. What is the cost of Mrs. White's *medical care?* And what are her *illness* costs?

To identify true cost requires using a definition of what cost is as a guide to measuring costs. The activity being measured must also be clearly defined. In this case two activities are measurable: the cost of *medical care* and the cost of *illness.* The cost of *medical care* refers to the size of resource commitment (in dollar terms) resulting from the use of medical services. Going back to Figure 3-4, this is measured by the flow of money received by the providers, as well as the administrative costs of the intermediaries. In Mrs. White's example, this is $800.

The cost of *illness* refers to the size of the resource commitment in dollar terms resulting from the illness. This is a broader concept; it incorporates medical care costs but also costs from any other resources resulting from the illness. In the case of Mrs. White, three days of work were lost, and so there was an additional cost of $180. The total illness cost was thus $980, and the medical care cost was $800. We refer to medical care costs as *direct costs* and foregone costs as *indirect costs.* In this case, $800 of the total costs of $980 were direct and $180 were indirect.

The reader might object, at this point, and say that the $180 was not a true cost, since Mrs. White never had the $180 in the first place. But this would be a mistaken notion of cost. As a nursing student the costs of your nursing education includes fees (say $2000 a year) and books and supplies (say $1000). But what about your time? If you weren't a nursing student, couldn't you have been working full time? If so, what would you be earning? Let us say you could have been working as a sales clerk for $15,000 a year. This $15,000 that you gave up is a cost to you, and even though it hasn't directly come out of your pocket, it is as real to you as if it did. You have, in fact, *given up* this $15,000 by going to nursing school. Therefore, in the light of the true meaning of the term *cost*—the amount of resources committed— your total costs are $18,000 per year.

We can also break down total illness costs by who bears the burden of the costs. In our example, Mrs. White bore $380 of the total burden of $980; $180 was borne indirectly and $200 directly. Of the direct medical care costs, $200 of the $800 were borne by Mrs. White. This breakdown is shown in Figure 3-7.

It should be noted that the $600 in costs that are reimbursed by intermediaries do, ultimately, fall on individuals. As will be recalled from the previous section, insurers' revenues come from premiums and governments' revenues come from taxes. Both premiums and taxes ultimately are paid for by individuals. At times it is difficult to pinpoint exactly on whose shoulders the costs fall. An employer's health insurance premiums are made at the expense of employees' money wages, though the employees may not fully recognize this. And Medicare's receipts for Part A

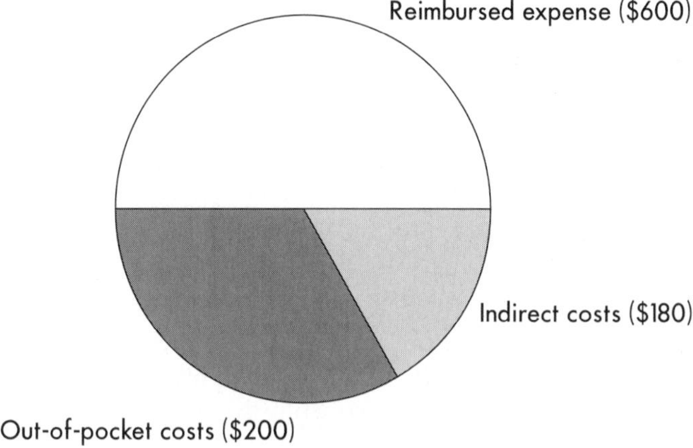

FIG. 3-7 Breakdown of Mrs. White's total illness costs.

come out of social security taxes, though, again, the payers may not fully recognize this. Nevertheless, *all* costs are borne by someone. And so when Mrs. White receives $800 in medical care for $200, she may at the time feel she is getting a bargain. But Mrs. White's husband has paid health insurance premiums, as have his co-workers, and the $800 has come out of their premiums.

The concept of costs can be used to explain the waste incurred by "flat of the curve" medicine, which was mentioned at the beginning of this chapter. To do this we introduce the notion of cost-benefit analysis. A cost-benefit analysis is a comparison of the costs of a particular activity with its benefits. Medical care is undertaken to improve health. The *benefits* of health can be measured in dollar terms as the dollar savings from reduced illness. Without medical care Mrs. White may have been unable to work for 10 days. Since with treatment she lost only 3 days of work, the medical care she received created benefits of 7 extra days of good health. The dollar value of these benefits can be roughly stated at $60 a day, or $420 in total.

Since the costs of medical care were $800, the benefit cost ratio was 420/800, or about .52:1. A ratio of less than one signifies that benefits were less than costs, and the activity was not worth it, from a strict dollar standpoint. This notion can be used to illustrate the wastage arising from "flat of the curve" medicine. If additional medical care is costly, but very little additional health results from this medical care, then the benefit cost ratio will be very low. Especially if the ratio is less than 1, we can say that the medical care has not yielded benefits equal to its costs. It is not that medical care is of *no* value, but that the benefits it creates, though they are positive, are less than the costs.

One particularly difficult problem arises in this analysis. If we take a "private" viewpoint, that of Mrs. White, we get a very different picture of the cost-benefit ratio from the "social" viewpoint, that of everyone. Mrs. White's private cost-benefit ratio, the ratio of her private or out-of-pocket costs to her benefits, is 420:200 or 2.1:1. And the lower her out-of-pocket costs (because of heavier insurance coverage), the more beneficial this ratio will be. From a social standpoint we get a different picture, however. It costs "society" (everyone, including Mrs. White) $800 to secure $420 in benefits. Clearly this is not cost beneficial. When analyzing costs and benefits, then, it is very important to distinguish the point of view being taken.

I must also add a very important reminder relating to benefit calculations. In many instances we do not have very good estimates of benefits. Employment benefits such as Mrs. White's are of limited use for calculating the benefits of those who are not currently employed, such as retired people, unemployed people, and the very young.

Take someone's (anyone's) grandmother. Let us say she is 70 years old and does not work, and suddenly she gets pneumonia. Hospitalizing her will cure her, but the cost is $3000. Since she does not work, the dollar value of employment benefits are zero. Is the cost-benefit ratio zero? Total money benefits are clearly greater than employment benefits; however, when we leave the concrete world of employment benefits and attempt to attribute dollar values to improved health from those who are not working, we encounter many problems. This is one area of economics where satisfactory solutions do not exist. Still, the resources are scarce and have alternative uses. Using resources in one way results in taking them away from another valuable use. Not having a sound measure of benefits merely makes the decision all the more difficult.

Actual data on the burden of disease allows us to determine what the actual distribution of costs are in a manner that is similar to those depicted hypothetically in Figure 3-7. In the United States in 1995 the total societal costs from heart disease were estimated as $60.6 billion. Of these costs indirect costs were estimated to be $8.9 billion and medical care costs at $51.7 billion. Of course, it should be remembered that heart disease largely affects the older population, and so most people with heart disease are retired. This means that indirect costs will be low in this illness group, relative to costs in areas such as motor vehicle accidents and violence.[5,8]

■ INCENTIVES IN HEALTH CARE

A dean of medicine in a large medical school once remarked that it would not make any difference whether you gave a hospital a lump sum of $40 million to operate or paid it $4000 a patient and limited the number of patients you reimbursed to 10,000. The total cost in either case, he remarked, would be the same. He was correct in observing that the total cost would be the same. But he was not correct in saying that it would not make any difference to the outcome. The incentive systems under the two types of reimbursement are radically different, and the outcomes will be different as well. Indeed, one of the most important lessons to be learned from economics is that an incentive system can affect the output (and outcome) of the system.

First, let us define what we mean by *output*. Output refers to the economic behavior of the consumer or provider. For the consumer, economic behavior refers to the quantity of medical care demanded. For the provider, it refers to the quantity and quality of medical care provided. When we say that incentives influence output, then we mean that these groups will behave differently—consume more or less, provide more or less quantity and quality—depending on the incentive system. As well, costs may be influenced by these behavioral differences, and *health outcomes* may differ.

What are the incentives that can affect behavior? Incentives consist of the rewards and penalties associated with any particular course of action. *Every* course of action taken by a consumer and provider has associated with it rewards and penalties. The consumer or provider will assess these and will choose the course of action with the greatest *net* rewards (rewards minus penalties). It is in this way that costs enter the picture. Costs to a consumer or provider are penalties. If a consumer or provider bears more costs for a particular course of action, then he or she will find that course of action less appealing.

We can now tie together the concept of flows and the concept of costs with the idea of incentives. Let us look at how all of these tie in with consumer incentives. As previously discussed, one of the key flows in the health care system is the out-of-pocket costs paid by consumers directly to the provider. Alternative policy and insurance arrangements can alter these flows, in that the co-payment can be increased (all the way to the point that the consumer pays the full cost of care) or decreased (all the way to the point where the consumer pays no cost). The key point in behavioral economics is that *it matters which option is chosen.* If the consumer bears a greater portion of the costs directly, then he or she will be penalized more for using medical care and will use less of it.

If Mrs. Smith has full insurance coverage, then for a particular episode of illness she might visit the physician four or five times. The rewards are there (improved health) but the penalties are not (no out-of-pocket costs). Now let us raise the out-of-pocket cost to Mrs. Smith to $20 a visit. The potential rewards from treatment are unchanged, but the penalties have increased. Mrs. Smith now finds going to the physician costly, and she will cut down on her visits. What has happened is that *the incentive system has changed her behavior.*

The analysis just described is the basic demand analysis of economics. It states that individuals will demand more of any commodity if the out-of-pocket price falls. Note that it is not the total cost that governs individual behavior, but the out-of-pocket price. It is this price that the client reacts to. The service can be very costly (e.g., intensive care), but if the service is insured or subsidized, then the individual will behave as if it is very inexpensive.

I have just shown how incentives can work on the demand side of the picture. They can also influence providers in terms of the quantity and quality of services that they are willing to provide. To illustrate that various incentive schemes will cause very different behaviors on the part of the providers, I will use an example of provider behavior in nursing education.

Not long ago the health economics course at Adirondack College of Nursing, a well-respected eastern institution, was being taught in a staid, routine manner by a part-time lecturer who had been teaching the course since 1969. The lecturer was being paid $2000 to teach the course, plus he was given a modest budget for course-related expenses such as supplies, travel, and honorariums for visiting speakers. His average cost summary for the years 1993–1994 are shown in Box 3-1; these figures are very close to what they were in 1969. In fact, everything about the course was similar to what it was in 1969.

This lack of dynamism in the course surfaced in 1994 when the college's nursing administration program came up for accreditation. As part of the accreditation process, a review of the program's courses was made by an external body of experts. The health economics course did not fare well in that review. The review team complained that the teacher had used the same lecture notes since 1969 and still (in

Box 3-1 Summary of Expenses for Health Economics Course Original Payment Method

Item	Expense ($)
Photocopying	400
Field trips (Saint Ives Hospital)	150
Honorarium for guest speakers	
Mr. Jack Spratt, Administrator, Fat City General Hospital	200
Miss M. Muffett, Director of Nursing, Tuffett Memorial Hospital	200
Computer time	150
Expense total	1100
Instructor's salary	2000
Total course expense	4200

1994) referred to the "new" Medicare and Medicaid programs, as well as the need for regulation to curb hospital cost inflation. Students who were interviewed professed to being bored by the lectures, though they praised the fact the examinations were easy to study for since they were the same from year to year.

The review team concluded that the course was "stagnant" and, in making recommendations, cited the "reimbursement" system as a major cause of the inertia. They asserted that there were no incentives for the professor to improve or update his course and that there were no sufficient resources to support updating.

The dean at Adirondack, whose objective included providing the very highest quality of education, took the criticisms to heart, though she questioned the means recommended by the committee to attain these ends. Being a full-time academic, she was under the impression that academics were motivated solely by the pursuit of truth, just as lawyers are motivated solely by the pursuit of justice and doctors solely by the pursuit of their clients' health. The dean argued that a good teacher will teach well under any payment system. Still, despite her reservations, she acquiesced and, with the help of a hospital administrator, designed a new reimbursement system for the health economics course.

The new reimbursement system chosen was called "cost plus" (which, because it was designed by a hospital administrator, resembled the pre-1983 formula used by Medicare and Medicaid to reimburse hospitals). According to this system the college would reimburse the lecturer for education-related expenses plus a percentage of those costs to cover the professor's salary. Since the ratio of educational costs to salary for the 1993–1994 period was about 1:2, the dean decided that this figure would be used in the formula. The final formula, then, was that the professor would be reimbursed education costs for speakers, supplies, travel, and so on plus an amount equal to twice these educational costs for his lecturing fee.

The system was initiated, and although the dean heard some rumblings of what was going on during the semester, she did not fully realize what had happened until she was presented with a bill (Box 3-2) of $117,000—one third of which was for course expenses. She immediately called in the health economics professor and protested. The professor explained each item, and tried to point out that he was trying to provide the students in Nurs Adm 103 with the very highest quality of education, and was grateful to the education system for allowing him to do so. He

Box 3-2 *Expenses for Health Economics Course Cost-Based Reimbursment Formula*

Item	Expense ($)
2 super deluxe VCRs	$ 3,000
1 set VCR tapes: "Health Care in the U.S."	3,000
Library trip to the British Museum to research Florence Nightingale papers	1,600
1 slide projector with sound system	800
Slide production	900
Supplies (gold Cross pens, etc.)	1,100
Trip to Bethesda, Maryland, NIH Library to research their nursing administration collection	800
Speaker: Stephen King on the pitfalls of nursing management	2,000
Speaker: Seinfeld and Elaine on the lighter side of nursing management	4,000
Speaker: George Bush on nursing management and international affairs	8,000
Speaker: Rush Limbaugh on what's right in nursing administration	$ 11,000
Speaker: General Schwartzkopf on nursing contributions to the Gulf War	5,000
Total direct expenses	39,200
Total salary (direct expenses × 2)	78,400
Total reimbursed	117,600

explained that the two super-quality VCRs were purchased ($1500 each) so that the students could view the PBS special series tapes ($1000) on the health care system. He explained that his trip to the British Museum ($1600) was expressly made to research the life and times of Florence Nightingale, which perked up students' interest in emergency care nursing. He defended his trip to the NIH library in Bethesda ($800) on the grounds that only there could he obtain materials pertinent to his lecture on the role of the federal government in nursing. When questioned about the relevance of the outside speakers, the professor stated that if one wanted to provide current and high-quality education, second-rate speakers simply would not do. So General Schwartzkopf was invited in to speak on the contribution of nursing administration to the Gulf War effort, Rush Limbaugh on what's right in nursing administration, and Stephen King on pitfalls in nursing management. And, if one wanted the best expert on nursing management and international affairs, who better to speak than Mr. Bush? Or Seinfeld and Elaine on the lighter side of nursing management? Although the point was well made, the dean felt that Adirondack's budget could not support such extravagance, so she sought a new funding formula.

The formula that followed, in the spring of 1995, was based on a simple fee schedule. A new instructor was presented with a basic fee schedule (Box 3-3) that specified a price for each "procedure" that the professor performed. This was much like a physician's fee schedule. For a short lecture (under 30 minutes) the professor was reimbursed $10, regardless of the size of the class. A longer (and more boring) lecture was funded $15. A separate fee was set for each student examined, with a $4

Box 3-3 Fee Schedule for Health Economics Teaching "Procedures"

Item	Fee ($)
Lecture (less than 30 minutes)	10.00
Lecture (over 30 minutes)	15.00
Examination, multiple choice	4.00
Examination, short answer, under 200 words per question	5.00
Examination, essay, over 200 words per question and over 4 questions	6.00
Term paper, less than 10 pages	12.00
Term paper, more than 10 pages and 50-item bibliography	16.00
Tutorial requiring only a minor clarification	6.00
Tutorial requiring a major clarification	9.00
Tutorial for a major miscomprehension	20.00

fee set for each student examined on a multiple-choice basis. In addition, fees were set for tutorials, beginning with $6 for a minor misunderstanding, $9 for a major misunderstanding, and $20 for a tutorial in which the student exhibited a major incomprehension.

The dean at Adirondack expected efficiency, and she got it. Lectures were generally short—very short, in fact, lasting about 10 minutes each. There was a multiple-choice examination after each class. In spite of this, there were a *lot* of major misunderstandings, and the students were continually lined up outside the professor's door for remedial tutorials. In fact, for each student in the 14 week course there were 21 multiple-choice tests and over 30 major misunderstandings. Again, the dean's preconception that truth would prevail was borne out, but *the manner in which the professor taught the truth varied.* And this variation was due to the fee schedule, or incentive system.

We might also hypothesize that, had the fee schedule differed, the behavior of the professor would have differed as well. For example, if the fee for a short lecture had been $5 and for a long one $30, the professor would have given more long lectures. Or had a multiple-choice test's fee been 25 cents and the fee for a long essay been $10, you would have seen a lot of long essays and not many multiple-choice tests. All of this would have been done in the search for truth and high-quality education! (It is not the goal that would change with the reimbursement method, but how that goal was sought.)

Regardless, the dean was not happy with the outcome, and again, in the summer session of 1995 the reimbursement system was changed (as was the professor). This time the new professor was reimbursed on a prepaid, per-student basis. This type of payment was very similar to that of HMOs. For each student taught, the professor was paid $40. If the professor brought in outside speakers such as Kramer or Oprah, he or she would have had to bear the cost out of his or her own budget. Unlike the case of cost-plus reimbursement, the penalty for incurring higher costs would have fallen on the professor. As one might expect, instructional costs fell dramatically (see the audited expense statement in Box 3-4. But the professor's promotional budget soared, with beer bashes, propeller beanies with the insignia "Nursing Adm 103 is A-OK," and spots on the college radio station. The dean was less concerned, however, because these expenses had to come out of the professor's $40 per capita payment.

Box 3-4 *Expense Summary for Health Economics Per Capita Reimbursement*

Item	EXPENSE ($)
INSTRUCTIONAL MATERIALS	
2 pieces of chalk (first broke)	$ 0.16
1 pencil to record names	0.11
1 paper pad	0.89
STUDENT RECRUITMENT	
1 recruitment session at Porky's	289.98
Color ad in Phi Kappa Theta News	99.00
20–30 second spot on WROK-1330	60.00
1000 propeller beanies with insignia "For an A-bsolutely A-ssured A-experience, Take Nurs Adm 103"	500.00
Distribution of beanies by the Greek Society	125.00
Total expenses	$1,075.14

As might be expected, enrollment in Nurs Adm 103 initially skyrocketed. But what of the quality of education? Did *it* remain the same? There will always be those naysayers who will say that quality deteriorated. But there are some who say that the students learned more this way, because every last one got an A in the course!

However, at the same time enrollment began falling in other courses. To counter these falling enrollments, instructors in these courses began clamoring for per capita payments as well. And those that got them also began to promote their courses. Soon the campus was filled with promotional signs for courses such as Nurs Adm 222 and Psych 239. And in early September, just before fall registration, meeting rooms at the local Jeffrey Amber Pub were booked solid by professors who were holding "course orientation" meetings.

Once again the outcome changed. Though the professor was still pursuing the same goal of quality education, each time the incentive system changed, the manner in which the course was taught changed as well. That is, the professors, who were in charge of resource use, used resources in different ways. By this time even the dean was becoming a believer that the reward-penalty system would affect resource use decisions.

At the beginning of this section I quoted the dean of a medical school who wondered what difference it would make to pay a hospital a flat sum of $40 million or pay it $4000 a client up to a maximum of 10,000 clients. The lesson of this section is, it would make a great deal of difference. Just as they worked at Adirondack, the various reimbursement schemes in the health care field work to influence delivery patterns. Depending on the specific rewards and penalties associated with a particular reimbursement system, health care providers will alter their delivery patterns accordingly.

Note that it is not necessarily a result of greed on the part of the providers that outcomes are determined in this way. A change in the incentive system makes it more costly to do things in a certain way, and discourages providers from behaving in certain ways. For example, providing a myriad of laboratory tests and x-rays is not necessarily bad, even if it is costly. It represents one way of providing health

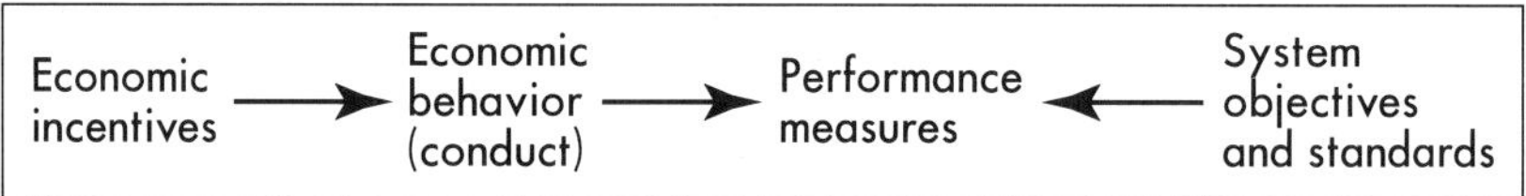

FIG. 3-8 Conceptual elements in an evaluation.

care, and if this manner of provision is rewarded (as it is under the cost-based and fee-for-service reimbursement systems) then it will be continued. Under prepayment, resource-intensive care results in the provider bearing the costs more directly and thus being penalized for providing resource intensive care. The provider will choose a less intensive mode of care under per capita payment. It is another question, and an open one, as to which type of care will be more effective in promoting *health*. Certainly this issue is also part of the evaluation of the various types of delivery, as is cost.

■ ECONOMIC ORGANIZATION OF MEDICAL CARE

Since 1966 the United State's health care system has gone through four phases, each of which has been associated with specific economic characteristics. In this section we will focus on the use of the concepts which we have developed in the previous sections of this chapter to understand the functioning and *performance* of these four phases. Central to understanding of system *performance,* then, lie the various incentives that have been adopted by the system.

What is meant by the performance of a health care system? Performance refers to the operation of the system in light of specific criteria, standards, or goals. As shown in Figure 3-8, performance has two sides: the setting of the standards themselves, in light of which the system's activities are to be evaluated, and the behavior (often called *conduct*) of the entities in the system, which as we have seen are significantly influenced by economic incentives. *Performance* refers to the comparison of actual conduct with the standards that have been established. It should be noted that in evaluating economic conduct we are really evaluating the incentives that influenced it. Remember that the economic conduct was influenced by these incentives in the first place. Although variables other than incentives may affect behavior, if we want to influence behavioral changes, incentives must be high up on the list of where to begin.

The first step in evaluating how the economic organization of a health care system has functioned, then, is to specify the social goals or objectives in light of which we are making our assessment. Three important criteria that can be used to gauge a system's performance are cost, consumer access to care, and quality of care. *Cost* comprises the efficiency with which providers deliver care (the unit cost of care) and the number of units of care provided. The goal of reducing cost is desirable in that, at lower costs, a given dollar will go farther in paying for more care and producing more health-related benefits. *Access to care* refers to the availability of care to consumers. Access has a number of economic characteristics, including the out-of-pocket price (which reduces access when this price is increased) and waiting and travel costs (which increase when availability or supply is reduced). Although access is a desirable trait up to a point, it should be remembered that there is a possibility of reaching the "flat of the curve" beyond which more care is not desirable. It should also be pointed out that total cost and access may at times be conflicting goals. We can increase availability by increasing supply and hence costs; in this case, we face a trade-off between these objectives and must make a choice as to how much of each we prefer.

The third policy goal is that of *quality of care. Quality* is a very elusive term and can refer to a number of characteristics. It usually is associated with resource intensity of care, but even that may not be accurate if resource intensity does not lead to improved outcomes (better health). We will define quality as relating to improved health outcomes, but it must be remembered that these are hard to measure in practice. To the extent that quality and resource intensity go hand in hand, then quality is a costly goal, and we are again faced with a trade-off of quality for costs. When quality and cost conflict with one another, we may not necessarily choose the highest quality of care; it may simply be too costly.

We turn now to an examination of four stages of the United States health care system since 1966, focusing on the role that incentives have played in these systems. When Medicaid and Medicare were instituted in 1966, the reimbursement systems established by Congress included fee-for-service payment for physicians and cost-based reimbursement for hospitals. Direct payments (e.g., co-payments and deductibles) for Medicare beneficiaries were reasonably low (the deductible for hospital care was $40—low by current-day standards), and premiums for those who chose the optional medical benefits coverage (SMI) coverage were also comparatively reasonable. As described previously, low co-payments, cost-based reimbursement for hospitals, and fee-for-service reimbursement for physicians encourage increased use and costs of the health care system.

These conclusions are summarized in Figure 3-9, with reference to our economic goals, which shows that the incentives of the post-1966 system were such that they encouraged greater costs, greater access, and greater quality. Of course, more of everything is not always better; greater accessibility and quality were achieved at the expense of greater costs, and greater costs are not well appreciated by those who bear them, primarily insurance premium payers and taxpayers. As well, there may be limits to how much access we want to achieve; if "flat of the curve" medicine is indeed a reality, then at some point increased access to health *care* adds little to health *outcomes.*

Not long after these incentives were put into place their inflationary tendencies were recognized. Although there was little disagreement as to the effects that these financial arrangements were having, there was considerable disagreement as to how to curb their inflationary effects. Introducing different incentives, such as higher out-of-pocket costs (deductibles or co-payments) would have curbed demand pressures, but this would have meant compromising on the goal of access. And cutting back on payments to providers (e.g., hospitals) would have meant less resources available for client care, which would have compromised on the quality goal. Initially Congress was not willing to compromise on either goal. Instead they introduced a series of regulations that were attempts to directly impose restrictions on providers to contain costs.

Regulation refers to direct attempts on the part of an authority to control the behavior of organizations. Regulation is conducted by a government-appointed agency that has been given the authority by the legislature to monitor and control

SYSTEM	CHARACTERISTICS	SYSTEM GOALS		
		COST	ACCESS	QUALITY
Pre-1970	Low out-of-pocket consumer prices; cost-based and fee-for-service reimbursement	↑	↑	↑
1970s	Same as above but with regulatory controls	↑	↑	↑
1980s	Increasing direct prices, prospective reimbursement, fixed physician fees	↓	↓	↓
1990s	Managed care and managed competition	↓	↓	↓

FIG. 3-9 Overview of economic characteristics of the health care system in four periods and their influence on goals of the health care system.

specific aspects of economic behavior of the regulated providers. For example, a regulatory agency may be given the authority to control the amount that hospitals spend on new equipment. The agency would review all new equipment spending plans and would approve those projects that fall within its guidelines. By setting very strict guidelines, the agency may curtail new spending on equipment.

Note that nothing in the regulatory process changes how much the providers *want* to spend. Regulation by itself does nothing to change the incentives of the providers. If the incentives are such that they encourage spending, imposing regulations will not discourage the desire for providers to spend more. What the regulation will do will be to disallow the providers from spending as much as they want to. However, depending on the incentives, the providers may seek ways of getting around the regulations.

One type of regulation that was introduced to curb rising health care costs was capital expenditure review. According to this type of regulation, a regulatory body is in charge of reviewing all new hospital expenditures for major equipment purchased and additions or renovations to the facility. Approval of the expenditure plans by the agency results in the issuance of a "certificate of need," certifying that the hospital's plans are in accordance with the regulatory agency's guidelines. The rationale behind this type of regulation is the belief that increases in hospital operating expenses are fueled by new equipment and plant. Thus one way to curb operating costs is to curb new equipment and facilities. Certificate of need regulation first appeared in New York state in 1964, but it was not until the mid-1970s that a full-scale federal effort at capital expenditure planning was undertaken with the passage of the National Health Planning and Resources

Development Act of 1974. According to this act regional health systems agencies were established to review all large-scale hospital capital expenditures.

The establishment of these agencies represented one additional step in a history of regulating the economic behavior of health care providers. But by the late 1970s the role of regulation in the economy in general was being questioned, and the effectiveness of capital expenditure review did not escape the growing scrutiny of the effectiveness of regulation. A study undertaken late in the 1970s[9a] raised considerable doubt about the effectiveness of certificate of need regulations in controlling capital expenditures in existing facilities. Federal funds for the national health planning effort were reduced and the national certificate of need effort was curtailed, along with a host of other regulatory efforts in diverse industries such as trucking and air travel.

From our perspective, our key point should be reemphasized. Certificate of need regulation did nothing to change the incentives the hospitals had to increase their operating costs. Throughout the 1970s hospitals were still being reimbursed on the basis of their costs, and so they still had incentives to expand these costs. The imposition of capital expenditure regulations simply amounted to the parachuting of an outside body to control a system that retained its inflationary tendencies. This is much like trying to contain the size of an expanding balloon by pushing in one of its sides. The balloon will keep expanding around the surface that is contained. In the same way, hospital administrators found their way around certificate of need regulations, thus reducing the attempts to contain hospital costs through regulation alone. As a result, in terms of the system goals of Figure 3-9, there was no difference in the performance of the pre-1970 unregulated system and the post-1970 regulated system *because the incentives were unchanged.*

Along with the growing disillusionment with regulation as a mechanism to control health care costs came an increasing interest in the role of incentives. Provider reimbursement schemes were receiving growing attention. In addition, the role of income tax regulations was gaining greater recognition. These income tax rules allowed health insurance premiums paid by employers to be treated as nontaxable benefits and allowed individuals to deduct premiums that they paid from their income for taxation purposes. It was contended that these income tax regulations were too lax and as a result encouraged overinsurance for health care expenditures. With very low direct prices people sought care to the point where they were on the "flat of the curve." It was contended that, with the failure of regulations to remedy the inflationary situation, incentives would have to be introduced.

Among the proposed incentive changes in the early 1980s was the limitation of tax-free insurance premium benefits.[2] It was felt that, if consumers had to directly bear a greater portion of the costs of health care insurance, they would shop around for less costly alternatives. HMOs were believed to be lower-cost alternatives, and a rationale for this proposal was that if consumers had to pay a greater share of their health insurance premiums, consumers would begin switching to lower-cost forms of insurance. At about the same time, faced with lower profits from recessionary times and foreign competition, United States businesses were also examining ways to lower their health insurance benefit costs.

The proposal to limit tax-free health insurance benefits never materialized, but faced with increasing deficits, several other policy initiatives did. Medicare sought to enroll at least some of its beneficiaries in HMOs, and to contain its hospital expenditures it initiated the prospective payment system by introducing hospital payment by DRGs in 1983. These initiatives, especially the latter, did help reduce Medicare's own costs, but several new issues have risen. First, concern has grown that, with the incentive to curtail resource use, hospitals have also contained quality of care. The degree to which this has occurred is difficult to measure and is largely unknown. Second, in their efforts to contain costs, hospitals have been less ready to treat nonpaying patients, those who have no insurance coverage from any source (roughly 14% of the population, or 34 million people) and who cannot afford to pay for the high cost of hospitalization. This latter problem has come to be known as the "indigent problem" and forms the focal point for health care reform.

Health Care Reform

Health care reform has been the dominant topic of health policy in the 1990s. It is concerned with attempts to change the payment mechanism from fee-for-service to capitation and to create an environment in which insurance plans and HMOs compete with each other to provide lower premiums. The former type of change has placed emphasis on managed care. The second type of change has been called *managed competition.*

One of the key factors in competition among health insurance plans has been the ability of the plans to pick and choose among potential insurees. Insurance providers would prefer to enroll customers who are healthier and who have less risk of illness and hospitalization. Insurers can and do use numerous markers of ill health (such as age, previous illness, and high blood pressure) to "rate" potential customers. The use of these markers leads to the selection by the insurance companies of low-risk insurees and makes it difficult for high-risk individuals to obtain insurance. Market reform is an attempt to force insurers to accept all risks, high and low, and to even out the premiums among all potential customers.

Market reform has been attempted in a number of states, but it has proved difficult to make health insurance markets conform to a competitive ideal. Insurers have every incentive to weed out high-risk customers, and the use of health status markers to do so is a common occurrence.

Among the possible regulatory proposals that were designed to curb these selection practices are designing a minimum benefit package so that everyone has at least a basic degree of coverage, mandating that employers provide this basic minimum coverage for all their workers and requiring all insurees pay the same premium rate. Such a system would indeed ensure that everyone had basic insurance and paid the same premium. However, every system that has been designed to date has considerable drawbacks. The system just outlined would require that all persons pay the same premium regardless of their risks. There would be no incentive for consumers to engage in healthy behaviors, such as nonsmoking, that might lower their risks. If consumers were rated according to risk, there would be such incentives. But then such a system would hardly be considered "fair."

CRITICAL THINKING *Activities*

1. **When might increases in health care not lead to increases in health status?**
2. **Identify the "cost" of providing free medical care to everyone whenever they want it. What policy goals would, and would not, be achieved by providing universal free care?**
3. **What payment system for hospital care would you prefer? What does your choice indicate with regard to your preference of policy goals?**
4. **What do you think will happen with regard to health care services and their provision in the next 10 years? How will persons of various ages fare? Who will pay?**

References

1. Angell M: Cost containment and the physician, *JAMA* 254(9):1203–1207, 1985.
2. Enthoven A: *Health plan,* Boston, 1980, Addison Wesley.
3. Goldfarb M: Who receives cesareans? Patient and hospital characteristics, HCUP Research Note No. 4. National Center for Health Services Research, September, 1983, DHHS Publication (PHS)84–3345.
4. Hahn B, Lefkowitz D: Annual expenses and sources of payment for health care services, National Medical Expenditure Survey research Findings 14, Rockville, MD, Agency for Health Care Policy and research, Publication 93–0007, November, 1992.
5. Health Insurance Association of America: *Source book of health insurance data 1995,* Washington, 1996, Health Insurance Association of America.
6. Letsch SW and others: National health expenditures, 1991, *Health Care Financing Review* 14(2):1-30, Winter, 1992.
7. Noseworthy TW: Resource allocation of adult intensive care, *Ann R Coll Surg Can* 21(3):199-203, May, 1988.
8. Rice DP and others: The economic cost of illness: a replication and update, *Health Care Financing Review* 7(1):1985.
9. Schwartz WB: The regulation strategy for controlling hospital costs, *New Engl J Med* 305(21):1249–1255, 1981.

9a. Salkever D, Bice T: Hospital certificate-of-need controls, Washinton, D.C., 1979, American Enterprise Institute for Policy Research.

10. Smeeding, TM, Straub L: Health care financing among the elderly: who really pays the bills, *J Health Polit Policy Law* 12(1):35–52, 1987.
11. United States General Accounting Office: *Health insurance coverage: a profile of the uninsured in selected states,* Washington, D.C., February 1991, GAO.

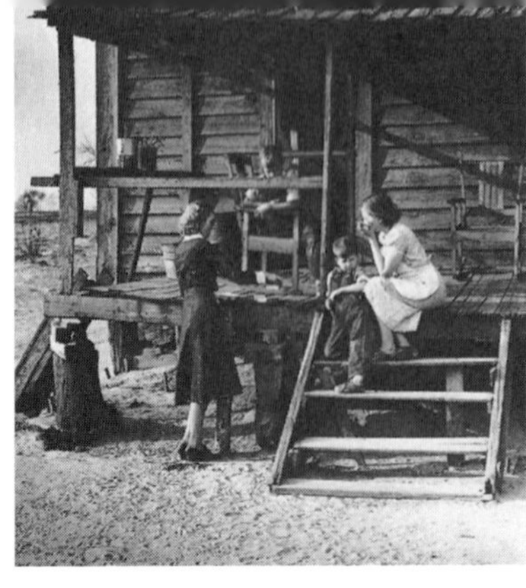

CHAPTER 4

Social Policy and Health Care Delivery

Shirley Newberry

OBJECTIVES After completing this chapter the reader should be able to:

- **Discuss the changes in health care delivery systems**
- **Explain what is meant by "the greatest good for the greatest number"**
- **Discuss the pros and cons of national health insurance and which countries mandate national health insurance**
- **List population groups that have special health care needs and how nurses can improve their skills to provide access to health care as needed**
- **Describe the role of the legislative, executive, and judicial branches of government as it relates to delivery of health care**

■ ACCESS TO HEALTH CARE

Access to health care in America has been a problem and will continue to be so until Americans decide whether health care is a universal right or a privilege. Today some Americans have the best care that medicine and technology can provide, and others cannot afford the medicine that would be prescribed if they could afford the physician's office visit. If one believes in the ethical canon "the greatest good for the greatest number," then every citizen should have basic minimum levels of health care. But who defines what is basic and minimum? A second question should be, "How fair is a system that allows everyone the basics, but allows only the rich to have access to high technology such as transplants, dialysis, and bypass surgery?" Can the nation afford to supply everyone with the level of care each individual may want? If not, who should be given access to the health care delivery system, who should decide, and how will this nation pay for that care?

Table 4-1 shows what percentage of their gross national products (GNPs) various nations spend on health care. The United States and South Africa are the only industrialized nations without national health insurance. Yet one of the biggest

TABLE 4-1

Health Expenditures as a Percentage of GNP: 1993

Gross National Product	%	Difference between 1987–1993
United States	13.2	+2.0
Canada	8.5	–.1
Germany	8.0	–.2
Japan	6.5	–.3
United Kingdom	6.1	0

From Organization for Economic Cooperation and Development, Health Data Bank

buyers of health care is the U.S. government. The United States spent 13.2% of its GDP on health care in 1992. Unlike the United States, these other countries provided health care coverage for all ages and many long-term services as well.

In 1992 the U.S. government spent $751.8 billion on health care, yet the care is fragmented and uncoordinated. Thirty-seven million Americans, about 15% of the population, are without any form of health insurance. Some are underemployed or work seasonally, some are between jobs, and some are excluded from health insurance policies. The greatest majority of the uninsured are the working poor—people who work but have incomes below the poverty level. The working poor earn monthly incomes averaging about $500, which makes them ineligible for welfare. The U.S. Census Bureau[31] estimates that 9 million adults work full time but earn less than $13,359, the poverty level. Two out of three workers have no employer- or union-subsidized health insurance. Of the underemployed and the unemployed, almost 60% are not covered by private or public insurance. This is in spite of the fact that the bill for Medicaid came to $20.3 billion in 1992. In addition to the working poor, the unemployed rely on Medicaid for their health needs. In the early 1990s the United States underwent a recession that caused a dramatic increase in unemployment, especially in higher-paid positions such as engineering and computer specialists, with accompanying income tax revenue losses. Most states have been in economic straits in addition to the national recession, and funds for Medicaid have subsequently been curtailed even as the demand for funds increased. Because of the aging of the American population, Medicare benefit payments have also been continually rising (Figures 4-1 and 4-2). This has been partly a result of the expansion of recipient eligibility for qualified poor people and the increased numbers who became eligible because of the recession.

Yet the United States must be cautious in implementing a solution to these problems. Now is a crucial time for the United States to learn everything possible from the experiences of other nations that have national health care systems. Problems such as inflationary costs, abuse of the system, and over-regulation are but examples. In Canada, for instance, physicians state that American clients who do not qualify for Canadian medical care are making illegal claims in significant numbers and abusing Canadian resources. This is a result of lack of stringent controls and lenient registration policies. Provinces are currently borrowing millions of dollars to address the predicament.

Even today the American taxpayer pays dearly for health care for illegal aliens inside U.S. borders. This is true not only because Americans are generous toward

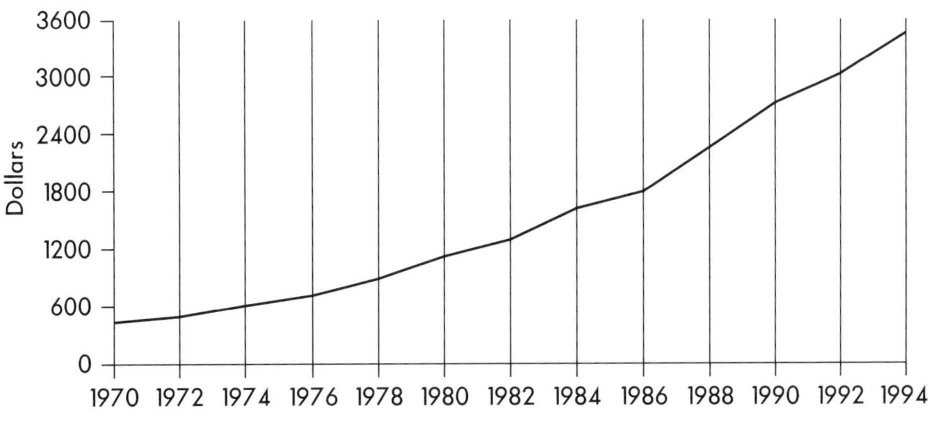

Source: Charts prepared by U.S. Bureau of the Census.

FIG. 4-1 Personal health care expenditures per capita: 1970 to 1994.

foreigners, but also because the government seeks to protect its own citizens from threat of disease and decreased welfare. The U.S. government is responsible for the health care of its citizens, and the U.S. Constitution obligates the government "to provide for the general welfare." In planning for national health coverage, projected budgets must take into account illegal aliens who cost government significant amounts but whose care does help protect the general welfare of U.S. citizens.

Managed Care

Health care delivery in the United States is changing rapidly. Whereas 25 years ago most people had indemnity insurance coverage, today most people who have health insurance are enrolled in some type of managed care plan. Managed care is an organized way of providing services and paying for them. Different types of managed care plans work differently and include preferred provider organizations (PPOs), health maintenance organizations (HMOs), and point-of-service (POS) plans. This system features increased capitation payments, increased provider risks, and a highly competitive marketplace for health care delivery systems. Approaches and outcomes in managed care will be differentiated by price, access, and quality.

Rationing of Health Care

Thirty years ago, making health care available to the poor and the elderly through Medicare and Medicaid appeared to be a first step toward a national health insurance program. In 1993 a task force to examine universal access and cost containment was selected and headed by the First Lady, Hillary Rodham Clinton. Americans have always been opposed to rationing, except in case of emergency, but more is being written about rationing health care than ever before. Rationing health care is certainly not a new concept; it has been practiced with varying degrees of intensity throughout time. The quality and quantity of health services in the United States have always been predicated on the person's ability to pay. Those who could

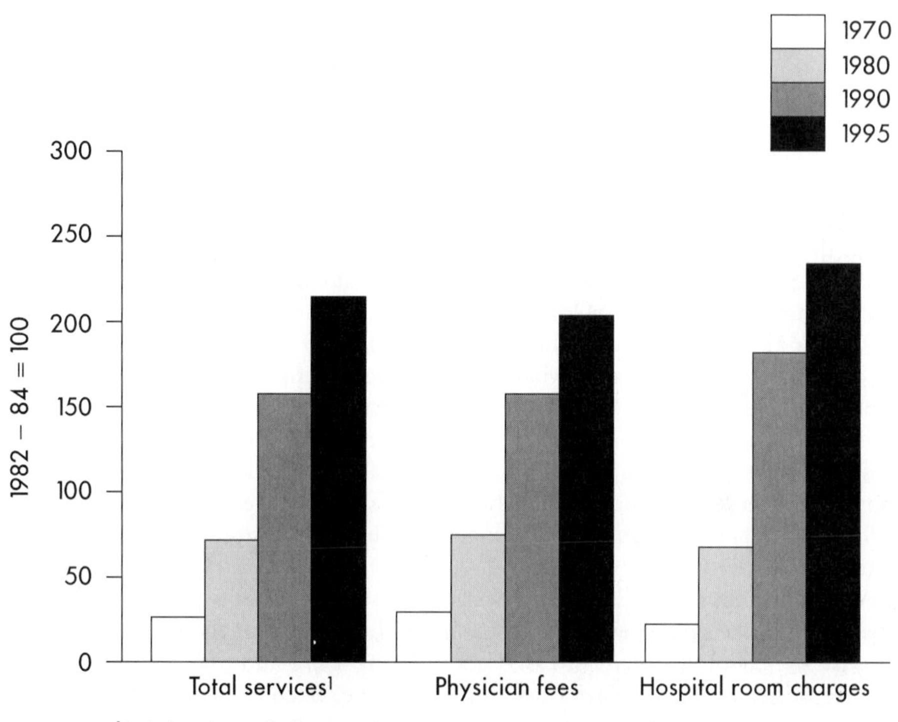

[1] Includes other medical care services.
Source: Charts prepared by U.S. Bureau of the Census.

FIG. 4-2 Consumer price indexes—medical services: 1970 to 1995.

afford the best received it. Heart transplants serve as an example to this; those with $150,000 have access to physicians and hospitals performing the procedure.

Rationing has also been based on other criteria. When kidney dialysis was new, access to the limited number of machines was determined by what were considered "objective measures." These measures include quality of life, potential contributions to the community, and age. Triage is in actuality another form of rationing. Using triage, those who are most critically ill take precedence over those who are not. Treating the most critically ill first is not, of course, the same as treating those most likely to recover, have a higher quality of life, or contribute to society.

Rationing health care is an accepted fact in industrialized countries such as Britain and Canada, where age limits determine access to high-technology procedures. In those countries, persons over the age of 55 are excluded from procedures such as bypass surgery and transplants. The trade-off is that all people have equal access to comprehensive personal health care. Does this make a difference? British life expectancy is slightly longer and infant mortality is lower than in the United States.[13] Canada also has a longer life expectancy and a lower infant mortality rate, despite spending 8.6% of its GNP on health, whereas the United States spends a staggering 13%.

Few health care professionals, particularly nurses, have spoken out on this topic. Yet they are the ones who will ultimately be involved in the outcome.

Client Self-Determination

In December of 1991 the Patient Self-Determination Act (PSDA), which was included in the Medicare Omnibus Budget Reconciliation Act, provided a mechanism (called an advance directive) by which clients can inform health care providers about the level of care they desire if they become incapacitated. The law contains several requirements, the first of which dictates that every competent adult entering an institution that receives Medicare or Medicaid reimbursement must be informed in writing about his or her rights under state law to refuse or accept treatment. Second, clients must be asked whether they have a living will or a durable power of attorney for health care (DPAHC), and the response needs to be documented in the chart. Each institution must make an effort to educate the public regarding these advance directives. Advance directives allow individuals to give direction about their care when they are unable to do so themselves. The DPAHC allows individuals to appoint a surrogate to make health care decisions for them when they cannot do so themselves.

Although these tools are empowering, several problems remain. First, the hospital is the last place where a client should be told about the legal instruments, because the client is already stressed about being there and may assume he or she is more critically ill than previously led to believe. Second, no universal protocol exists regarding who shall inform the client. The clerk admitting the client to the hospital must ask whether a document exists. If one has not been completed, it is necessary for staff to provide the actual instruction. The registered nurse or social worker is the person so designated in most hospitals. Actually, nurses are in a unique position to inform the client, since people generally view nurses positively and entrust them with intimate personal information, perhaps even more readily than they trust other health professionals. The optimal place, however, for persons to be educated about their rights and about advance directives is either in the physician's office as the normal part of a history and physical or in the home. When conducted by the person's physician, the discussion begins a relationship that will become crucial at the end of life. In the development of the mandate regarding advance directives, many physicians were resistant. As a result, federal legislation was passed that gave hospitals the responsibility for its implementation.

It is encouraging to learn that advance directives seem to be popular with the aging population. Aged people are beginning to face their own mortality, and numerous surveys have indicated that they do not want their lives extended if the quality of that life is seriously impaired. Younger people often resist the opportunity to sign an advance directive even though the majority of court cases adjudicating the issue of the "right to die" have been related to young brain-injured adults.

Although advance directives are based on humanitarian ideals, they can become tools for rationing since care extending beyond insurance coverage ultimately becomes the responsibility of the family or the government. Neither entity is able to pay for endless care for hopeless cases. As more studies are being completed, the value of client self-determination becomes even more evident. In grassroots movements across the country, people are expressing their belief that the quality of life is infinitely more important than the quantity.

A further use of the PSDA is to force primary caregivers to present all aspects of care of treatment with full disclosure, so that the client can accept or refuse medical treatment. Of course, the doctrine of informed consent was also supposed to accomplish that same condition, but each state enacted its own legislation. Now it is a federal decree. It is possible that this could have prevented the misuse of approximately 800 people during the Cold War of the 1940s and 1950s. During this period the U.S. government conducted radiation experiments on humans who were not adequately informed so as to make a rational decision. Some radiation experiments were designed to determine the use of radioisotopes to diagnose or cure disease. Others were less legitimate, such as injecting plutonium into a person with relatively short life expectancy, or using semicomatose brain-tumor clients to determine how much uranium it took to induce kidney damage. Many of the exposed persons were veterans, soldiers, prisoners, or hospital clients. Officials knew that what they were doing was ethically wrong but did it anyway, using the wartime rationalization that morality is a luxury when facing a foe lacking morality itself.

As of 1994 the Departments of Energy, Defense, and Veterans Affairs and the National Aeronautics and Space Administration have been ordered to search the files to locate all records of human experimentation and radiation testing. One such experimentation was the Tuskeegee experiment, which took place during the 1940s and 1950s. In this experiment black men who suffered from syphilis were placed in a study and not given treatment that was available to cure their disease. In May of 1997 President Clinton made a personal apology, from the citizens of the United States to those few remaining survivors of the experiment for their mistreatment.

■ QUALITY AND ALLOCATION OF HEALTH CARE

In 1971 Elliot Richardson, then Secretary of the U.S. Department of Health, Education and Welfare, testified that:

> In general our critical health problems today do not arise because the health of our people is worsening, or because expenditures on health care have been niggardly, or because we have been negligent as a nation in developing health care resources, or because we have been unconcerned about providing financial protection against ill-health. We must look elsewhere. I should like to suggest that our present concern is a function of two broad problems. The first is the inequality in health status and care, and in access to financing. The other is the pervasive problem of rising medical cost.[26]

Although that statement is more than 25 years old, little has changed, and it is still applicable. The government, with the introduction of prospective payments and DRGs, is still spending approximately 13% of its GNP on health care. In 1991 hospitals had a total of $180 billion in revenues, 8% more than in the previous year.[31] It is estimated that hospital profits will continue to grow at a rate of 10% or more per annum.[19] According to the Health Care Financing Administration, hospitals consume 38% of the health care budget and physicians accrue 19% of the budget. Incomes of the medical and allied health community have not decreased either. What remains is a two-tiered system, in which those with the ability to pay have different health care and access to that care than those with limited ability to pay. According to Congressman Ronald Dellums in his introduction to the Health Service Act (1979):

> We have in the country today a health delivery system where the quality of health care received is determined by race, language, national origin, or income level. Health is a commodity to be bought and sold in the marketplace; it is not viewed as a right of the people; a service to be provided by the government. However, financing is not the only problem facing the people when it comes to the delivery of health care. Other, equally important problems are the maldistributions of health manpower, the unequal access to services, the unreliable quality of care, and the lack of public control over health care. No matter how much we guarantee the payment of services to the people, it is of little comfort to them if there is no one around to provide the service.[8]

Within days of Hillary Rodham Clinton's appointment as chair of a task force to examine health care reform, the leadership of the American Nurses Association was called to the White House to confer about the nation's health. Their input revolved around the issues laid out in Nursing's Agenda for Health Care. Those issues center around universal access to a continuum of services, with the priority placed on preventive care. This should place nursing on the front lines, because nursing can provide primary care to clients and focus on preventive modalities. Once economic barriers are removed, nurses will finally be able to do that which has been their professional forte.

In order to devise a system that all Americans would be willing to invest in, it will be necessary to resolve the polarity created by different values. Systems based on explicit values such as Canada's and Germany's provide affordable, high-quality health care for all. Explicit values can assist in reaching agreement on what the system should look like, what can be got out of the system, and what trade-offs must be addressed. If universal access is the driving value, then the decisions made must focus on prevention while curing what can be cured and mitigating symptoms through treatment or pain relief. Presently, access is subordinate to autonomy and choice, with health care professionals and clients given the right to choose whom to serve, whom to select as a provider, what fees to charge, and what care plan, if any, to select. Choice—or lack of it—is still the biggest fear among Americans.

If universal access becomes the top priority, then every citizen will have access to some health care, but not unlimited access to every service that may be beneficial. One way to ensure that treatment is cost effective is to examine the outcomes of each treatment. Research indicates that surgery for the early stages of prostate cancer may not be the best way to manage the disease. Rather, the best may be no treatment at all, since the disease spreads so slowly in older-age men that most die of other causes before the tumor becomes lethal. A further study examined the need for bypass surgery found in one group of people, some of whom were treated medicinally for heart disease and some of whom received bypass surgery. The outcomes were similar. The difference is in the number of cardiac procedures done. In the decade of the 1980s 772,000 procedures per year were done, while during the early 1990s 1,890,000 procedures per year were completed—more than twice the earlier number. When technologic advances are made, professionals tend to use them rather than the lower-cost alternatives. Instead of less costly x-rays, MRIs or CAT scans are done. Technology-driven costs may soon lead decision makers to pit ethics against economics. The question is whether Americans should have access to the wide array of technologic tests and treatments regardless of the cost or whether health care dollars should be rationed and spent on the basis of who receives the greater benefit. These issues must be addressed by any plan for reform.

The balanced budget act and tax reforms of 1997 did postpone the inevitable insolvency of the Medicare trust to the year 2002. The issues have not gone away, and reform in the current system is underway. Numerous health care reform proposals have been discussed during President Clinton's terms of office. No single plan has met with sufficient support for adoption. Some features of the Clinton reform plan are likely to be implemented, including financial incentives aimed at steering people towards provider networks of managed care such as health maintenance organizations (HMOs) or preferred provider organizations (PPOs). Such networks are designed to contain costs but limit the choice of physicians who serve as primary caregivers. Fee-for-service remains an option so individuals can keep their private physicians. Either option must provide the same basic benefit package, including coverage for preexisting conditions. The benefits include hospital and physician services, some mental health services, and prescriptions. Worker's compensation is proposed to be included in the basic package, as well as some tort reforms to reduce malpractice litigation. A single standardized insurance form is proposed. A cap on administrative costs must be part of the formula to operate as effectively as the Canadian plan, which covers 25 million people. More specifically, Canada employs fewer administrators than Massachusetts Blue Cross, which covers only 2.7 million people. American hospitals spend 20% of their budget on billing administration, compared to 9% in the Canadian system.

The method of paying for any plan is probably the biggest problem of all. Government employer mandates and limits on physician fees, along with stricter controls on hospitals, are already meeting resistance. Increased taxes are anathema to conservative legislators. An energy tax appeals to everyone but people from energy-producing states. Taxing or capping entitlements gains some supporters, but large blocks of voters are campaigning in opposition. Those lobbying for the elderly want Social Security and Medicare left untouched. Farmers want their subsidies, the sugar industry wants theirs, and the oil industry theirs.

Abuses of the system must most certainly be addressed. It is estimated that $200 billion dollars of the $800 billion spent is wasted on useless or overpriced treatments as well as bloated bureaucracy. The General Accounting Offices estimates that about 10% of the total health care budget goes to the cost of fraud—paying for unnecessary tests, services never rendered, falsified DRG codes, and inflated bills for supplies and medical devices. This must all be considered by the health care task force in the decision-making process. Until necessary decision making is completed, this nation will spend $800 billion on health care while 37 million of its citizens have no access to the system.

In an effort to control health care costs and to provide universal coverage to its citizens, some states have proceeded to organize their own reforms. Hawaii is notable among all the states because its program has been in place the longest and now covers 98% of its population. Monthly premiums there are the lowest of the 50 states and are paid for by employees and employers. The state pays for anyone not covered by an employer. Hawaii attributes its success to the facts that insurance rates are based on the total community rather than individual companies and that their citizens are healthier because they seek preventive care.

The Oregon plan will eventually cover all residents either through employer-based insurance or Medicaid. To control costs, services deemed less than essential will be excluded from coverage under a priority-ranking system developed by the residents of Oregon and their lawmakers. Treatments for extremely premature babies and certain transplants will not be covered, since they ranked low on the system. However, basic care such as immunizations and prenatal care will be available to every Oregonian. Many people were angered at this rationing system since they believe everything could be covered if taxes were raised on upper-income residents of Oregon. Defenders of the Oregon plan say rationing already exists but that it is now only the rich who have access to any and all procedures while the poor have access to none. Oregon recently received the Medicaid waivers necessary to institute their plan. California, Connecticut, Michigan, and Washington are all working toward state health reform. But so is the United States. Over the past 30 years national legislation related to health care reform has been proposed and failed to secure passage because of heavy lobbying efforts by insurance companies, the business community, and the American Medical Association.

While Congress debates reform, other states have enacted legislation that helps small employers group together and purchase insurance as a body. Even cities are looking for a solution. Rochester, New York is a prime example; at a time when the nation is struggling to tame a health care system plagued by increasing costs and numbers of uninsured persons, Rochester has a viable system. Through a cooperative effort the city's employers, insurers, and medical providers worked out a model that covers all residents. Rochester is unique in that one large employer employs the majority of residents, and there is a single dominant provider. This cuts down on administrative costs and paperwork, ultimately resulting in lower premium costs.

Political and Social Systems and Their Impact

Because so much of the funding for health care comes from the government through laws that are enacted, one must be acquainted with the political and social system that shapes the legislation. This country has a two-party system, but that says little about the shades of political and social philosophy that mold the thought process of legislators. Although Republicans are presumed to be more conservative than Democrats, many beliefs overlap at the center of each party. A review of the voting record on any social issue will indicate the extent to which centrists of either party cross over to join like-minded legislators of the opposition. The latest Medicare expansion was supported by an overwhelming majority of both parties in the House and Senate, but it was no giveaway program because it was designed to be financially self-supporting. It was therefore acceptable to liberals and conservatives from both parties. With the latest discussion of budgetary issues, caps on Medicare and Medicaid, as well as a means test for Social Security, have gained support from centrists of both parties.

To find actual differences in political beliefs, one must look at the extremes of each party, because they more accurately reflect what the public believes the party stands for. The stereotypical ideology attributed to the Republican Party is that of the conservative, "less government intervention is best government," business-oriented, rich man's party, whereas Democrats are supposedly for the working man, government intervention, and legislation to address social ills. Actually, this summary reflects the conservative versus the liberal belief. Each party has a range from conservative to liberal, and the voter needs to be well informed of the philosophic stance of each candidate, as well as party affiliation. However, to vote in an election one must declare a party affiliation, be an independent, or decline to state; the latter two choices eliminates one from primaries. Demographics indicate that the majority of Democrats are working people, minorities, and people living in large cities. Republicans tend to come from the Midwest farm land, deep South, and mid-Atlantic states and, increasingly, are younger members of the white-collar labor force.

The Constitution assigns Congress all legislative powers on the national level; therefore Congress enacts laws, the president executes laws, and the Supreme Court interprets the law. The president has the right to veto a law, but Congress may override the veto. Each state in the Union has a similar system to enact, execute, and interpret state laws.

Both state and federal legislators are representatives of the electorate and, to survive elections, they must demonstrate their ability to enact legislation and secure resources that are beneficial to their constituents. The Senate is the smaller federal body because each state is allowed only two senators, whereas a state's population determines its representation in the House of Representatives—the most populous states receive the most representation. A bill must clear both houses before being sent for presidential signature.*

A bill enacted into law must also have an appropriations bill to have funds necessary for putting the program into effect. Traditionally the House of Representatives has the power to originate tax bills, and it assumes the power to initiate appropriation bills also. Each January the president submits to Congress a budget that contains the programs for the year. The budget reflects the president's political and social philosophy. Decisions related to the federal budget are based on a variety of political, social, and economic issues. Each government agency wants a larger part of the budget, yet dividing the limited funds among the competing forces is necessary. Which agency gets the largest cut depends on the president's vision of the country's needs, based on personal philosophy and ability to gain support of the legislators. After Congress reviews and revises the president's budget, it is returned for presidential signature. Under President Reagan the Department of Defense received the largest share of the budget, with sizable cuts coming out of the Department of Health and Human Services. To meet increased defense spending Congress reduced the budget for Medicare and Medicaid by $13 billion.

By assessing the political and social philosophy of the majority of the legislators and the president during the period of 1980 to 1984, one sees that a conservative

---

*The way in which a bill becomes a law is beyond the scope of this chapter. For more information see Mason D, Talbott S: *Political action handbook for nurses.*[20]

budget was appropriated. The Republicans, for the first time since 1954, gained control of the Senate and increased their numbers to 192 in the House. By adding 30 conservative southern Democrats, the Republicans counted on at least 212 votes to the Democrats' 243, some of whom joined the conservative coalition. Under the Program for Economic Recovery the Reagan administration replaced many of the federal health care grant programs with unrestricted block grants to the states. The health planning system that had attempted to contain health costs and ensure proper distribution of services was dismantled. Funding to the states was cut 25%. The theme of the recovery program was that a safety net be provided for the truly needy, but no one defined the terms.

In 1988 voting resulted in the election of another Republican president, George Bush, and a change to a Democratically controlled legislature. The 101st Congress contained 262 Democrats and 173 Republicans in the House and 56 Democrats and 44 Republicans in the Senate.

President Bush, in campaign promises, stated that he planned no major changes in the governing of the country. Analysts believe that the majority of voters supported Reagan's policies and therefore voted for Bush. The following issues led to this support:

1. Peace
2. National security
3. Economic prosperity
4. Concerns about higher taxes
5. Crime

Although most Americans reported satisfaction with the general state of national affairs, they were not satisfied with the state of the health care system. No major changes occurred, although discussion about some form of national health care cropped up with increasing regularity. Polls by the Gallup and Harris organizations, completed in 1989, indicated that 75% of Americans favored the concept of national health insurance. However, the budget remained a largely conservative one, with no massive infusion of dollars for social problems.

In general, since 1960 major legislation for health and human rights has been enacted by a Democratic president and a liberal Democratic Congress. Bills such as the Civil Rights Act, the Food Stamp Act, the Health Manpower Act, and the Nurse Training Act were initiated in the 1960s. Under Republican presidents in the 1970s funding for these were expanded, and the Women and Infant Children (WIC) program was funded, as was the Sudden Infant Death Syndrome and Child Abuse prevention program. Curtailment of funds for social policy became noticeable in the early 1980s, when disillusionment with previous policies, an escalating inflation rate, and increased taxation caused a conservative backlash. As a result of this backlash, in the 97th Congress of 1981 only 46 senators and 236 congressman had 4 or more years of experience.[17] A similar situation occurred in the election of 1992. Voters unhappy with the recession, corruption in government, and gridlock in Congress decided to vote for change.

When communism collapsed in 1992, the Soviet Union was financially bankrupt and posed little threat to the safety of the United States. The American voter looked toward home and found a recession. "Trickle-down economics" had not trickled, 12 million people were unemployed, and Congress was gridlocked and wrapped in layers of misdeed and corruption. Voters were dissatisfied, not necessarily with their own legislators but with the government in general. The Democratic theme was "change," whereas the Republicans promised 4 more years. However, the wealthiest 20% of the population received the highest percentage (43.7) of income ever recorded. Four more years were not inviting. Governor Clinton promised a national health program, a middle-class tax cut with increased taxes for the rich, and a deficit reduction plan.

With the election of 1992 one third of the Senate was up for election, yet the Democrats gained only one seat. But they gained the White House with the election of Bill Clinton. In the House the Democrats fared less well, with only 174 seats to the 260 Republicans. Although the shift in relative strength was small, it was still a year of upheaval. Voters were angry about a secret vote on a congressional pay hike and overdrafts written on the Congressional Bank, and voted to unseat 19 incumbents. Fifty-four women (one a nurse), 40 blacks, 19 Hispanics, 6 Asian Americans, and one Native American were elected to Congress, changing the face and color of Congress. Fourteen states had term limitations imposed on their legislators. Many baby boomers were now in seats of power, and the following issues were deemed important:

1. Crime
2. Health care
3. The economy
4. The national deficit

The Supreme Court may also acquire a conservative or liberal inclination depending on the justices' points of view regarding the interpretation of the Constitution. Presidential appointments to the court are based on judicial experience, political involvement, and philosophy. Strict constitutional constructionists tend to be conservative and to be appointed by conservative presidents. However, once appointed to the court, most justices appear to migrate toward the center so that few ideologues have been on the recent courts. Former President Reagan appointed the first woman justice to office, Sandra Day O'Connor. The Reagan court was, for the most part, strictly constructionist and conservative.

Former President Bush appointed David Souter and Clarence Thomas to the court, further enhancing the strict constructionist and conservative nature of the court. With the nomination of Ruth Bader Ginsberg to replace Justice Byron White, President Clinton had his first opportunity to change the complexion of the court toward either the liberal or centrist view of legislation. Judge Ginsberg has had a distinguished career and was a leader in early women's issues.

Because Justices of the Supreme Court rule on the constitutionality of the law, it is vital to the nation's stability that their decisions remain constant over time. If that stability were absent, every contested law would be argued and modified or changed endlessly, as is the case with the issue of abortion.

Pro-Life versus Pro-Choice

In 1973 the Supreme Court, in Roe v. Wade, ruled that any state laws prohibiting or restricting a woman's right to abortion during the first 3 months of pregnancy were illegal. This resulted in conflicting ethical and social opinions. The pro-life movements claim that conception marks the beginning of new life and that any action to terminate that life is analogous to murder. Pro-choice activists claim that each woman has the right to determine what happens to her body, and if she chooses to have an abortion, it is her legal right to do so. For some, life must be regarded as sacred and termination of life at any point is a crime. Others believe that although abortion is distasteful, there are circumstances, such as incest or rape, in which it is justifiable. Some believe that early termination of a deformed or defective fetus is acceptable. Others believe that any early termination, during the first trimester, is acceptable, but late termination is not.

The pro-life group cites various religious beliefs that do not allow interference with the procreative process and views abortion as tantamount to infanticide. The group works ceaselessly to repeal the Supreme Court decision. Unfortunately, in the last few years, some fanatics have bombed abortion clinics and, in general, acted in ways that have detracted from the overall ethical stance of the group.

Those who argue in favor of abortion emphasize a woman's control over her own body. They explain that the quality of life is as important as the right to life and suggest that the quality of life for an unwanted baby is minimal. However, most people do not support abortion as a form of birth control and have negative feelings about abortion after the fifth month for any reason except the mother's safety.

In its 1989 decision in Webster v. Reproductive Health Services, the Supreme Court narrowed the federal interpretation of the right to abortion. With this decision the court upheld the constitutionality of a Missouri law that sharply restricted the availability of publicly funded abortions, and also required physicians to test for viability of a fetus at 20 weeks. Although this appeared to narrow the focus of Roe v. Wade and invite individual states to address the issue of abortion, it did not overturn Roe entirely. The results of this decision are still to be explored, and other states' cases remain to be heard. In a poll conducted in 1993 by Time/CNN, the majority of Americans supported abortion in some form, whether it be unrestricted or with special circumstances, and this issue crossed party lines. One fact has emerged: both pro-life and pro-choice movements are becoming more vocal, and each side threatens to have abortion become a key issue in the coming elections. The debate continues in 1997, with the legislators busy arguing over the Partial Birth Abortion issue.

Health Promotion and Disease Prevention

It is a paradoxic government that pays farmers to grow tobacco, warns citizens of its dangers, and supports medical care for those who choose to use tobacco. It is a paradox that this nation spends billions of dollars to treat diseases arising from environmental pollution, poor nutrition, stress, and toxic waste yet spends very little on prevention. Streams, lakes, and oceans are giving clear messages that we are irreparably damaging the food chain, yet we are doing nothing about it. Science has eradicated smallpox and prevented polio, diphtheria, and whooping cough, but it cannot cure the common cold. Since antibiotics have come on the scene, organisms have been evolving to become more resistant. Antibiotics can cure many infections but viruses and bacteria, such as MRSA, are becoming more deadly and more common.

In the past, Medicare and Medicaid reimbursed the health delivery system for illnesses incurred, not for maintenance of health. Medicine does not equal health, yet physicians earn considerable salaries, vast prestige, and millions of research dollars, whereas those involved in prevention garner little recognition. In fact, the physician who knows less about the whole client may have more status and collect larger fees (for example, the cardiologist versus the family practitioner).

Another paradox is that whereas illness can be defined and measured by morbidity and mortality tables, health is more complex and often defined as the lack of illness. Although life expectancy rates are increasing, this is not because of better health but because bacterial infections are no longer always fatal, nor are there wildfire pandemic diseases such as the bubonic plague. But the world is seeing increases in diseases such as cholera and typhoid as a result of contaminated water supplies; measles epidemics are increasing as a result of lax vigilance on immunizations; sexually transmitted diseases are escalating; malnutrition is worldwide. The problem is not lack of treatment modalities but the lack of commitment to health.

Widespread problems arise from lifestyle problems, stress, poor diet, smoking, the use of alcohol and other drugs, lack of exercise, and pollution. The surgeon general's office estimates that as much as half of U.S. mortality is due to unhealthy behavior or lifestyle, and 20% to environment factors. Thus, although the population looks to medicine to cure disease, the true cure lies in behavior changes that are difficult to accomplish. It seems easier to cope with a coronary bypass than to eat sensibly, exercise regularly, and abandon smoking.* Humans engage in magical thinking, believing that they will know when they are about to become ill so that they can then give up the behavior that is causing it. It seems less expensive to tolerate filthy waterways and polluted air than to restore the environment to healthy levels.

As with other health issues, this nation does not have a social policy that can shape the manner in which public funds are distributed. At present public funds are invested largely in illness, with minuscule amounts (less than 1% of the health care budget) distributed between health promotion and disease prevention. Yet while all other consumer prices increased by 3.1% in 1991, medical costs escalated by 8.7%.[29] In the long run, prevention may be the best investment, with fewer dollars needed and more people served—in other words, "more bang for the buck." The Public Health Research Group estimates that $100 billion is spent each year on preventable illnesses, yet today we have an "armamentarium of preventative principles that work and work well. Prevention holds significant promise for problems as diverse as stroke, immune disorders, and a huge range of chronic, debilitating diseases from pernicious anemia to osteoporosis."[4]

Nor have the health care professions served society well. Ivan Illich states that by transforming pain, illness, and death from personal challenge into a technical problem, medicine expropriates the potential of people to deal with their condition in an autonomous way.[15] Physicians and nurses have done little to teach consumers how to stay out of the system, to manage their own wellness, and to live healthier lifestyles.

---

*The death rate for coronary heart disease (CHD) in the United States has declined approximately 50% since 1970, but CHD remains the leading cause of death for both men and women, accounting for 489,340 deaths in 1990.

In the past nurses did not see health care as an area of expertise, but their vision has changed. In 1991 *Nursing's Agenda for Health Care Reform* was published and established nursing as the premier profession working toward health care, not medical care, for all Americans. Wisely, the discussion and planning that led up to the *Agenda* involved all the major organizations within the profession, with each taking responsibility to inform its membership. The *Agenda* is only 22 pages long but covers a multitude of subjects. To summarize, the basic components are to:

1. Enhance access to services by delivering primary health care in community settings
2. Seek consumer responsibility for personal health and self-care
3. Ask for the most cost-effective providers and therapeutic options in the most appropriate settings

In the plan, managed care would be required in public access facilities, with incentives for citizens having private plans to utilize managed care. It calls for policies based on outcomes and effectiveness of treatments. A major effort must be utilized to eliminate unnecessary or duplicative bureaucratic and administrative controls. The keystone of the plan is having appropriate services delivered in appropriate settings by the appropriate provider. The appropriate provider might well be a nurse.

Hillary Rodham Clinton wrote, "As informed providers, nurses are in a unique position to educate health care planners, legislators, and community leaders about immunizations and prevention activities as important aspects of personal health care. Your support is vital."[7] This is a hallmark period for nursing if it accepts the challenge and responsibility of health promotion and disease prevention.

The power that is the potential of health care reform will not be easy to achieve. Already the American Medical Association (AMA) has raised the old argument that nurses are not qualified to render primary care. In late 1993, at the AMA interim house of delegates, a report was released opposing autonomy for advanced practice nurses. In the report, inaccuracies were used to attack the high-quality, cost-effective primary care that advanced practice nurses deliver. The fight over who delivers primary care under health reform is truly a fight over economics. Physicians want to keep control over the billing practice that prohibits nurses from billing autonomously. At present the nurse must submit a bill through a physician. The physician submits the bill to the insurer for care he never gave and then pays the nurse as though she was an employee. As of 1992 the average physician's salary was $170,000. The average advanced nurse practitioner's salary was $43,000. Billing practices are one major cause for that discrepancy.

For decades nurses have delivered health care in areas that doctors were not interested in, such as inner cities and rural areas. Physicians had all but abandoned general or family practice, seeking instead lucrative specialty areas. Now that health care reform is shifting from high technology toward prevention and primary care, in which nurses have had years of success, physicians want the turf back. Historically, physicians opposed any form of health care reform; but now that the public has demanded changes, physicians have accepted the inevitable and are rallying to at least control those who deliver the care. Nurses must support the organizations that will mount the legislative battles to secure consumer choice. Health care reform requires a professional qualified to delivery primary care, wise enough to refer complicated problems, and cost effective. To many, that spells *nurse*.

School Health

The World Health Organization (WHO) defines *health* as the state of complete mental, physical, and social well-being, not just the absence of disease. Certainly this is a holistic view encompassing all the factors that contribute to the quality of life. With this definition school systems could design health programs from kindergarten through college. In the primary grades schools focus on prevention with programs for immunizations and hearing and eye checks, but all too often the programs are underfunded. School nurses are almost always the first to be discharged when budget cuts are made. Health promotion in schools is either ignored or relegated to a small portion of the curriculum borne by the already overburdened primary teacher. With content as complex as substance abuse, HIV infection, and sex education, the primary source of information should be a nurse who has had educational preparation to impart that information. In addition, the school nurse can spot signs of alcohol or other drug abuse and intervene at an early stage.

Health education should not stop in the primary grades. High school and college students can profit from classes on healthy lifestyles and how to achieve them. Certainly it is important for students to learn how the health care system works. In addition, they need to learn about health insurance, selecting a primary care provider, use of generic drugs, how to get a second opinion, and how to get good care within the hospital.

Sex Education

Parents are often so busy with their own work schedules they are not involved with their children's school system to any large degree. Teachers complain that no one is available in the home to assist students with homework or study. Yet when content regarding sex information is discussed, parents are at PTA meetings and at school board meetings in full force. All too often parents demand to be the sole providers of sex information to their offspring. This information is frequently inadequate, incorrect, and given too late.

Children with little information regarding their sexual health are having their own children in epidemic proportions. Teenage pregnancies are altering millions of lives and costing the government billions of dollars a year in subsidies. Sadly, the statistics bear this out. At least half of the girls and 60% of the boys in America are sexually active by the age of 17, with about half of those becoming active before the age of 15. One million teens become pregnant each year, with a 41% abortion rate. The government spent $21 billion dollars to subsidize teenage mothers and their children. There is a lack of adequate information regarding birth control, whether it be in the form of abstinence, the pill, or other forms of contraception. Besides increases in teenage pregnancies, sexually transmitted diseases among teenagers are increasing, including HIV infection. There is serious concern about funding effective ways to alter the sexual behavior of teenagers.

This is another example of a failed social policy. Because American culture is traditionally conservative in sexual matters, sex was once a forbidden topic. Currently we are bombarded with sexual images in commercials and movies. Television is a major purveyor of sex, vividly demonstrating intense love scenes. However, the same medium that extols the thrill of sex cannot advertise contraception. Children learn the excitement of sexual activity but not the possible sequelae—unwanted pregnancy and disease. Nowhere in our culture is systematic information available regarding human sexuality, disease transmission, pregnancy, and contraception. In this area the public operates under puritanical rules while allowing permissive sexual display. Prevention is always the least expensive form of intervention. This nation needs a policy that encourages sex education beginning in the primary grades and continuing through high school and college. Contraceptive information should be available so that sexually active teens can learn how to protect themselves. Moral issues should be addressed in homes and places of worship while schools disseminate information.

Stress Reduction

Modern society is fast-paced and complex, with rapidly changing social and cultural norms. People are placed in competitive arenas where success is the order of the day; sometimes the competition comes from within. Wherever its source, the feeling engendered can be overwhelming. Work, play, and particularly human relations can disrupt the internal sense of harmony and peace, producing stress. All stressful situations are not harmful; anticipation of a long-awaited kiss can produce the same physiologic response as a minor automobile accident. Heartbeat increases, blood pressure elevates, and "butterflies" invade the stomach, resulting in the stress response. Some stress is necessary in life to motivate people to accomplish tasks, confront challenges, and pursue goals so the individual can grow and change. Some people thrive on stress, whereas others become ill. Certain diseases such as ulcers, colitis, asthma, eczema, psoriasis, and migraine headaches are thought to be stress induced. The physiologic response to stress activates the nervous and endocrine systems, releasing epinephrine, norepinephrine, and other catecholamines.

Scientists propose many theories regarding the causes of stress. Some believe it is the accumulation of life events—such as marriage, divorce, becoming widowed, even Christmas or taking a vacation—that can induce feeling of stress.[14] Others suggest that personality characteristics and stress are related. Cardiologists Friedman and Rosenman[9] conducted studies of people they called type A and found that they were constant hurriers and highly competitive, worked on multiple tasks at one time, were aggressive, and hated waiting in lines. They often had higher incidence of heart disease than their peers who had a more relaxed approach to life. On the positive side, behavior that reduces the effects of stress on the physiologic system can be learned.

Because stress-related illness involves mental processes, it is possible to exert control over the processes. Change in a disruptive situation such as work or interpersonal relationships may be possible. Seeking counseling may assist in the search for alternatives to high-stress situations. By eliminating stressors in the environment or by controlling reactions to the stressors, one may achieve a healthier lifestyle. Even more convincing is the fact that health care is the responsibility of the individual, and decision making is under individual control. Also, relaxation techniques often reduce the physical response to stress. Biofeedback is one form of relaxation that is proven effective on stress management. Meditation is a centuries-old form of relaxation that is simple, inexpensive, and effective. Meditation requires a comfortable chair, a quiet room, freedom from distraction, and a 20-minute period of time, preferably twice a day. To meditate, one simply becomes comfortable and clears one's mind of extraneous thoughts. A mantra, or single-syllable word, helps keep focus. "Om" or "won" is often used, but any word will do.

Stress reduction techniques are easily taught and certainly within the nurse's realm, yet nurses rarely initiate such teaching. If nurses believe in health promotion and primary prevention, they will address the issue of stress control by learning and teaching techniques that will assist clients.

■ BASIC LEVELS OF CARE: FOR WHOM AND BY WHOM?

Perinatal Care

An expectant mother with no prenatal care is three times more likely to have a low birth weight baby than a woman who receives prenatal care. Despite evidence that early prenatal care assists in protecting against low birth weight and infant death, nearly one out of four pregnant women in this country receives no care in her first trimester.[21] A disproportionate share of these mothers have low incomes, less than a high-school education, or are very young. More than a million teenage women become pregnant each year and are at particular risk of having low birth weight babies. In addition to this problem, 14 million women of reproductive age have no medical insurance to cover maternity care.

There are 3.4 million women who are just above the poverty level and therefore do not qualify for Medicaid. The poorest one fifth of American families are headed by African American women whose disposable income has dropped. Inadequate prenatal visits, according to the Centers for Disease Control and Prevention (CDC), are associated with maternal anemia and low birth weight, and subsequently with diminished intellectual and physical development in babies. The most prominent factor in infant death is low birth weight (less than 2500 grams), and it is associated with more than half of all infant deaths. African American babies have twice the risk of being born weighing less than 2500 grams. The March of Dimes' statistics indicate that babies weighing less than 5½ pounds are 40 times more likely to die during their first month of life and 5 times more likely to die before their first birthday.

The United States currently ranks eighteenth among nations in infant mortality. The National Academy of Sciences Institute of Medicine estimates that the United States spends $3.3 billion annually on neonatal intensive care. This authority states that this extraordinary financial cost could be reduced by two thirds by adequate prenatal care. The Institute of Medicine in Washington, D.C. estimates that for every $1 spent on prenatal care, $3.38 could be saved in neonatal intensive care costs.[16] As far back as 1971 it was noted that low birth weight infants are highly susceptible to neurologic developmental handicaps and have a higher risk of developing illness throughout childhood.[9] So for every $1 spent on prenatal care, an additional $6 could be saved if all costs associated with caring for disabled children are included.[33]

Although infant mortality rates seem to be declining, the perception may be misleading. Infant deaths in the first month of life are down; however, deaths during the following 11 months are increasing. It appears that high technology and skills of nursing and medicine in neonatal intensive care units save premature and low birth weight neonates, whereas lack of supportive services precludes adequate care in the next critical months.

Of great current concern is the ever-increasing number of babies being born with AIDS or with cocaine or alcohol addiction. According to the CDC, about 2000 babies were born with HIV infection in 1991.[21] Of the 339,250 AIDS cases in the United States recorded by the CDC between 1981 and September 1993, 4906 cases were of children under 13 years old. The mothers of 4328 of these children either had HIV or were at risk of acquiring the disease. Additionally, around 300,000 infants were perinatally exposed to cocaine or related substances in 1991. The long-term consequences, such as fetal alcohol syndrome (FAS), congenital anomalies, or behavioral or learning deficits, are inestimable.

In 1994 more than 90% of pediatrics AIDS cases reported to the CDC identified perinatal transmission as the route of infection. Any nurse who cares for children should anticipate dealing with pediatric HIV infection, thus indicating the importance of understanding the mode of transmission, symptoms, treatment, and management of the illness. Nurses can play a central role in delivery of health care for this population by combining excellent clinical and interpersonal skills with sensitivity and respect for children. In addition, they can educate and support the children and caretakers and have a tremendous impact on their quality of life.

Elderly

Since 1900 the percentage of 65-year-old persons in the U.S. population has tripled, and it continues to rise dramatically. The older population, defined as those 65 years of age or older, numbered about 33 million in 1994. They represent approximately 12.7% of the U.S. population. The elderly population will more than double between now and the year 2050, to 80 million.[31] Most of the growth will occur between 2010 and 2030 when the "baby boomer" generation reaches their elderly years (Figure 4-3). The baby boomer cohort was born between 1946 to 1964, reflecting an exceptionally high birth rate following World War II. Life expectancy in 1900 was 47 years; it jumped to 68 years in 1950 and rose steadily to 76 years in 1991. For women life expectancy in 1991 was 79 years, and for men 72 years. This improvement in life expectancy improved for all race/sex groups. In 1994 elderly women outnumbered elderly men by a ratio of 3 to 2. As age increased, the age difference continued to grow. By age 85 and older the difference reaches 5 to 2. It becomes apparent that whereas most elderly men are married, most elderly women are not.

In 1992 the poverty rate of the 65- to 74-year-old group rose to 11%; it rose to 16% for those 75 years and older. Elderly women had a higher poverty rate than men. Elderly African Americans had a rate of 33%, and Hispanics had a rate of 22%. In contrast, the median income for the elderly population rose to $14,548 for men and to $8189 for women.

Medicare provides, and limits, access to health care for the majority of the elderly in America. The majority (70%) of older Americans consider themselves to be in good health, with fewer than 30 days per year in which activities were restricted because of illness or accidents. However, most older persons have at least one chronic disease, and some have multiple health problems. In 1991, of the 2.2

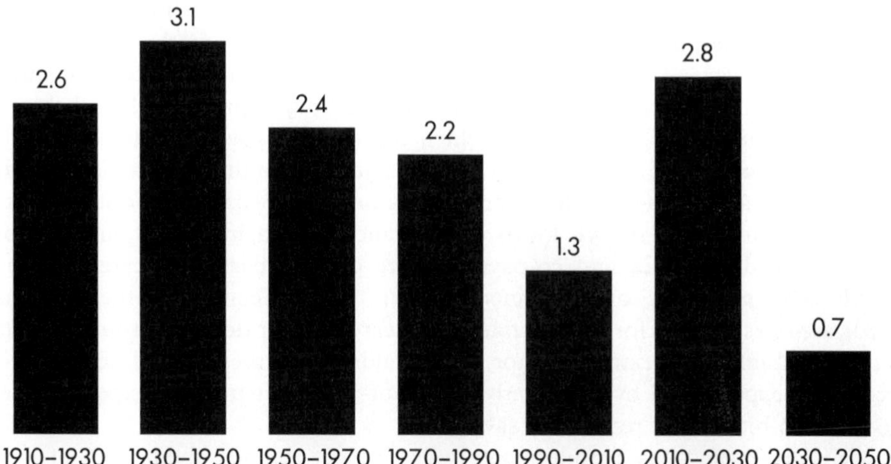

FIG. 4-3 Fifteen years from now, elderly population growth will explode.[31]

million Americans who died, 1.6 million were elderly. The leading causes of death included heart disease, cancer, and stroke.[2]

The elderly account for 36% of the total health care expenditure of the United States. On the other hand, out-of-pocket expenses rose to $1666 per person in 1992, which means that each older person must underwrite about 25% of their yearly health care costs because higher deductibles and a decrease in the amount of reimbursement are now a part of the Medicare program. In 1992 older persons spent almost $12 billion to meet cost-sharing (deductible or co-insurance) requirements. Relatively well-off persons may purchase Medigap insurance to cushion against the huge expenses that Medicare does not cover. Those elderly citizens who live at or below the poverty level can afford no such cushion.

As of 1994, Medicare Part A helped pay for four types of medical care: inpatient hospital care, inpatient skilled nursing care, home health, and hospice care. Medicare pays everything but the first $696 for the first 60 days of the hospital stay; this is called a *deductible* and is a one-time charge for any stay during a benefit period. For days 61 to 90 there is a $174 daily co-payment that the client pays out-of-pocket. If the client must go to a skilled nursing facility immediately following an acute hospital stay, then Medicare will pay 100% for the first 20 days. From days 21 to 100 the client must make a co-payment for $87.00 per day. Physicians' charges are covered only while the client is in an acute-care facility. The skilled care admission has five conditions attached, and all five conditions must be met. These are (1) the medical conditions require daily skilled nursing or rehabilitation services that can be provided only in a skilled nursing facility; (2) there was a minimum 3-day acute hospital stay; (3) the skilled care admission followed the acute admission within a short time; (4) the skilled care is for the condition that was treated in the acute hospital; and (5) a medical professional certifies that the treatment is necessary. Medicare does not pay for custodial care; the client must need daily skilled care.

Medicare Part B helps pay for physicians' services, outpatient hospital care, diagnostic services, medical equipment, ambulance service, and other services such as drugs (that cannot be self-administered) and transfusions. The cost for this is $100 per annum (per year). Then there is a 20% co-payment charge for all charges that are provided "on assignment," which means the provider charges only the Medicare-approved fee. If the provider charges more, then the balance between the Medicare fee and the service fee charged by a provider becomes an out-of-pocket expense. Although these two forms of insurance are an invaluable aid to most retirees, the deductibles and co-payments are often a barrier to care for those elderly who must live only on income from Social Security. Remember that Medicare does not pay for routine foot or eye care, nor for dentures, routine dental care, dental fillings or extractions, or hearing aids. Since these are all health needs frequently experienced by the elderly, their out-of-pocket medical expenses often take a deep bite out of retirement savings.

Medicare, which has a multibillion-dollar budget, spends about 30% of it on clients who have less than 1 year to live. This money is primarily spent in high-technology areas using life-extending techniques on clients who, if given a choice, would probably prefer to remain at home receiving available comfort and support measures. With the new changes in Medicare coverage, that may soon be a possibility. As health care consumers become more open in their communication with family and physicians, they can guide the level of care they wish to receive by means of living wills and living trusts.

In a time when the aging population is burgeoning, it is poorly protected against the cost of chronic illness. Although some of these costs are covered under Medicare Part B, with the shifts from in-hospital care to outpatient care the overall costs can become impossible to manage on fixed incomes.

In 1983 the exploding costs of health care caused significant changes in Medicare payments within hospitals. Under the Prospective Payment System hospitals were offered incentives to shorten the length of stay for Medicare recipients. Length of stay was predetermined by a diagnostic-relating grouping (DRG) so that an average number of days for a specific disease was determined; hospitals were then reimbursed for the predetermined stay rather than for the actual number of hospitalized days. Therefore if a DRG designated a 5-day stay and the client was discharged earlier, the hospital could still keep the difference. This has had significant impact on Medicare beneficiaries by increasing early hospital discharge. Also, because of increased deductibles, many clients are more ill on admission. Common DRGs with the sharpest decline in length of stay were hip and femur procedures, joint replacements, fractures of the hip or pelvis, and cerebrovascular disorders.

Early discharge has lead to a proliferation of home health care agencies. More clients are discharged to skilled nursing facilities and require more acute care in those facilities. According to Health Care Financing Review,[12] clients discharged with large length-of-stay reductions increased their use of skilled nursing facility (SNF) care by 83% and increased their use of home health care by 102% between

1982 and 1987. In addition, the increase of day surgery has led to increased demands on home health care. Because Medicare focuses on acute care, home health care is provided as a follow-up to an acute episode rather than for chronic care. Medicare provides limited coverage in skilled nursing facilities, with very rigid requirements. It is available only after a hospitalization, limited to 100 days per benefit, and applies only to around-the-clock skilled care. Such shifts in coverage expose older people to continually rising financial liability.

To the extent that older Americans must forego health services because they cannot afford it, they are denied access to care and deprived of even the basic quality of health they could enjoy. Access to health is denied to many others as well. Increasing reports regarding migrant workers, undocumented aliens, and the homeless indicate that they receive little or no care, thereby jeopardizing their health and the population at large.

Poor, Migrant Workers, Homeless

In the United States poor people are more ill than nonpoor people. African Americans, Hispanics, Native Americans, migrant workers, and the homeless are more ill than suburban, white, white-collar-employed persons, and they get less medical care. At least 37 million people have no insurance to pay for their health care. Some are ignored by the system and some encounter barriers when attempts are made to receive care. Lack of information, lack of transportation, inability to pay, a complex bureaucratic system, and language differences can all be barriers to the health care delivery system.

The homeless number in the millions across the country. About 25% of the homeless are young people, with minority groups being disproportionately represented. Families with children constitute another 30% and present multiple problems such as inadequate nutrition, schooling, immunizations, and basic safety. An additional 30% of the homeless are mentally ill, drug and/or alcohol dependent, or have AIDS. There are numerous reasons for their plight. Rising rents, low-paying jobs, and the loss of affordable federally subsidized housing, along with the deinstitutionalization of the mentally ill, have all contributed to the problem. Some persons who might be able to afford monthly rent cannot afford the 2 months' advance rent required by many apartment owners.

There is another relatively unidentified homeless population. These are the single parents and their children who are displaced through divorce or economic circumstances. They can be found living in the homes of friends and relatives, not necessarily on the streets. They are not counted in the census as homeless but can be deemed just that, not having a permanent home for a short or even long period.

Currently in the United States there is a new type of homeless persons: those made homeless as a result of a natural catastrophe such as fire, flood, hurricane, tornado, or earthquake. Unfortunately, during 1993 and 1994 these phenomena occurred with regularity. This group of people would probably be deemed the temporarily homeless.

A further way to view the homeless is through the arrangements for living on a daily basis. There are the street homeless, who abide there over a 24-hour period. Another group may be called the emergency-housed homeless, who may find shelter for the night but must leave in the morning. The final category is the sheltered homeless, who have a limited time within a shelter, usually 30 to 60 days, to find employment and a permanent home.

Bollini and Siem[5] defined a *migrant* as a person who in moving crosses boundaries for a change of residence intended to be permanent or of substantial duration. It is believed that only one out of three persons who migrate actually settle for good in the new location. The article also points out the difference between refugees and migrants. Migrants move for economic reasons, whereas refugees move for political reasons.

Health can be affected by the stresses of migration, including separation from family and friends, disruption of social support networks, and adaptation to the new set of cultural norms, roles, and responsibilities. Psychologic and social stresses often lead to poor health and family problems. These are compounded by difficulties obtaining health care, including inadequate access, linguistic obstacles, and cultural and economic barriers.[5]

Migrant workers tend to belong to large families. Half of the workers are less than 25 years old, with a life expectancy of 49 years. Although it is illegal, children often work in the fields to supplement the family income. Because work is episodic and the families travel to crops that are ready for harvest, schooling is limited and fewer than 50% complete the ninth grade. Health problems include the following:

1. Tuberculosis
2. Parasitic diseases
3. Pesticide poisoning
4. Multiple pregnancies with little prenatal treatment

Such illnesses contribute to high infant mortality, and high morbidity and mortality among the rest of migrant population.

Most Americans assume that Medicaid pays health care costs for the majority of the poor; actually only about 31% are covered. Research has shown that 5 million people annually report that they do not seek medical care because they cannot afford it. Medicaid is a joint federal-state program designated specifically for the poor. Because each state administers its own program, resulting in essentially 50 different programs, eligibility requirements and coverage differ from state to state. At a minimum, those who qualify include the following:

1. People in welfare programs
2. Those enrolled in Social Security Supplemental programs
3. Those enrolled in Aid to Families with Dependent Children (AFDC)

Each state sets its own welfare criteria. Therefore many underprivileged people slip through the cracks. The following are some of the reasons for lack of aid:

1. No eligibility for welfare
2. No permanent address
3. Fear of deportation
4. Lack of understanding of the complexities of the system

Many public health nurses complain that underprivileged people find it difficult to access the right agency through the bureaucratic maze, and nurses themselves can well understand clients' problems.

Literacy and language problems foil attempts to fill out forms or understand instructions. Health teaching becomes impossible because directions are poorly comprehended. Nurses' own values often conflict with the realities faced each day by the poor and the homeless. Sterile techniques for dressing changes become impossible when one lives on the street with a cardboard box for a shelter. When directions are not followed, medications are taken incorrectly, or treatments are not completed as prescribed, the fault may be lack of money, language, or literacy rather than poor compliance.

The severe restrictions that inhibit access to health care have lead the majority of citizens of the country to call for health care reform. Although seemingly uncertain about the form it should take, the American public is convinced that it needs some form of universal coverage. The business community feels overly burdened with the rising costs of health care insurance, health care providers feel abused since so little of their care is fully reimbursed, and physicians complain about malpractice costs and the lack of reimbursement from the government for Medicaid patients. Additionally, downsizing of industry and a poor economy have caused highly educated workers to be caught in a web, with the loss of a job often followed by the loss of health insurance. All of this has led to widespread agreement that something must be done. It also began the serious search for a comprehensive health plan, with cost controls based on limitations in the type of procedures covered (in other words, rationing).

AIDS

Access to adequate health care has also been denied people with AIDS. The debate on financing AIDS services will assuredly include the issue of budgetary constraints and unequal access. According to the CDC, African Americans (174,562) and Hispanics (73,721) accounted for 48% of all AIDS cases as of September 1995. Many of these patients rely on publicly sponsored health services. Even those fortunate enough to have health insurance ultimately run out of benefits. In recent years only two fifths of the poor have qualified for Medicaid; therefore it cannot be viewed as a panacea. The system has not taken the necessary steps to anticipate the needs of people with AIDS. Catastrophic health insurance remains a future dream for people with AIDS, as well as for people who have cancer.

In 1988 64,506 cases of AIDS were reported in the United States, with 36,255 known deaths. In 1992 the number of cases approached 300,000.[32] The mortality rate is about 56% (Figure 4-4).

In 1993 a new definition for AIDS was developed that added about 90,000 new cases to the growing list of patients. The definition now has four new indicators to add to the previous 23: cervical cancer, pulmonary tuberculosis, recurrent pneumonia, and a drop in the level of CD4 T cells to 200 per cubic milliliter. This new definition will be beneficial to women since many had died of AIDS before the appropriate diagnosis was made. Women constitute the fastest-growing group of people with AIDS in the United States. Using the latest procedure to diagnose cervical cancer, more women will be tested for HIV infection and treated for that as well. Meanwhile, in statistics quoted by the CDC, teenagers are being exposed to the virus at a rate much faster than previously believed, and girls are more frequently the victims (Figure 4-5).

AIDS has to a large extent been treated as a political issue rather than a health problem. AIDS activists call for increasing funds for research and treatment, citing homophobia for the lack of adequate funding. However, the greatest increase in

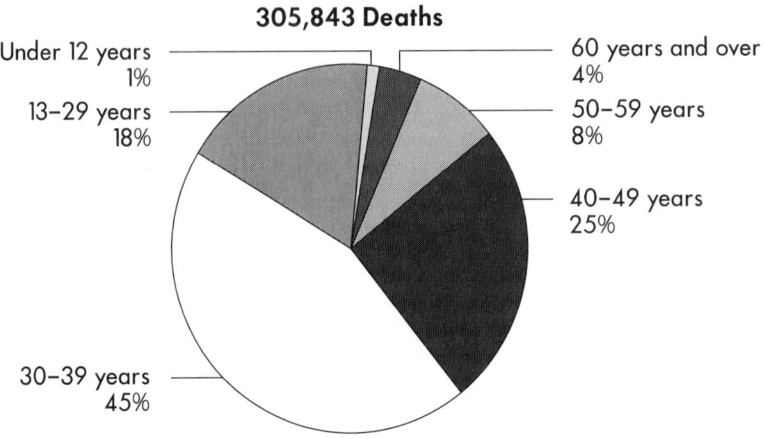

Source: Chart prepared by U.S. Bureau of the Census.

FIG. 4-4 Distribution of AIDS deaths, by age: 1982 through 1995.

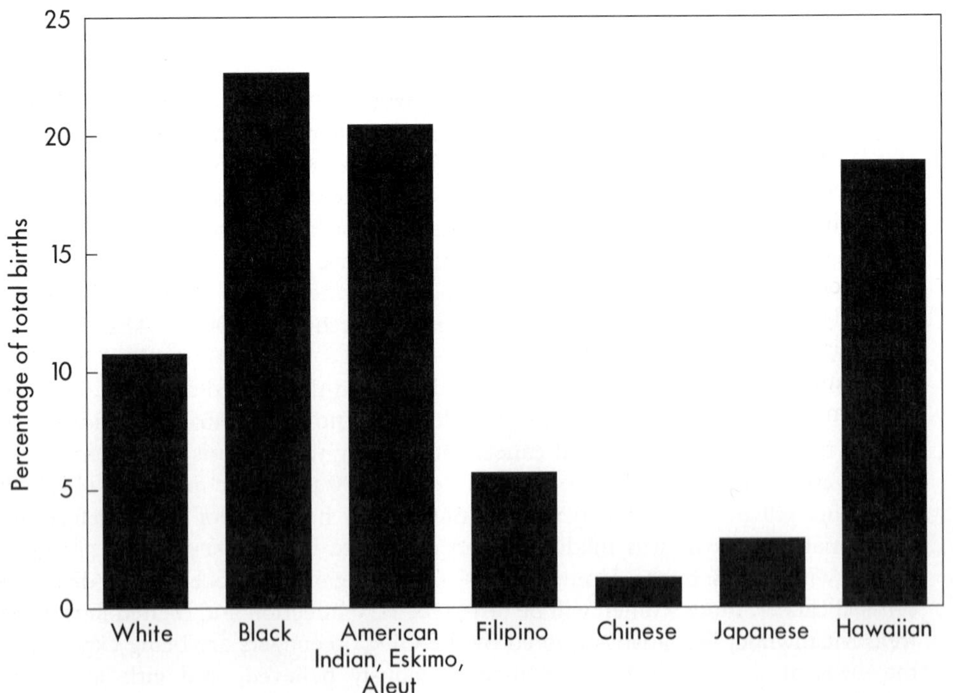

Source: Chart prepared by U.S. Bureau of the Census.

FIG. 4-5 Births to teenage mothers as a percentage of total births, by race: 1993.

rates is among heterosexual contacts, most specifically among adolescents. According to WHO, the ultimate way to control the epidemic will be to prevent infections in young people who are sexually active. AIDS must not be a political issue; it is a deadly disease for which there is currently no cure. Research, funding, and treatment must be examined within this context.

A group with increasing importance is children with AIDS. Almost 6000 pediatric cases were reported in 1996. In 1994 more then 90% of infant HIV cases reported to CDC were obtained by perinatal transmission. HIV transmission results from exposure to blood and body secretions. It is not a highly contagious disease if the proper precautions are taken. Former U.S. Surgeon General C. Everett Koop recommended that monogamous relationships, the use of condoms, and avoidance of dirty needles will protect the majority of persons. Health care personnel are cautioned to use standard precautions against blood and body secretions. CDC cites universal precautions as the most effective way health professionals can protect themselves from contracting the disease.

Unfortunately, AIDS victims are faced with discrimination at various levels throughout this country. Health care personnel, families, and whole communities discriminate. Potential victims are afraid to come forward for testing, many refuse to disclose their sexual contacts, and some have lost jobs and homes based on a positive HIV test. Until people address the issue openly, it will be impossible to solve many of the problems associated with the care and treatment of AIDS patients.

Mental Illness

Although a person with mental illness has limited coverage under some health insurance policies, and no coverage under many, mental illness is a big-budget item costing $9.4 billion a year. This cost is an out-of-pocket expense for some or is provided by local and state government. With the deinstitutionalization of the mentally ill since the 1960s, many have been cared for through county outpatient clinics, some have been placed in halfway houses, and some have become homeless. Incapacitated, unable to work, and unwilling to join the "system," the homeless mentally ill populate parks, street corners, grates, and public buildings of every inner city in America. This problem poses many ethical questions. Are the mentally ill capable of making their own health care decisions? Should society allow them freedom of choice or, for their own welfare, should the mentally ill be placed in protective environments and given the health care they need? Who should decide? The individual? The family? The government? Should there be some minimal standard of living to which we are all entitled and subsequently accept?

Since suicide was the ninth leading cause of death in the United States in 1994 and clients with serious mental illness occupy such a great number of hospital beds, nurses in all settings must be able to recognize clients with psychiatric emotional disturbances and meet their special needs.

Women's Health

In years past women were considered the hardier of the sexes because they lived longer and had lower incidence of heart disease, ulcers, and lung cancer. But this perception has changed. In past decades women had limited choices and most became wives and mothers; but with the women's movement came wider choices and increased stresses. Today women contend with the same problems that men have faced in the workforce—desire to advance, earning adequate income to support the family, and achieving status from work. In addition women often work 8 hours at one job and then work another few hours at home. Some women must decide whether to forego children for careers; others worry about child care. With the increase in smoking, stress in the work setting, and a polluted environment, women are rapidly approaching men in stress-related illnesses.

Prevention of illness is the best defense against the health care industry.

Primary care provision and health assessment/health promotion/disease prevention services are needed for women of all ages. This includes education and counseling services. For women, the need for childbirth/fertility counseling, injury prevention counseling, assessment of work-related health risks, and assessment of immunization status is called for. When counseling women it is a perfect opportunity for education, assessment, and referral regarding immunization of their children also. Other areas of concern include:

1. Smoking cessation
2. Safe-sex habits and counseling
3. Screening high-risk populations for HIV
4. Screening for abusive relationships (domestic abuse)
5. Physical exercise habits
6. Mental health care
7. Dental care

Although prevention for men and women is essentially the same, there are a few differences. Women need regular breast examinations and Pap smears, and perhaps regularly scheduled mammograms. Men need prostate checkups on a regular basis. In addition, a baseline electrocardiogram is probably a good idea for anyone over 40 years old. The greatest barrier to routine checkups is the lack of coverage for preventive examinations, which leads to out-of-pocket expenses of several hundred dollars.

Substance Abuse

Although death from infectious diseases declined as a result of antibiotics, a new group of health problems has arisen—respiratory diseases such as emphysema, chronic bronchitis, and lung cancer caused by tobacco use and abuse. Social problems such as alcoholism and drug addiction have made front page news as movie stars and sports figures join the ranks of street people in "doing drugs." Cocaine was considered a recreational drug until the first 21-year-old athlete died of a massive heart attack after cocaine use. Nationally approximately 700,00 infants each year are perinatally exposed to illicit drugs, not including alcohol. The cost of care to these infants for the first 5 years of life averages $63,000. The consequences are low birth weight, developmental lags, and behavioral problems. Frequently these children are also victims of other child abuse or are abandoned, often in newborn nurseries.

As a nation we seem to be victims of our own destructive behaviors. A recent study about teenage behavior notes the increase in substance abuse and sexually transmitted diseases. Teenage girls have the additional problems of pregnancies, eating disorders, and depression. Since young women often have no health insurance, they rarely seek medical help. Often their own misconceptions about the "ideal look," fostered by the media's portrayal of physical perfection, heads young women toward such self-destructive behaviors as anorexia or bulimia. These can lead to death or at least produce severe malnutrition, which in itself damages the heart and/or the bone structure. Young men resort to steroids to gain the body conformation displayed in magazines or to improve performance in competitive sports. Solutions to some of these problems lie outside the traditional medical system. Better health education about human development, emphasis on critical thinking so that young people can analyze the messages with which they are bombarded, more and better access to school nurses, and better role models at home are fairly low-cost investments toward developing healthy men and women.

Yearly, smoking contributes to 130,000 deaths resulting from lung cancer, 170,000 deaths resulting from cardiovascular diseases, and 60,000 deaths resulting from respiratory diseases other than cancer. In 1984 Surgeon General C. Everett Koop stated that pollution from secondhand smoke in homes and the workplace can contain more contaminants than is permitted by most occupational and environmental regulations. Yet the same government that warns about the dangers of smoking provides subsidies to farmers who grow tobacco. The tobacco industry was forced to place warnings about the dangers of smoking on each package of cigarettes; meanwhile they spend $2.5 billion advertising their product. In the past few years nonsmokers have become aggressive in securing their right to a smoke-free environment. Many localities have ordinances prohibiting smoking in public buildings and mandating smoke-free areas in restaurants and in the workplace. In 1988 smoking was banned on airline flights of 1 hour or longer within the borders of the United States. During the 1990s in-flight smoking on international flights has been banned.

Another lifestyle problem, alcohol, contributes to the untimely death of citizens through cirrhosis of the liver, esophageal hemorrhage, cancer, and suicide. Include the numbers of deaths and maimings resulting from automobile accidents caused by drivers under the influence of alcohol and the statistics are staggering. An estimated 17,700 alcohol-related traffic fatalities and 355,000 traffic injuries occurred in 1992.[22,23] Alcohol-related accidents cost $46.1 billion in 1990, including $5.1 billion in medical expenses.[6,25,28]

The incidence of family violence and work and school absenteeism is escalating. There is no evidence that drinking alcoholic beverages in moderation is harmful to health, but there is overwhelming evidence that abuse of it can cause significant physiologic damage to the brain, the liver, and the gastrointestinal tract. Advertisements lead people to believe drinking is sophisticated, that chic and up-and-coming executives use it to become successful, or that it is wonderfully relaxing to have a drink after work. For some that may prove correct. For others it is deadly. Ads never show the deadly aspects of drinking.

Social policy that bans advertisements glamorizing cigarettes and alcohol needs to be developed. Laws regarding smoke-free environments and the legal ages for purchase or use of cigarettes and alcohol should be strictly enforced. Mandatory jail sentences for drunk drivers should be enacted and enforced in every state.

Physicians and nurses need to have substance abuse content added to their curricula so they can diagnose and counsel at the early phase of a problem. Education regarding hazards of substance abuse must become part of every schoolchild's learning. Nurses must begin to shape social policy so that it focuses on health promotion and prevention issues rather than on restoration. Here is a void that nurses can fill with their knowledge and expertise, and thus contribute to the health of the nation.

■ COMPETING SOCIAL ISSUES

Despite the fact that government has interceded in many areas of life, it normally is considered inappropriate for it to encroach too far into family life. Because the family represents personal freedom, the government has established very few laws regarding marriage, divorce, or childrearing. In general there are laws for the protection of women and children, particularly in the area of family dysfunction. The government has traditionally defined the family as two parents and children. All other family structures were seen as deviant. Much has changed over the past decades, and there are now multiple forms of family structures, without much policy to assist in their support.

Single-Parent Families

Divorce used to be a social stigma, and women with children had few skills to enable them to consider divorce as an option. Now divorce no longer stigmatizes the family, and the majority of married women with children are already in the workforce. Somehow the image of the "perfect" family is retained—two kids, mom in the kitchen, and dad in the office. Yet the increases in divorce rates and numbers of single-parent families cause growing concern over family breakdown. Single-parent households account for 15% of American families. By age 18 nearly half of the children in the United States will have lived a period of time with a single parent.[28] Single parenthood is seen as a transitional state, but all too often, especially past age 30, remarriage does not occur. A recent study indicates that fewer than one fifth of unmarried head-of-household women remarried within a 5-year period. Single parents are classified in one of the following ways:

1. Widowed
2. Divorced
3. Separated
4. Unmarried

However they are classified, single parents and their families suffer as a result of the public image of the perfect family.

In the perfect family the man brings home the money needed to support the family. The latest study by the Joint Select Task Force on Changing Families (1989) indicates that only 15% of families live in this traditional mode. Today most mothers, 62% nationally, work outside the home. Even though society knows the perfect family image is not reality and that even two-parent families need the mother's salary to live at middle-class levels, the myth remains that women work for pin money. Thus, although often doing the same work, women earn less than men—about 70 cents to every dollar men earn. This also applies to women who are heads of the household. The result of this form of discrimination is that three out of five poor children come from single-parent families.

Working mothers have problems other than money. Job structure is usually inflexible and long, leaving little time or energy for homemaking and mothering. Just getting the children to the dentist or physician is a major problem because their hours conflict with the wage earner's hours. Child care is expensive and in short supply. Many single mothers have informal arrangements with grandparents, other relatives, or neighbors. School-age children may become part of the "latch-key kid" solution to child care because they are unattended from the time school lets out until the parent comes home. Single parents, because of job- and home-related time constraints, have little time for social interaction and may feel socially isolated.

Although lip service is paid to "equal pay for equal work," overwhelming evidence shows that it is not happening. This has increased the numbers of the working poor. Low-paying jobs often do not offer health care insurance but pay enough to prevent the family from qualifying for Medicaid. Childhood diseases may become a nightmare from which no budget can recover. No one else is available to care for the sick child, so the parent is forced to stay home to provide care while sacrificing the much-needed paycheck. Sadly, many childhood diseases are preventable with proper immunizations, which are not universally administered in this country.

Public policy that affords children access to free or affordable health care is needed, resulting in primary prevention rather than tertiary intervention. Most industrialized nations have health coverage for all children; the United States does not. Also needed are enforceable laws that do not tolerate fathers avoiding child support.

Child care is another social policy issue that has been overlooked. One option that government can take is to award tax breaks to companies that have in-house child care facilities. School districts could combine after-school activities at schools with a low fee, which would afford children the protection of supervised play. Stricter enforcement of child care regulations would preclude molestation scandals, which are becoming more prevalent in child care facilities.

With the signing of the Family and Medical Leave Act, February 1993 marked a small change in the government's position vis-a-vis families. This act requires employers with 50 or more workers to allow up to 12 weeks of unpaid leave annually for the birth or adoption of a child, for a serious personal illness, or for the care of a seriously ill child, spouse, or parent. Some believe this bill is long overdue, since many European countries have had similar laws for decades. However, this Act was locked in a political battle that pitted Democrat against Republican, the most salient argument being how business might be harmed. With the election of a democratic president the bill, which had previously been passed by Congress but vetoed by the president, was almost the first to be enacted in the new term.

■ ALTERNATIVE FAMILY STYLES

Divorce and Remarriage

Divorce rates are rising continuously in the United States. Divorce affects each member of the family because children are deprived of the constant interaction with both parents, and their divorced parents are concerned about finances, social relationships, and diminished time to meet family needs. When the single parent remarries, children from a previous marriage are often added to the family unit. There is little to guide blended families to resolve the complex problems remarriage brings. Even language is not supportive, because *stepmother* and *stepchild* are viewed as pejorative terms. What does a child call a parent's new spouse? Is it permissible for a stepparent to discipline children? Whose? His, hers, theirs? Step roles must be achieved rather than ascribed. Stepparents must earn love and respect; it is not automatic, because they are not the child's biologic parents. After remarriage, the incidence of failure to provide child support increases, and the law is lax in enforcing the natural father's obligations. However, there is currently a strong movement toward stricter enforcement and computerized vigilance through state and federal tax rolls.

The problem is complex and no direct relationships are established, but at this time in our history sexual abuse of children is also on the increase. Children in blended families commonly complain that other children are being treated better. Problems in remarriage and blended families are widespread, and each family has its own myriad of smaller or larger ones. Additionally, there are no social norms to assist the family in achieving the new roles required in the blended family. The fact that the divorce rate in remarriage is higher than the divorce rate in first marriages attests to this problem.

Living Together

During the 1980s cohabitation increased rapidly as society began to accept it as an alternative to marriage. In a national sample the majority of couples questioned believed that living together was a prelude to marriage. For many it was an attractive alternative to marrying again. During the last census the government developed an acronym for this phenomenon, *POSSLQ,* which stands for person of the opposite sex sharing living quarters. In that census 1.8 million couples were living together, more than double the number obtained in the previous census.

Traditionally, couples who chose to live together came from the very poor; now, however, another class has joined them—well-educated urban professionals and the somewhat less-educated previously married. The legal system has not resolved the legal ramifications involved in long-term cohabiting relationships. From this arrangement serious economic and social complexities have just begun to be addressed. The case of Marvin v. Marvin, involving property rights distribution between Lee Marvin and Michelle Triola-Marvin, his long-time live-in partner, indicated that the law was beginning to address what has become a societal norm. Seventeen states now recognize de facto marriages as having nearly the same rights as de jure marriages.

Homosexual Families

The alternative family lifestyle that has accrued the most stigma is the homosexual family. Homosexuals are "coming out of the closet" in ever-increasing numbers. Their problems are much more societal than legal. Numerous laws have been passed ensuring their civil rights, but society retains a largely negative prejudice against this group, making it more difficult for them to achieve their rights. Homosexual parents have difficulties obtaining custody of their children. They are not considered fit adoptive parents. Recent studies show that some lesbians have taken the step to have donor insemination and are becoming a nontraditional family unit. Society is outraged when persons in long-standing homosexual relationships seek the sanctity of marriage. With the advent of HIV infection, homophobia may well continue to increase rather than decreasing to allow homosexuality to become an acceptable alternative family style.

■ CARE FOR FAMILY MEMBERS

The Sandwich Generation

Aging parents live with their adult children for the following reasons:

1. Death of a spouse
2. Limited resources
3. Chronic illness
4. Emotional dependence

The burden of caring for aging parents often falls on women, traditionally the eldest daughter. However, approximately 60% of these women work outside the home. Increasingly the middle-age generation is sandwiched between aging parents and young adult children. They are faced with the problems of their own careers and marriages and the problems encountered by their children and by their parents. Emotional and financial resources may be strained by the needs of both ends of the generational lifespan, resulting in conflict and guilt when the needs of one intersects the needs of the other.

Taking care of an elderly parent not only involves taking care of the physical needs, it also includes psychologic and spiritual issues in reversing the roles of parent and child. In addition, it can be a challenging task to get to know a parent again while adjusting to their changing condition.

Adult Day Care

Most elderly persons live full and meaningful lives. Some become debilitated by disease and must reside in long-term care facilities. Others are primarily independent and need only supplementary home care. In addition, increasing numbers of frail elderly are being cared for by their aging children. Often caregivers are gainfully employed, not ready for retirement, and must face the problem of how to care for a parent who cannot be left home unattended for long periods.

Day care centers may help the older adult remain independent. They offer activities such as arts and crafts, exercise, health education, continuing education, and reality orientation and remotivation. Nutritionally balanced meals are served for a nominal cost. Day care can fill a void in the older person's day. It can also provide a secure and nurturing environment while the caregiver continues to work. Some centers are allied with agencies such as the following:

1. United Way
2. Red Cross
3. Nursing homes
4. Acute-care hospitals

Some centers are associated with nursing homes or acute-care hospitals but are separate entities and are self-supporting. Some day care centers are particularly innovative; they combine child care with adult day care, giving both generations the opportunity to spend time together. Surrogate grandparents have the warm love of the children, and the children have a "family" during day care hours.

Problems arise from costs and transportation. Most centers try to keep costs at a minimum, because almost everyone has a limited budget. If the caregiving family covers the cost, there are no tax incentives, no write-off, and no tax shelter. Elderly parents who live with a child and who receive Social Security afford no tax advantage to the caregiver. The costs of food and shelter, as well as of day care, must be underwritten by the family.

Long-Term Care

Nursing homes provide a vital function in the overall health care system. Although thought of as permanent homes for the elderly, they also serve many short-term functions such as rehabilitation. The following three levels of care are offered by nursing homes:

1. Skilled nursing—for persons who need intensive 24-hour supervision and treatment by a registered nurse or other skilled rehabilitation service
2. Intermediate care—for persons who do not require intensive care or treatment, but who, because of their mental or physical status, require care above the level of room and board
3. Custodial care—for persons who can no longer attend to their personal needs and need supervision with activities of daily living such as eating and hygiene

Intermediate and custodial care are paid by Medicaid or private funds, whereas Medicare covers the cost of acute and skilled care only.

Nursing homes charge a daily rate, depending on the level of care, that can add up to $2000 to $3000 a month. Medicare covers 100 days of long-term care for each benefit period, if it follows an acute illness, but there is a deductible for days 21 to 100. Furthermore, there must be a 60-day hiatus after the 100 days is exhausted before readmission from a hospital to a nursing care facility is permitted. Some private insurance companies provide long-term care insurance and some provide Medigap insurance, but these vary in amount and kind of service. Medicaid insurance is available for low-income persons and for persons who have exhausted their resources paying for long-term care. Because Medicaid payments are much lower than private pay or Medicare, many long-term care facilities limit the number of admissions or do not accept Medicaid clients at all. Some states use a policy called *deeming.* A couple living together has funds that are considered (deemed) available to pay each other's medical bills. Therefore the Medicaid applicant must deplete the spouse's assets before receiving coverage. Even if the spouse's name appears on a pension or Social Security check, it is not a joint income, but must be used to pay for the Medicaid care. This may cause the healthy spouse to become impoverished to maintain long-term care for the Medicaid client. Now some states split income and assets in half when determining a spouse's eligibility.

In 1990 Medicare covered less than 3% of the $35 billion spent on nursing homes. Families financed aid for more than half, $18 billion, with Medicaid picking up the rest of the bill. Contrary to popular belief, only 5% of the elderly population is in long-term care facilities at any given time. Much of skilled nursing care costs goes toward rehabilitation. Although the stereotypical picture of long-term care is of very old and senile people, in reality clients recuperating from accidents, strokes, and complicated surgeries also receive skilled nursing care. Except for the family, Medicaid is the only source of funds for custodial care, and the numbers of custodial care admissions are increasing. High technology, although giving and maintaining life, has not improved the quality of life. Therefore victims of irreversible head trauma, degenerative muscle and nerve diseases, Huntington's chorea, and Alzheimer's disease, after depleting all other resources, including those of the family, find themselves in long-term care facilities. There, at any given time, one may see a mix of chronic debilitating physical diseases, vegetative states, and psychopathologic diseases. Caring for these persons requires caregivers with special sensitivities and motivations since few rewards are otherwise likely.

Long-term care is fraught with problems that stem from a lack of coordinated policies, goals, and methods. No well-defined standards of care provide minimum protection for clients. There is a serious shortage in the numbers of nursing homes, so that even those who qualify find it difficult to find a vacancy.

Qualified, licensed personnel have typically been less available to provide health care in nursing homes. Often the staff consists of aides who have a few months of limited training and are paid minimum wages. Supervision is either lax or lacking. Because of repeated accounts of client abuse and neglect, cruelty, and violations of whatever health and safety rules that exist, most states have commissions investigating complaints. Further, physicians and R.N.s have generally avoided the responsibility of the care and treatment of nursing home clients. Nursing home care is considered a low-status job for registered nurses, who tend to choose intensive care and acute hospitals.

Nursing home administrators list problems within the system: overwhelming red tape, confusing rules, insufficient funds, and skyrocketing costs.[27] Medicaid pays less than $25 per day for care of its beneficiaries, which must cover the total care required by the client.

Because long-term care facilities are in short supply, and also to control escalating costs, alternatives to institutionalization had to be found and financed. Many programs can assist the client to stay within the community, such as home health care, day care, respite care, and homemaker and nutrition services.

Home Health Care

Home health care comprises a provision of skilled nursing services by licensed nurses; rehabilitation services such as physical, occupational, or speech therapy; and personal care such as bathing, eating, and ambulation. Home health care agencies pioneered the pricing of nursing services because they always considered nursing care a revenue-producing center, unlike hospitals, which include nursing service in room and board charges.

A health professional or a multidisciplinary team determines whether an individual's need warrants the provision of home care. The four types of agencies generally involved in the delivery of home care are public agencies, visiting nurses, agencies operated by hospitals, and proprietary agencies. Because agencies are growing rapidly and there are a variety of providers, the quality of services vary.

Cost savings resulting from the provision of home care services provide incentives to use those services. Recent studies estimate that the average cost of 1 hospital day is $500, whereas the cost of 1 home care day ranges between $45 and

$110. In another study, Visiting Nurses Service of New York demonstrated that AIDS patients could be cared for at home for $800 a day, whereas the costs of hospitalization would be $3000 a day.

Instituting the DRG system led to shorter hospital stays as a result of fixed hospital reimbursement from government and third-party payers (insurance companies). Clients are discharged "sicker and quicker." The flood of still–acutely ill discharged clients encouraged the growth of the home health industry.

Between 1980 and 1990 home health care spending grew 440%; the largest increase occurred between 1989 and 1990, when spending on home health care increased 47% to $4.4 billion.[30] The major identified problem with home health is quality control. Quality assurance tools that measure client outcomes, an adequate surveillance system, and a monitoring mechanism that surveys client benefits from treatment are not standardized. Providers of care, accreditation agencies, and legislators must work together to ensure the adequacy of care.

Barhydt-Wezenaar[3] proposed that the new focus of the home as a setting of choice will enhance the quality of life of those who receive care. Furthermore, self-care at home decreases iatrogenic infections and allows the client a greater degree of freedom. However, home care is increasingly complex as a result of early discharge under the DRG system, and it is common to deliver care to a respirator-dependent client at home. Nurses are delivering home care to clients on chemotherapy, intravenous hydration, intravenous antibiotic therapy, and parenteral and enteral nutrition. Clients are taught self-care of parenteral feedings, kidney dialysis, and Hickman catheters. Often little time in the hospital is available for the necessary teaching to provide the client with the requisite skills for the task. However, with home health a licensed nurse can follow up on the level of knowledge and skill that a client and family has.

To receive home health coverage under Medicare, the beneficiary must meet the following criteria:

1. Be homebound
2. Required skilled nursing or therapy
3. Have physician certification
4. Be cared for by an authorized agency
5. Be reevaluated every 2 months

If a physician approves the plan of treatment, a home health aide and medical supplies can be included. Fortunately, home health nurses are knowledgeable in the intricacies of Medicare's prescribed care planning and charting and can assist the client and the physician in gaining the best compensation for the treatment needed. Even with the best documentation, benefits are often denied as part of government cost cutting.

Under Medicaid there are fewer restrictions. A wider range of health and personal services is available if ordered by a physician. These can include personal care services such as assistance with dressing, hygiene, and meal or housekeeping tasks. These services are subject to review every 60 days.

Homemaker and housekeeper services are provided under Title XX directly through a county department of social services or provider agencies. Because of the cost-saving factors, many private insurers provide home health protection with their policies.

Hospice

The modern hospital with all the marvelous technologic advances is the best of worlds and the worst of worlds. Many lives are saved by the latest medical breakthrough. However, many lives are prolonged needlessly by the very same methods. Often the higher the level of technology, the more dehumanizing the treatment may seem to the client and the family. For persons with terminal illnesses, the emotional cost of hospitalization is exceeded only by the enormous financial burden. Society is beginning to understand and accept that death is a normal process and therefore does not require the sterile, efficient machinery offered in an acute care setting. Because many people do not want their dying postponed by machines and because of the government's interest in cost saving, alternatives to hospital care for the dying have become more acceptable. One alternative is hospice, which has the following as its philosophy:

> Dying is a natural process whether or not resulting from disease. Hospice exists neither to hasten nor to postpone death. Rather, hospice exists to affirm life by providing support and care for those in the last phases of incurable disease so they can live as fully and comfortably as possible.[24]

Hospice is specifically for clients and their families who have decided to forego treatment that focuses on curing a terminal disease. Instead they choose to receive pain relief, palliative care, and emotional support at home. Hospice care provides or arranges for the following:

1. Nursing and physician services
2. Social work
3. Pastoral counseling
4. Psychologic services
5. Therapies ranging from physical to pharmaceutical
6. Home health aides
7. Homemakers
8. Equipment and supplies

To be truly effective hospice must be the key part of an interdisciplinary service. Hospice must be available 24 hours a day, 7 days a week. Its goal is the provision of comfort and peace in the familiar setting of the client's own home.

Hospice addresses physical, psychologic, spiritual, and social needs of the client and the family. Pain relief is a primary task, whether it be physical or psychologic. Removing the client's fear of pain through proper management is essential. Working with the nurse and physician, the client can be taught to anticipate and administer the appropriate treatment to alleviate physical pain. The client and the family need assistance with acceptance of the dying process and in dealing with the stress that the knowledge of dying engenders. The nurse is the client advocate in providing care that leads to a comfortable, pain-free atmosphere. The nurse facilitates interaction between client and family so that adequate physical and psychologic caring is shared.

Although the hospice movement is usually associated with cancer, persons with other terminal diseases such as amyotrophic lateral sclerosis, AIDS, and end-stage renal or cardiac disease are also using the service. Hospice is paid for by Medicare if the client is eligible; through private insurance; and, in some states, by Medicaid. Because both government and private insurers view hospice as a valuable and cost-cutting service, it has moved into the mainstream of health care delivery.

Summary

The U.S. government has no Bureau of Family and few laws regarding family life, but its authority is felt in subtle ways. Because of its size and influence the federal government has a great effect on family life. Tax policies regarding home mortgage deductions, credits for child care, and deductions for dependent children directly influence family life. Legislation regarding aid to dependent children, Medicaid, Medicare, and school lunch programs influences the lives of low-income families. Tax breaks afforded the affluent influence the monetary gifts given to offspring. Although one may argue that government policy is too little in many areas, unfair in some, and too much in others, the general consensus is that a successful family perspective is one that affords the greatest freedom yet protects individual environments so that children and the less fortunate are protected.

Futurists predict that health care will consume an even larger portion of the nation's income. Payers will attempt to hold down health care spending through cost sharing or rationing. Americans fret over the spiraling costs of health care and now seem willing to pay more taxes to gain health insurance not limited to the work place. If current needs are not met, demands for future needs will be even greater. One solution may be to closely examine the biomedical model, which has been ineffective in the areas of stress, substance abuse, infant mortality, the aging population, chronic diseases, and wise use of technology. Public policy will need to include nurses as primary caregivers and recipients of third-party payments. Nursing has demonstrated the cost effectiveness of home care, primary care, and the value of prevention over restoration of health. It is time for nursing to become involved in policy formation to provide care for the least advantaged, as well as for those who are fortunate enough to have adequate health coverage.

Certainly some public policy has never been successfully resolved. The issue of national health insurance is a problem that continues. Bioethical concerns regarding life-and-death genetic engineering, fetal transplants, and rationing of health care will continue into the 2000s. The American people are becoming involved in these issues through a rapidly growing grassroots movement. Community health decision projects are indirect agents of change. Through public forums, people come together to think about and discuss their own health beliefs and values in an attempt to influence public policy. Community health decision groups exist in Oregon, California, Iowa, Illinois, Maine, and Washington. Each is successful in influencing public policy on health care issues related to distribution of block grant funds, access to health, and health insurance. These projects may be the wave of the future, and "we, the people" may indeed resolve the remaining difficult health care decisions rather than await government action. The primary social aspects that concern Americans today are listed in Box 4-1.

Box 4-1 Social Concerns of Americans

Drug abuse
Cost of medical care
Federal budget deficit
Unemployment
Crime
Loss of manufacturing jobs
Alcoholism
Plight of farmers
AIDS
Poverty
Smoking
Pornography
Threat of nuclear war

CRITICAL THINKING *Activities*

1. **What factors are in favor of or against national health insurance? What is your position?**
2. **What are major obstacles to access to health care in the United States?**
3. **What underserved populations are a societal concern in the United States in today's society? In what ways?**
4. **How can nurses affect the health care delivery systems to improve access to adequate health care?**

References

1. American Association of Retired Persons: *Aging in America,* Washington, D.C., 1988, American Association of Retired Persons.
2. American Association of Retired Persons: *A profile in older Americans,* Washington, D.C., 1988, American Association of Retired Persons.
3. Barhydt-Wezenaar N: Home health and hospice. In Jonas S, ed: *Health care delivery in the United States,* ed 3, New York, 1986, Springer.
4. Berger S: *What your doctor didn't learn in medical school,* New York, 1988, William Morrow.
5. Bolhni P, Siem H: Health needs of migrants, World Health 48:20-21, 1995.
6. Centers for Disease Control and Prevention (CDC): Economic impact of motor-vehicle crashes—United States, 1990, *MMWR* 42:443, 1993.
7. Clinton H: Nurses in the forefront, *Nursing and Health Care* 14(6):286, 1993.
8. Dellums R: The Health Service Act, H.R. 2969, *Congressional Record* 125(33), 1979.
9. Friedman M, Rosenman R: *Type A behavior and your heart,* New York, 1971, Knopf.
10. Gartrell N and others: the national lesbian family study, *J Orthopsychiatry* 66(2):272, 1996.
11. Harrington C, Lempert L: Medicaid: a public program in distress, *Nurs Outlook* 36(1):6, 1988.
12. Health Care Financing Association: *Health Care Finance Rev* 9(3):68, 1988.
13. Hiatt H: *Medical lifeboat,* New York, 1987, Harper & Row.

14. Holmes T, Rahe R: The social readjustment rating scale, *J Psychosomat Res* 11:213, 1961.
15. Illich I: Medical nemesis. In Lee P, Brown N, Red I, eds: *The nation's health,* San Francisco, 1980, Boyd & Fraser.
16. Institute of Medicine: Preventing low birth rate, Washington, D.C., 1985, National Academy of Sciences.
17. Kalish B, Kalish P: *Politics and nursing,* Philadelphia, 1982, Lippincott.
18. Kaufman R: Abortion. In Hiller M, ed: *Medical ethics and the law,* Cambridge, MA, 1981, Ballinger.
19. Kimball M: Hospital Medicare profits collapsing, *Health Week* 2(3):1, 36, February 1, 1988.
20. Mason D, Talbott S: *Political action handbook for nurses,* Menlo Park, CA, 1985, Addison-Wesley.
21. National Center for Health Care: Statistics Organization: *National vital statistics system,* Hyattsville, MD, 1990.
22. National Center for Statistics and Analysis: *Fatal accident reporting system file, 1992,* Washington, D.C., 1993, U.S. Department of Transportation, National Highway Traffic Safety Administration.
23. National Highway Traffic Safety Administration: *Traffic safety facts 1992: alcohol,* Washington, D.C., 1993, U.S. Department of Transportation, National Highway Traffic Safety Administration.
24. National Hospice Organization: *Hospice principles and standards,* Washington, D.C., 1979, National Hospice Organization.
25. Office of Plans and Policy, National Highway Traffic Safety Administration: Saving lives and dollars: highway safety contribution to health care reform and deficit reduction, Publication no. DOT-HS-808-047/NPP-32, Washington, D.C., 1993, U.S. Department of Transportation, National Highway Traffic Safety Administration.
26. Richardson E: Health care crisis in America, 1971, testimony before the Subcommittee on Health of the Committee on Labor and Public Welfare, U.S. Senate, Feb. 22, 1971.
27. Rowland D: Meeting the long-term care needs of an aging population. In Schramm CJ, ed: *Health care and its costs,* New York, 1987, Norton.
28. Shorr A, Moen P: The single parent and public policy. In Skolnick A, Skolnick J, eds: *Family in transition,* ed 4, Boston, 1983, Little, Brown.
29. Spector M: Searching for the best medical care money can't buy, *The Washington Post* National Weekly Edition, December 25-31, 1989.
30. Thompson KD: Hot industries for small businesses, *Black Enterprise* 23(8):61, March 1993.
31. U.S. Bureau of the Census: *Statistical abstract of the United States,* Washington, D.C., 1966, U.S. Bureau of the Census.
32. U.S. Centers for Disease Control and Prevention (CDC): HIV/AIDS surveillance report, Atlanta, 1,3,8, July 1992.
33. U.S. Department of Health: *Healthy people 2000,* DHHS Publication N. (PHS) 91-50213, Washington, D.C., 1990, U.S. Printing Office.

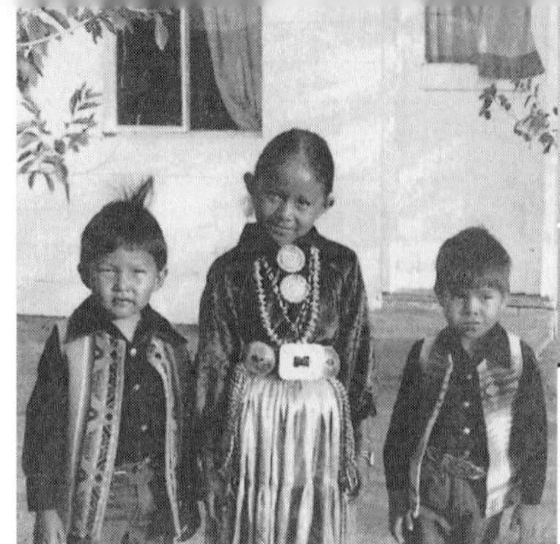

CHAPTER 5

Cultural Influences on Nursing

Kem B. Louie

OBJECTIVES

After completing this chapter the reader should be able to:

- **Define culture and how it manifests itself**
- **Describe the changes in American society since the melting pot theory was predominant**
- **List some physiologic and physical characteristics that nurses must assess accurately when caring for various ethnic peoples**
- **Identify some ways in which cultural beliefs and values of an individual may alter a nurse's plan of care for that individual**
- **Give several examples of how a nurse can achieve a desired goal for a client while staying within the context of that person's cultural patterns, beliefs, and values**
- **Make a general overall cultural assessment of an individual, family, and group**
- **Describe the reader's own cultural beliefs, values, and behaviors that can affect nursing care if not recognized and accounted for when caring for a client of another culture**
- **Define the goal of transcultural nursing**

The world is a global community. The advent of satellite technology has made communications faster and more readily available; news is transmitted around the world as quickly as it was once relayed across the backyard fence. Modern transportation makes access to remote corners of the earth an everyday occurrence; jet travel takes hours, whereas more primitive modes of travel used to take weeks and even months. Not only are people around the world more aware of each other, but they are also intermingling to a greater extent as immigrations and migrations make the world a giant mobile society. The ultimate outcome of these

You and I
We meet as strangers, each carrying a mystery
within us, I cannot say who you are.
I may never know you completely.
But I trust that you are a person in your own
right, possessed of a beauty and value that are
the Earth's richest treasures.
So I make this promise to you:
I will impose no identities upon you, but will
invite you to become yourself
without shame or fear.
I will hold open a space for you in the world and
allow your right to fill it with an authentic
vocation and purpose. For as long as your search
takes, you have my loyalty.

Author unknown

changes is an increased merging of the global population, which brings with it demands for new cultural understandings.

Nursing is one of the frontline professions that keenly feels the impact of this diverse population shift. It is no longer sufficient to practice an ethnocentric nursing protocol and expect it to meet needs universally. Each culture has a set of values and beliefs that are inextricably intertwined with health-related behaviors. Nurses are developing and utilizing cultural knowledge and skills that would promote understanding of health care practices in transcultural situations.

■ SOCIETAL FACTORS AFFECTING DEVELOPMENT OF TRANSCULTURAL NURSING

The social programs of the 1960s made a significant impact on nursing. Nurses began to see more Medicare and Medicaid clients whose income was below poverty level.

Minority groups traditionally have been among the poorer segments of the population. As poorer people receive more health care as a result of increased social welfare funding, ethnic minority groups are often recipients as well. Increased participation of ethnic minority groups in the health care system brought a new awareness of their needs to the nursing profession, which in turn added impetus to finding ways for better understanding of their cultural needs.

A second social factor that brought pressure on nursing to address multicultural needs was the rapid influx of immigrants. During the 1970s an average of half a million immigrants entered the United States legally each year. Two minorities in particular added considerable numbers to the American population: 15 million Spanish-speaking persons and 3.5 million Asian Americans. Previously African Americans were the only minority of significant number.[24] During the 1980s over 6 million immigrants legally entered the United States. Of this number, approximately 600,000 were from Europe; 2.5 million were from Asia; over 1.5 million were from Mexico, Central America, and South America; and 150,999 were from Africa.[33]

Immigration of peoples with birthrates different from those of ethnic groups already residing in the United States has produced a change in ethnic composition. The white European population decreased 6% between 1980 and 1990, while the African American population increased by 13.2% and persons of Hispanic origin increased by 53%.[31] Population projections show an acceleration in this trend, with the white European population composing approximately 69% of the total population, African Americans 14.5%, Hispanics 6.5%, and Asian Americans 9.9% by the year 2025.[20]

Over the past 25 years transcultural nursing has emerged as a formal area of study and an explicit practice in nursing with a definite set of goals and purposes. A variety of societal factors, including the advent of Medicare and Medicaid, the rapid influx of immigrants, and the civil rights movement, has influenced the direction of nursing toward multicultural interests.

As the need for a better understanding of ethnic-minority cultural values became evident, educators addressed their problem by incorporating transcultural content into nursing curricula on the undergraduate and graduate levels. Nurses, who shared a common interest in advancing the field of transcultural nursing, joined forces and organized national conferences, societies, and councils.

Technical advances continue to bring peoples of the world closer, creating a greater demand for nurses who understand other cultures. Nurses have made marked progress in the past two decades toward seeking a better understanding of other cultures. In view of the size and complexity of the world, however, the challenge still lies before nurses, who have only just begun the task.

■ MEANING OF CULTURE

Culture is an accepted set of values, beliefs, and behaviors shared within a social group.[30] Culture influences the ways in which people express themselves, as well as the foods they eat, and establishes the rules—spoken and unspoken—within which people operate.[19]

Many variations exist within, and between, cultures. Each person may belong to more than one subculture within a major culture. For instance, over 254 million people in the United States[12] form the American culture, and within this culture numerous subcultures share common characteristics within the group but not necessarily American culture as a whole. Although born in the same country, teenagers living on farms in rural Iowa may find it difficult to relate to teenagers raised on the streets of Los Angeles; they may speak the same language but have so many diverse experiences and perspectives that they cannot relate to one another.

Culture is like a template used as a pattern to make duplicate copies. Members of a society attempt to preserve the status quo for the next generation by replicating their values, beliefs, and behaviors, much as a template would be used to make copies. Imagine, however, a template made of soft cardboard. After multiple tracings the edges begin wearing and the new copies differ somewhat from the previous ones. After a while the original template is discarded and the copies, each of which has taken on its own unique variations, are used as new templates. Imagine also that periodically someone introduces a variation of the template that is thought to be superior to the old one, resulting in a new line of copies that develop their own changes over time. For many reasons, the templates of culture develop variations that result in changes from one generation to the next, as well as in a multiplicity of subcultures.

■ CULTURAL DIVERSITY

The United States has been described as a melting pot in which diverse groups from all over the world gather and are encouraged to forsake many of their native traditions and become homogenized as Americans. In the past those who attempted to retain native beliefs, customs, and language were often scorned, ridiculed, and otherwise made to feel like misfits.

Fortunately, the melting pot theory is slowly changing to appreciation and acceptance of other cultures, described by some as the *stewpot theory.*[11] In stew each ingredient is enhanced and becomes more flavorful as a result of exposure to the distinctive flavors of the other food items. The mingling of cultures can be likened to the stewpot. When each individual culture is allowed to exist and, more importantly, is appreciated and valued for its unique contribution to society, the cultural stewpot will become more "flavorful." One's perspective on the world in general and one's own culture in particular will be broadened and enlightened when an appreciation is gained for cultures different from one's own.

The melting pot theory also presumes that all cultures that change over time acculturate into the larger or dominant group and become Americans. *Acculturation* is a term that means a cultural group unconsciously adopts the attitudes, beliefs, and traditions of another group. Acculturation is a process of normal change when two cultures interact. Acculturation may not be considered desirable by some groups, and varying degrees of acculturation exist. Some groups may have the outward appearance of acculturation to Western values, such as wearing dress suits, speaking English, and eating fast foods, but when they are in their homes traditional languages and behaviors are expected. Spector (1991) suggests the concept of "heritage consistency" as a means of assessing the degree of maintaining their traditional heritage.

Others have used the term *cultural relativism.*[8a] This is the understanding of the cultural group and members in their own view rather than the view of the larger culture. All behaviors are relative to the context from which they are learned. Each member of any culture is understood and known by its unique characteristics, values, and beliefs.

Timely and appropriate nursing care is not always instituted because of a basic lack of knowledge about other cultures. Frequently health care workers learn only one perspective of managing care. Branch and Paxton[10] noted that ethnic persons of color receive less than optimal nursing care when nurses lack basic knowledge of culture. For example, recognizing cyanosis in a client with dark skin can be a challenge for nurses who have worked with clients who have light skin. Nurses should be taught assessment skills for noting signs and symptoms such as cyanosis and jaundice in persons of all skin colors.

Nurses must be aware that certain disease conditions are prevalent in certain population groups and relatively nonprevalent (or even absent) in others. For example, phenylketonuria is a chronic condition that is especially prevalent in infants of European descent. It occurs rarely among African Americans. On the other hand, sickle cell anemia is found only among African Americans.

Cultural factors that affect an individual's illness and care and thus are a concern of nursing services include the following:

1. Client's role and status in the family
2. Social, material, and professional support
3. Family and group treatment of clients with chronic illness
4. Identification and interpretation of symptoms of illness
5. Acceptable manifestations of pain and discomfort

For example, young Amish men are taught to be stoic in the face of excruciating pain, whereas Philippine women have what appears to be a very low tolerance for pain.

Cultural factors also influence the ways in which people interact with health care professionals. Cultural and ethnic differences influence differences in delivery of health and social service. However, while considering group differences within the larger cultural (ethnic) group, one must also be aware of individual differences within the groups.

■ CULTURAL BELIEFS

Cultural beliefs that may appear strange and unfounded to persons from other cultures can be deeply rooted and greatly influence behavior. Some beliefs produce positive effects, and others produce negative ones. Certain beliefs of the Masai women of Kenya, Africa, are examples of those that produce beneficial effects. Because the Masai are primarily nomadic herdsmen, they acquire very few material possessions. Their simple grass-thatched dwellings are furnished with little more than the skins stretched and preserved from their herds. The only beds available are animal skins laid on the bare ground. The women believe that laying a newborn baby on this hard surface may cause the baby's head to become misshapen. To prevent this problem from occurring, the women in the tribe take turns, night and day, holding newborn babies throughout their first week of life.[22]

Health care workers know that one of the primary causes of neonatal deaths in third world countries is hypothermia,[21] of which the Masai women are unaware. The women hold newborns to protect their heads from hard surfaces, but it is probably the 98.6° human incubator effect that is the beneficial factor. Regardless of the rationale behind the belief, the fact remains that the end result is a positive one since babies thrive better when they are held during the first week of life.

On the other hand, some of the Masai beliefs can be quite detrimental. One belief contends, for instance, that if a woman eats very little when she is pregnant, she will have a small infant, which will ensure an easy delivery. Pregnant women are, therefore, encouraged to eat nothing but a porridge made of maize. The end result may indeed be a small infant, but one who has not had the advantage of good prenatal nutrition. An additional effect of this nutritional deprivation is the physical depletion of the mother, which results in an inability to sustain successful breast-feeding.[21] It is obvious that this belief has negative effects in this situation.

In other cases beliefs have neither obvious positive nor negative effects; they are simply used to explain the unexplainable. For example, a common belief among mothers living in the *bateys,* or sugar cane fields, of the Dominican Republic is that of *mal de ojo,* or the evil eye. One of the mothers relates an event in which her 2-month-old daughter was taken to the small store on the batey by an older sister. A woman who was also shopping at the store said, "Be careful, don't let the baby fall down. Give her to me. I will hold her while you shop." When the woman took the baby, she exclaimed, "What a beautiful baby. She's such a beautiful child." The mother relating the story went on to explain that this interaction, the verbal admiration or *mal de ojo,* caused the infant to become seriously ill. When the baby arrived home, the mother immediately discovered it had a high fever, a cold, and diarrhea. She contended the baby was very healthy before going to the store. She said she believed the only reason the baby survived the spell was because the *curandera,* or local healer, was consulted and invoked a "friendly" spirit to deal with the evil spirit cast by the *mal de ojo.*

Mothers in this culture protect their children by tying red rags or red strings around their children's wrists. It is commonly believed that ordinary people, male or female, in addition to persons with supernatural powers, can be born with the power to give *mal de ojo.* It is believed they are not necessarily evil people; they are simply victims themselves, because they cannot rid themselves of the power.

A nurse in this culture discovers that it is extremely important to be aware of this belief. Verbal admiration of a child, which is highly valued in some cultures, could be viewed in other cultures as a threat to the child and render the nurse powerless because of the mother's fears. In that case, a nurse who maintains a sincere but strictly professional interest in a child will likely earn the trust of a mother more quickly than one who tries to create a more personal relationship by admiring a child.

■ CULTURAL VALUES

Cultural values refer to the powerful, persistent, and directive forces that give meaning, order, and direction to the individual, family, or group actions, decisions, and lifeways.[17] Values are beliefs about which one feels strongly and will go to great lengths to preserve. Values vary significantly from culture to culture and are sometimes diametrically opposed. The wide diversity of some commonly held values is illustrated in Box 5-1. If persons from a variety of cultures were given this questionnaire, some would strongly agree with the beliefs listed on the left, whereas others would strongly agree with the opposite view listed on the right of the box.

Those who view their own culture as superior and reject all other cultures as being underdeveloped, inferior, or second-class hold a belief called *ethnocentrism.* The problem that evolves from ethnocentrism is not necessarily the belief that one's own culture is the best. As a matter of fact, this belief would usually suggest one has adapted well to a specific culture.[31] The problem occurs when the health care professional attempts to impose personal values on others, believing not only that one's own way is the best way, but also believing it is the *only* way. Ethnocentrism can be extremely limiting in the health care field because the nurse who holds this belief may assess and plan intervention for the client, as well as evaluate the effectiveness of what was done, based on personal perceptions and values without taking into account the perceptions and beliefs of the client. Health care managed in this way often fails from the beginning because of the lack of communication and understanding between the health care worker and the client.

Box 5-1 Cultural Values

Directions:

Circle 1 if you strongly agree with the statement on the left. Circle 2 if you agree with the statement on the left.		*Circle 3 if you agree with the statement on the right. Circle 4 if you strongly agree with the statement on the right.*
1. Preparing for and influencing the future are important parts of being a responsible adult	1 2 3 4	Life follows a preordained course; the individual should follow that course
2. Vague and tentative answers are dishonest and confusing	1 2 3 4	Vague answers are sometimes preferred because they avoid embarrassment and confrontation
3. Punctuality and efficient use of time are reflections of intelligence and concern	1 2 3 4	Punctuality is rarely important and should be subordinate to such concerns as maintaining a relaxed atmosphere, enjoying the moment, and being with family and friends
4. When in severe pain, it is better and more appropriate to remain stoic	1 2 3 4	When in severe pain, it is better to vent the discomfort vocally and physically
5. It is presumptuous and unwise to accept a gift from someone you do not know well	1 2 3 4	It is an insult to refuse a gift when it is offered
6. Addressing someone by their first name shows friendliness	1 2 3 4	Addressing someone by their first name is disrespectful
7. Direct questions are usually the best way to gain information	1 2 3 4	Direct questioning is intrusive, rude, and potentially embarrassing
8. Direct eye contact shows interest	1 2 3 4	Direct eye contact is intrusive
9. Ultimately, the independence of the individual must come before the needs of the family	1 2 3 4	The needs of the individual are always subordinate to the needs of the family

Modified from Renwick GW, Rhinesmith SH: *An exercise in cultural analysis for managers,* Chicago, Intercultural Press.
In Thiederman S: Ethnocentrism: a barrier to effective health care, *Nurs Pract* 11(8): 54, 1986.

Parenting and child-rearing behaviors are based on cultural values and may differ from those of the nurse. For example, several cultures believe that it is appropriate to sleep with their infants and young children to give them a sense of security and trust.[10b]

Cultural values sometimes change significantly and then come back full circle to previously held values. Breast-feeding is an example of this change in the United States. In pioneer days women breast-fed because it was the only practical option they had. With the advent of bottles and readily available formulas, however, bottle-feeding grew in popularity and breast-feeding fell into disfavor. However, as the benefits of breast-feeding, for both mother and baby, become more widely publicized, breast-feeding is once again highly valued in the United States.

■ CULTURAL HEALTH ISSUES

Since culture permeates and influences every facet of a person's actions, it is understandable that health and treatment are determined to some extent by cultural beliefs and practices. For instance, members of Jehovah's Witnesses are opposed to blood transfusions. As another example, it is known that the numbers of reported cases of AIDS/HIV disease are dramatically increasing in some ethnic and minority groups.[8] Sociocultural attitudes and values may affect whether treatment or prevention of a specific condition is accepted or rejected. For instance, some cultural beliefs are fatalistic, causing individuals to believe they have no control over their own destiny; other beliefs would affect specific practices such as the use of condoms. In some countries, long-held traditions of polygamy or multiple sex partners rapidly promulgate new cases of AIDS. "Since various cultures have diverse beliefs and attitudes about intimacy, sexuality, health, illness, medical treatment, drug use, and death, the challenge is to understand the nature of the cultural differences of others. Care providers and educators need to be aware of this diversity to respond with culturally sensitive behavior."[8] The stance of the ANA is that "the provision of skilled, knowledgeable, and compassionate nursing care that respects client conscience and integrity, cultural values, beliefs, relationships, and the right to make choices" should be upheld by the profession.[8]

■ CROSS-CULTURAL COMMUNICATION

Communication is a continuous process whereby the person conveys ideas and messages to another. This can be accomplished through verbal communication, written communication, gestures, facial expressions, body language, space or distance between the two individuals, and other symbols. Communication, particularly in nursing, has a therapeutic effect in caring for others. This process of communication becomes even more important when caring for a client from a different culture who speaks a different language than does the nurse.

According to Giger and Davidhizar,[11a] various factors influence communication:

1. Physical health and emotional well-being
2. The situation being discussed and the meaning it has
3. Distractions to the communication process
4. Knowledge of the matter being discussed
5. Skill at communication
6. Attitudes toward the other person and toward the subject being discussed
7. Personal needs and interests
8. Background, including cultural, social, and philosophic values
9. The senses involved and their functional ability
10. Personal tendency to make judgments and be judgmental to others
11. The environment in which the communication takes place
12. Past experiences that relate or are related to the present situation

The most obvious communication barrier is for the non–English-speaking client. It is important to be aware of misunderstandings because of language barriers. Orque[28] relates a case in which an English-speaking nurse gave a non–English-speaking client preoperative instructions. The nurse explained the way in which povidone-iodine should be used to prepare the area preoperatively; the client nodded and smiled, indicating she understood. Unfortunately, the client had not understood, and drank the bottle of solution rather than applying it topically. Fortunately the error was discovered immediately, and appropriate measures saved the client's life. Demonstrations followed by return demonstrations are usually a more appropriate way of validating understanding across language barriers than relying solely on spoken language. Ideally, of course, both nurse and client speak the same language.

Generally, when the client does not speak English it is common to call for an interpreter. Louie has noted several ways to effectively communicate with a client using an interpreter:[18a]

1. Explain the reason for the interview and the type of questions to the interpreter. This information will assist the interpreter in eliciting general or literal responses, essay or short answers from the client.
2. Introduce the interpreter to the client. If possible, allow some time for them to become acquainted.
3. Speak directly to the client and allow the interpreter to translate. Do not interrupt the interpreter or client when either is speaking.
4. After the interview, spend some time with the interpreter to share information about the nonverbal communication and ease of obtaining information from the client.
5. Whenever possible, arrange for clients to speak to the same interpreter each time they are interviewed.

The nurse needs to be aware that certain cultural groups have different styles and types of feedback in the communication process. For example, some members of cultural groups prefer to engage in small talk before formal questions are asked. Other members may respond with a yes, a nod, or a smile, but this does not indicate understanding. Nurses have commonly interpreted this as compliance and understanding. The smiling and nodding are gestures of respect for the nurse and avoidance of confrontation. Nurses need to develop other measures of a client's understanding rather than just a verbal response or gesture.

Other different communication preferences include voice qualities, intonation, rhythm, speed, pronunciation, and the use of silence. Asian Americans and Native Americans generally use a softer volume in their speech. American nurses generally are known for speaking at a rapid pace and using medical jargon. Silence also has cultural meanings for many groups. For example, English and Arabic persons use silence for privacy, and Russian, French, and Spanish persons use silence to denote agreement. Some traditional Asian Americans view silence as a respect for elders.

Other nonverbal communication misunderstandings have occurred because of the lack of understanding to the meaning of touch, facial gestures, eye movements, and body postures for members of cultural groups. Touching in various cultures can convey power, affirmation, empathy, communication, frustration and anger, intrusion into privacy, sexual arousal, and cordiality. It is important that the nurse use touch judiciously.

■ CULTURAL COMPETENCE

The term *cultural competence* has several meanings, and there is no consensus regarding them.[18a] The standard goal of caring for clients whose cultural background is different from the nurse is cultural competence.

Campinha-Bacote, in her culturally competent model, categorizes four components: cultural awareness, cultural knowledge, cultural skills, and cultural encounter.[10a] Cultural awareness involves the respect for clients from diverse cultural

TABLE 5-1

Cultural Sophistication Framework

	Culturally Incompetent	Culturally Sensitive	Culturally Competent
Cognitive Dimension	Oblivious	Aware	Knowledgeable
Affective Dimension	Apathetic	Sympathetic	Committed to change
Skills Dimension	Unskilled	Lacking some skills	Highly skilled
Overall Effect	Destructive	Neutral	Constructive

From Orlandi M: Cultural sophistication framework. In Orlandi M, Weston R, Epstein L: *Cultural competence for evaluators,* (OSAP Cultural Competence Series) HHS Pu. (ADM) 92-1884, 1992, U.S. GPO.

backgrounds. Cultural knowledge is the ability of the nurse to gather cultural information from the client. Cultural skill involves the ability to make a cultural assessment. Cultural encounters are skills to which nurses interact with clients in cross-cultural situations.

Orlandi has defined cultural competence as "a set of academic and interpersonal skills that allow individuals to increase their understanding within, among, and between groups. This requires a willingness and ability to draw on community-based values, traditions, and customs and to work with knowledgeable persons from the community in developing focused interventions, communications, and other supports." Orlandi views cultural competence as multidimensional, involving aspects of knowledge (cognitive dimensions), attitude (affective dimension), and skill development (skills dimension). The Cultural Sophistication Framework (Table 5-1) describes the three dimensions of cultural competence along a continuum of cultural incompetence, cultural sensitivity, and cultural competence. This framework allows the individual to assess what he or she needs to work on to become culturally competent. It is important to recognize that with each different cultural group the process of cultural competence is required. Nurses must identify the cultural group(s) in the community in which they provide care and assess their level of cultural competence.

The American Academy of Nursing Panel (1992) suggested the following general principles for culturally competent care:

1. Acknowledge the client's situation and be sensitive to the need to have culturally specific content
2. Respect cultural norms, values, and communication/time patterns
3. Provide support for the cultural client to implement (if possible) his or her own solutions to care
4. Develop interpersonal competence and sensitivity on the part of the nurse

■ CULTURAL ASSESSMENT

A specific means of communicating cultural beliefs, values, and behaviors that are important in health care is through a formal cultural assessment. Cultural assessment places the nurse in a better position to meet the client's needs by enabling the nurse to understand cultural factors that influence people's health behaviors. If

Box 5-2 Assessment of Cultural Variables at Three Levels

	Beliefs	Customs	Values
Client			
Nurse			
Health care facility or agency			

culturally specific care is not achieved, clients become unhappy, uncooperative, and ultimately withdraw from the relationship. Remember that maintaining the dignity of the persons involved requires treating each as an equal who brings important and relevant cultural beliefs to the relationship. *Culture* is defined as a system of values, beliefs, and customs that an individual learns while growing up in the environment; it is largely an unconscious learning process.

Persons of different cultures define health in different ways. They also describe disease causation in different ways. They may describe a disease as having natural causes or as having supernatural causes, such as spirits or other phenomena. The Navajo, for example, theorize that illness has natural causes, whereas another tribal group explains the illness of a child as being caused by envy of an adult who admires the child (a result of what they label the "evil eye"). It is necessary that nurses be cognizant of the way in which the client is culturally conditioned to view his or her condition of illness.

Compliance with nursing and medical protocol also depends on the acceptance or way in which people deal with chronic illness and/or defects. A congenitally malformed child who is considered a shame and hidden from public view is not likely to keep appointments when parents feel the lack of acceptance and support from their social group or health care professionals. Nurses must learn to identify cultural variables and be able to alter nursing care interventions so that they are congruent with the client's cultural belief patterns.

Making Cultural Assessments*

Rather than impose personal cultural care values on others, the professional nurse is an active listener and analyst who develops appropriate care plans based on the insights, knowledge, and beliefs of other cultures. The problem in implementing this philosophy is the inclination of nurses to use their professional and culturally determined personal values and beliefs to give care to others.

Beliefs, customs, and values are variables at three levels: the client, the nurse, and the health care facility or agency (Box 5-2). When one is incongruent with any other, the incongruencies must be resolved. The format in the box can be used to measure the degree of congruency or incongruency. Following this format, the nurse may begin to plan nursing action and interventions.

Perhaps one of the greatest mistakes nurses make in working with culturally different persons is transferring expectations based on their own cultural background. This is easy to do and makes one feel secure, but the outcome may be a

*Parts of this section were contributed by Toni Tripp-Reimer.

Box 5-3 Parts of a Cultural Assessment

Values	Beliefs	Customs	Social Group Factors
Health	Health	Communication	Family structure
Nature of humanity	Health maintenance	Verbal	Religion
Human nature	Illness	Language	Politics
Time	Cause	Speed of talking	Education
Activity	Diagnosis	Style	Economy
Relationships	Treatments	Nonverbal	Health systems
	Religious	Touch	Formal
	Other	Space, interpersonal	Informal
		Silence	Alternative practitioners and facilities
		Eye contact	Ethnic identification
		Decision making	History
		Religion	Art
		Food	Physical environment
		Family roles/behavior	Other
		Death, dying	
		Other	

failure to obtain desired behavioral results. Another mistake is that of making generalizations about culturally different groups. Groups have subgroups whose core beliefs may be shared but whose language, customs, beliefs, and values may differ significantly. Subgroup ideas about the cause and cure of illness and health may or may not be shared. For example, there are over 500 tribes among Native Americans and over 25 subgroups of Asian Americans.

When language barriers are present it is difficult to ensure that clients are given care within the standards of the Patient Bill of Rights. For example, informed consent is not possible when the health care team and client speak different languages. The client may have a different set of beliefs regarding the meaning of a procedure based on values. An interpreter may be the only means of communicating. Because of fear and differences in values, it may be necessary to keep the number of procedures to a minimum for culturally different clients.

A culture is composed of a group of persons with a shared set of beliefs, customs, and values that dictates behavior common to the group. For a cultural assessment, a systematic study must include these factors.

A number of cultural assessment tools have been developed for use by health care professionals. Some are short and specific, whereas others are lengthy and comprehensive. Whether nurses choose to integrate cultural assessment in the nursing process or to conduct a specific and separate assessment should depend on the health problem and clinical setting. Regardless of how it is accomplished, cultural assessment should be included in the provision of health care. Guidelines are listed in Box 5-3.

The importance of accurate assessment of individual families and groups in planning nursing and overall health care cannot be overemphasized. The planning of residential communities often does not accommodate cultural preferences, and consequently nursing and health care are affected. Persons of certain European nationalities—for example, Czechs, Hungarians, Rumanians—may prefer to live in their own homes, but when that is not possible they are likely to accept long-term care facilities much more readily than persons of Amish or Greek origin. When working with clients of a given background, it is necessary as well to understand how families of these clients feel. If their feelings are not congruent, then additional factors must be worked out.

One example is that of nursing home planning. Adjustments can be made within the environment to stimulate the preferred living situation of persons for whom the facility is the least desirable care option. Amish clients may prefer an area of the building where clutter and noise of radios and TV are less. The nurse caring for a person from that culture should, as part of the nursing care plan, make a goal of providing an environment in which mechanical technology and its noise output are kept to a minimum. As client advocates nurses must be creative about making such adaptations. In suggesting actions, nurses can make life more satisfying and humanistic; for example, the Amish nursing home resident can benefit from short leaves of absence to a family farm to check on a horse or other animals. Restrictions from all that is meaningful can cause a client to become belligerent.

Psychiatric nurses who work with depressed clients need to look for insights into the cause of the depression by obtaining data specific to the cultural background of the client. For some ethnic groups, such as African Americans and Asian Americans, depression is expressed by complaints of physical and bodily discomfort rather than affective expression. For example, a young Greek man is depressed because he thinks he has betrayed the family's status of honor by moving his father to a nursing home. Cultural data make the nurse alert to social factors that may be the basis for depression and other conditions. This is useful in making an assessment and planning nursing interventions.

Nurses must include a cultural assessment in nursing care plans and while caring for individuals, either well or ill. Factors to consider are individual but are also influenced by cultural factors. Some factors to identify are whether the individual is a part of a cultural group that is predominantly made up of nuclear families, isolated individuals, or extended families. Also consider whether the society is male-dominated, female-dominated, or egalitarian. One must be aware of the difference between being strong and being dominant. For example, women demonstrate strength to preserve family life, but they are not necessarily dominant. Further, the nurse must recognize the overall characteristic, in this case male/female dominance, but remember that individual variations occur within the predominant pattern.

Basic cultural data include the following ethnic variables:

1. Religious preference
2. Pattern of family makeup (eating patterns, food preferences)
3. Patterns of caring for health

This knowledge can provide all the information that the nurse needs in many situations. When the client is inexplicably noncompliant with a recommended plan of care, knowing how to explore cultural data in greater depth is necessary to explain the client's behavior.

Box 5-4 Process of Cultural Assessment

	Beliefs	Customs	Values
DATA COLLECTION General content Ethnicity Degree of affiliation Problem content Diabetic diet Pregnancy Intervention			
DATA ORGANIZATION General content Problem content Intervention			
DATA INTERPRETATION General content Problem content Intervention			

Cultural assessment tools have been devised by numerous nurses. However, the goal here is to assist the student-reader to gain awareness of cultural patterns and differences and, as a professional nurse, apply them to the assessment of clients. Assessment models have been developed by Orque, Brownlee, Black, Tripp-Reimer, Admodt, Leininger, and Branch. Included here is a basic assessment format (Box 5-4).

After the nurse identifies the client's ethnicity, degree of identification with ethnic roots, religion, and decision-making process, the next step is to obtain more specific data. To do so, pertinent questions must be answered. Appropriate questions for obtaining cultural information about specific health problems are provided in the following six sample questions:

1. What do you think caused your problem?
2. How did it start?
3. How bad/serious is your illness?
4. How does your sickness work?
5. What treatments do you think will make you well?
6. What frightens you about your sickness?

Before planning nursing actions or interventions the nurse needs further information that is designed to obtain cultural data. The following six sample questions can be useful:

1. Is your situation good or bad?
2. Have you had this problem before, and what do (did) you do for it?
3. What should a person do if he or she has this problem?
4. What are you planning to do about your situation?
5. How should a person in your situation (with your sickness) be treated by your family?
6. How should people in the community treat you?

Values have been categorized into the following four aspects:

1. **Time** is *past, present,* and *future;* cultural groups vary in the emphasis placed on one versus the others.
2. **Personal activity** orientation of a culture has emphasis on either *doing* or *being.* An example of the former is a culture that emphasizes personal accomplishments. A culture that is being-oriented values a person simply for existing; for example, being a link between generations.
3. **Relationship orientation** can be broken down into several categories; in societies such as Russia and Israel, a *collateral* pattern of rational behavior predominates because individuals are concerned with others on a lateral plane as members of their own groups; other societies stress the importance of *lineage,* and kinship is emphasized in terms of maintaining lineality, usually stressing that the males carry the major responsibility for lineage.
4. **Orientation of the individual to nature** describes how the culture views *humanity* and *nature,* and what has major emphasis; for example, nature over humanity, humanity over nature.

An aspect of nursing care is concern for nutritional status. Cultural differences within the mainstream of American society affect nutritional status. Persons born in the United States have profound differences in food habits depending on ethnic origin, socioeconomic status, beliefs, and religious background. These habits can serve as risks to good health. Persons of Scandinavian origin tend to prefer cheese and fish, Mexicans tend to eat cornmeal and highly spiced foods, and Asians tend to like fish and vegetables. To determine nutritional balance in a person's diet, have clients keep a 7-day dietary record of all foods eaten; at the end of that period review the record for congruency with the requirements of a well-balanced diet.

Religious affiliation also influences food intake and nutritional status. Orthodox Jews eat only kosher foods of a certain kind that are prepared according to Jewish law. Some conservative Christian denominations sponsor frequent church suppers or potluck meals, which are heavily concentrated with high-calorie desserts, salads, and macaroni dishes that have little meat.

The nurse receives verbal or nonverbal messages from clients that indicate both whether an assessment is accurate and whether the nursing care provided is congruent with that client's expectations. In other words, by being attentive to what the client communicates, the nurse and/or health care facility can tell whether it has appropriately crossed cultural lines. When actions and messages are culturally acceptable to the client, then the client, nurse, and facility can proceed on the same wavelength.

One behavior that may be observed when providing care to culturally different people is *passive obedience.* This may be explained in various ways, but could result from a belief by the client that the nurse or other health care worker is an authority figure or an expert. The Southeast Asian person is apt to cope with uncertainty and authority in the same way—by being passively obedient. Instead of asking questions when uncertain, such a person may conceal lack of knowledge by being obedient or compliant.

Sometimes when clients are labeled as noncompliant, it is because of an inaccurate cultural assessment by the nurse or other health workers. The client may not understand or may be unable to accomplish expectations. Noncompliance among persons of different cultures may have bases associated with cultural perceptions of the client. Reasons for lack of compliance with planned care, in the case of a Vietnamese refugee, may be disappearance of the symptoms, inconvenience, and lack of precedent for continuing the regimen. This lack of compliance is reinforced when there is a relative lack of other supports such as family and social encouragement, absence of knowledge about treatment of asymptomatic conditions, and the precedent of traditional self-care and self-medication.

Refugees, in general, tend to seek care from health care providers because they feel alone, are alienated socially, and other sources of institutional support (school, church) are not available to them as a result of language and various barriers. They form a bond with people who demonstrate a caring attitude.

In the past several years nurses have become increasingly aware of a lack of professional training to prepare them for cross-cultural experiences. Some learn by doing as they travel to new environments and live with people in cultures different from their own. Some have frustrating experiences in other cultures as a result of a lack of understanding. Out of this frustration, however, has emerged a movement to become better informed about cultural beliefs through formal nursing education and interactions.

One of the pioneers in this new area of transcultural nursing was Madeleine Leininger. In 1955 she founded the field of transcultural nursing as a formal area of study and practice. Working as a psychiatric clinical nurse specialist in a guidance home for disturbed children in Ohio, Leininger observed the children's different reactions to nursing activities. Because they came from diverse cultural backgrounds such as African American, Spanish American, Jewish American, and Appalachian, she began looking at the association between their backgrounds and their actions.

Leininger was one of the first nurses to seek additional academic preparations through graduate study in anthropology at the University of Washington in 1959. She conducted fieldwork in New Guinea to become the first professional nurse to complete a doctoral program in cultural anthropology. In 1968 she organized the Committee on Nursing and Anthropology of the American Anthropological Association. The primary goal of this committee was to "help nurses and anthropologists work together to incorporate anthropological knowledge into nursing curricula."[17]

Leininger saw the critical need to prepare nurses in anthropology to develop the new field of transcultural nursing. Transcultural nursing is the branch of nursing that focuses on comparative study and analysis of cultures with respect to nursing and culturally determined health-illness practices, beliefs, and values. The goal is to develop a scientific and humanistic body of knowledge to provide caring, culturally based nursing care. Under her leadership educational programs in transcultural nursing began to develop. In the late 1960s and early 1970s she encouraged a core of nurse educators and practitioners to acquire a background in anthropology to assist in the development of the new discipline of transcultural nursing. She was instrumental in establishing the first transcultural nursing courses at the University of Colorado and, since then, has provided leadership in establishing graduate programs in transcultural nursing in several other universities.

As health care workers became involved in cultural settings different from their own, the following problems were identified:

1. Lack of knowledge about diversities in cultural beliefs and practices
2. Health care personnel difficulties in identifying relationships between social structures and health systems
3. Cultural shock, or feelings of helplessness and disorientation felt by the health giver, leading to ineffectiveness
4. Cultural imposition, or the imposition of the health worker's beliefs on another cultural group, resulting in distrust and, many times, failure of proposed health interventions

■ HISTORY AND EVOLUTION OF TRANSCULTURAL NURSING

Transcultural Nursing and Curricula

During the early 1970s several nurse-anthropologists encouraged the Western Commission on Higher Education in Nursing to help faculty members in schools of nursing develop cultural concepts in nursing curricula. By 1975 the word *culture* was appearing in nursing philosophies, objectives, and course descriptions of various schools. Several articles have since been published that give guidelines for including transcultural content in curricula.[9,17,23] In 1972 the University of Washington initiated a master's degree program in transcultural nursing, and Pennsylvania State University started a similar program in 1974. A more recent program is the Nursing School at Wayne State University. The University of Utah approved a master's degree program in transcultural nursing in 1977, and later that same year initiated the first Ph.D. program in the field. By 1984 four master's and five doctoral programs focused on transcultural nursing, while over 20% of the baccalaureate and associate degree programs included courses or material on transcultural nursing.[18] Most schools have added cultural concepts in varying concentrations to their curricula since that time.

The University of Miami School of Nursing, which emphasizes transcultural nursing, has emerged as one of the leaders in providing educational opportunities for nurses interested in cultures other than their own. Their undergraduate and graduate nursing programs incorporate a transcultural nursing curriculum. A $1 million endowment established funding of the William R. Ryan Distinguished Chair in Transcultural Nursing, as well as a Transcultural Nursing Research Institute.

The impetus for providing multicultural content in nursing continues to increase. In 1976 the ANA adopted the following statement as part of its Code for Nurses: "Consideration of individual value systems and lifestyles should be included in the planning and health care for each client."[1] ANA's Standards of Nursing Practice further indicate that health status data should include cultural background.[7] NLN supplied guidance for those responsible for providing nursing curricula by affirming in 1977 that "the curriculum is based on the philosophy, purposes, and objectives of the program and recognizes the contribution of nursing and other disciplines toward meeting the health needs of a diverse and multicultural society."[25]

In addition to transcultural nursing, some nurses also pursue degrees in related fields. Between 1965 and 1972, 28 nurses obtained graduate degrees in anthropology. By the late 1970s an estimated 55 nurses in the United States held master's degrees, and 45 had doctoral preparation in anthropology.[17] Appreciating cultural diversity, nurses recognize the need to shape nursing to meet the population's cultural needs, rather than expect the entire population to conform to their own ethnocentric model.

Even though nurses displayed a long-time interest in transcultural nursing, the events of the 1960s and 1970s added impetus for formal organization. Nurses' interest in transcultural nursing certainly was not generated in a vacuum; rather it emerged simultaneously with concerns in society at large. Interest in transcultural nursing and its relevance to care and health increased. Care behavior in transcultural nursing was later reflected in the organization of the Annual National Caring Conference, first held in 1978.

Transcultural Nursing Organizations

In 1974 a national transcultural conference on communications and culture was held at the University of Hawaii School of Nursing. That same year, under the leadership of Leininger, plans for a series of transcultural nursing conferences were initiated, with the objectives of bringing together nurses, anthropologists, and other social scientists who had expressed an interest in shaping the field of transcultural nursing. The first National Transcultural Nursing Conference was held in 1974 at the College of Nursing at the University of Utah. Subsequent conferences were held annually through 1978, with Leininger serving as conference chairperson. The first three conferences were organized around the life cycle, and the presentations focused on specific age categories. The fourth conference departed from the life cycle framework and focused on cultural change and ethics related to nursing care.

Subsequent conferences resulted in a desire to organize ongoing activities and interactions; this was formalized in the founding of the Transcultural Nursing Society in 1975. Originally initiated at the University of Utah, the Transcultural Nursing Society became independently and legally incorporated in 1981; it presently has a membership of around 400.[15] The official semiannual publication of the Society, the *Journal of Transcultural Nursing,* was initiated in 1989.

Soon after the Transcultural Nursing Society was organized, a group of nurses began to express concern for the ethnic composition of the nursing profession itself. In 1977 the Division of Nursing of the U.S. Department of Health and Human Services conducted a survey with the ANA to determine racial and ethnic composition of the registered nurse population. The study indicated that 6.2% of all registered nurses with active licenses were of an ethnic minority background.[6] Soon after the release of this report, the 1980 ANA House of Delegates reaffirmed ANA's commitment to increasing ethnic minorities in the nursing profession by adopting resolution number 52, which addressed the "recruitment, retention and graduation of minority persons in baccalaureate and higher-degree programs in nursing."[6]

About the same time, the ANA Commission on Human Rights sent a questionnaire to all ANA members who had identified themselves on their membership applications as members of an ethnic minority group.[3] Responses to the questionnaire indicated these members wanted to become more involved in their professional organization but felt it did not allow them to do so. The Human Rights Commission members proposed the formation of a council to provide direction in the development of programs on human rights concerns and to increase the responsiveness of nurses to cultural and ethnic variances among patients.[4] To obtain an indication of level of interest in their proposal, the commission surveyed its members at the 1978 and 1979 conferences. Approximately 130 members expressed an interest in joining a council that would focus on cultural and ethnic concerns.[3]

Nurses' interests in intercultural affairs were officially recognized by ANA in 1980 with the establishment of the Council on Intercultural Nursing. Approximately 30 ANA members applied for membership in the council at that time, and plans were made for election of an executive committee later that year. This council, initially under the chairmanship of Mildred Cox, was directly accountable to the ANA's Commission on Human Rights. Short-term goals adopted by the newly elected Council Executive Committee focused on involvement in national legislative issues concerning human rights and the dissemination of information regarding human rights issues to the membership at large.[2] In the first *Council of Intercultural Nursing Newsletter*, which was published in February/March of 1981, Chairperson Cox noted:

> While we have needed such a council over the past year, it is most apparent at this time that the number of ethnic minorities comprising our patient population is ever increasing. Nurses by necessity will be in the forefront of promoting safe and effective health care. Efforts of the council will be to focus on developing a mechanism to bring this about—to share with constituent nurses.[6]

In 1984 ANA moved the council from the Human Rights Commission to the Cabinet on Nursing Practice and changed the name from the Council on Intercultural Nursing to the Council on Cultural Diversity in Nursing Practice. The purpose of the move was to focus the attention of the council on the improvement of nursing practice through incorporation of cultural awareness. In addition, the council accepted as its 1984 goal the commitment "to promote the development of nursing curriculum models to provide culturally specific nursing care."[5] The focus of the Council broadened over the next decade, and by 1993 position papers had been prepared on career mobility for ethnic minorities in nursing as well as racism in nursing. They also developed guidelines for addressing issues of culture and cultural diversity in Informed Consent documents.

The membership roster for the Council on Intercultural Nursing reveals a wide variety of culturally diverse surnames.[13] Membership of ethnic minorities on the Council was undoubtedly encouraged by the original inquiry of interest that was targeted at nurses of ethnic and cultural minority backgrounds. This was further encouraged by ANA activities in the early 1980s that focused as much attention on the ethnic nurse as on the ethnic client.

Sensitivity to multiethnic issues in the workplace continued to increase and resulted in the adoption of a resolution by the 1993 ANA House of Delegates to collaborate with other nursing organizations to identify and promulgate strategies to promote diverse and multicultural nursing in the workforce. According to the resolution report, "Recent anecdotal evidence suggests that the nursing workforce environment mirrors the stresses and frustrations experienced in multiethnic and multicultural communities in the larger society. Reported incidents by nurses ranging from experiences of feeling isolated, verbal abuse from their colleagues, prejudicial work assignments, to actual physical violence resulting in injury, have been received.[8]

The Board of Directors of ANA gradually assumed an increasingly visible role in highlighting the health needs of the emerging ethnic majority. An informational report, submitted to the 1993 ANA House of Delegates by ANA President Virginia Trotter Betts, delineated the ANA's strategy in this area as being threefold: "to increase access to health care of minorities; to increase access to education for minorities, and to broaden the ANA's representation and work in minority communities."

The substructure of the entire ANA Congress of Nursing Practice was subsequently reviewed, with recommendations for major restructuring as it related to developing trends in nursing practice. The purposes of the restructuring were to advance the principles of *Nursing's Agenda for Health Care Reform* and to advance standards and public policy on the national level. The new Council configuration adopted by the ANA Board eliminated the Council on Cultural Diversity per se and instead integrated cultural awareness issues into all of the newly formed Councils.

Transcultural Nursing Research

Research and the acquisition of a sound knowledge base are crucial to the development of transcultural nursing. The primary goal for health personnel working in transcultural settings is to determine the dominant culture values, priorities, and characteristics of the cultural group, and then ascertain how best to provide for the needs of people.

As early as 1960 nurses began to use the ethnoscientific method to address a lack of knowledge in nursing. Encouraged by Leininger, nurses began a rigorous system to collect carefully documented statements of the indigenous people's views about *their* health care system.[16] According to Leininger,[14] advantages of the ethnoscience approach include the following:

1. A more accurate picture of a cultural group
2. An emphasis on importance of viewing health care from the client's viewpoint
3. Data for a sound basis for prediction studies and generalizations
4. Generation of nursing theories
5. Reduction of intuitive nursing

Nightingale once suggested, "in beginning new things we commence with the easier, and having mastered that, proceed to the more difficult."[26] Leininger believed ethnoscientific methods also should be implemented first on a small scale by studying one or two cultures in depth and then by following up with field studies. The knowledge base gradually expands as more in-depth studies are conducted and a variety of cultures is compared and contrasted. Tripp-Reimer[32] suggests that one of the reasons for lack of progress in this area is that cross-cultural research is conducted in a horizontal manner; in other words, one culture described, then another culture, and then another. Instead, she says, knowledge should be linked vertically; in other words, studies should be replicated or hypotheses retested so that the knowledge base can become more substantive.

Ultimately this classification and testing of transcultural knowledge "should generate new theories, different practices and clues for the prevention of illness."[16] Variables to investigate should include biophysiologic, genetic, environmental, social, and general cultural ways.[17]

In some of her later writings, Leininger recommended, in addition to the ethnoscience approach, the following methods:[17]

1. Participant observation
2. Descriptive survey
3. Experimental and control-group laboratory
4. Hypothesis testing
5. Paradigm and model

While nurses were organizing professional interest groups and defining the domains of the new subspecialty *culture,* society was not stagnant. Government decisions, grassroots pressures, and shifting populations were all changing and ultimately added impetus to the transcultural nursing movement.

■ SUMMARY

Nurses accept and respect the dignity of all individuals as they are, regardless of the setting or circumstances. In present American society few nurses are limited to caring for people exclusively from backgrounds that parallel their own. In the past, Native Americans, African Americans, Hispanics, and persons from Northern European cultures composed the major groups with which nurses interacted in daily practice. With the recent great influx of Asians, South Africans, persons from the Middle East, and now persons from the former Eastern Bloc, nurses are challenged to learn how to meet cross-cultural health care needs and foster communications.

One mistake a nurse can make is to generalize. For example, nursing care to the Native American cannot be planned and provided universally to all Native Americans without consideration of subgroup differences created by tribal differences.

The nurse should remember that cultural assessments and judgments are relative, based on experience, and experience is interpreted by persons based on their own cultural values and beliefs. One stereotypes people unconsciously on the basis of one's own value systems. Therefore, when performing a cultural assessment it is important not to stereotype, because persons in a cultural group may be more acculturated to the dominant society rather than their group of origin.

Significant changes in U.S. demographics require nurses to provide culturally competent care. Theories from anthropology and other fields are important, but each nurse must establish a foundation that has a nursing perspective. Transcultural nursing is developing knowledge through research and experience with ethnic cultural groups.

CRITICAL THINKING *Activities*

1. **Describe your own background in cultural terms using the three major categories of data (beliefs, values, customs).**
2. **Describe a situation you have encountered in which you feel you could have given better nursing care had you known the client's cultural background better.**
3. **Review briefly the history of transcultural nursing in the United States.**
4. **Ways to learn more about other cultures:**
   1. **Ask students from other cultures**
   2. **Speak to cultural community resources (e.g., churches' ethnic associations, community groups)**
   3. **Read about different cultures**

References

1. American Nurses Association: *Code for nurses with interpretive statements,* Kansas City, 1976, American Nurses Association.
2. American Nurses Association Commission on Human Rights, Council on International Nursing: *Executive Committee meeting minutes,* December 5–7, 1980, American Nurses Association.
3. American Nurses Association Commission on Human Rights: Historical background (unpublished).
4. American Nurses Association Commission on Human Rights: Guidelines for Council on Intercultural Nursing (unpublished).
5. American Nurses Association Council on Cultural Diversity in Nursing Practice: Operating guidelines (unpublished), 1984, The American Nurses Association.
6. American Nurses Association: *Council on Intercultural Nursing Newsletter,* 1(1), Feb./March 1981, American Nurses Association.
7. American Nurses Association: *Standards of nursing practice,* Kansas City, 1973, American Nurses Association.
8. American Nurses Association: *Summary of proceedings, 1993 House of Delegates,* Washington, D.C., 1993.

8a. Andrews MM, Boyle JS: *Transcultural concepts in nursing care,* ed 2, Philadelphia, 1995, Lippincott.

9. Branch M: Models for introducing cultural diversity in nursing curricula, *J Nurs Educ* 15(2): 7–13, 1976.
10. Branch M, Paxton P: *Providing safe nursing care for ethnic people of color,* New York, 1976, Appleton-Century-Crofts.

10a. Campinha-Bacote J: *The process of cultural competence: a culturally competent model of care,* ed 2, Ohio, 1994, Transcultural CARE Associates Press.

10b. Canuso R: Co-family sleeping: strange bedfellows or culturally acceptable behavior? *Cultural Diversity* 3: 109-111, 1996.

11. Donders JG: African Institute lecture, Notre Dame University, 1987.

11a. Giger JN, Davidhizar RE: *Transcultural nursing: assessment and intervention, St Louis, 1991, Mosby.*

12. Johnson O, exec. ed: *Information please almanac,* New York, 1993, Houghton Mifflin.

13. Johnson C: Data on ethnic nurses, *Council on Intercultural Nursing Newsletter* 1(1), Feb./March 1981.

14. Leininger M: Ethnoscience: a new and promising research approach for the health sciences, *Image* 3(1): 22–28, 1969.

15. Leininger M: Personal communication, June 11, 1993.

16. Leininger M: *Transcultural health care issues and conditions,* Philadelphia, 1976, F.A. Davis.

17. Leininger M: *Transcultural nursing: concepts, theories, and practices,* New York, 1978, Wiley.

18. Leininger M: *A decade of growth, discovery, and recognition,* paper presented at the Tenth National Transcultural Nursing Society Conference, Boston, October 1984.

18a. Louie KB: Cultural competence. In Allen K, ed: *Nursing care of the addicted client,* Philadelphia, 1996, Lippincott.

19. Major JL: Developing cultural sensitivity, *Calif Nurse* 83(2):5, 1987.

20. Mattson MT: *Atlas of the 1990 census,* New York, 1992, Macmillan.

21. Morely D: Personal interview, July 6, 1988, London, England.

22. Muntere A: Personal interview, July 18, 1988, Kenya, East Africa.

23. Muillo-Rohde I: Cultural diversity in curriculum development, Paper presented at "Chautauqua 76," sponsored by the Colorado Nurses Association, Vail, Col., July 1976. In Leininger M: *Transcultural nursing: concepts, theories, and practices,* New York, 1978, Wiley.

24. Naisbitt J: *Megatrends: ten new directions transforming our lives;* New York, 1982, Warner.

25. National League for Nursing, Council of Baccalaureate and Higher Degree Programs: *Criteria for the evaluation of baccalaureate and higher degree programs in nursing,* Pub. No. 15-1251 (ed. 5), New York, 1983, National League for Nursing.

26. Nightingale F: Suggestions on a system of nursing for hospitals in India. In Seymer L, compiler: *Selected writings of Florence Nightingale,* New York, 1954, Macmillan.

27. Orlandi M: Cultural sophistication framework. In Orlandi M, Weston R, Epstein L: *Cultural competence for evaluators,* (OSAP Cultural Competence Series) HHS Pu.(ADM) 92-1884, 1992, U.S. GPO.

28. Orque M: Orque's ethnic-cultural system: a framework for ethnic nursing care. In Orque M, Block B, Monrroy L: *Ethnic nursing care: a multicultural approach,* St. Louis, 1983, Mosby.

29. *Rand-McNally road atlas,* 1986, Library of Congress No. 79-62950.

30. Spradley B: *Community health nursing: concepts and practice,* ed 2, Boston, 1985, Little, Brown.

31. Thiedeman S: Ethnocentrism: a barrier to effective health care, *Nurse Pract* 11(8):56–59, 1986.

32. Tripp-Reimer T: Research in cultural diversity: directions for future research, *West Nur* 6(2):253–255, 1984.

33. United States Bureau of the Census: *Statistical abstract of the United States,* ed. 112, Washington, D.C., 1992.

Additional References

American Academy of Nursing Expert Panel Report: Culturally competent health care, *Nurs Outlook* 40(6):277–283, 1992.

Louie KB: Cultural issues in psychiatric-mental health nursing. In Lego S, ed: *Psychiatric nursing: a comprehensive reference,* ed 2, Philadelphia, 1996, Lippincott.

Orlandi M: Defining cultural competence: organizing framework. In Orlandi M, Weston R, Epstein L: *Cultural competence for evaluators,* DHHS Publ. #(ADM)92-1884, 1992, U.S. Government Printing Office.

Spector RE: *Cultural diversity in health and illness,* ed 3, Norwalk, CT, 1991, Apple-Century-Crofts.

U.S. Bureau of the Census: *Population projections of the U.S. by age, sex, race & Hispanic origin: 1992–2050,* Washington, D.C., 1992, U.S. Government Printing Office.

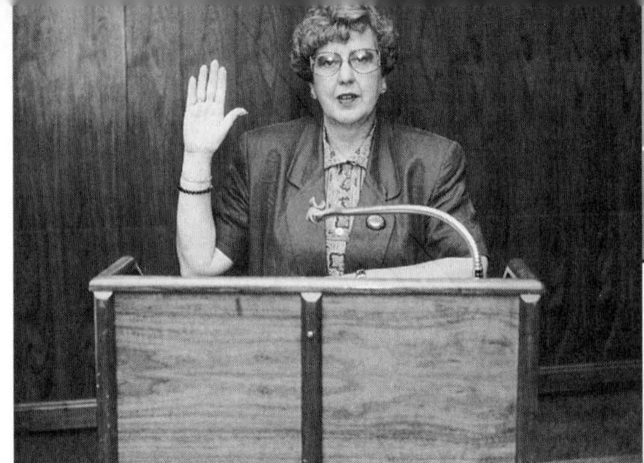

CHAPTER 6

Legal Aspects of Nursing

Cheryl Hall Harris

OBJECTIVES After completing this chapter the reader should be able to:

- **Identify three major sources that provide laws**
- **Differentiate between statutory law, common law, and administrative law**
- **Distinguish between criminal law and civil law and give examples of how each may be breached by the nurse**
- **Identify at least three areas within the category of civil law and provide explanations of each**
- **Define the difference between negligence and malpractice**
- **Explain how a complaint case moves through the court system**
- **Define liability**
- **Identify and describe three types of professional liability insurance nurses may carry**
- **Discuss some areas out of which lawsuits often originate, such as informed consent, do not resuscitate (DNR) orders, physician orders, and documentation**

In a civilized society, a system of laws promotes order, protects the rights of citizens, and provides the framework for a wide variety of relationships. Laws help establish order within a society for the common good of all. In today's complex world, with advancing technologies and an array of societal problems, legal issues are an important aspect of life. For nurses in practice within the current health care system, knowledge of basic legal concepts is vital.

Nurses have been legally accountable for their actions for many years, and current trends regarding the legal ramifications of nursing practice compel nurses to learn the legal aspects of their field. Many contemporary nurses are functioning in more autonomous roles in which liability exposure increases in proportion to their level of independence. In addition to the altruistic motivation of providing the highest quality care to their clients, nurses need to understand the parameters of nursing practice within their state and country as governed by nurse practice acts and standards of care established by organizations and their employing institution. As nurses adopt the role of client advocate, they should promote concepts of client rights. Finally, nurses must be aware of legal implications of nursing practice because present-day society is litigious, and an increasing number of nurses have been named as defendants in malpractice lawsuits.

Malpractice lawsuits continued to increase during the past decade, but now their numerous ramifications are serving as catalysts for bold tort reform that will affect future practice. Partially driven by the need for health care reform and partially as a result of the fact that very few claims that are filed prove to be actual malpractice, new directions are deemed necessary. Examples are greater use of mediation and other conflict resolution techniques to decrease the incidence of filing lawsuits, increased risk management activities that identify adverse client occurrences, and correction of potential problems resulting in decreased malpractice claims. Some states are considering "no-fault" systems in which adverse client outcomes are not related to health care worker negligence. In such a system a central "pool" of funds assists in treatment and management of increased health care problems for the individual who was adversely affected.[15] Moves are also underway to limit awards in malpractice cases. No one can be certain, in this time of extensive health care reform, exactly how malpractice reform may affect nursing practice, but these changes are certain to have direct implications for nurses.

■ LEGAL CATEGORIES

The legal system can be divided into two categories: criminal law and civil law. Criminal law relates to a violation of law. In criminal cases an individual commits a crime, faces trial in the criminal court system, and, if convicted, expects some form of punishment. The purpose of the punishment is to discourage others from committing the same crime, as well as to punish the person who violates the law. Civil law deals with disputes over legal rights and duties of individuals in relation to one another. In a civil action compensation or damages may be awarded to the injured person from the other person(s) who caused the harm. It is possible for nurses to be in a situation that involves both civil and criminal laws. This may result because civil and criminal components are included in both statutory and common law.[12]

For example, Horsley[20] describes a case in which a home health nurse overstepped nursing boundaries. A Visiting Nurses Association (VNA) nurse, Mary was assigned to visit a client under emergency circumstances, when a physician believed the client might have suffered a cerebrovascular accident (CVA). In her initial assessment, Mary reported the symptoms to the physician, who diagnosed a transient ischemic attack (TIA) and prescribed medication to decrease the client's blood pressure. Mary continued to provide care.

A month later Mary received an emergency call from the family. She notified neither the VNA nor the physician, but rushed to the client's home to examine him. She assessed his condition as another TIA and then made a severe error; she instructed the client to take the remaining portion of the medication, even though she still had not contacted the physician. This constitutes the practice of medicine, which is illegal because Mary was not licensed to do so. Unfortunately, the client suffered a massive CVA that night, and continued to have weakness and aphasia nearly 2 weeks later when he was released from the hospital. This client charged Mary with professional malpractice. Horsley reminds nurses that no matter how autonomous the environment in which they practice, they must never diagnose, prescribe, or direct treatment.

Criminal Law As It Relates to Nursing

There are instances in which a nurse breaks a law and is tried in the criminal court system. An example of criminal activity involves a nurse who misappropriates controlled substances, whether for her personal use or to sell to others. This circumstance usually includes falsification of records to cover the misdeed.

In *State of New Jersey v. Winter,* a conviction of manslaughter was judged against a nurse who had transfused incompatible blood into a client, concealed her conduct, and falsified the records. The client died of a transfusion reaction.[26] Northrop and Kelly further note, "In some jurisdictions, alterations of a medical record or creation of a false medical record is a misdemeanor in itself."[26]

The expanded role of the nurse, including anesthetists, midwives, practitioners, and clinical specialists, has led to development of new statutes and regulations, as well as increased legal exposure. One of the important areas of clarification involves legal distinctions in the definition of nursing practice as opposed to medical practice. In most instances additional education and/or certification in a specialty are required for a nurse to practice in this extended capacity. "Some states have specific advanced practice laws authorizing nurse practitioner practice . . . Many state laws require that nurse practitioners be certified by the applicable professional association."[13] Practice laws carefully define the scope of nursing practice within these specialized fields.

Besides specified expanded roles of nursing, there are specialty areas of practice, such as the recovery room after surgery. For example, in *Laidlaw v. Lions Gate Hospital,* a client was taken to the recovery room still unconscious from an uneventful cystectomy. The charge nurse was alone because her staff nurse had left the unit for a work break. At the time Ms. Laidlaw was taken to the recovery room three other clients were under the charge nurse's care. When the charge nurse rendered care to another client and accepted a phone call, she left Ms. Laidlaw unattended. The client stopped breathing and, after resuscitation, suffered permanent brain damage that required lifelong care.[11]

In the court decision the hospital was found not liable because the unit had an appropriate number of staff, although they were not present at the time. The anesthesiologist was not liable because there was no evidence that the physician knew that there was only one nurse in the eight-bed unit. Both nurses were found negligent, the charge nurse because she allowed the staff nurse to leave, and the staff nurse because she did not consider the client load with anticipated arrivals of other clients. In the decision, the legal opinion held that a recovery room is a highly specialized area requiring the nurse to provide "frequent and careful observation of

Box 6-1 Procedure Pattern for a Civil Case

1. A person (*plaintiff*) files a complaint against another person (*defendant*).
2. The complaint includes allegations of wrongdoing, which the plaintiff must prove.
3. After the complaint is "served" to the defendant, litigation procedures begin.
4. Pretrial exploration of the facts are completed by both sides. This may include witnesses to support the allegations or defense.
5. The trial begins with selection of a jury. Then the plaintiff and the defendant state their positions, often with attendant corroborating evidence.
6. After all the information is revealed, the jury deliberates and makes a decision.
7. If one of the parties believes the decision is in error, they may elect to appeal the decision by taking it to a higher court.

patients who are under the influence of anesthesia." Further, a "close scrutiny and ever-present watchfulness were required in this room, and the patient is entitled to expect the same."

Cases such as this one delineate the scope of nursing practice.[11] Similar future cases will further define the role of nurses in specialty areas.

Civil Law

Areas of civil law that affect nurses include tort law, contract law, antitrust law, and other civil laws such as employment discrimination and labor laws. Only tort law will be discussed in this chapter, although the other areas are important as well.

Tort Law

"A tort is a wrongful act committed by one person against another person or against a property. The purpose of tort law is to make the injured person whole again primarily through monetary compensation or damages."[1] In *intentional torts* (for example, false imprisonment, or assault and/or battery) the injured party may seek damages for personal injury and punitive judgment against the person who caused the injury. In an intentional tort the injured person must prove that there was actual intent to harm. In an *unintentional tort* (for example, professional negligence), there is no intent to cause harm. In a negligence case no punitive damages are sought.

Cushing[11] defines the difference between negligence and malpractice: *negligence* pertains to a person's failing to do something that a reasonable and prudent person would do, or doing something that a reasonable and prudent person would not do. *Malpractice* involves professional wrongdoing or remarkable lack of skills in performing expected professional duties.

A civil case is heard before a judge and a jury unless the plaintiff waives that right. A procedural pattern ensues after a civil case is initiated (Box 6-1). In the initial stages of a negligence suit the complaint must contain the following four distinct elements:

1. A statement that the defendant has a duty to perform in a certain manner
2. An allegation that there was a breach of that duty
3. A statement of proximate cause (that the error caused a problem)
4. A demand for compensation to cover damages

Common cases of negligence include foreign objects (such as sponges) left inside a client, burns caused by equipment or solution, falls that cause injury to a client, serious inaccuracies in administration of medications, and failure to exercise reasonable judgment.[9]

■ IMPORTANT LEGAL CONCEPTS FOR NURSES

Many key legal concepts are important for nurses to understand. As nursing practice evolves, these fluid concepts are refined and changed. For example, many standards of care are well defined and of long standing, but as the practice of nursing develops with new areas of specialization, new standards are formulated to address these changes. These legal concepts apply to all areas of nursing practice and are not restricted to any specific segment.

Standards of Care

Standards of care exist to provide guidance to nurses in practice and to define appropriate levels of quality client care. Nurses are expected to know and follow these standards of practice, which are developed from a number of sources, including state legislatures that produce Nursing Practice Acts to define the parameters of nursing practice within their jurisdiction. In 1991 the American Nurses Association Congress of Nursing Practice adopted Standards of Clinical Nursing Practice that include standards pertaining to nursing process such as assessment, nursing diagnosis, evaluation, and so on. These standards also include professional performance criteria such as maintaining competency, continuous quality improvement, ethics, and peer review. Congress also recommended the development of practice guidelines as a course of action for nurses to follow.[1] The Joint Commission on Accreditation of Health Care Organizations (JCAHO) publishes yearly standards that included those pertaining to nursing practice.[1] Finally, the employing institution usually has a carefully defined system of policies and procedures that regulate the performance of specific nursing tasks and duties.

Within the context of standards of care, one emerging trend that causes concern for nurses is the use of unlicensed assistive personnel (UAPs) as additions to a nursing staff. Important legal considerations include the requirement that duties performed by a UAP must not involve client care responsibilities that require a license to perform. In addition, adequate supervision and appropriate training and orientation of UAPs is extremely important.[5] To ensure quality nursing care, nurses must address these issues.

In the event of a claim of malpractice, one important issue will include whether the nurse followed the expected standards as defined by these sources. It is possible that all of the standards of care applicable to the situation may be introduced as evidence to determine whether the nurse met the criteria. Therefore it is important for nurses to determine the standards that apply to their specific area of practice.

Reasonably Prudent Nurse

The practice of nursing not only requires a high degree of education and knowledge but also involves the use of common sense. If a nurse's performance is in question, those functions will be measured against the norm of how another comparably

Box 6-2 Key Elements for Informed Consent

1. The consent must be given voluntarily by a mentally competent adult. The client should not be coerced into giving consent.
2. Clients must understand exactly what they are consenting to. If a client speaks a foreign language or is deaf, an interpreter must explain the consent.
3. The consent should include risks to the procedure, alternative treatments available, and prognosis if the treatment is refused.
4. The consent is usually written, to provide a record of the transaction.
5. Consent to treatment for a minor is usually given by the parent or legal guardian, but, increasingly, children who are at least 7 years old are included in the decision-making process.

educated nurse, within an equivalent setting, using good judgment, would have acted in the same situation. Naturally, nurses within specialized areas of practice who have received additional education will be required to perform a higher level of care than nurses who have not received additional training.

Kelly discusses how in many cases physicians testify as expert witnesses regarding whether a nurse functioned according to standards of care.[26] Kelly asserts that professional nurses should serve as expert witnesses whenever standards of care are in question in any nursing malpractice case. This is the position adopted by The American Association of Nurse Attorneys and represents an emerging trend.[26] In addition, Rabinow[29] believes that, as the nurse's role in assessment of client conditions becomes more recognized, nursing assessment may become a focal point for lawsuits in the future.

Informed Consent

Many procedures performed within the health care setting, such as surgery, require consent from the patient. Each person has the right to authorize or refuse medical treatment. As Berry and her colleagues note, "Informed consent necessitates real respect for the autonomy of others, not simply the provision of a mandated act."[4]

Although the physician is legally responsible for obtaining a client's consent, nurses are often involved. Rabinow[29] asserts that as physicians assign increased responsibility for client teaching to nurses, the nurse will also experience increased obligations for obtaining informed consent.

There are several key elements in ensuring that the client actually gives informed consent (Box 6-2). An extremely important component of obtaining consent involves assessing the client's capacity to either consent or refuse permission for the procedure. The primary issue is whether the client is capable of understanding the medical conditions, the risks of treatment or nontreatment, the risks and benefits of the proposed intervention, and any alternatives that may prove beneficial. Capacity to decide often becomes a subjective assessment of the health care provider.

Ellis and Harltey[14] suggest that nurses must obtain consent for nursing measures. For example, if a nurse enters a client's room to administer an intramuscular medication, the nurse should inform the client of the intended procedure. If the client turns over to receive the injection in the buttocks, that constitutes implied consent.

Informed consent and minors. A recent legal development involves the rights of minors, also known as "children's rights." Historically, children were presumed to be the property of their parents, who were given full authority to make all decisions about a minor child less than 18 years of age. The 1992 case of Gregory K., who chose to sue his mother for divorce and to be adopted by his foster parents, serves as an example of acceptance of children's rights to make decisions for themselves, based on their level of competency.[33] If you consider that children are developing decisional capacity, then they would be increasingly involved in making health care treatment decisions based on their ability to comprehend situations and the factors involved in informed consent. Future trends suggest increased involvement of minors in making health care treatment decisions.

Consent to experimental treatment. Protocols for studies that use human subjects for experimental purposes must pass a stringent review process by an institutional review board before they are approved. When experimental drugs and some techniques are employed, the Federal Food and Drug Administration is also involved in the review process. If a client enters such a study, a highly detailed consent form is presented for signature, and the client has the right to withdraw from the study at any time. In an effort to improve techniques for maximizing client understanding and minimizing opportunities for coercion to participate in clinical trials, nursing leaders suggest that research investigators should impose a time interval between the time that information about a clinical trial is given and when the client makes a decision to participate. Other recommendations included the use of videotaped explanations of the study protocols so that clients can review them as often as desired before making their decision.[4]

Originally children were not allowed to participate in research because the Helsinki Declaration of 1957 strictly forbade anyone under the age of 18 from being used for research. However, with new cancer treatments and other experimental options, children are often asked to participate in research protocols. In 1988 The American Academy of Pediatrics recommended that young people who are older than 13 should grant consent for participation in clinical trials. Furthermore, researchers suggest that competent children who are younger than legal age for giving consent should be asked to give assent when their legal proxy decision maker grants lawful consent.[4]

Submitting such cases to a court for decision is relatively commonplace. However, current trends find most health care providers attempting *not* to employ such drastic measures unless all other avenues have proven unsuccessful. For example, in an instance where a Jehovah's Witness family produces a small premature infant, the health care providers draw as little blood as possible to prevent the necessity for blood transfusions, within limits that appropriate treatment permits. In an effort to be sensitive to a family's religious beliefs and to understand the importance of supporting those belief systems, institutions are making an increased effort to abide by parental wishes so long as the minor does not suffer untoward results.

Right to Privacy and Confidentiality

Clients who enter the health care system have a right to privacy of their personal lives. As society relies more heavily on computerized information and health care institutions computerize client records, clients become more apprehensive about possible invasion of privacy. In particular, clients who are infected with HIV are concerned that their privacy be maintained because of possible repercussions if that information becomes available to outside sources.

As health care agencies begin to use computers to keep records, they must develop policies and procedures to ensure the confidentiality of all computerized information. A system of identification and authorization codes will help maintain the integrity of computer data.[3] Security devices must be checked periodically to ensure confidentiality is maintained. Severe sanctions should be brought against persons who abuse their access to confidential computerized information. One other risk with computerized records is the possibility that the system may not function correctly or that important data may be lost. Steps should be taken to decrease risks caused by computerized records management.[15]

Facsimile transmission of client records affords other opportunity for a breach in confidentiality. Institutions should develop policies and procedures regarding the use of this means of transmitting information, such as locating facsimile equipment in a secure location with access limited to authorized personnel. When sending confidential information, obliteration of identifying names and numbers would be a reasonable precaution to prevent an inadvertent breach of privacy by accidentally sending the fax to the wrong fax number.[18]

Other persons directly involved with a client should have access to client records. But if information is given without consent of the client or legal guardian, a nurse can be held liable. Many health care institutions and agencies have rigorous policies about issues of confidentiality and the right to privacy. Nurses must be aware of these policies to avoid a breach of confidentiality.

■ DOCUMENTATION

Health care records for each client should provide a complete and accurate representation of all care delivered to the client, including diagnostic tests and their results, physical procedures, assessments of condition, and any therapy ordered and received. Nurses are involved in this extremely important aspect of client care. If there is a malpractice lawsuit, written documentation of a client's care may literally determine the outcome of the case.[3] An important legal presumption regarding documentation is that if something was not documented, it was not done. Keeping this legal presumption in mind, both the routine and more complex aspects of client care ought to be documented.

Important elements of appropriate nursing documentation[3] include the following:

1. Accuracy—a client's record must never be falsified; entries should be dated, timed, and written in sequence as events occur
2. If an error is written, it is marked through with a single line, and the word "error" written and initialed; do not erase or obliterate the error
3. Completeness—it is important to record all nursing and health care interventions and their outcomes
4. Nursing charting should be objective, with factual data
5. Documentation must be legible and permanent

Quality Assurance

Quality assurance is a program adopted by an institution that is designed to promote the best possible care. These systems include ongoing education of staff, evaluation of staff performance on a routine schedule, and an audit of selected activities on a regular basis. If a problem surfaces, efforts will be made to correct it.[25] For example, a nursing service department develops the expectation that every client will have an individualized nursing care plan within a certain period after admission. Using a system of routine monitors, they determine whether the expectation is being met. If clients do not have nursing care plans, the department works to correct that problem.

Risk Management

Risk management is usually related to quality assurance and may overlap functions; however, it is designed to identify problems and to evaluate and correct problems to decrease the possibility of financial loss to the institution or individual. Typically, risk identification involves a specific client-care problem such as an unusual incident. A medication error, a client who falls, or an IV that infiltrates and leads to further complications are examples of unusual incidents.

In a system of risk management, an incident report is filed describing the error. After the report is completed, it is analyzed by a risk manager who looks for possible trends within a nursing unit or the entire institution. If a trend is noted, corrective actions are initiated to decrease occurrence of the problem, and then an evaluation of effectiveness of these activities is completed. Bowyer predicts an increase in risk management in the future, because it not only decreases liability but also benefits health care.[25]

Floating to Another Unit

In many health care institutions nurses are required to work in settings other than their normal area of practice. The practice of "floating" nurses from one unit to another usually results from inadequate numbers of staff. As the current staffing crisis in nursing increases, this problem may intensify. If nurses are floated to areas where they do not feel qualified, they may want to submit a formal "Assignment Despite Objection" (ADO) note to the supervisor.[31] The best way to deal with a potential conflict over this type of situation is to present ideas for solutions, such as requesting a restricted set of duties within the role required. For example, if floated to an intensive care setting, a nurse might assess vital signs and give medications—tasks with which the nurse is familiar—but another nurse might closely supervise and perform tasks that the floating nurse is not comfortable in doing, such as caring for a central line. Another solution to problems caused by floating is to cross-train nurses in specialized yet related areas, such as nurses who are assigned to Intensive Care Units, Emergency Room, Postoperative Recovery Room, and so on. The shared orientation and education will increase the number of nurses who can perform competently in all areas.[1]

Nurses who perform outside of their accustomed area of practice may do harm to a client. Creighton[10] describes a case in which an obstetric nurse, floated to an emergency room, administered a markedly increased dose of lidocaine to a client.

The client suffered cardiac arrest and subsequent irreversible severe brain damage. The hospital and the nurse were named as defendants in the lawsuit, which the plaintiff won.

Short Staffing

Clients have the right to competent nursing care, with adequate numbers of appropriately educated nurses. Health care institutions and nurses have an obligation to provide competent staff to address the needs of clients and to meet standards of care of any given client's condition.[15]

Staffing ratio guidelines based on the level of acuity of the clients have been established by JCAHO. If required to accept an assignment to provide care for more clients than is reasonable, a nurse should write a protest to the supervising nurse. Although this protest would not relieve the nurse from responsibility if a problem ensues, it would demonstrate that the nurse was attempting to act in good faith. Nurses should not refuse assignment in such a situation and leave the area, because this could lead to a charge of abandonment by the clients.[19]

Managed Care

An emerging trend in nursing involves the development of managed care designed to decrease the costs of health care. Nurses who have been confronted by "redesign" and fiscal management requirements are concerned that the *quality* of care not diminish secondary to the decreases in staff, elimination of nursing units, use of UAPs, and other cost containment initiatives. The legal risks of managed care are currently under scrutiny. Some of the areas to watch include:

1. Premature discharge of clients
2. Staff reductions that diminish the amount of time nurses can spend in assessment, planning, and providing care for clients
3. Cost containment as it relates to standards of care set by the nursing profession and licensure bodies

The implementation of managed care principles raises ethical and legal issues for nurses to consider.

If nurses are asked to implement what they consider an unsafe practice in the name of cost reduction, Mahlmeister[23] suggests asking these questions:

1. Is the planned practice, action, or act lawful?
2. Does the planned action or act violate a published standard? Consider the standards of care that relate to nursing practice such as those from the State Nurse Practice Act, ANA Standards of Practice, and policies and procedures of the health care institution.
3. Would the planned action or act violate the ANA Code of Ethics? Nurses may need to consult with either the Ethics Center of the American Nurses Association or their own institution's ethics committee to determine whether an ethical concern is present.

Mahlmeister suggests that every nurse be familiar with the *ANA Code of Ethics,* the *ANA Guidelines for Reporting Incompetent, Unethical or Illegal Practices,* and the Nursing Practice act of their state. "With a working knowledge of these important guidelines, nurses can determine when and where to draw the proverbial line in the sand."[23]

Decreasing Risk of Malpractice Lawsuits

Even when the societal climate continues favorable towards initiation of lawsuits, nurses can take some actions to decrease risk.[12] Generally, clients want to be considered as individuals and not just as a number. Therefore any nursing activity that helps to personalize care will set a positive nurses-client relationship. Formulating individualized nursing care plans is a way to accomplish this goal.

If the client believes the nurse is trying to render the best possible care, the client is less likely to sue, even if unforeseen circumstances arise and some problem develops. Nurses must be sensitive to client needs and try to respond in a timely fashion. As Rabinow[29] affirms, "A patient-centered attitude will go a long way toward minimizing your liability."

Naturally, following accepted standards of care and attempting to give the best possible care is the best means of decreasing risk. Nurses must continually update their education and maintain competency in their area of practice, as well as maintain good rapport with their clients.

Liability Insurance

If named as a defendent in a malpractice lawsuit, the costs incurred in a nurse's defense may be exorbitant. The legal climate of our society is changing slowly, but the number of lawsuits initiated continues to be high, as are the size of monetary awards and the fees that some attorneys generate. An emerging trend involves a dramatic increase in the number of lawsuits initiated against nurses, with no current sign of a shift in that practice.[15] To address this situation, some state legislatures are drafting laws that permit awards covering only actual losses and cost of care, thereby eliminating awards for intangible factors such as pain and suffering.[12]

With this emerging trend, nurses are encouraged to carry individual malpractice insurance to help defray the costs of defense. The American Association of Nurse Attorneys, Inc. (TAANA) recommends that "all professional nurses engaged in the practice of nursing should be insured against liabilities to third parties arising out of their professional practice." Aiken[1] suggests that in looking for an individual liability policy, nurses need one that covers injuries resulting from their professional services, not medical incidents. She also advises the "occurrence basis policies are preferable to claims-made policies."

The following are three types of professional liability insurance:[25]

1. *Individual professional liability*—insures the individual nurse for any professional actions performed at any time or any place; the nurse should look for several elements, such as coverage period, limits on coverage, and the authority to select an attorney
2. *Institutional liability*—provides coverage for nurses if they are acting within their scope of employment in their institution
3. *Commercial liability*—covers partnerships, corporations, or business ventures

Baldwin-Mech[3] suggests that nurses should be sufficiently protected by individual policies or institutional policies before they practice nursing. Frequently individual policies are available from professional organizations such as the ANA. Ford[16] describes a lack of professional liability insurance as the "Ultimate Malpractice

Pitfall." He relates, "If you're ever sued and found liable for damages, your insurance may be all that stands between you and serious financial hardship."

Physician Orders

Physicians are responsible for directing medical treatment, and nurses are obligated to follow physicians' orders for medical treatment unless they believe that the orders are in error and would cause harm to the client. If a nurse performs a medical order in question, both the nurse and the physician could be liable. "The courts increasingly have begun to recognize that the scientific knowledge base on which nursing relies increases the duty nurses owe to the health care consumer."[10] In the event a nurse questions a medical order, the physician continues to confirm that order, and the nurse still believes it is inappropriate, the supervising nurse should be notified. The supervising nurse should help resolve the questionable order.[17]

Physician's orders should be written; oral orders are not recommended because of increased possibility of error. The legal editor of *Nursing '89* wrote a review letter in which a nurse accepted a verbal order from a resident physician. When the attending physician questioned the order, the resident denied having given it. Therefore the nurse appeared to have acted without authority. The legal editor suggested that a nurse accepting a verbal order should have another nurse listen and then cosign the order as verification.[22] If an oral order is necessary during an emergency situation, it should be written and signed within 24 hours if possible.

Advance Directives

Several landmark legal cases and federal legislation have led to the development and use of advance health care treatment directives. Advance directives provide a means for individuals to make their decisions clear, while they are still competent, about health care treatment they desire in the future. Clients diagnosed as being in a persistent vegetative state, such as Nancy Beth Cruzan, have provided impetus for the development of advance directives and have further defined issues of withholding and withdrawing treatment. Diagnostic criteria to determine brain death have been established to assist in decision making.

An advance directive may be oral or written, with the latter being preferred. Of equal importance in many instances is naming a Durable Power of Attorney for Health Care Decisions who serves as a surrogate decision maker when the individual becomes incompetent through coma or other means. Advance directives clearly provide information about a client's health treatment choices to ensure respect for that individual's autonomy and to allow health care providers to honor those personal directives without involving the courts. In a personal communication in 1995 from Patricia Murphy, R.N., Ph.D., C.S., F.A.A.N., a bereavement ethicist at Beth Israel Hospital in Newark, New Jersey, she described how in that institution they give every client an Advance Directive form upon discharge. Since the clients have just been hospitalized, they are more likely to discuss with family members future treatment they may or may not wish to have in the event they are readmitted to the hospital.

On December 1, 1991 the *Patient Self-Determination Act* became effective. This federal legislation requires that hospitals, home health agencies, skilled nursing facilities, hospice programs, and prepaid organizations must advise clients of their legal rights to make an advance directive and to make health care decisions, including refusal of treatment as well as attempting treatment. One clear and powerful intent of this legislation is to encourage health care providers to enhance client autonomy and self-determination through education of professionals, clients, and communities.

Under this law several key components are required:[15]

1. Clients must be offered written information and summaries of the institution's policies about their rights under state and federal law to accept or refuse treatment and to make advance health care directives.
2. Written documentation in the client's record must indicate whether the client has made any advance directives.
3. It is illegal for institutions to discriminate against a client on the basis of whether the client has completed an advance directive.
4. Institutions must comply with all state and federal law requirements about advance directives.
5. Institutions must provide staff and community education on advance directives.

Advance directives should be placed in the client's medical record, preferably always in the same place in each client's chart. Although legally nurses cannot act according to a client's advance directive without a physician's order, if a physician orders a treatment, the nurse is subject to legal liability for providing treatment without consent if the nurse is aware of the client's advance directive. "This places the nurse in a serious legal and ethical dilemma."[15] Currently many nurses and clients express frustration about physicians who will not honor advance directives. Future trends may include some type of enforcement that will require physicians to comply with advance directives and some means to address the "double bind" for nurses.

Because each state's statutes are different, it is imperative that health care professionals learn what is operative in their area. There is agreement that the client is the true "captain of the ship" and has the legal right to determine the course of care. Because of that, nurses can no longer be satisfied with only following physicians' orders and must teach clients about their rights, advocate for their wishes, and be active on committees that serve to meet the client's needs. Life-and-death decisions are complex and therefore need educated and caring professionals willing to grapple with the complexities to serve the client well.

Do Not Resuscitate Orders

Historically, when his or her heart has stopped beating, a client has been declared dead. However, in modern health care institutions resuscitation for cardiac and pulmonary arrest is commonplace. When a *code* to prevent death is required, an entire system of emergency and extraordinary care is initiated to return a client to a viable state. Our technologic advances have led to dramatic and emotional decision-making situations.[25]

In many intensive care settings, Do Not Resuscitate (DNR) orders are common, and most hospitals have policies to address this important issue. Physicians are responsible for writing DNR orders, although the decision to receive life-sustaining measures rests with the clients.[22] Kelly presents key elements, proposed by a

Box 6-3 Key Principles for a DNR Order

1. Statement of policy of the institution that resuscitation will be initiated unless there is a specific order to withhold resuscitative measures
2. Statement from the client regarding specific desires
3. Description of the client's medical condition to justify a DNR order
4. Statement about the role of family members or significant others
5. Definition of the scope of the DNR order
6. Statement about the initiation of the DNR order
7. Delineation of the role of various caregivers

Modified from Northrop CE, Kelly ME: *Legal issues in nursing,* St. Louis, 1987, Mosby.

number of professional organizations, that should be included in a DNR order (Box 6-3).[25] A DNR order provides some clear-cut and specific actions to be withheld. The ethical components to deciding these and other cases are frequently reviewed by hospital bioethics committees.

Hospital DNRs on individual clients may require updating every 72 hours, for example. Rigid protocols delineate how a DNR is assigned and who participates. Nurses are often involved in the dilemma of an expiring DNR or in caring for clients whom they feel should have such status. Currently some humane-thinking professionals, and the public in various states, are taking radical steps to ensure individuals a graceful end to life when it is those individuals' willful desire. Some scholars and clinicians are promoting a reversal in current procedure; rather than approaching these situations with DNR orders, only those clients with a "To Be Resuscitated" order would receive CPR. If such an order were not explicitly stated in physician orders, DNR would be automatic. Ethical, social, economic, and other factors currently mandate that our society analyze the overwhelming task of maintaining persons on life-support machinery.

The Patient Self-Determination Act (PSDA), enacted in 1991, requires that all hospitals, long-term care facilities, HMOs, and other health institutions that receive federal funding must inquire whether a client has completed an Advance Health Care Treatment Directive. These documents, which supplant Living Wills in the breadth of their scope, have enabled clients to make their treatment wishes known, both in refusal of treatment and in treatment options that they wish continued. It is perhaps of equal value for the client to name an agent as Durable Power of Attorney for Health Care (not routine Durable Power of Attorney) to make sure the client's values and directives are followed in the event the client is unable to speak for himself or herself. The Nancy Cruzan case led to the drafting of the PSDA.

■ PERINATAL NURSING

In perinatal nursing nurses see effects of their care on both mothers and their infants. Technologic advances have altered this field immeasurably over the past two decades, and new techniques are being developed continuously. Advances in genetics, perinatal diagnosis, fetal surgery, and techniques of newborn intensive care have increased chances for infant survival. However, societal problems such as drug abuse, spread of sexually transmitted diseases, and low rates of prenatal care and immunization among the poor keep infant mortality rates at a high level in the United States.

In some cases, maternal-fetal conflicts arise when treatment of the fetus requires that an invasive procedure be performed on the mother. The case of Angela C. illustrates this issue. Angela was a young pregnant woman who had successfully battled bone cancer in her youth. During her pregnancy she developed lung cancer, which was treated with chemotherapy. At 26 weeks' gestation she exhibited severe lung dysfunction and eventually became comatose. Before that event she had expressed a desire that her fetus not be delivered surgically. Her husband and parents concurred with her decision. However, the hospital obtained a court order to perform a cesarean section to deliver the fetus. The fetus died a few hours later. Angela died 2 days after learning that her baby had died. Later legal action filed against the hospital resulted in a favorable decision for Angela's family members. Other cases of maternal-fetal conflict considered by the courts have included forced monitoring, testing of pregnant women for drug use, and compulsory amniocentesis.[15]

Maternal Drug Use

One of the most alarming trends to affect perinatal nurses is the rise of drug use among pregnant women. Alcohol, tobacco, and various sedatives have been used for many years, but the increase in numbers of pregnant women who use cocaine and other illegal drugs complicates treatment and nursing care of these women and their infants. The negative effects of maternal drug use on children may produce problems for a prolonged period, perhaps a lifetime.

Experts agree that most drug users are actually *polydrug users;* that is, they use more than one substance at a time. Frequently the effects of a drug such as crack cocaine will be extended with other drugs such as PCP. Also, sometimes several drugs, such as alcohol and cocaine, are used together to enhance the effect. Another alarming aspect of today's societal drug use is that "Thousands of women from middle and upper socioeconomic groups are addicted to this drug [cocaine] of the 1980s."[8]

In some health care facilities nurses assist addicted clients in entering drug treatment centers. If a mother refuses to do so, then her baby may be removed from her care and placed in protective services or foster care. Although there may be clinical indications for testing for substance abuse, this practice has legal ramifications. Women with positive drug screens have been prosecuted for risking injury to a minor. Many health care institutions have resisted establishing consent requirements for drug screening because they believe this practice would result in women refusing to be screened and clinical care being compromised.[9] However, the woman's right to privacy is jeopardized by routine screening.

Sexually Transmitted Diseases in Pregnancy

Of the more than 20 sexually transmissible diseases, two present serious ramifications because they are incurable and because they cause irreversible congenital effects: herpes and AIDS. Public health officials indicate that the number of infected women continues to rise.[30] The effects of these diseases may prove life-threatening to the newborn.

Many sexually transmitted diseases must be reported to local health departments. The CDC[7] has issued guidelines for reporting that stress the importance of preserving privacy for the client while promoting public good by disclosing information about the infection. Incidence statistics are compiled using this reported data. Because reporting this information is mandated, the nurse is immune from a claim of breach of confidentiality if she reports the information. Other than official reporting of these diseases, confidentiality still applies.[25]

Contact tracing is a difficult issue that arises in caring for clients with AIDS. This program requires the cooperation of the client identified as a carrier: the client is asked to reveal names and addresses of any sexual or drug-sharing partners. In such instances the carrier, or *index case,* is asked to incriminate close associates. Current laws do not compel the infected person to provide such personal information, which represents a significant invasion of privacy.[16,32] This topic will be discussed later.

Abortion

Rarely has a subject led to as much public debate and level of sentiment as the issue of abortion. Two diametrically opposed camps exist: those who believe that the mother has a right to privacy in matters concerning reproduction, and those who believe that once conception has occurred, the baby has a right to be born. The monumental U.S. Supreme Court decision *Roe v. Wade* in 1973, along with several other decisions dealing with abortion during that year, established the rights of women to have an abortion and to be free from government intrusion.[10] Since that time the debate has raged unabated.

Individual states continue to legislate or regulate various components of abortion, such as funding of the procedure for women who otherwise would not have access or adding the necessity of written spousal notification.[9] The U.S. Supreme Court continues to hear cases dealing with the constitutionality of state legislation during almost every term.

Impaired Newborns

In newborn intensive care units (NICUs), technologic advances have led to legal dilemmas for nurses. In the early 1980s "Baby Doe cases" involving lack of treatment for some handicapped infants resulted in regulations requiring the reporting of such situations to a hotline number as abuse and neglect. This established an important trend.

In 1984 the U.S. Congress enacted legislation that mandates treatment unless (1) the infant is irreversibly comatose, (2) providing treatment only prolongs inevitable dying, and (3) the treatment would only prove futile regarding survival of the infant and was considered inhuman in itself.[24] The American Academy of Pediatrics Bioethics Committee[2] recommends that decisions be made on each individual case and that bioethics committees should be established to assist in the decision-making process.

Before these discussions, health care workers in the NICUs struggled with the ethical and moral issues involved in these decisions. Current trends suggest that they also need to be concerned with legal implications.

▪ HOME HEALTH CARE NURSING

Home health care is a rapidly expanding field of practice for nurses. Not only are clients discharged from the hospital with more complex short-term high-technology care needs, but many more clients with chronic health problems are treated as outpatients. For example, clients on peritoneal dialysis or extended intravenous chemotherapy may be treated at home with sporadic nursing assessments. Infants are sent home who require continuous ventilatory support or central-line total parenteral alimentation, and an increasing number of care needs are now relegated to home care. This trend is likely to continue.

With the changing dynamics in acute health care, where clients are sent home to recover more quickly, pressures rise for those who provide home health nursing. Home health agencies should develop clear policies and procedures for care provided and establish risk management programs to identify and correct possible problems for the practitioners who work for them.[6]

Home care nurses must be sure their practice remains within the scope of nursing, effectively document all levels of care, and receive authorization from a physician for all medications and treatments. If home care nurses question a physician's order, they should notify their agency supervisors and follow appropriate channels to clarify the proper course of action.[21]

Hospice Nursing

As federal legislation regulates home health care, so is hospice nursing regulated. Hospice nursing addresses issues for clients who have no reasonable prospect for a cure for their disease and who are expected to die within 6 months.[25]

Basic legal concerns surround such issues as pronouncement of death. New Jersey passed a law allowing professional registered nurses to determine client death, make legal pronouncement of death, and sign a death certificate. The procedure includes notification of a physician, who also signs the death certificate, but the nurse is permitted to specify events surrounding last sickness and details of death.[25] Other states have adopted variations of this, and it will probably establish a precedent for practices that are more practical and realistic to the setting.

■ MEDICAL-SURGICAL NURSING

A number of legal issues affect nurses who practice in the area of medical-surgical nursing. Many malpractice lawsuits are initiated as a result of incorrect administration of medication, client falls, and other errors. However, within the scope of this chapter only two trends will be discussed.

Critical Care Nursing

As the incidence of malpractice litigation increases, nurses involved in critical care nursing will also probably experience a higher rate of malpractice claims brought against their highly specialized area of practice. Nurses who pursue this field must receive additional training and maintain competency in their skills. The American Association of Critical Care Nurses (AACCN) has standards of care that guide nursing practice in this area.

In this technologically advanced field reliance on medical equipment is very important. If equipment malfunctions, it must be checked and repaired if necessary. Although critical care nurses are expected to possess mechanical aptitude, most hospitals have biomedical equipment departments to routinely check equipment and respond if a problem arises.

■ AIDS

Care of patients who are HIV-seropositive or who have developed AIDS may change significantly if the new treatment options identified in late 1996 continue to hold the promise they initially suggest. Care providers explain that rather than being an automatic death sentence, AIDS may become a manageable chronic disease given appropriate treatment.

Acquired immune deficiency syndrome (AIDS) was first described in 1981. Since that time its incidence has increased at an alarming rate. New populations of individuals infected with HIV include women and children in increasing numbers, with African American and Hispanic individuals making up a disproportionate share of AIDS patients. An estimated 1.5 million Americans are carriers of HIV, with large numbers of those people expected to develop AIDS. Another alarming statistic, provided by a joint study of the American College Health Association and the Centers for Disease Control and Prevention (CDC), reveals that nearly 1 of every 500 college students is infected with the AIDS virus.

The CDC provides current information and statistics about the number of HIV-challenged patients as well as those who have developed AIDS. As of 1996, the cumulative number of AIDS cases reported to the CDC is 573,800. The number of women infected (86,070) has risen to 15%, a dramatic doubling during the previous 2 years. The increase is expected to continue. The Public Health Service projects that this epidemic will continue to rage in our country and around the world. The Americans with Disabilities Act makes it illegal to discriminate without cause against persons infected with HIV/AIDS.

In December 1991 the Occupational Safety and Health Administration (OSHA) issued regulations that require that universal precautions be observed with all clients. The use of personal protective clothing, appropriate signs and labels, education, and other stipulations are designed to reduce the risk of exposure to bloodborne pathogens such as hepatitis B virus (HBV) and HIV. Given the severity of the disease and the current lack of a cure, many legal issues surround this devastating disease.

Although some states require mandatory testing of certain populations of individuals, there are legal concerns about this practice. The potential for discrimination and the necessity of informing a client who tests positive (even though the testing may have been done without obtaining consent) are only two of the legal implications of this practice.

Nondiscrimination

In 1990 Congress passed legislation (the Americans with Disabilities Act) that, among other provisions, extends civil rights protection to persons with AIDS. Discrimination against those who are HIV-infected is prohibited by law. Any institution that receives federal funding (including Medicare or Medicaid benefits) is also required to treat clients with HIV.

Partner Identification

The issue of partner notification presents a dilemma for health care workers. When a person is diagnosed as HIV-positive, others may potentially be infected through sexual contact or sharing of needles during illegal drug use. One basic public health infection control measure is to notify partners who may have contracted the disease through contact with the infected person.[28] Historically this technique has been used to help control outbreaks of smallpox, scarlet fever, and gonorrhea or other sexually transmitted diseases. Currently parents are notified if their school-age children are exposed to chicken pox or other contagious diseases. Everything possible is being done to identify contacts of HIV-infected persons, but there is no effective legal power to implement fast and accurate action.

Potterat and his colleagues[28] state that partner notification in relation to HIV-positive status or AIDS has produced several objections, including the following:

1. It is too expensive
2. Because there is no known cure, there is no reason to notify
3. It may lead to discrimination or stigmatization of infected individuals

We argue that none of these objections is valid. Estimated cost of notification is approximately $2 million at an annual case rate of 100,000. Although this is expensive, it is not prohibitive, and benefits from the expected decrease in infection rate would justify the cost. Also, even though there is no cure to date, there are life-prolonging compounds, and any method of relaying information about the disease should decrease the incidence of HIV transmission. Finally, the current laws regarding confidentiality would help decrease discrimination, and U.S. public health departments have a long and distinguished track record for protecting patient confidentiality.

■ SUMMARY

Legal issues are a major component in contemporary nursing in all areas of practice. Nurses must be informed about the legal implications of their actions and continue to update their information as situations change. Throughout contemporary society the evolution of societal thought, and the legal ramifications of that thought, continue to affect the practice of nursing.

CRITICAL THINKING *Activities*

1. **What are common legal issues that affect nurses practicing in medical-surgical nursing?**
2. **What are common legal issues that affect nurses practicing in home health?**
3. **What are common legal issues that affect nurses in critical care?**
4. **How can you prepare to serve as an expert witness in a case when a nurse's practice is in question?**

References

1. Aiken TA, Catalano JT: *Legal, ethical and political issues in nursing,* Philadelphia, 1994, FA Davis.
2. American Academy of Pediatric Committee on Bioethics: Treatment of critically ill newborns, *Pediatrics* 74:306, 1984.

3. Baldwin-Mech A: Quality assurance and documentation. In Northrup CE, Kelly ME, eds: *Legal issues in nursing,* St. Louis, 1987, Mosby.
4. Berry DL, Dodd MJ, Hinds P, Ferrell BR: Informed consent: process and clinical issues, *Oncology Nurs Forum* 23(3):507-512, 1996.
5. Blouin AS, Brent NJ: Unlicensed assistive personnel: legal considerations, *JONA* 25(11):7-8, 21, 1995.
6. Brent NJ: Risk management and legal issues in home care: the utilization of nursing staff, *JOGNN* 23(8):659-665, 1994.
7. Centers for Disease Control and Prevention (CDC): 1993 revised classification systems for HIV infection and expanded surveillance case definition for AIDS among adolescents and adults, *MMWR* 41, no. RR-17, 1992.
8. Chasnoff IJ: Perinatal effects of cocaine, *Contemp Ob/Gyn* 29(5):163-179, 1987.
9. Cohn SD: *Malpractice and liability in clinical obstetrical nursing,* Rockville, MD, 1990, Aspen.
10. Creighton H: *Law every nurse should know,* ed 4, Philadelphia, 1981, Saunders.
11. Cushing M: *Nursing jurisprudence,* Philadelphia, 1988, Appleton & Lange.
12. Cushing M: When the courts define nursing: what it is, and what it does, *Am J Nurs* 87(6):773, 1987.
13. Dodell D: Update: impact of the expanded AIDS surveillance case definition for adolescents and adults on case reporting—United States, 1993, *Health Info-Com Network Newsletter* (Internet: mednews@asuvm.inre.asu.edu), March 18, 1994.
14. Ellis JR, Hartley CL: *Nursing in today's world: challenges, issues and trends,* ed 3, Philadelphia, 1988, Lippincott.
15. Feutz-Harter SA: *Nursing and the law,* ed 5, Professional Education Systems, 1993.
16. Ford RD, Haston L: *Nurse's legal handbook,* Springhouse, PA, 1985, Springhouse.
17. Gostin L, Curran WJ: Legal control measures for AIDS: reporting requirements, surveillance, quarantine, and regulation of public meeting places, *Am J Public Health* 77(2): 214-218, 1987.
18. Grant AE: Facsimile transmissions, *Can Nurse* 92(4):47, 1996.
19. Hemelt MD, Mackert ME: *Dynamics of law in nursing and health care,* ed 2, Reston, VA, 1982, Reston.
20. Horsley JE: Short staffing means increased liability for you, *RN* 44(2):73, 1981.
21. Horsley, JE: The new risks of home care, *RN* 52(1): 59-61, 1989.
22. Legal Column Editor, *Nursing '89* 19(5), 1989.
23. Mahlmeister L: When cost-saving strategies are unacceptable, *Ped Nurs* 22(2):130-132, 1996.
24. Moreno J: Ethical and legal issues in the care of the impaired newborn, *Clin Perinatal* 14:345, 1987.
25. Nolan K: In death's shadow: the meanings of withholding resuscitation, *Hastings Cent Rep* 17(5): 9-14, 1987.
26. Northrop CE, Kelly ME: *Legal issues in nursing,* St. Louis, 1987, Mosby.
27. Patch FB, Holaday SD: Effects of changes in professional liability insurance on certified nurse-midwives, *J Nurs Midwifery* 34(3):131-136, 1989.
28. Potterat JJ and others: Partner notification in the control of human immunodeficiency virus infection, *Am J Public Health* 79(7): 874-876, 1989.

29. Rabinow J: Where you stand in the eyes of the law, *Nursing* 19(2): 34-42, 1989.
30. Rocerto L, Maleski C: *The legal dimensions of nursing practice,* New York, 1982, Springer.
31. Rushton CH, Hogue EE: Confronting unsafe practice: ethical and legal issues, *Pediatr Nurs* 19(3):284-288, 1993.
32. Wilson D: An overview of sexually transmissible diseases in the perinatal period, *J Nurs Midwifery* 33(3): 115-128, 1988.
33. Wingert P, Salholz E: Irreconcilable differences, *Newsweek* Sept 21, 1992.

Suggested Readings

American Nurses Association: *Standards of clinical nursing practice,* 1991.

Derse AR: HIV and AIDS: legal and ethical issues in the emergency department, Emerg Med Clin North Am 13(1):213-221, 1995.

Feutz-Harter S: *Nursing and the law,* Eau Claire, WI, 1993, Professional Education Systems.

Fiesta J: Long term care update, *Nurs Management,* 27(7):26-28, 1996.

Fiesta J: *The law and liability: a guide for nurses,* ed, 2 New York, 1988, Wiley.

Handbook of living will laws, New York, 1987, Society for the Right to Die.

Infante MC: The legal risks of managed care, *RN* 59(3):57-59, 1996.

Meisel A: Barriers to forgoing nutrition and hydration in nursing homes, *Am Law Med* 21(4):335-82, 1995.

Smith MH: Legal obligations to human immunodeficiency virus—seropositive patients and health care providers, *J Professional Nurs* 11(3):183-191, 1995.

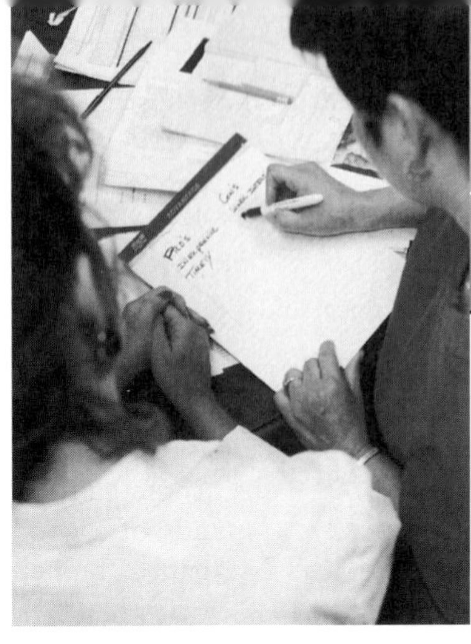

CHAPTER 7

Ethical Decision Making and the Role of the Nurse

James H. Husted, Gladys L. Husted

OBJECTIVES After completing this chapter the reader should be able to:

- **Examine the relationship between nursing and bioethics**
- **Discuss nursing's need of bioethics**
- **Analyze dilemmas according to various ethical theories**
- **Describe the benefits that nurses gain through a bioethically guided practice**
- **Illustrate why bioethics ought to be a practice-based ethic**
- **Examine the ways in which the traditional ethical systems lead to harmful and unjustifiable bioethical decisions**
- **Describe the importance of context in the interaction of nurse and client**
- **Discuss the role of probabilities in reaching ethical certainty**
- **Explain the unique role of nurses in bioethical decision making**
- **Discuss the role of interdisciplinary bioethics committees**

■ WHO NEEDS ETHICAL THEORY ANYWAY?

Everyone assumes that all people believe in and value the same things. The fact of the matter is that people do not always agree with each other; people do not always understand each other. They do not share the same experiences. They do not evaluate their experiences in the same ways. They communicate with each other in vague generalities. They do not have the same purposes. They do not work toward the same goals. This makes ethical conflicts all too frequent. When persons interact, they sometimes find themselves in disagreement. When they disagree, their disagreements cannot be resolved through their personal values. This is true for all persons, not just nurses. The values that motivate the actions of the valuer do not serve to resolve disagreements unless persons share the same values. The parties to an agreement on which interaction is based seldom share the same personal values.[17]

As with every science and every art, ethics arose when thoughtful persons began to examine the world about them and their activities in it—activities they had taken for granted. People counted long before founding the science of mathematics. People grew crops before they initiated the formal study of agriculture. They made decisions and choices, on the level possible to them, concerning their lives and the lives of others for millennia before meditating on ethics.

During the golden age of ethical philosophy (Greece, circa 350 BC) *ethics* was defined as the science of a good human life. At some times and in some cultures ethics was better or worse—more or less appropriate to the demands of a good human life—than at other times and in other cultures. Over the span of human history the appropriateness of ethics to human life has waxed and waned.

From the beginning individuals began to meditate on different aspects of the world and their relationship to it. With the advent of language, two or three together would discuss this topic. Eventually some individuals, notably Confucius in the eastern world and Socrates in the western world, came to devote their lives to meditating on the need for wisdom in the practical objectives of human action. A belief that the progress of ethical thought has been an uninterrupted advance would be a very misguided belief. Since that time no human study, with the possible exceptions of astrology and the conjuration of ghosts, has ever made slower progress than the study of ethics.

Different ethical theories still in vogue today have arisen in times and in circumstances very different from today. Perspectives on the meaning and purpose of ethical deliberation have changed over time. Many ethical theorists have a general mindset on ethics but no clear definition of the subject, and no orientation on the function of ethics in relation to the needs of a good human life. This makes it possible for a bioethicist, perhaps in a moment of uncontrolled enthusiasm, to declare, "Medical ethics must stop being case oriented and become institutionally oriented. We bioethicists must stop approaching problems from a philosophical perspective and adopt a political science perspective."[7]

In the health care setting technologic advances, an increase in the awareness of cultural differences and individual rights, a greater level of sophistication in the general public leading to a spate of law suits, and political interference in health care matters has far outstripped the ability of the traditional ethical systems to maintain justice and harmony between health care professionals and clients. If, and as, concern for the individual humanity of clients withers, nurses will take a stand or pass into history.

The expansion of managed care has raised a number of ethical and moral issues in the evolving health care marketplace. Health care providers have been highly concerned about the dominant shift from quality to cost in the health care marketplace. Dr. Franzblau draws a unique comparison between the economic and political pressure facing today's physicians and the incredible role physicians played under Hitler in Nazi Germany. Dr. Franzblau is not suggesting we are like Nazi Germany, but cautions society to remember what happened when an honorable profession was perverted for a political purpose.[19] Whenever the purposes of a profession become changed to serve political ends, the profession has become "perverted." This perversion can gradually or quickly redefine the profession. And then a profession that had served human needs becomes an instrument to serve arbitrary political whims.

■ WHAT'S IN IT FOR THE NURSE?

Nurses, as professionals, need to establish themselves, and nursing, as a necessary and valuable part of the health care setting. If other health care professions are mastering ethical decision making while nursing is discussing abstract ethical theory, then nurses place themselves at a significant disadvantage. If, on the other hand, nurses can develop a greater skill at ethical decision making than other health care professions, this enormously enhances their value as individuals and the value of their profession.

By mastering ethical decision making a nurse increases her* client's well-being, strengthens the profession of nursing, and establishes for herself a status at least equal to any other health care professional.

If the profession of nursing is not to be perverted then the client must always be the center of a nurse's ethical concern. The nature of the nurse and the nature of the client are internally related. A change in the presidency from one person or one political party to another does not affect what a nurse is. The nature of nursing is unaffected by changes in the weather or in television programming. But without a client or the prospect of working with sick and injured persons as clients, a nurse is not a nurse. She is an unemployed person. If she gets a job as a bookkeeper she is no longer unemployed, but she is still not a nurse. In the same way, without a nurse or other health care professional a client would simply be a sick or injured person. A client who is not the client of a health care professional is not a *client.*

A nurse who does not hold her client as the center of her ethical attention is, on the ethical level of her practice, not functioning as a nurse. A nurse is "the agent of a patient, doing for a patient what he would do for himself if he were able."[15] A client is the proper center of a nurse's ethical attention because a client makes a nurse what she is. The nature of a nurse is *defined* in terms of a client.

If bioethics adopts a political science perspective it may be that a nurse's only ethical responsibility will be mindless obedience. Until that day, which hopefully will never come, nurses have ethical responsibilities. These responsibilities involve a high degree of awareness of the clients under their care. In return something is in it for a nurse. There is the opportunity to be a nurse.

And there is more in it than this. Just as a client is the beneficiary of his interactions with a nurse, a nurse is the beneficiary of her interactions with a client. Through these interactions a nurse establishes a basis for her objective worth as a human being, and increases her right to pride in herself.

■ BUT DOES A NURSE REALLY *NEED* TO CONCERN HERSELF WITH ETHICS?

Every human being holds and practices an ethical system. Every nurse, right now, at this moment, is practicing an ethical system. For any given person—any given nurse—her ethical system is simply the way she guides her actions in situations

---

*We predominantly use the pronoun "she" to designate the nurse. This is, we hope, justified by the fact that over 90% of nurses are women. On the other hand, we almost invariably use the pronoun "he" to designate the client. This is not because the majority of clients are men, but simply for the reader's ease of understanding.

where there is a significant potential for benefit or harm. The only question is: Is a nurse aware of the nature of her "ethical system"—is it under her conscious control?

No one ever took up bowling or bridge or horseback riding hoping to bowl or play bridge or ride horseback badly. Frustration at the difficulty of a study may lead one to be content to become inept and clumsy at it, but no one ever *sets out* to perform less than adequately in a pursuit that interests her. Why then should one be content to learn nursing badly? It is inconceivable that any nurse would be content with a superficial knowledge of, and skill at, the technical aspects of nursing. Dozens of journals are published whose purpose is to enable a nurse to perfect and increase her skill as a nurse. These journals answer a felt need of nurses to attain excellence. Yet it is possible to master the technical aspects of nursing with great skill while, nonetheless, learning the art of nursing badly and performing ineffectively in it. Nursing is a very intersubjective art. The ability to act logically and appropriately on an intersubjective level in a health care setting is the entire spectrum of a nurse's bioethical effectiveness.

Nurses are in an excellent position to promote the agency of patients and their families in considering courses of action and coming to decisions—possibly decisions regarding alternatives that will enhance their lives. "Nurses are able to identify alternatives for patients when they can see no options in a situation."[11] For a nurse the analysis of a bioethical dilemma always involves the analysis of a person. Often it involves nothing more than this.

"For a nurse to interact with a patient in an objectively justifiable manner, she must have some understanding of the person she is interacting with. . . . Even where a nurse does not have an explicit awareness of the elements of human personality . . . she cannot avoid this awareness on an implicit level. She acquires it simply through her internal dialogues."[16]

In a nurse the lack of this ability, whatever other ethical knowledge she may possess, is more than a mere failure; skillful and effective ethical action on the part of a nurse is a reasonable and justified expectation on the part of a client. When two people interact in an ambiance as fundamental and as intimate as the nurse/client context nothing can replace a commitment to the ethical standards of that context. It is perfectly reasonable for a client, in this circumstance, to assume that his nurse will be deeply concerned about the intersubjective—the ethical—aspects of their relationship. As we will discuss later, a concern for anything else, including an extrinsic ethical theory, undermines a nurse's bioethical actions.

■ TRADITIONAL THEORIES OF ETHICS

Traditional ethical theories are probably the most commonly studied and discussed. Over the centuries the question has been: What ultimately determines ethical behavior—good outcome or good intent? Adherence to the first approach have been labeled *consequentialist,* while the second is associated with *deontology.*

Deontologic

Deontology, or *nonconsequentialism,* is a theory of ethical inquiry that views actions as right or wrong not because of their consequences or the type or amount of good produced but because of their right-making characteristics such as fidelity to promises, truthfulness, and justice. The grounds for these principles, or "rules" of conduct, may arise from divine revelation, intuition (instinctual belief), common sense, or social contracts. The philosopher Immanuel Kant (1724-1804) believed the rules of conduct must be autonomous choices by the one acting in the situation.[18] Although the rules may come from a divine or societal source, they must be freely chosen by the participants in any decision-making situation.

As with all theories, deontologic theories do have problems. Paramount is the question of how to handle the conflicts that arise among different deontologic obligations. Who decides which rule to follow? God? As interpreted by whom? Society? By which members?

Deontology regards only those actions that are motivated by an ethical *intention*—the intention to do one's duty—as justifiable ethical actions.

In summary, deontology is the theory that an agent's ethical actions must be guided by rules and motivated by a sense of duty. It holds that the consequences of an action are irrelevant to the ethical quality of an action. The theory recognizes no good as an absolute good but the desire to do what one ought to do—that which constitutes one's *duty.*

Consequentialist

Consequentialist theories entail the belief that *good* is defined by the consequences of any action. The focus of this theory is the result or effects of a person's action. The most well-known consequentialist theory is that of *utilitarianism.* Classical utilitarianism, as advocated by the English philosopher John Stuart Mill (1806-1873), recommends those actions that produce the most good for those persons or groups affected by the actions; that is, those actions that have the most utility, or usefulness.[23] (Applied to societies, utilitarianism has been identified with promoting the greatest good for the greatest number.) Theories of utility require an evaluation of the benefits or harms that may occur. Benefits are results that are advantageous, or "good." Harm involves an injury, or "hurt."

No theory, though, is without problems. One obvious problem with utilitarian theories is that of how to define *good.* Every nurse has a different definition of what is good. Consequentialism "is based more on the collective good rather than on the value of the individual. Consequences are evaluated in terms of usefulness, cost-effectiveness and efficiency so that the greatest good for the greatest number is realized . . . the end justifies the means."[8]

The consequentialist desires to bring about the best possible *consequence* simply because it is the best possible consequence. It is a reaction against the barren formalism and essential irrelevance of deontology. It is not necessarily a successful reaction. At best, attention to consequences without a well-ordered and real-life concern for how and why these consequences are going to be brought about, who is going to be affected by these consequences, and what further consequences will flow from the initial consequences may produce absurd and tragic consequences. With consequentialism it is often the case that the solution to one problem is a second problem.

Principle-based ethics, or deontologic theory, appeals to duties or obligations to determine the rightness of a moral decision, whereas consequential ethics, or utilitarian theory, appeals to outcomes to determine the rightness of a moral decision. Many nurses who study ethics quickly conclude that moral decision making based on either principles or consequences may not provide an adequate answer.[3]

■ CASUISTRY AND CONTEXTUALISM

Casuistry

A third framework, which is growing in interest and attention, is that of contextual reasoning. Contextualism has grown out of earlier casuistry frameworks. Casuistry and contextual reasoning are built on the experience of specific clinical cases of moral conflict. Casuistry is based on a belief that the best humans may achieve in ethics is "for good-hearted, clear-headed people to triangulate their way across the complex terrain of moral life and problems."[28] In other words, it rejects a rigid compliance with absolute principles, which is believed to reflect an unrealistic search for clear-cut answers.

In contextualism the client is at the center of the process of decision making. It is assumed that by working through actual cases involving similar moral conflicts, future conflicts might be more easily resolved by referring to analogous cases that have become "paradigm cases." In other words, paradigm cases serve as "rules of thumb" to follow for correct conflict resolution. These "paradigm cases serve to illuminate other cases, using argument by analogy. [It is the practical experiences of those dealing in client care that is valued.] Thus casuistry is rooted in traditions and practices, not in pure reason or a special faculty of moral intuition."[4]

In practice the knowledge gained from contextual reasoning would grow incrementally as the number of cases referred for ethical consultation grows. With this history, careful evaluation by practitioners of the guidelines and criteria from these previous cases will then assist in deciding the appropriateness of the care and treatment provided in any specific future case. In using this contextual orientation of casuistry, we do not look to universal principles to provide concrete answers for moral conflict. It is the totality of the situation that is of importance: the medical facts of the case, the persons involved, the extenuating circumstances, and, possibly, guidance from theory.

However, one of the problems associated with casuistry centers on what ideals guide its development. Does one simply do what the majority has done in the past? If we look only to traditional practice to help resolve moral conflict, we may discover that traditional practice is incomplete, not always evaluating all possible solutions. And with the fact-changing world of health care, new conflicts may appear for which paradigm cases may not exist. Additionally, traditional practice may include outdated beliefs, such as the female nurse being subservient to the male physician.

Casuists reject notions of universal principles as being too vague and too inflexible to have any practical application to the realities of human existence. They believe that such an absolutist stand obstructs compromise when principles conflict, making resolution not only difficult but sometimes impossible. The more reasonable casuists believe that experience with situations leads to the accumulation of knowledge, which allows for the ordering of cases and the subsequent creation of a paradigm. Casuistry in this sense then becomes a summary of experience regarding particular instances, lending insight and guidance to decision making.[6]

On a very basic level a casuistic method is essential to ethical decision making. An ethical dilemma cannot be analyzed in a vacuum. One must call upon the resources of experience.

Casuistry is a valuable, even irreplaceable, means of analyzing ethical dilemmas. But no method of analyzing dilemmas is identical to resolving a dilemma. Casuistry differs from the other ethical systems in this. Deontology tells one what to do—in other words, what one's duty is. Consequentialism does the same. It tells one to bring about the best consequence—the greatest good for the greatest number. Logically casuistry cannot do this. It is a logical fallacy to declare, "This is the action that ought to be taken now, because this is the action that brought about a good result in the past." It is the same fallacy as declaring, "George was sitting at the kitchen table at this time yesterday, therefore George is sitting at the kitchen table now today." In neither case does the limited knowledge that is appealed to justify the conclusion that is drawn.

Despite the claims of casuists, casuistry and contextualism are not the same. For less reasonable casuists, analysis consists entirely in an appeal to the past. Contextualism appeals to the present situation and the knowledge one has of it. A dilemma is what it is because, here and now, it is all the things and only the things that is itself. This has no necessary connection to the past. The past, taken as tradition, is an incompetent guide.

Universal principles—for instance, the greatest good for the greatest number—taken as rules or duties, at best, may very well be (and almost always are) too vague and inflexible to be useful. But some *contextual* standard of judgment is absolutely necessary to the contextual analysis of a *present* ethical dilemma. Otherwise there would be no way of judging the quality of the resolution of the present case. In fact, there would be no way of judging the quality of the resolution of a *past* case. It is not valid to judge that the past case had a desirable and justifiable resolution unless you have some way of knowing this—some way other than looking at cases even further back in time, ad infinitum.

It is reasonable to attempt to bring about a consequence similar to a consequence that was brought about by specific actions in a similar dilemma from the past only if that consequence can be shown to be a desirable consequence. And it can *only* be shown to be a desirable consequence according to a standard of judgment other than a further past case.

Casuistry invites subjectivism and rationalization. It produces a powerful incentive to do whatever one wants to do as long as one does not do that which is obviously unacceptable.

Contextualism

The ethical actions appropriate for a nurse to take in any given circumstance depends on three things. It depends on the relationship of agreement that her role as a nurse creates between herself and her client. Secondly, it depends upon the specific aspects of her client's situation, including his desires and purposes. Finally, it depends upon the knowledge and abilities that she is able to bring to her action. These things can be identified only within the context of their present circumstances.

The nature of the relationship between a nurse and a client implies the nature of the interaction that ought to take place between them. The ethical nature of their relationship articulates the quality of this interaction. For a nurse to meet its ethical demands she must, at a minimum, maintain her objective awareness of her client's circumstances. That she will is implied by the understanding under which they interact.

More than this, a nurse ought to act to ensure that her client has the objective awareness that he needs in order to deal with his circumstances. This awareness and fidelity to the understanding that grounds their interaction, are implied by the relationship that binds them together. If a nurse bases her action on responsibility to an abstract duty, or the benefit of a majority, or the circumstances of another situation, she does not maintain an objective awareness of her present client's circumstances. Nor does she allow her client to act with objective awareness. He has no way of knowing that she is interacting with him according to a duty, a responsibility to a majority, or the structures of a previous dilemma. Therefore in shattering their relationship she violates the standard of fidelity to their relationship.

Nurses have a long history of implicit contracts and promise keeping with clients. We establish relationship with our clients in which we jointly agree to work for the accomplishment of shared goals for their care.

Felt obligations to ethical standards other than the implicit contracts nurses make with patients act in direct conflict with a nurse's professional commitment. If a nurse is motivated by, for instance, something outside the context of her patient, she has abandoned the ethical contract she has with her patient. She has set up, or allowed to be set up, a contradictory state of affairs. Her commitment will be to this patient. But, at the same time, the ethical center of her attention will be something other than this patient. This is an impossible situation. When a client is struggling to regain his health and well-being and a nurse is acting to accomplish her duty, or to provide the greatest good for the greatest number, or when she places herself under the sway of tradition, it cannot be said that nurse and client are working for the accomplishment of shared goals. These various theories tend to take the nurse out of the context and put her under the power of subconscious processes and emotional states. In this condition a nurse cannot be clearly aware of her client. There is a difference in kind between these two forms of awareness.

Research on nurses' moral reasoning, based on Kohlberg's model, has revealed that nurses sometimes do not obtain the expected score. In one study, for example, it was found that the nurses' years of experience were related negatively to moral reasoning. How can these low scores be explained? One explanation is that nursing experience may increase the use of context in moral reasoning. Contextualism, or sensitivity to details of a particular situation, according to Kohlberg, limits a person's ability to apply universal principles, and *as such, exists at a lower level of moral reasoning* (emphasis added).[21]

It could not be said better: The more a nurse takes her profession seriously, the more she fails her ethical obligations as outlined in the traditional ethical systems. The more experience and knowledge she gains, the more she remains aware of what she is doing and why she is doing it—the greater her value to her client—the more blameworthy she becomes.

Charity requires that we pass this by with only the observation that, in making this discovery possible, Dr. Kohlberg has revealed that he has not the gift of self-awareness or, perhaps, that he lacks a sense of humor.

■ FREEDOM FROM ETHICAL THEORY

Deontologists and consequentialists may both be wrong. They cannot both be right. The intention of an action is not the same thing as the consequences of an action—the changed conditions that the action brought about. The consequences of an action are not the same as the intention of the action—the reason why the action was taken. If the intention behind an action alone determines its moral value, then the consequences of an ethical action do not. If the moral value of an action is determined solely by the consequences of the action, then the intention behind the action does not determine its moral value.

Some agents, consciously or unconsciously, base their ethical actions on a beneficent intention. Other ethical agents, consciously or unconsciously, predicate their ethical actions on optimum consequences. Between these two there is, probably, little difference to be observed in their ethical behavior. Some ethical agents are not consistently motivated by either intention nor consequences. The behavior of these agents, probably, does not differ much from the behavior of the other two. Finally, no ethical agent is, or could be, motivated by both intention and consequences, each taken in isolation.

Since contemporary ethical theory has little determining influence on behavior it seems that an argument can be made that no one, including nurses, *needs* ethical theory. But, as we shall argue, nurses do need ethical theory.

■ PROFESSIONAL BENEFITS OF NURSING

A person facing the choice of a career has many options. The choice she makes will ultimately be decided by the values she holds. A person will probably opt for the profession that promises to incorporate the greatest number of the values that she is seeking.

If she made a conscious decision to become a nurse then, all things being equal, she became a nurse because she wanted to promote the survival of clients, to ease their suffering, to increase their well-being, and to enhance their lives. Either this or no specific value prompted her to become a nurse. Whatever the reasons she *became* a nurse, she can accomplish these things through *being* a nurse. Through her profession she can make her life a great adventure and herself a person to take pride in. If this is not her motivation she will do many of her clients great harm, if only in preventing them from interacting with a dedicated and professional nurse. And she will do herself significant harm.

If a nurse is concerned with ethical decision making both she and her client gain. If she is not, both she and her client lose. This is why she ought to be concerned with the ethical aspects of nursing. The fact that a nurse incorporates ethical concerns into her practice and functions as a dedicated nurse does not, in itself, ensure her success and happiness. But it helps stack the deck in her favor.

All interaction takes place for two or more people to benefit from the actions of each other. But what if a nurse interacts with a client? Other than a salary, what benefit does she gain from this interaction?

All the benefit of realizing those values that inspired her to become a nurse.

If nursing is not a profession that motivates and inspires a nurse, then it makes her professional life dismal. It ought not to be dismal. If her expectations are not unreasonable, a nurse can ease suffering and bring strength and comfort to others *and to herself.* Nursing can enhance the life of a nurse as much as it enhances the lives of clients.

■ THE ETHICAL POWER OF CONTEXT

"In ethics everything is contextual and the context of every action is unique and unduplicable, with the result that even a small difference between two situations may yield a difference in our moral verdict."[14] What one should do usually, or in general, is not the same thing as what one should do in a specific case. A number of contextual backgrounds surround every dilemma. It is these contextual backgrounds that produce the complexities of the dilemma. In the health care setting these may include such things as the possibilities afforded by a client's condition, the skills of the professional staff, the stage of technical development, and the availability of resources.

All of these play a part, but the bioethical dilemma proper consists of those aspects of the situation that are directly under human control, those aspects of relevant knowledge that are presently available, and the aptitude of these to serve the well-being of a client.[16]

The Nurse's Context

Two aspects of every context are interrelated: the first is the context of the situation the nurse faces—those objects in, and the structures of, the situation that are relevant to a nurse's purpose. The second is the context of knowledge she brings to and obtains from the situation.

The *context of the situation* is the interwoven *aspects* of a situation that are fundamental to understanding the situation and to acting effectively in it. The *context of knowledge* is a nurse's *awareness* of the relevant aspects of a situation that are necessary to understanding the situation and to acting effectively in it. These aspects are asymmetrically related to each other. The objects and structures of the situation are what they are whether or not the nurse has knowledge of them. They are independent of the nurse's knowledge. But whether the awareness and beliefs of the nurse are knowledge depends entirely on these objects and structures.

The nurse is often motivated by preconceptions in her mind, which she brings to a bioethical dilemma. Or she is motivated on a purely affective level by the situation facing her. If she moves away from one of these extremes it is apt to be to the other extreme. What is needed is to move into and gather motivation from both aspects of the context.

In bringing together the context of the situation and the context of her knowledge a nurse actualizes a notable ethical accomplishment. She brings together and integrates ethical intention and consequences. She intends, through the actions she takes, to bring about appropriate consequences. The consequences she acts to bring about are consequences that she has a reason, over and above the consequences themselves, to intend to bring about.

It is natural and appropriate that a nurse have an emotional reaction of some sort to every ethical dilemma. But a too-intense or inappropriate emotion can deflect responsible action. A nurse's responsible and justifiable ethical action requires understanding. It requires that she understand the context of the situation and the context of the knowledge she already possesses, not emotionally but conceptually.

Her understanding cannot be an emotional response. An emotional response is not an act of *understanding.* Yet one emotion is essential to a nurse's effective ethical decision making. That is the emotion of *caring.* Without caring ethical interaction would have no fuel. Caring is the essential principle to guide bioethical analysis.

Other than caring, in the broad assortment of common dilemmas a nurse faces she has no right to bring any other emotion into her ethical decision making until she can clearly discern the difference between conclusions and decisions she makes on the basis of acute contextual analysis and those she reaches that are based on her emotional responses to conditions. "Although the ethical concerns of . . . nurses are permeated with compassion, . . . answers must come from thoughtful reflection, too."[20]

The nurse's context, as such, is the interweaving of her awareness and the aspects of the situation of which she is aware. It is this interweaving of her consciousness and the situation—of intention and a determination on appropriate consequences—that makes understanding and effective ethical action possible. Through the connection between these contexts, that which is intelligible in a situation becomes understood in a nurse's awareness.

A nurse who understands through an interweaving of these contexts understands as well as any person can understand. Any ethical action she takes that is appropriate to this understanding is, in principle, perfectly justifiable.

The Health Care Context

In the health care context, justifiable ethical action is action appropriate to the nature of the context. The health care context is an interweaving of contexts—the context of a health care professional and the context of a client. It is an intertwining of the nurse's circumstances and the client's circumstances. It is an interplay between the client's experience of his present circumstances and the nurse's knowledge of his circumstances.

The health care context is formed by all of the diversity to be found in the health care setting. "Diversity is evident everywhere in nature and can bring richness to our world. Not understanding diversity can negatively affect our abilities as practitioners and leaders. Success is really predicated on understanding not only diversity but also how different types of individuals can work together more effectively. . . . How the understanding of these differences can assist us as leaders and practitioners."[27]

A nurse's context begins at the client's bedside, but it extends throughout the entire health care system.

■ IS THERE AN ETHIC OF THE HEALTH CARE SETTING?

It is a notorious fact that the practice of nurses who study the traditional ethical systems is unaffected by this study.

This fact is not at all strange. If the traditional ethical systems were ever relevant to the vital complexities of the health care setting, which is doubtful, they certainly are not now. Not only are they not relevant, they are, perhaps in the majority of cases, totally inappropriate. The obvious demands of humanity's distilled ethical wisdom, such as the prohibition of murder, child abuse, rape, and theft, are essential backdrops to the health care setting as they are to any human situation.

But these demands do not depend on any ethical system. Murder is not wrong because it violates a rule. Child molestation is not wrong because it works against the greatest good for the greatest number. These prohibitions were norms recognized and practiced universally long before the foundation of formal ethical systems. A professional ethic has nothing to say about these offenses. If someone *needs* to be told that theft is wrong and prohibited by her professional ethic, she will pay little attention to that ethic or any ethic.

■ PRACTICE-BASED ETHICS

Murmurings are being heard among nurses of the need for an ethical system derived from, and therefore appropriate to, the health care setting—a practice-based ethic. In terms of ethical theory, nursing is coming of age.

If nurses can take the small step of embracing a practice-based ethic they will elevate themselves and their profession over and above health care professionals who conduct their practice according to the empty rituals of the traditional ethical systems. In a crucial area of biomedicine they will create a benefit for themselves and all of their future clients. They will produce the inestimable benefit of knowing why they are doing what they are doing, and they will make themselves aware of how they are doing it. If nurses can understand and function under an ethical system specifically appropriate to the health care setting while other health care professionals are engrossed in irrelevant ethical speculations, nurses, on a very crucial level of biomedical practice, acquire a significant excellence.

What will be the final form of a practice-based ethic?

It will be an ethic whose defining terms have to do with the condition of a client and the practice of nursing. Unless it is misnamed, this alone can qualify as a practice-based ethic.

A practice-based ethic must pursue the study of ethical action through an examination of the meanings of terms relevant to the interaction of biomedical professionals and clients and the purposes of the health care setting.

Principles and norms will have virtually no part in a practice-based ethic. Rather, a nurse's attitude of caring in relation to a client is the overarching principle and norm of such an ethic.

The nature of an ethical system is determined by its center of attention. Under deontology a client's ethical dilemma leads a nurse's awareness to a duty. Under utilitarianism it leads to the greatest good for the greatest number. Under casuistry it leads to tradition. In the same way a practice-based ethic will lead the nurse's awareness to the situation of her client.

A nurse is, most fundamentally, an agent—the agent of a client, doing for the client what the client would do for himself if he were able. A practice-based ethic in nursing, then, must be the ethic of one person acting as the agent of another person. It must be an ethic of actions implied by the nature of the health care setting. It is the natural ethic of a nurse acting for a client—a client being one who has, through incapacity, sickness, or injury, lost the power to take those actions for himself that he would take if he were able.

One example of an explicitly practice-based ethic is symphonology. Whenever a nurse is practicing her profession, she is interacting with clients. The actions she takes is her practice. This interaction, directly or indirectly, always takes place on the basis of mutual agreement. The term *symphonology* comes from a Greek word meaning *agreement.* "[Symphonology] focuses on the nurse/patient agreement . . . . It differs from [other systems] in [its] emphasis on the strength of the relationship . . . It was designed to assist the nurse in making justifiable ethical decisions."[9] The nurse/client agreement is normally unspoken. Yet, although it is implicit, it is an agreement that is made consciously. A nurse and her client are always, to some extent, aware of its existence. According to their understanding of it, it shapes and colors everything they do.

An agreement is a shared state of awareness on the basis of which interaction occurs. A shared state of awareness produces the intelligibility and understanding that interaction requires. Successful interaction requires intelligibility and understanding. The health care setting produces few ethical demands that cannot be met by successful interaction. A practice-based ethic is an ethic whose standard is the shared state of awareness that produces this success.

This implies several further standards—a recognition of and respect for the nature of the person with whom one has made the agreement. One does not interact successfully with another person if one does not know that other person and the purposes that motivate him.

This shared state of ethical awareness is structured by the expectations and commitments of each participant. The entire practice of nursing, including its ethical aspects, is created by the agreement that establishes a professional relationship between a nurse and a client. The orientation of their agreement centers entirely upon the role of the nurse, the situation of the client, and the practice of nursing. A symphonologic ethic places the client and his situation at the center of practice.

A nurse's practice is her process of executing the actions she has agreed to execute. A practice-based ethic simply dictates that her ethical responsibility is to do what she has agreed to do—not what is demanded by a duty, what society expects, what is traditional or what anyone except her client expects her to do, but simply what she has agreed to do. Even the expectations of her client must be limited. A client has no right to make unreasonable demands—demands not in the role of a nurse. And he has no right to expect anything that violates her nature as a human being.

Nothing is unusual about the nurse/client agreement. Everyone, in any situation, has a responsibility to do what she has agreed to do. A nurse has an interweaving of agreements with her client and the health care system, and a responsibility to follow through on these agreements. But no agreement is as central to bioethics as the nurse/client agreement. Indeed, the validity of every agreement arises because of the triangular relationship between the client, the health care system, and the nurse. The central agreement of everyone involved in the health care system, and the standard of ethically right and wrong, is the agreement that everyone in the health care system has with the clients who enter that system. Symphonology, like any practice-based ethic, is contextual. It is a system of standards to motivate a nurse to take actions in relation to a client, to help her discover what is the best action to take, and to make it possible for her to explain how her actions were appropriate to her professional purpose. These standards are preconditions of the nurse/client agreement. They also serve as lenses to enable a nurse to understand her client and to interact with the choices he makes for himself.

To make an agreement a person must have some *reason* to make the agreement. Otherwise she would never conceive of the idea of making the agreement. For her to have this reason the person with whom she makes the agreement must differ from her in some significant way. A nurse's recognition and acceptance of a client's difference—his uniqueness—is one of the natural standards of a practice-based ethic. This, in common with every standard, is because a recognition of and respect for whatever is necessary to the nature of persons making an agreement is itself an agreement. Before one makes an agreement with another person one must recognize the fact that he is a person—one must, in effect, agree to the fact that he is a person.

A client must be able to conceive of and carry through long-range plans and purposes. There is no such thing as an agreement made for the split second. The recognition and acceptance of a client's power to take purposeful long-range actions is also a standard of a practice-based ethic.

An agreement between two persons exists only if each is objectively aware of the terms of that agreement. Interaction on the basis of objective awareness must be a standard for a practice-based ethic. It is an agreement implied by the existence of the professional/client agreement, the agreement that establishes the relationship and the interaction between the nurse and the client. When nurse and client interact each has a right and a responsibility to know what she is doing. To make an agreement the client must have rightful control of his time and effort—the time and effort necessary to make the agreement. He does not lose that rightful control in entering the agreement; he retains it. It is a natural standard of a practice-based ethic.

Every agreement is made between two people to realize some benefit or to avoid some harm. Acceptance of the benefit-seeking nature of human beings is a standard for a practice-based ethic. It is certainly appropriate to the ethical interaction of any health care professional and her client.

A Nurse's Fidelity

For an agreement to exist between persons it must be possible for them to exercise fidelity to the agreement, and they must actually exercise that fidelity.

Who a client is—the character structures that make him a unique person—he is by right. Whenever one person makes an agreement with another, she agrees to recognize the right of the other person to be who he is. Otherwise their relationship would be characterized not by agreement but by aggression.

The Nurse/Client Relationship

A nurse is an individual living a specific role in the health care setting. A client is, in relation to a nurse, one who has a need to interact with a nurse.

A client needs a nurse simply because the client lacks the power to take action. He lacks the physical or mental ability, the knowledge, the motivation, or the emotional stability to take action. For any one or a combination of these reasons the client needs a nurse. This is why a nurse takes the role of agent for the client and does for the client what he would do for himself if he were able.

When the ethic of the nurse/client relationship is practice-based it is symphonologic in a fundamental sense. It is formed by the agreement that binds them together and the implications of this agreement. Their agreement is unspoken but essential to the relationship.

A nurse walks into a client's room or into a client's home. The client is in some version of a bed. Right there the agreement is set up:

"You are my client. I will be your nurse."

"You are my nurse. I will be your client."

Their discovery of each other is sufficient to produce the agreement. They immediately recognize the facts that have brought them together.

The agreement arises when a nurse, in effect, accepts a client's invitation to be his nurse and a client accepts a nurse's offer to be his nurse. It is formed by the expectations and commitments of each. Each makes a commitment to satisfy the expectations of the other when these expectations are implied in the nurse's profession and the client's situation. These expectations and commitments establish the ambience of the relationship between a nurse and her client.

It establishes the boundaries of the justifiable and the unjustifiable in ethical interaction.

It establishes what each party has a right to expect from the other within their interactions.

A nurse, as a nurse, is not a marriage counselor, a secretary, or an expert in family relations or childrearing. She is not the ultimate decision maker in matters concerning a client's way of living. She is not many things. Above all she is not an intuitive and infallible judge of good and evil.

The role of a nurse is a role of agency. She is the agent of a client. Her role includes utilizing her technical and therapeutic skills, educating her client concerning facts he needs to know about his condition, counseling her client, and, when necessary, making demands for her client and protecting him in the health care system.

Above all she ought to develop and exercise the ability to serve as custodian of the virtues—the moral resources and personal strengths—her client needs to bring to bear on his condition. This she does when she uses the bioethical standards as a link between herself and her client. She does this when she recognizes the standards as ethical preconditions of their relationship. She does it when she interacts with him and facilitates his acting guided by the bioethical standards as lenses upon his character structure. Two things are crucial in their relationship: her understanding of him, and his understanding of himself.

If her ethical system is practice-based, if it is derived from the nature of her profession, a nurse will derive practical benefits from bioethics. If these practical benefits are necessary to the success of a nurse in her profession then she needs bioethics.

When a nurse and a client are related through an agreement, and the agreement is honored, they form a harmonious union. Where the agreement is lacking or broken there is no harmony and no union. The nurse's actions imply that she regards the client as possessing no value. And, in fact, in relation to her client, a nurse then possesses no value.

In the nature of things, a nurse derives practical benefits from practice-based ethics. Such an ethic allows a nurse to develop the virtues of a nurse. The development of her virtues as a nurse enables her to develop her virtues as a person.

These virtues are necessary to her success as a nurse. Therefore a nurse needs a practice-based ethic.

■ VIRTUE ETHICS AND THE VIRTUOUS NURSE

For every ethical agent some mindset—some ethical attitude—is inevitable. No one can face the world without some orientation toward it.

For most ethical agents this mindset is very unstable. Most ethical agents do not know why they are doing what they are doing; they have no objective purpose. They simply follow their duty or their assumed responsibility to a greater number. They submit to what they assume is demanded by social conventions. They hold no final goal that their actions are oriented toward. Therefore their actions are unpredictable and vacillating. They swing from an intense ethical enthusiasm for some problems to an attitude of ethical indifference to others. At certain times they may approach every problem, however minor, with excessive ethical fervor. At other times they are unmoved by an interest in any ethical dilemma.

It is impossible to practice a traditional, ritualistic ethic and not fall into one of these mindsets. No one ever knows for certain where his or her duty lies. No one ever knows for certain how to bring about the greatest good for the greatest number.[15]

Perhaps the most ancient system of ethics is the system known as *virtue ethics.* It can be traced back to ancient Egypt circa 7000 BC.

Before the flowering of philosophic ethics in ancient Greece the term *virtue* meant excellence. For instance, the virtues of a horse are its swiftness and endurance. The virtue of a physician is his ability to heal. The virtues of a wrestler are his strength and skill. The virtue of an artist is his ability to portray. In its classic sense, the virtue of a person came to mean all those excellences that arise from the person exercising control of her actions through reason.[5]

For the Greek philosopher Aristotle, virtue is the intention and capability of doing the right thing, at the right time, for the right reason, in the right way, and to the right degree. This is reminiscent of "the five rights" of giving medications. It may be the source of the idea of the five rights. Aristotle thought of virtue as a kind of art. This art arises from habits of action—actions that bring about good results. These habits of action become a second nature. In becoming a second nature they form settled character-structures.

The virtue or excellence of a living thing is a form of well-being or power. It is the power, possessed by the living thing, to sustain its life as the kind of thing it is. Virtue, then, is a form of health.[22]

The ethicist Benedict Spinoza describes virtue thusly: "[R]eason demands . . . that every person . . . would desire everything that really leads man to greater perfection, and absolutely that everyone should endeavor, as far as in him lies, to preserve his own being."[10] This is, of course, the ethical motivation of every client, and it is what the health care setting is all about.

■ CARING VERSUS PRINCIPLISM

One framework for ethical reasoning is that of the care perspective. This framework is only in the beginning stages of development, and various authors have considered it as everything from an ethical theory, another principle of bioethics, and a moral value to a stance one takes to ethical decision making.

An orientation arising from care is "characterized by a view that the primary moral concern is one of creating and sustaining responsive connection with others."[12] The care orientation is most often defined in contrast to the principlist orientation. Where the principlist perspective values impartiality and detachment when arriving at ethical decisions, the care perspective stresses that each situation is unique and requires sensitivity to others' needs and to the dynamics of particular relationships. Persons, from a care perspective, are viewed as interdependent in relation to others. Moral conflict resolution is a process of dialogue to understand the particular needs of the persons involved.

If caring is well directed it fulfills the promise a client hopes to find in the health care setting, whereas principlism—an ethic of norms and principles—must have a different, and very possibly a contrary, outcome. Such an approach implies that a nurse's ethical concerns are related primarily to norms and principles and are only secondarily related to a client's concerns. It also implies that, under various circumstances, the ethical concerns of a client are in conflict with the ethical concerns of a nurse. This makes the client into a sort of moral enemy to the nurse against whom she must defend herself behind the shield of principles.

Caring, as an outcome, and as productive of outcomes, is quite obviously desirable. It is possible to define *caring* from the aspect of outcomes.

The most effective interaction between a nurse and client—the best outcome caring can have in their interrelationship—is when their interaction maximizes the activity of a client on his own behalf. When a client cannot act on his own behalf, a nurse's action still ought to maximize the benefit the client can realize. A nurse ought to do "for a patient what the patient would do for himself if he were able" and *as* he would do for himself if he were able. For instance, if, from an attitude of caring, a nurse exercises agency for her client, she will act toward him with an attitude of compassion. In this she expresses the fact of her humanity. There is no doubt that a client cares for himself and the outcome of his actions. And, being human, if he were able it is virtually certain that he would act with compassion for himself. The nurse will act with empathy and compassion, not from guidance by an external norm or principle, but through thinking of what it is to be a nurse, a client, and a human being. She can easily define actions that are caring from this perspective.

■ EXPERTISE IN NURSING

"[S]killful ethical comportment will deteriorate to a merely competent level if we apply norms and principles to complex practical situations where we have the potential for skillful recognition of patterns and intuitive responses. Strategies of adjudication and the search for certitude through the application of norms and principles, though comforting, do not produce expert skillful ethical comportment."[1]

A nurse, expert in the ethic of the health care setting, is one who has observed clients and their situations and derived an explicit understanding of her relationship to them. An expert nurse, generally speaking, will have an informed idea of why her client acts as he does. At a high level of expertise, if he does not act as she would expect him to act, she will be able to discover why.

There is a way to master this art. The first step is for a nurse to differentiate between two aspects of her own personality. The first aspect is those qualities she shares in common with all human beings just by virtue of the fact that she is a human being. This will include, for instance:

1. Her desire to continue living.
2. Her propensity to act toward things in the outside world with desire and aversion.
3. Her inability to understand and evaluate her circumstances immediately and infallibly—her need for experience and analysis.

The second aspect of her personality is her idiosyncratic characteristics—those qualities that are peculiar to her and that other people do not necessarily share. These will include:

1. Her choice of an occupation.
2. Cultural beliefs that she accepts or rejects.
3. Her attitude of fear toward certain objects and pleasure toward others.
4. Certain actions she has taken that she recalls with pride and other actions she recalls with regret.

The next step in attaining expertise in bioethical action is to accept the fact that these idiosyncrasies are idiosyncrasies. Although one has a right to make them part of one's own character, one has no right to expect them to be part of the character of another person.

Then, to become proficient in ethical interaction, the nurse will approach any problematic situation with this knowledge. After rigorously taking her idiosyncrasies out of consideration, a nurse can ask herself *how* she would decide and act in her client's situation. To understand her client's choices and actions she can ask herself *why* she would decide and act in this way.

If under his circumstances she would not act differently than her client, then she has discovered his motives. If she would act differently then she must ask herself what idiosyncrasies underlie his motives—what factors cause him to act as he does. Following this, her task is to accept or, under unusual circumstances, to deal with these idiosyncrasies.

Why did her client choose a certain value?

1. Because, given the fact that he is a human being, it is an understandable choice.
2. Because of a personal idiosyncrasy of the client—an idiosyncrasy that does not clash with the needs of his human nature.
3. Because of a personal idiosyncrasy that does clash with the needs of his human nature.

Given the first two motivations, a nurse has an obvious responsibility to support the action of her client and to act as his agent. If, on the other hand, his motivation is of the third variety, a nurse has no responsibility and no right to support him in his action. The practice of making these differentiations puts a nurse on the level of expertise in bioethical decision making.

An ethical decision maker is very much like a pool player. An unskilled pool player merely attempts to put a ball into a pocket. An unskilled decision maker decides what is best and acts on it. A skilled pool player sets up shots and tries to put the ball into a pocket while leaving the cue ball in such a position that it will be easy to make the next shot. A skilled decision maker makes decisions purposefully.

A skilled nurse makes decisions based on the purposes of her client and on what is necessary to accomplish them. A skilled decision maker does not exert intense mental effort to make arrhythmic ethical decisions, but masters the process of bioethical decision making as a skill.[15]

■ CASE

Following is a case specifically designed to illustrate the point made by Benner and others.[1]

Alice Marshall arrives for her 11 to 7 shift and, following report, begins to make her rounds. She finds one of her clients, Beth Reynolds, agitated and in severe pain.

Alice knows from caring for her before that 7 years ago Beth's 2-year-old son was kidnapped. To this day Beth and her husband have no idea as to the fate of their son—whether he is alive or dead.

Beth, now age 42, is in the hospital undergoing treatment for ovarian cancer. In all probability she will be sent home to die once her physician, Dr. Ackerman, has successfully controlled her pain.

Beth has been alert and still able to get around, although she is weak. She has a living will that states that, among other things, she does not want to be connected to a machine nor to have CPR performed. In line with her wishes, Dr. Ackerman has written a DNR order.

Alice knows from report that, in addition to her morphine drip, Dr. Ackerman has ordered another drug to better control Beth's pain. Alice gives Beth the drug by IM injection. Within minutes of giving the drug Beth has what Alice believes to be an anaphylactic reaction and goes into respiratory arrest. At the moment that she arrests a close colleague of Alice's rushes into Beth's room to tell Alice that a call has just been received from Beth's husband. Their son has been found alive and well.

Alice has every reason to believe that this colleague is reliable. Given all and only the facts laid out in this context, what is Alice's best course of *ethical* action?

■ METHODS OF ANALYZING ALICE'S DILEMMA

Alice, in her analysis of this dilemma, will evaluate the "good" (allowing Beth to know the facts of her son's fate before her life is over) that will be made possible by resuscitating Beth versus the "hurt" (resuscitating Beth only to compel her to go through the dying process again).

Consequentialism

Alice may call upon consequentialism—a desire to bring about the greatest good for the greatest number. One obvious problem with this approach is the problem of how consequentialism will define *good.* Alice may leap to the conclusion that resuscitating her will provide Beth's life with a more desirable history. Or she may have an irresistible insight into the fact that resuscitating Beth would constitute an undesirable harm. Every nurse has a different definition of what is good.

Also, Alice will have to consider the good provided to Beth's husband and son in knowing that Beth died knowing, or not knowing, her son's fate. In addition to this she will have to consider the potential benefit and harm to herself if others disagree with her decision. Different persons in administration have different ideas of what is and what is not good.

Casuistry

If Alice believes that she has sufficient time to analyze the situation that she and Beth share through casuistry, it is very likely that she will find no relevant prior cases to refer to.

If she perseveres she can choose from her past experience any case whatever according to her subjective and more or less arbitrary inclination. When she examines the case it will not be by any process of analysis, properly called, but through her present preconceptions. She will find what is similar and what is relevant through a process of rationalization. But what she will find will be similar and relevant only to these subjective preconceptions.

If Alice decides to resolve Beth's case by what was done in a previous dilemma, then she faces the problem of how she knows that what was done in the prior situation was the best thing, or even a responsible thing, to do.

If she has no standard by which she can judge that the best thing was done in the previous dilemma, then it is probably better that she does not act on the basis of it. If she has a standard of judgment by which to judge that the actions taken in the previous situation were appropriate, then she has unknowingly abandoned decision making through casuistry. She is not resolving her present dilemma according to the standard of past experience. She is resolving it according to the *standard* by which she judges this past experience.

Deontology

If Alice appeals to deontology to resolve her dilemma she may recognize her duty to protocol and follow the DNR order. Or she might recognize a duty to her client, in which case she may choose to ignore the DNR order.

If she chooses (although a chosen duty is, strictly speaking, no longer a duty) her duty to Beth then, again, she is faced with the problem of competing ideas of the good.

If her action is to be an ethical action then she must follow her duty. It is her duty to follow her duty, and it is impossible to know what her duty is. Her duty lies on either side of a tossed coin. This provides little guidance.

Symphonology

If she turns to a practice-based ethic to bring about a professionally responsible and justifiable result, she will begin by attending to Beth's situation. She will refer to what she has learned of Beth's purposes and desires. She will then use this knowledge to gain an understanding of prior statements Beth has made and actions she has taken. This must be done, of course, without intruding her own personal values onto Beth.

When she makes a decision for Beth she ought, at least, to consider the following facts concerning human values and the communication that would probably occur between herself and Beth if communication were possible.

She has no definite knowledge of what Beth would want in these final hours of her life. Therefore she might best refer to what she knows of what most people would want in these circumstances. In this way she can determine, with the highest probability, what Beth would want. And then, as Beth's nurse, she can, within the context of her knowledge, do for Beth what Beth would (according to the highest discoverable probability) do for herself if she were able.

If a significant preponderance of people in Beth's circumstances would want to be resuscitated, then it is probable that Beth would want to be resuscitated. If they would not want to be resuscitated, then it is probable that Beth would not want to be resuscitated.

Alice is not given the opportunity for ballistic accuracy here. But a practice-based ethic provides a very great deal of guidance for Alice. The DNR is a subagreement of the nurse/client agreement. It is an agreement that never would have been made in the absence of the nurse/client agreement. It was an agreement as to the best way to fulfill the terms of the original nurse/client agreement—given Beth's context of knowledge of her situation when the agreement was made. But a radical change has occurred in Beth's situation, and this knowledge is no longer *knowledge.*

The overarching agreement that establishes a nurse/client relationship between Alice and Beth is, on Alice's part, an agreement to act for Beth's well-being—the best state she can enjoy. Not to resuscitate Beth would violate this agreement. A very significant preponderance of persons in Beth's circumstances would want to be resuscitated. The probability that Beth would want to be resuscitated is very high. The probability that she would prefer dying without knowing of her son's fate is very low.

Therefore the original nurse/client agreement overrides the specific agreement on the DNR, or any subagreement. The subagreement on the DNR, in relation to the nurse/client agreement, becomes a mistake, just as many times choices and decisions prove to be mistakes in need of alteration with changing circumstances.

Whatever decision Alice makes, she will not make it with absolute certainty. But absolute certainty is not the greatest benefit a nurse can bring to a client. It is often said that the greatest value a nurse can bring to a client is her concern—her caring. A nurse cannot be caring and careless—caring and indifferent—at the same time. Nothing will make her careless more quickly and more completely than a feeling of perfect certainty. An agreement between a health care team and a client often provides this certainty to a careless nurse. A caring nurse will always maintain toward her client's situation an attitude of suspended doubt. If a nurse is to be caring and careful about her client's welfare she will have to avoid the comfort of certainty. She will accept the possibility, or even the probability, that her patient's situation might change. She will not be compulsive, but she will entertain the possibility that an easy judgment might be mistaken.

Alice is not given the opportunity for ballistic accuracy here. But she can act with a high degree of certainty. This degree of certainty will allow her to act with perfect bioethical responsibility. It is sufficient to completely justify Alice's action.

A radical change occurred in Beth's life situation. She was unable to think, choose, and act in response to this change. Yet there are strong reasons to believe she would have responded had she been able. Beth can act, but only through Alice. If it were a thoughtful friend rather than a nurse beside Beth's bedside, and the friend were able, it is quite predictable that this friend would act to resuscitate her.

In acting for a client a nurse acts as a friend. If one analyzes what it is to be a friend, one will deepen one's understanding of what it is to be a nurse. "[I]nstrumental friendship may prove useful as a metaphor for nurses to expand the meaning of caring."[25]

Alice has no sufficient knowledge of the specific character structures that make Beth who she is—not a sufficient awareness to allow her to judge with perfect certainty the status of Beth's desire. But from her life experience, her experience of herself and other people, she knows that, even under these circumstances, most parents would want to complete their life knowing of the happy fate of their son.

Given the amount of time Beth had spent wondering about the fate of her son, and given the emotional effort she had invested in concern for his fate, it is quite unlikely that she would be indifferent to his fate now.

If resuscitating Beth would be a harm it would be relatively minor harm. If Beth would want to be resuscitated to discover the fate of her son it would be a benefit—a major benefit in the whole history of Beth's life, and certainly the greatest benefit possible here and now.

Alice owes Beth fidelity to her professional agreement. That agreement would necessarily include Alice's courageous application of an objective analysis to Beth's situation. Under these circumstances Alice, as a human being and as a parent, would want to be resuscitated. There is no reason for Alice to provide less for Beth than she would want for herself.

Alice has done all she can do, in the context of all her knowledge, to ascertain her best course of action. Although she does not enjoy the perfect certainty that communication with Beth would give her, it is massively probable that Alice ought to resuscitate Beth to inform Beth of the discovery of her son.

As a professional Alice owes this to Beth. As a professional, and as a human being, Alice owes this to herself.

■ A PROFESSIONAL ETHIC AND THE PROBLEM OF CERTAINTY

"Nursing is a vital and an integral part of the health care system. Nurses have more continuous and, perhaps, more intimate contact with people than any other health care professional. Nurses are privy to patients' and family members' fears, hopes and regrets. This position, therefore, offers unique privileges and responsibilities."[8]

Between nurse and client a special relationship has been set up without a rational basis for trust. There is no prior friendship, or even acquaintance. In addition, the values and dangers involved can be much more vital and fundamental than those involved in ordinary interactions.

A professional ethic does not have to do with good and evil, or right and wrong. That is part of the ethic of the man on the street. A professional ethic does not control a professional's relationship to God, society, or the legal system. It controls her relationship to the health care system on the one side and her client on the other. Her ethical relationship is established by the expectations of the health care system, her client, and her commitments to them. She has fulfilled her part of the ethical relationship if, and only if, she has lived up to the justifiable expectations of the health care system and her client and met her commitments to them.

Whatever a professional's relationship to God, society, or the legal system, she needs a way to guide her actions in relationship to her profession and her clients. Her professional ethic should not conflict with these other relationships. But her profession is a distinct, and important, part of her life. To this end a professional ethic is necessary.

A client does not come into the health care setting for good or evil, much less for right or wrong. He comes in for life, health, and well-being. This is the ethical standard of a biomedical professional's role—the life, health, and well-being of her client, in all the areas in which they interact, and to whatever extent this is possible—but always within the confines of what is possible. Bioethics is an ethic outlining a biomedical professional's role in promoting the life, health, and well-being of a client.

Ethical certainty is possible in a biomedical setting. But it is not possible to enjoy an absolute certainty. The only certainty a nurse can enjoy is a contextual certainty—whatever certainty is possible in a limited time and a limited context.

Certainty is only possible to the extent that:

1. One has relevant facts available as evidence pointing toward a decision—the context of the situation.
2. One has relevant knowledge to apply to these facts—a context of knowledge.

This is unfortunate, but it is the way the world is set up. An attempt to escape awareness of the situation, or to evade one's knowledge, cannot change this. Irrelevance is not a solution to the problem of certainty.

■ ROLE OF INTERDISCIPLINARY ETHICS COMMITTEES

One avenue that may be of help to health care providers in deliberating over ethical conflicts is the hospital ethics committee. The current trend is for an increase of ethics committees and a process of ethics consultation to be available to staff and clients with ethical problems. The purpose of institutional ethical committees usually is to:

1. Review or write institutional policies based on ethical considerations.
2. Deliberate about complex cases and, at times, to make recommendations to the proper person.
3. Educate staff and the community.[2]

Since ethics committees are of recent origin, they will differ in the specifics of their makeup and role as a result of the environment in which they were created and the length of time they have been in existence. Some committees keep a very low profile in the institution, meeting only rarely and performing few case consultations or educational programs. Others, which have been in existence for a decade or more, are known for their active education programs, the formality and extensiveness of their consultation role, and the respect they engender among their colleagues.

Membership will vary from committee to committee, but most are interdisciplinary, including membership from medicine, administration, nursing, social work, the clergy, ethical philosophers, lawyers, and the local community.

However, each member of the committee should be free of a personal agenda. He or she ought to be able to deliberate without prejudice on the basis of what is justifiable—what best serves the rights and well-being of individual clients.

Decisions are often shaped and polished best by the friction of discussion, and, generally speaking, the more viewpoints available the better. However, two types of members will hinder the work of the committee and predictably produce harm to clients.

1. Those who cannot come to an ethical decision.
2. Those who immediately have the answer to every ethical dilemma.

Deliberations are all too often clouded by tradition, individual vanity, dogma, and gut reactions.

One type of person, whatever his possession or lack of other qualifications, who will facilitate the work of the committee is one who has been in the client's situation and, thereby, has first-hand knowledge of it. This type of person is referred to as a *native.*[26]

The following questions need to be considered during bioethical deliberations:

1. Is this actually a bioethical dilemma?
2. Can this dilemma be resolved at the unit level or should this be taken to the ethics committee?
3. What assumptions are being made about the rights of the individual?
4. What ethical decision-making model or theory will be used to help guide the bioethical deliberations?
5. Is the resolution to the bioethical dilemma such that it will be difficult to take action on the decision?

If the answer to #5 is *yes,* the committee should consider the following:

1. What are the constraints that are making it difficult?
2. In what ways can these constraints be mitigated?
3. Is this a situation in which the benefit/harm ratio requires that action be taken immediately, or is it one that would permit deferring action at this time?

Further questions of concern are:

1. Who should serve as chair of the committee? Why?
2. What are the policies under which this committee will function?
3. What arrangements can be made for clients, families, and "natives" to sit in on the deliberations of the committee?

Until recently, nursing has been underrepresented on most ethical committees. However, as the role of nursing has grown throughout the health care institutions, their visibility on ethics committees has increased to include more middle management and staff nurses. With the inclusion of diversified nursing representation, the particular ethical concerns of the clinical bedside nurse are more readily recognized and addressed.

In some instances nurses within a hospital or agency have developed their own nursing bioethics committee that encourages (1) the education of nurses in bioethical decision making, (2) discussion of ethical issues unique to nursing, and (3) the involvement of nursing in institutional ethical concerns, policy making, and committee work.

■ SUMMARY

What is the role of the nurse as bioethicist? To argue for rules or to offer insights? To further the goals of the institution or to defend client autonomy? To call attention to the formalities of the health care system or to place sound analysis at the service of the client?

"Ethics is a process of analyzing the appropriateness and effects of human action."[13]

A nurse can learn what is and is not ethically appropriate through memorizing what others tell her. This will take place long before she becomes a nurse. Or she can learn what is and what is not ethically appropriate to a nurse after she becomes a nurse. She can do this only through a serious analysis of the ethical dilemmas of nursing and only if her analysis continues to the point of understanding.

"As the twenty-first century approaches, much of nursing practice time entails processing complex health-care situations. Assisting individuals and families to resolve profound, value-laden questions related to their lives has become a common intervention in nursing practice."[11] This is not possible with the ethics of childhood—the ethic of the "man on the street." A nurse can reason from her client's situation *to* a contextual ethical judgment or she can reason *from* abstract memorized preconceptions to a decision that ignores her client's situation.

For the ethical systems that predated bioethics, ethics has to do with what one does. For a practice-based ethic, ethics also has to do with the reasons why one does it and the way in which one does it—with self-respect, a respect for rights, and a recognition of the character structure of one's beneficiary.

An ethically effective novice nurse acts *for* a client. An ethically effective expert acts *with* a client. A nurse ought to work for a client's self-interest while remembering that a client's self-interest is not always identical to his pleasure or convenience. She also ought to remember that her client's self-interest is seldom identical with the pleasure or convenience of third parties who disagree with his decisions.

For every ethical duty or principle there is always another duty or principle to supplement or replace it. For every good and every number there is always the possibility of a greater good or a greater number. For every exercise in casuistry there is always the possibility of more cases to consider. For none of these is there an end point—a time when one can say, "Ethically, I ought to have done X. I did X. I did everything I ought to have done."

With practice-based ethics this is not the case. As well as providing standards of behavior, a practice-based ethic provides goals of behavior. If one ought to act according to a client's right to freedom or his right to control his life—his time and effort—or to bring about any other benefit for a client, and one does this, then one has done what one ought to do. One has done what one has agreed to do, and grand irrelevant gestures are unnecessary.

CRITICAL THINKING *Activities*

1. **How does a nurse benefit nursing by mastering bioethics?**
2. **How does a nurse benefit herself by mastering bioethics?**
3. **How does an understanding of the client facilitate bioethical analysis and decision making?**

Note: Portions of this chapter are from the second edition of this book and were contributed by J. Anne O'Neil. We hope she approves of the use to which we put her work and thank her for her contribution.

4. **Choose a bioethical dilemma from your own practice. How would you analyze it in terms of the different systems?**
5. **How can a reasonable application of casuistry contribute to expertise in bioethical decision making?**
6. **What are the aspects of the bioethical context, and how does a nurse integrate them?**
7. **Why is neither intention nor consequences in isolation an adequate guide to bioethical decision making?**
8. **How does a practice-based ethic differ from the traditional ethical systems?**
9. **Why is the client the central ethical concern of the health care system?**
10. **What is the role of the nurse/client agreement in bioethical interaction?**
11. **How does "What most people in this circumstance would want" facilitate bioethical analysis?**

References

1. Benner P, Tanner CA, Chesla CA: *Expertise in nursing practice,* New York, 1996, Springer.
2. Corsino BV: Bioethics committees and JCAHO patients' rights standards: a question of balance, *J Clin Ethics* 7(2):177-183, 1996.
3. Crigger NJ: Universal prescriptivism: traditional moral decision-making theory revisited, *J Adv Nurs* 20:538-543, 1994.
4. DeGrazia D: Moving forward in bioethical theory: theories, cases, and specified principlism, *J Med Philosophy* 17:510-513, 1992.
5. Den Uyl DJ: *The virtue of prudence,* New York, 1991, Peter Lang.
6. Dimmitt JH, Artnak KE: Cases of conscience: casuistic analysis of ethical dilemmas in expanded role settings, *Nurs Ethics* 1:200-207, 1994.
7. Emanuel EJ: Medical ethics in the era of managed care: the need for institutional structures instead of principles for individual cases, *J Clin Ethics* 6:335-338, 1995.
8. Gibson CH: Underpinnings of ethical reasoning in nursing, *J Adv Nurs* 18:2003-2007, 1993.
9. Greipp ME: A survey of ethical decision making models in nursing, *J Nurs Sci* 1(1-2):51-60, 1995.
10. Gutmann J, ed: *Spinoza's ethics,* New York, 1949, Hafner. (Original work published in 1675).
11. Hartman R: Identifying opportunities to ask patients about their treatment wishes, part 2: ethical analysis, *Leadership Dimension* 12:322-326, 1993.
12. Hamric AB: Measuring the care perspective: a measurement protocol, Unpublished manuscript.
13. Hogstel M: *Geropsychiatric nursing,* St. Louis, 1990, Mosby.
14. Hospers J: *Human conduct: problems of ethics,* New York, 1972, Harcourt Brace Jovanovich.
15. Husted GL, Husted JH: *Ethical decision making in nursing,* ed 2, St. Louis, 1995, Mosby.
16. Husted GL, Husted JH: The bioethical standards: the analysis of dilemmas through the analysis of persons, *Adv Pract Nurs Q* 1(2):69-76, 1995.

17. Husted JH, Husted GL: Personal and impersonal values in bioethical decision making, *J Home Health Care Pract* 5(4):59-65, 1993.
18. Kant I: (J.H. Paton, trans.). *Groundwork for the metaphysics of morals,* New York, 1964, Harper & Row. (Original work published 1785).
19. King CS: Managed care: is it moral? *Adv Pract Nurs Q* 1(3):7-11, 1995.
20. Kinion ES, Jonke NL, Paradise N: Descriptive ethics and neuroleptic dose reduction, *Perspect Psychiatr Care* 31(2):11-14, 1995.
21. Lutzen K, Nordin C: Modifying autonomy—a concept grounded in nurses' experiences of moral decision-making in psychiatric practice, *J Med Ethics* 20:101-107, 1994.
22. McKeon R: ed: *The basic works of Aristotle,* New York, 1941, Random House.
23. Mill JS: *Utilitarianism,* London, 1863, Oxford Press.
24. Deleted in proofs.
25. Rawnsley M: Of human bonding: the context of nursing as caring, *Adv Nurs Sci* 13(1):41-48, 1990.
26. Siegel B: Going native, *Hastings Center Report* 23(1):46, 1993.
27. Straka DA: Look for so much more! *Adv Pract Nurs Q* 2(2):79-81, 1996.
28. Toulmin S: The tyranny of principles, *Hastings Center Report* 11:31-39, 1981.

PART TWO

Nursing Education

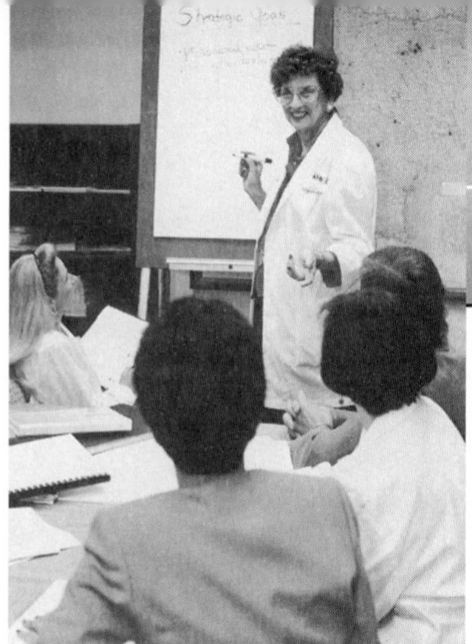

CHAPTER 8

Nursing Education

Judith A. Halstead, Diane M. Billings

OBJECTIVES After completing this chapter the reader should be able to:

- **Discuss societal changes that affect nursing education today**
- **Describe how state government establishes and regulates standards for nursing practice**
- **Describe how the federal government influences nursing education at the national level**
- **Discuss the influence of health care reform on nursing education**
- **Describe the differences between practical nurse, nurse, diploma, associate degree, and baccalaureate degree nursing education programs**
- **Discuss master's degree programs in nursing and the practice roles the master's degree graduate is prepared to perform**
- **Discuss the various types of doctoral education for nurses and the practice roles the doctoral graduate is prepared to perform**
- **Discuss the concept of educational mobility in nursing education and how these strategies are implemented**
- **Describe the various curriculum designs and instructional delivery systems that are used to promote educational opportunities in nursing**
- **Discuss the various issues that affect the future of nursing education**

Health care needs of the twenty-first century will require increased numbers of nurses who are prepared to practice in a community-based health care delivery system. The nursing profession is responding to the demands of today's radically changing health care environment by developing nursing programs and curricula that will provide learners with the competencies necessary to provide cost-effective, quality health care in a managed care environment. The purposes of this chapter are to recognize the dynamic context in which nursing education programs develop, differentiate the types of nursing programs, explain the concept of educational mobility, and identify alternative curriculum models created to meet the needs of an increasingly diverse population of nursing students. The chapter also discusses alternative delivery systems for making nursing education accessible. It concludes by raising issues for further dialogue about the future of nursing education.

■ EDUCATIONAL PREPARATION FOR NURSING PRACTICE

Context of Nursing Education

Nursing programs are an outcome of a dynamic relationship with the social, educational, legislative, economic, and professional forces present in contemporary society. Nursing and health care will emerge in the year 2000 in forms and patterns unlike those of previous decades. Nurse educators must therefore be responsive to the contextual changes in society and develop nursing programs that prepare graduates to contribute to society as informed citizens and professionals.

Social context. The social context in which nursing programs are embedded has major implications for the development of program curricula. In the United States, for example, substance abuse, domestic violence, homelessness, and poverty have become increasingly commonplace. Lack of health care, inadequate educational support, and joblessness continue to affect the quality of life experienced by many Americans.[45] Changing demographics also affect society. For example, the number of elderly persons has increased, and so has cultural, racial, and ethnic diversity.[43,45] The aging population increases the demand for a health care system that emphasizes the prevention and treatment of chronic illness.[22] The increasing multiculturalism present in society demands a health care system sensitive to the needs of a diverse population. Furthermore, the epidemiology of health problems in America has changed as society copes with such prevalent communicable diseases as tuberculosis, AIDS, sexually transmitted diseases, and other health problems caused by a polluted and shrinking environment.

To meet the challenging health care needs of society, sweeping health care reforms have been proposed and implemented. Development of a collaborative, community-based health care system that emphasizes health promotion and disease prevention and is affordable and accessible to clients has become a national priority.[19,22,62,65] Changes brought about by health care reform will continue to have a significant impact on the roles of nurses in the health care system and the types of competencies and skills nurses will be required to possess. To be responsive to the needs of society, curricula in nursing education programs must reflect these social trends and prepare nurses with the appropriate cognitive, affective, and psychomotor skills.

Educational context. In addition to the effect of societal issues on nursing education, a discussion of the context of nursing education must address the current educational issues facing postsecondary education and nursing education. Postsecondary education, particularly higher education, has been criticized for graduating students unprepared for the future and for maintaining curricula that perpetuate a lack of purpose and learning.[9] As a result of such criticism, higher education has been under close scrutiny from consumers, legislators, and the business world, with an accompanying demand for increased accountability for improving student learning.[43] Through curriculum revision, colleges and universities have responded to criticism from the public and the demand from state commissions on higher education to be accountable and assess learning outcomes. Curricula are being revised to prepare individuals, with a liberal education along with a major area of study, who are capable of demonstrating such characteristics as critical thinking and problem-solving skills, a commitment to independent learning, adaptability, and creativity.[43] Such curricular revision will enable higher education to produce graduates who are informed citizens capable of contributing to an increasingly complex, information-driven society.

Nursing education programs must be responsive to the curriculum changes occurring in higher education and the mandate for change in nursing curricula. In addition to debates about differentiation between professional technical nursing practice and preparation for entry into practice, nurse educators are raising questions about what learning is, what should be taught, how it should be taught, and how performance and outcome can be assessed. At all levels of education, nurses of the future must be prepared to practice in a community-based health care system and provide nursing care to diverse cultural populations. As with other higher education curricula, nursing curricula are being revised with an emphasis on the development of critical thinking skills, collaborative abilities, and shared decision making.[2,56] As nurse educators question historical models of curriculum development and urge reform of both undergraduate and graduate education, new patterns in nursing curricula are emerging to integrate theory and practice, to redefine learning, and to use teaching-learning strategies that best facilitate learning as nurses move from novice practitioners to expert clinicians.[3,56]

Legislative context. Nursing education is influenced by legislation at local, state, national, and international levels. Such legislation defines nursing practice and nursing education and sets standards for determining who will be the practitioners of the profession. At the state level, state boards of higher education have responsibility for planning and recommending numbers and types of programs, whereas state boards of nurses' registration and education establish standards for licensure and quality of nursing education programs, qualifications of faculty, and curriculum requirements. State legislation also regulates nurse practice acts. Legislation in North Dakota, for example, specifies separate licensure for two categories of nurses, the technical and the professional nurse. In North Dakota a baccalaureate nursing degree is required for R.N. licensure, whereas an associate nursing degree is required for L.P.N. licensure.[37] This is the only state that currently requires a baccalaureate nursing degree for R.N. licensure.[2,23,48,56,74]

State legislation also regulates the advanced practice roles of nurse practitioners, clinical nurse specialists, nurse-midwives, and nurse anesthetists. For example, legislation has been enacted in many states that grants advanced practice nurses prescriptive privileges and eligibility for third-party reimbursements for services.

Federal legislation, in turn, influences nursing education at the national level. Examples include funding nursing research, providing student financial assistance, and funding innovative nursing education programs. Nursing education is also influenced by the development of federally legislated changes in health care policies.

Economic context. Closely related to legislative forces, economic forces affect nursing education by influencing the supply and demand for nurses, salaries, and health care delivery systems. Staffing patterns, utilization of nurses in differentiated practice, and employment opportunities contribute directly to the recruitment of students into educational programs, as well as influence the numbers and geographic location of these programs. For example, over the years the use of nurse practitioners to provide primary health care to clients has proven to be cost effective. With the increasing emphasis on a primary health care delivery system, many more nurse practitioners are needed. Nursing education programs have responded to meet this demand by increasing the number of master's degree programs that prepare nurse practitioners.[22]

Professional context. Also important are the professional forces and organizations that are shaping the direction of nursing education programs and curricula. These forces are related to the marketplace, practice environment, and strategies for effective use of nurses with varied educational preparations. The work of two nursing organizations can be traced to demonstrate the relationship of nursing's professional organizations and development of nursing education programs.

In 1965 the American Nurses Association (ANA) proposed two entry levels for the practice of nursing: the technical nurse, with an associate degree as educational preparation, and the professional nurse, with the baccalaureate degree as educational preparation. In 1984 ANA reaffirmed its position on the baccalaureate degree in nursing as entry for practice and in 1985 voted to support two categories of nurses, the technical and the professional, with education in associate and baccalaureate programs, respectively.[4] At the same time the National Commission on Nursing Implementation Project (NCNIP), composed of a governing board representing a variety of nursing and health care organizations including the American Association of Colleges of Nursing, American Organization of Nurses Executives, the National League for Nursing (NLN), and ANA, was established for the purpose of implementing recommendations for earlier studies[74] by identifying trends and establishing consensus for action to affect the future of nursing.[55] In 1987 NCNIP identified characteristics of professional and technical nurses of the future and established a timeline for changes in the educational system, developed a model for describing nursing care systems that are cost effective and ensure quality, explored how nursing research can be used to influence public policy, and advocated an information system to ensure timely access to data for education, practice, and research.[21,54]

Nursing specialty organizations have affirmed the ANA position and the direction established by NCNIP. For example, in 1989 the American Association of Critical Care Nurses identified competence statements for the technical and professional nurse in differentiated practice.[39] The American Association of Colleges of Nursing (AACN) recently issued a policy statement identifying the baccalaureate degree as the minimum requirement for professional nursing practice.[3] The issue of differentiated practice has yet to be resolved. However, because of proposed changes in the health care delivery system, it is anticipated that there will be a greater need for nurses prepared at the professional level. It is estimated that by the year 2000 the United States will need twice as many nurses prepared at the baccalaureate level as will be available.[31] The differentiation of the roles and responsibilities of nurses based on educational preparation will become necessary to effectively meet the needs of clients. Nurse educators will be responsible for designing educational programs that produce the appropriate mix of nursing personnel.[2,22,31]

It is in these contexts, then, that nursing programs are designed to prepare graduates with the knowledge, skills, and values to practice in a complex and changing health care arena. The educational preparation of nurses is described below.

Nursing Programs

Nursing educators are responsible for developing nursing curricula to ensure adequate numbers and categories of nurses prepared to meet the current and future health care needs of society. As health care reform in the United States continues to evolve, it has become apparent that nursing programs must produce broadly educated graduates capable of providing care in a variety of settings.[3,31] Increased numbers of advanced nurse practitioners are also necessary to provide community-based primary health care.[56]

In the United States nursing programs prepare nurses as *technical nurses* (practical nurse, diploma, and associate degree programs), and *professional nurses* (baccalaureate degree, master's degree, and doctoral degree programs). These programs differ in education base, curriculum, educational setting, accrediting agency, and professional organizations that advocate their interests. Graduates of these programs differ as to the type of roles and practice settings in which they prepared to function as nurses. Each program is described below.

Practical nurse programs. Practical nurse programs prepare students to become licensed practical nurses (L.P.N.s) or licensed vocational nurses (L.V.N.s). The graduates give client care under the direction of a registered nurse or other licensed health professional.

The first practical nurse program was offered in 1892 as a 3-month training program by the YWCA in Brooklyn, New York; others followed in the 1900s. Later, world wars created a demand for nurses who could be quickly trained, and the number of practical nurse programs increased. In 1941 the schools formed an Association of Practical Nurse Education and began accrediting schools of practical nursing in 1945.

Educational setting. The practical nurse program is typically offered by a vocational or technical school. The program may also be sponsored by high schools, hospitals, or community colleges.

Entry requirements. Requirements are a high school diploma or demonstrated high school equivalency. Other requirements may be stipulated by the educational institution.

Educational base. The curriculum builds on introductory content in the biologic and social sciences. These courses may carry college credit or may be integrated into the curriculum.

Curriculum. The course of study is typically 12 to 18 months and includes courses with a focus on acute and chronic illness, rehabilitation, maintenance of health, and prevention of disease. Heavy emphasis is on clinical practice. Graduates from L.P.N./L.V.N. programs are prepared to give care, under the direction of a registered nurse or licensed physician, to clients whose care plan is well established, and in structured settings such as long-term care or acute-care hospitals, homes, outpatient settings, or physicians' offices.

Licensing examination. After graduation from the L.P.N./L.V.N. program the graduate is eligible to take the National Council for Licensure Examination-Practical Nursing (NCLEX-PN). The L.P.N./L.V.N. is then licensed for employment as a practical/vocational nurse.

Accrediting agencies and professional organizations. The Council on Practical Nursing of the NLN is currently responsible for accrediting L.P.N. programs. Other accrediting agencies may be involved in the accreditation process for the technical school in which the practical nurse program is located. Several professional organizations such as the National Association for the Practical Nurse Education and National Federation of Licensed Practical Nurses are active in advocating quality education and informing the public about the role of practical nursing in nursing service.

Diploma programs. Diploma programs prepare students to become registered nurses. The programs are typically associated with a hospital, but more recently are affiliated with a college or university. The programs prepare graduates for technical nursing practice in a variety of health care settings.

Diploma schools of nursing were the primary educational agent for educating nurses during the 1800s and early and mid-1900s. The schools were patterned after the Florence Nightingale training school model. The first school in the United States was the New England Hospital for Women and Children. Linda Richards was its first graduate, in 1873.

As a result of studies, commissions, and position papers[4,55], the setting for nursing education programs shifted to colleges and universities. The number of diploma schools and entrants in diploma schools has steadily declined since 1960. As of 1996, 121 diploma schools were accredited by the NLN; three more diploma schools were scheduled to close.[24]

Educational setting. The hospital is the primary educational setting for the diploma program. Cooperative arrangements are usually established with a community college or university to provide general education courses in the biologic and social sciences.

Entry requirements. A high school diploma is required for entry into a diploma school. Some schools use scholastic aptitude tests such as the SAT and nursing aptitude tests as admission guidelines.

Educational base. The diploma program is based on a foundation of general education courses in the biologic and social sciences. Generally these courses are offered by a college or university with credit transfer arrangements with baccalaureate or master's degree programs.

Curriculum. The curriculum is designed to prepare nurses for direct patient care and includes courses in nursing management and home health care. The curriculum can be completed in 2 to 3 years. Heavy emphasis is placed on clinical practice. The graduate of a diploma program is expected to demonstrate the following competencies:

1. Provide nursing care for individuals, families, and groups by using the nursing process

2. Provide for the promotion, maintenance, and restoration of health, and support and comfort to the suffering and dying
3. Use management skills, including collaboration, coordination, and communication, with individuals, families, and groups with the other members of the health care team
4. Assume a leadership role within the health care system
5. Teach individuals, families, and groups based on identified health needs
6. Function as an advocate for the consumer and the health care system to improve the quality and delivery of care
7. Practice nursing based on a theoretic body of knowledge, ethical principles, and legal standards
8. Evaluate nursing practice for improvement of nursing care
9. Accept responsibility and accountability for professional development
10. Use opportunities for continuing personal and professional development
11. Participate in health-related community services
12. Use critical thinking in professional practice[61]

Licensure. Graduates from diploma programs take the NCLEX-RN and are licensed as registered nurses.

Accrediting agencies and professional organizations. Diploma programs are currently accredited by the Council of Diploma Programs of NLN. Professional organizations representing the interest of diploma programs include NLN and ANA.

Associate degree programs. Associate degree programs prepare students to become registered nurses. The curriculum is offered in a community college or senior (4-year) university and prepares the graduate for technical nursing practice. The goal of associate degree nursing programs is to prepare registered nurses who provide direct client care.[59]

The associate degree program originated in 1952[72] and was the first planned approach to nursing education based on organized research. The development of the program was influenced by (1) the need for additional nurses in the work force and (2) experience from the cadet nurse training program that indicated that registered nurses could be educated in less than the 3 years of the typical diploma program. The first associate degree nurse (A.D.N.) program was conducted in the Cooperative Research Project in Junior and Community College Education at Teachers' College, Columbia University, under the direction of Mildred Montag.[53] The purpose of the program was to prepare technical nurses who could assist professional nurses. The curriculum was designed to increase the science base and decrease the practice base, which was to be provided in the employment setting. Although originally intended to serve as a terminal degree, most A.D.N. programs now serve as a base for R.N. mobility programs.[72]

Educational setting. Associate degree programs are offered primarily by community and junior colleges. They may also be offered in vocational colleges, senior universities, or free-standing degree-granting institutions.

Entry requirements. Applicants to associate degree programs must meet the entry requirements of the college or university in which the program is located. The requirements typically include graduation from high school or the equivalent college preparatory curriculum and evidence of scholastic aptitude. Entry requirements for

L.P.N.-to-A.D.N. programs may include licensure as an L.P.N. and clinical practice experience.

Educational base. Associate degree education is based on a general education course. The courses meet degree requirements of the college or university and include biologic and social sciences. Approximately half of the curriculum (usually 25 to 30 credits) is composed of general education courses.

Curriculum. Two curriculum patterns prepare graduates for the A.D.N. degree. The first is a generic or basic curriculum. The second pattern is an L.P.N.-to-A.D.N. program that provides mobility for graduates of L.P.N. programs and accepts credit and experience for previous learning.

The A.D.N. curriculum builds on the base of general education courses in the biologic and social sciences and includes nursing courses in adult and child health, maternity nursing, psychiatric and mental health nursing, legal aspects of nursing practice, ethical issues, and professional roles. Community health concepts may also be included.[45] The curriculum can be completed in 2 academic years (around 60 credits). Associate degree graduates are expected to assume three basic roles in their nursing practice: provider of care, manager of care, and legitimate members of the general health care team. To assume these roles, the associate degree graduate is prepared to demonstrate the following knowledge, skills, and attitudes: clinical competence, critical thinking, accountability, commitment to caring, collaboration and organizational skills, knowledge of legal and ethical standards, communication skills, advocacy, respect for other health care professionals, and commitment to professional growth.[59]

The nursing practice of a graduate from an associate degree program is directed toward providing care for clients across the lifespan, with an emphasis on adult clients. A.D.N.s are prepared to meet the acute and chronic health care needs of clients in practice settings that have specified policies and procedures and where professional guidance is available. A.D.N.s may practice in acute and long-term care settings.[59]

Degree granted. The degree is granted by the institution of higher education in which the associate degree program is located. The degree may be an Associate of Science in Nursing (A.S.N.), Associate Degree (A.D.), or an Associate of Applied Science (A.A.S.).

License. The graduate from an associate degree program is prepared to write the NCLEX-RN examination. In most states the A.D. graduate is licensed as a registered nurse.[28] In North Dakota, however, the A.D.N. graduate is licensed as a licensed practical nurse under state legislation for differentiated education and licensure.[37]

Accrediting agencies and professional organizations. Associate degree programs are currently accredited by the Associate Degree Council of NLN. The institution of higher education may also be accredited by an appropriate technical or college accrediting agency.

Professional organizations promoting the interests of associate degree nursing include NLN, ANA, and NCNIP. The National Organization for the Advancement of Associate Degree Nursing was formed in 1986 to support associate degree education and nursing practice. The organization endorses registered nurse licensure for the associate degree graduate.

Baccalaureate nursing programs. Baccalaureate nursing programs set in colleges and universities are designed to prepare graduates as generalists in professional nursing practice. Baccalaureate graduates are caregivers, client advocates, agents for change, consultants, casefinders, teachers, and leaders. Bachelor of science in nursing (B.S.N.) graduates care for individuals, groups, families, and communities, and are prepared to give nursing care in structured and unstructured settings. The B.S.N. degree may be earned in a 4-year college or university with a major in nursing or after completing an associate degree or diploma program and completing the postdiploma/A.D.N. baccalaureate nursing curriculum.

Baccalaureate programs began in the early 1900s; the University of Minnesota established the first nursing major in the undergraduate program in 1919. In the early years of baccalaureate education, programs were 5 years in length: 2 years for the college courses and 3 years for the nursing curriculum. Momentum for the program increased when an ANA paper in 1965 specified a baccalaureate degree in nursing as the minimum education necessary for entry into practice of professional nursing.

Educational setting. Baccalaureate nursing programs are offered in senior (4-year) colleges and universities. Free-standing independent degree-granting programs, usually supported by a health care agency in cooperation with a senior university, are alternative settings for the baccalaureate nursing program. These programs are affiliated with a college or university, but the degree is granted from the program itself.

Entry requirements. Students entering baccalaureate nursing programs must meet requirements of the college or university and the school of nursing that include high school graduation with college preparatory courses in English, chemistry, biologic sciences, and mathematics. The college or university may also stipulate admission tests such as the SAT or ACT and specify a high-school grade point average. Some schools of nursing admit or certify students only to the upper-division major. In these instances students must complete and demonstrate success in lower-division prerequisites. It is also possible for R.N.s who are graduates of an associate degree or diploma program to enter a baccalaureate program to acquire a B.S.N.

Educational base. The baccalaureate curriculum is founded on a strong base of liberal arts and sciences. These courses are selected to develop a person who has a liberal education, which includes inquiry, literacy, understanding numerical data, historical consciousness, science, values, art, international and cultural experience, and in-depth study of one concentrated area.[1,20,51] The liberal arts and sciences foundation makes up approximately 60 credits of the 120-credit curriculum.

Curriculum. The two types of curricula preparing students for a B.S.N. are the generic curriculum and the postassociate or postdiploma (two-plus-two, registered-nurse baccalaureate, or second-step) curriculum.

The generic curriculum builds on prerequisites in arts, sciences, and humanities.[74] The majority of courses are offered in the last 2 years of the program (with a few courses in the sophomore year) and include content in the following:

1. Theory
2. Research
3. Care of adults, children, and the childbearing family

4. Psychiatric and mental health nursing
5. Interpersonal skills and group dynamics
6. Community health
7. Nursing management
8. Professional concepts with an emphasis on critical thinking, decision making, and problem solving

The postassociate/diploma programs build on the associate degree (or diploma) curriculum of the registered nurse and are designed to move the student from a predominantly technical focus in nursing to a more professional orientation.[77] General education courses are supplemented by selected liberal arts courses and include senior-level courses in nursing leadership and management, community health, group dynamics, interpersonal skills, professional concepts, nursing theory, nursing research, and health assessment.

The graduate from a baccalaureate program in nursing is prepared to perform the following:[57]

1. Provide professional nursing care, including health promotion and maintenance, illness care, restoration, rehabilitation, health counseling, and education based on knowledge derived from theory and research
2. Synthesize theoretic and empirical knowledge from nursing, scientific, and humanistic disciplines with nursing practice
3. Use the nursing process to provide nursing care for individuals, families, groups, and communities
4. Accept responsibility and accountability for the evaluation of the effectiveness of her own nursing practice
5. Enhance the quality of nursing and health practices within practice settings through the use of leadership skills and a knowledge of the political system
6. Evaluate research for the applicability of its findings to nursing practice
7. Participate with other health care providers and members of the public in promoting general health and well-being
8. Incorporate professional values and ethical, moral, and legal aspects of nursing into nursing practice
9. Participate in the implementation of nursing roles designed to meet emerging health needs of the general public in a changing society

Degree granted. The degree granted is a B.S.N. (Bachelor of Science in Nursing), B.N. (Bachelor of Nursing), or B.A. (Bachelor of Arts) in Nursing.

License. The graduate from a baccalaureate program in nursing is eligible to write the NCLEX-RN examination. Registered nurse graduates from B.S.N. programs have registered nurse licenses. In 1988 the Council of Baccalaureate and High Degree Programs of NLN voted to support differentiated licensure.[15] This would create two licensing examinations, one for a baccalaureate degree with a major in nursing, and one for nurses educated with an associate degree in nursing. As of 1997 differentiated licensure examinations have not been developed.

Accrediting agencies and professional organizations. Baccalaureate nursing programs are currently accredited by the Council of Baccalaureate and Higher Degree Programs of NLN. Colleges and universities in which the programs are based are accredited by higher-education accrediting bodies. Professional organizations influential in baccalaureate nursing are ANA, NLN Council of Baccalaureate and Higher Degree Programs, NCNIP, and the American Association of Colleges of Nursing (AACN). In 1996 AACN indicated an intention to become the accrediting agency of baccalaureate nursing education, replacing NLN in this capacity. This issue is unresolved at the time of this writing.

Master's degree programs. Master's degree programs in nursing prepare nurses for advanced practice roles in nursing. The programs prepare nurses with a functional focus of administrator, clinical specialist, nurse practitioner, nurse midwife, and nurse anesthetist. Master's degree programs in nursing were originally developed to meet the need for educators and advanced practitioners.[69] With the current emphasis on the delivery of primary health care, master's degree programs that prepare nurse practitioners are increasing in number.[60]

In the mid-1960s a need for primary care practitioners was identified, and certificate programs were developed to prepare nurses as nurse practitioner, pediatric nurse practitioner (PNP), and family nurse practitioner (FNP).[12] Over time these programs have moved into academic settings and have been incorporated into Master of Science in Nursing (M.S.N.) programs. Graduates of these programs now receive a certificate as a nurse practitioner and the M.S.N. degree.

Educational setting. Master's degree programs are offered in colleges and universities with graduate programs. The master's program is usually located in schools with baccalaureate nursing programs.

Entry requirements. Requirements for admission to most M.S.N. studies include graduation from a B.S.N. program. Other admission criteria may include R.N. licensure and evidence of scholastic ability as measured by qualifying examinations such as the Graduate Record Examination (GRE) and grade point averages from undergraduate study. For schools with a generic M.S.N. program, admission requirements may include B.S. or B.A. degrees in a field other than nursing. R.N.-to-M.S.N. programs require graduation from an associate or diploma program and licensure as a registered nurse, and in some instances evidence of professional accomplishments and demonstration of knowledge equivalent to a B.S.N. degree.

Educational base. The baccalaureate degree in nursing is the educational base for the M.S.N. degree. The base includes the liberal arts and sciences courses of a baccalaureate degree and, depending on the curriculum, a baccalaureate in nursing degree or equivalent competencies.

Curriculum. There are three major curriculum models for obtaining the M.S.N. The common model is that of the postbaccalaureate curriculum. Courses build on the liberal arts and sciences and nursing curriculum of baccalaureate programs. The curriculum consists of core courses in nursing issues, research, statistics, and nursing theory; courses in the specialty major (such as medical-surgical nursing, critical care, psychiatry, and maternal-child health); and courses in a functional role (for example, education, administration, and practitioner.) The typical curriculum includes 30 to 45 credit hours.

A second curriculum for obtaining a M.S.N. is the generic M.S.N. The generic M.S.N. provides the first degree for entry into the practice of professional nursing. In this model the curriculum builds on the arts and sciences background of a baccalaureate degree and includes nursing courses of the baccalaureate curriculum and that of the postbaccalaureate master's degree. Students may or may not earn the B.S.N. en route to the M.S.N.[34]

A third route to obtaining a M.S.N. is becoming increasingly popular as nurses seek educational mobility. In this curriculum registered nurse students with an associate degree or diploma enter the R.N.-to-M.S.N. curriculum. Credit is awarded for previous knowledge in clinical nursing courses. Nursing research, professional concepts, issues, and statistics are taught at the M.S.N. level, with "bridging" content for the courses in the baccalaureate curriculum. The remainder of the curriculum is similar to the M.S.N. curriculum.

The graduate from a M.S.N. program is prepared to perform the following:

1. Incorporate theories and advanced knowledge into nursing practice
2. Demonstrate competence in selected role(s)
3. Identify researchable nursing problems and participate in research studies that influence nursing practice
4. Use leadership, management, and teaching knowledge and competencies to influence nursing practice
5. Assume responsibility for contributing to improvement in the delivery of health care and influencing health policy
6. Assume responsibility for contributing to the advancement of the nursing profession.[58]

Degree granted. Graduates from master's programs receive the M.S.N. or M.A. (Master of Arts). Several schools offer a Master of Nursing Science (M.N.Sc.), Master of Public Health, or Master of Education.[25]

License and certification. Graduates from a generic M.S.N. program are prepared to write the NCLEX-RN; most graduates of the M.S.N. programs are previously licensed as registered nurses. Some schools of nursing prepare graduates for a specialty practice, and graduates may write certification examinations or nurse practitioner examinations in the specialty as an outcome of the degree.

Accrediting agencies and professional organizations. M.S.N. programs are currently accredited by the NLN Council of Baccalaureate and Higher Degree Programs. NLN, ANA, and AACN advocate the interest of M.S.N. curricula. The requirements of certifying agencies of advanced practice nurses also influence curriculum design in M.S.N. programs.

Doctoral programs. Doctoral programs prepare nurses for roles as academicians, administrators, advanced clinical scientists, researchers, consultants, and independent practitioners. Doctoral degrees in nursing may be professional degrees (Ed.D., D.N.S., N.D.) or research degrees (Ph.D.).

The first doctoral program in nursing was offered at Teachers' College of Columbia University in 1924, with the first graduate being awarded a doctorate in nursing education (Ed.D.) in 1932. Other doctoral programs developed slowly, and the next school to offer a nursing doctorate, a Ph.D., was New York University in 1934.[63] During the 1960s doctoral programs in nursing science (D.N.S.) were established in response to the need for nursing scientists and academicians. The professional degree (D.N.S.) was developed at this time as a result of lack of (1) prepared faculty, (2) a well-defined knowledge base, and (3) a research record required to establish research degrees.[50] In the 1970s there were four doctoral programs with a nursing major, expanding to 27 in the mid-1980s.[25] As of 1993, 54 schools of nursing had doctoral programs.[60]

Educational setting. Doctoral programs in nursing are offered in colleges and universities with graduate programs in nursing. The school of nursing may be aligned with the university and follow an academic model for doctoral education, or it may be located in a health sciences setting with a professional-model focus.[35]

Entry requirements. Admission requirements to doctoral programs are set by the nursing program and the college or university. They may include completion of an M.S. program, evidence of scholastic achievement, and admission examinations such as the GRE. Evidence of professional accomplishment and writing skills may also be required. Entry requirement for the nursing doctorate is a B.S.

Educational base. Doctoral programs in nursing build on the education base of advanced arts, sciences, and nursing of the M.S.N. program. Depending on the educational setting, the educational base for the program may follow an academic model or a professional model.[5,35]

Curriculum. There are four types of nursing doctoral programs: the Doctor of Nursing Science (D.N.S.) or the Doctor of Science in Nursing (D.S.N., D.N.Sc.); the Doctor of Philosophy (Ph.D.), which is the most common; the Doctor of Education in Nursing (Ed.D.); and the Nursing Doctorate (N.D.).[27,33,50] The curriculum design of the doctoral degree depends on the purpose of the program, program objectives, and the degree granted. A typical plan includes 90 credits, with an inquiry component (statistics, research methods) of 15 to 18 credits, a concentration in nursing major (theory development, substantive focus courses) of 30 to 35 credit hours, and an external cognate minor, related to the area of concentration in the major, of 12 to 15 credits. Other credits for the degree are obtained from elective and dissertation credits.

The doctorate may be combined with other fields of study, such as the Ph.D.-L.L.B. degree, combining nursing and law, or the Ph.D.-M.B.A., combining nursing and business. More than 90 credits may be required to obtain dual degrees.

The D.N.S. or D.S.N. is a professional terminal degree that prepares graduates for practice. Core courses provide a base for advanced nursing knowledge and practice, clinical specialization, and interdisciplinary leadership. The research focus is on communication, use, and interpretation of findings of research rather than generation of new knowledge.

The Ph.D. is an academic degree that prepares graduates to conduct basic research and develop and test nursing theory. The emphasis of the program is the discovery of new knowledge and ability to conduct research. Courses focus on clinical scholarship and the design and testing of theory.

The Ed.D., the least common type of nursing doctorate, is an applied degree that emphasizes preparation in nursing education.[63] Graduates are prepared for scholarship and research, but the emphasis is on application of knowledge rather than generation or dissemination. At this time only one school of nursing offers the Ed.D.

The generic doctorate, the N.D., is a professional degree that is based on a baccalaureate education.[49] The curriculum prepares the graduate for generalist practice and interdisciplinary collaboration. The research focus is on interpretation or reinterpretation of nursing knowledge. Some educators advocate the N.D. as the degree for entry into practice.

Graduates from doctoral programs are prepared to function in advanced nursing roles. Educational outcomes depend on the type of program, although outcome differences are often negligible.[5]

Degrees granted. The degree granted depends on the type of educational program the student attends. The degree may be a Ph.D., D.N.S., D.S.N., D.N.Sc., Ed.D., or N.D.

Licensure. Graduates from the N.D. are eligible to write the NCLEX-RN. Graduates from nursing doctoral programs are already licensed.

Accrediting agencies and professional organizations. As of 1996 there is no accreditation specifically for doctoral programs in nursing. The graduate programs of a university, however, are accredited by its higher education and accrediting body. Nursing doctoral programs are monitored by peer review and judged by the quality of the faculty and graduates. Several professional organizations assume responsibility for advocating doctoral education. AACN and NLN also have committees supporting the interests of doctoral education.

■ EDUCATIONAL MOBILITY

As previously discussed, there are six types of educational nursing programs. Although each is designed to attain specific educational and professional outcomes, graduates from one program can, and are often encouraged to, seek degree and career opportunities requiring subsequent education. The movement to another degree program is referred to as *educational mobility.*

Educational mobility facilitates multiple points of entering the profession of nursing, as well as career advancement through additional education without loss of credits from previous education. For example, an individual may enter the nursing education system as an L.P.N. in an associate degree program, exit with an A.D.N. degree, and at a later date reenter the system in an R.N.-to-M.S.N. program and obtain an M.S.N. or doctorate in nursing.

Nursing programs have been developed for mobility from L.P.N. to A.D.N., L.P.N. to B.S.N., A.D.N. to B.S.N., R.N. to B.S.N., R.N. to M.S.N., and B.S.N. to doctorate. Nursing programs are also being developed to facilitate education for graduates with bachelor's degrees in other disciplines into an M.S.N. program (B.S. or B.A. to M.S.N.).[41] Each mobility program is developed according to the philosophy of the school of nursing, employs a variety of curriculum patterns, and uses a variety of mechanisms to award credit for the previous education. The concept of educational mobility is supported to recruit qualified individuals into the nursing profession and encourage preparation for advanced practice roles.

One major advantage of educational mobility is that a number of options for nursing education exist. The options fit student educational interests and abilities, career plans, and financial work commitments. Another advantage of a mobile nursing education system is that students can graduate with one degree and be employed while earning another degree. Employers and many health care organizations support the concept of educational mobility because employees can be quickly prepared for the workforce; additional education can be obtained while the employee is working.

Mechanisms for Educational Mobility in Nursing

Educational mobility can be promoted by articulation and advanced placement. Nursing programs may incorporate one or more of these strategies to facilitate mobility.

Articulation

Articulation refers to a process in which nursing programs cooperate to plan programs that minimize duplication of learning experiences.[10] The curriculum is designed so that one program is a base for another. For example, a B.S.N. program may be designed to build on the background of an associate degree or diploma curriculum. The credits and course work for one program are included in the entry and degree requirements for the next program. In articulated programs there is little or no duplication of previous learning or loss of program credits.

Advanced Placement

Advanced placement is a procedure for recognizing previous learning.[60] Advanced placement can be accomplished by transferring credit, establishing course equivalency, and awarding credits for previous learning.

Credit Transfer

Credit transfer involves transferring credits from one nursing program to another. The credits in general, liberal, and nursing education are used as degree requirements in subsequent programs. Programs not based in a college or university, such as L.P.N. programs or diploma programs, may have affiliation agreements with a college or university and incorporate these courses in curriculum, with the intent that the credits be accepted by a junior or senior university if the graduate wishes to continue education.

Credit transfer agreements may be established to ensure mobility between specific programs. Although credit transfer preserves credits earned, it does not eliminate the need to complete other education and nursing credits required in the curriculum. Credit transfer for nursing credits is less common than for general or liberal education credits.

Education mobility can also be facilitated by estabiishing *course equivalency.* Courses from one nursing program or college or university can be reviewed by the nursing program accepting the credits to determine whether a course in one program is equivalent to a course in another program. Course equivalency can be established on a course-by-course basis, or a blanket equivalency can be awarded for courses reviewed by faculty.

Credit for Previous Learning

When course comparability cannot be established by credit transfer, some nursing programs have developed mechanisms for validating previous learning and awarding comparable credit for advanced placement. Two ways of establishing credit for previous learning are by testing and by portfolio.

Testing assesses knowledge, skills, and aptitudes and may be accomplished by administering standardized examinations developed for the purpose of promoting educational mobility such as those offered by NLN or ACT.[8] Schools of nursing may also use teacher-made examinations written by nursing faculty. These examinations may be developed for didactic courses, as well as to evaluate clinical proficiency. Passing the examination awards credit for the course.

The portfolio is another mechanism for awarding credit for previous learning. A portfolio is a completion of evidence of achievement that provides a vehicle for assessment of competencies and educational outcomes.[44] The portfolio is presented to a faculty review board for review of the materials to assure course comparability. Evidence may include the following:

1. Work experience
2. Formal courses
3. Examination scores
4. Continuing education experience
5. Letters of reference detailing competency

The portfolio is submitted as evidence of meeting course or program objectives and is reviewed by faculty for verification of meeting requirements. Portfolio acceptance confers credit for nursing or general education course work.

Transition Courses

When nursing curricula are not designed for direct articulation, nursing programs have developed specific courses to provide content missing from previous learning, to "bridge" the student into the program. These bridge, or transition, courses are developed specifically for each curriculum and for students in the mobility program. Transition courses offer students opportunities to assess learning needs, obtain peer support, and prepare for nursing role transition. On completion of the transition courses, students may receive credit for nursing courses and then move into the additional content of the curriculum.

Outcomes of Educational Mobility Programs

Evaluation of mobility programs supports that these curriculum designs are cost effective.[76] Mobility programs produce graduates who meet program outcomes, enlarge the pool for entrants into baccalaureate and higher degree programs, and ultimately improve the quality of nursing care for the consumer.

■ ALTERNATE CURRICULUM PLANS IN NURSING EDUCATION

As the needs of employers change and as nursing students become older, have previous educational experience and degrees, seek educational mobility, and often live at a distance from the nursing program offering the degree, schools of nursing are developing alternative curriculum plans to meet the needs. The alternative patterns of curriculum and instruction include flexible curriculum designs, creative delivery systems, and cooperative arrangements with health care agencies.[32]

Curriculum Designs

Flexible curriculum designs are developed to facilitate diversity of educational opportunity and overcome barriers of distance and time.[26,32,52] These curricula are often competency based and focused on outcomes, and they emphasize student involvement and responsibility for learning. These plans may include external degree programs, competency-based programs, accelerated programs, and expanded programs.

External degree programs. An external degree is a degree awarded for study that does not take place within the typical structure of a classroom, but rather takes place outside of the classroom and is self-paced. Competencies are developed independently by students through a variety of off-campus experiences.[70] The outcome of learning is assessed through standardized criteria and referenced performance examinations, which may have cognitive, affective, and/or psychomotor components. One example of an external degree program is that of the New York Regents External Degree Program, which offers both associate and baccalaureate degree programs in nursing.[46] External degree programs have also been developed for graduate programs.

Proponents of external degree programs cite emphasis on professional practice, self-direction, use of adult education principles, accessibility, and match with learning style as advantages of this curriculum design. On the other hand, external degree programs have been criticized for the decreased contact with faculty and student peers, lack of academic rigor, and unsupervised clinical practice.

Competency-based curricula. Competency-based education involves the definition of specific knowledge, skills, and aptitudes (competencies) to be demonstrated. Instructional strategies are selected to facilitate learner attainment of competencies. Evaluation strategies are developed to indicate the criteria for successful performance and are used to measure outcomes in multiple modes and contexts. Competency-based curricula foster development of individual competence and can be self-paced for learners with varied needs.

Accelerated programs. Accelerated programs offer the nursing major in a compacted time frame. These programs are developed to facilitate educational mobility and to expedite entry into the workforce. Courses are offered in a sequence that is convenient for the learner and can be completed without delay of disrupted course sequence. Course work that might typically be completed in 2 calendar years (four semesters) can be completed in 12 to 18 months.

Expanded programs. Nursing programs have been developed to accommodate the needs of learners who wish to study at a slower pace. In expanded programs the learner can enroll in part-time studies over a longer period. The curriculum is developed to encourage options for students who are unable to enroll in the typical full-time course sequence.

Cooperative programs. Cooperative programs refer to the integration of classroom study with practical experience.[26] Cooperative programs offer students opportunity for clinical practice, income or tuition reimbursement, and simultaneous employment. These programs extend the nursing program to the practice setting and maximize use of clinical facilities and clinical preceptors. Benefits also accrue to the cooperating agency, which gains student service and recruitment potential. Examples of cooperative programs include *internships, preceptorships,* and *work-study.*

Internships. Internships are based on a physician education model that bridges the gap between education and practice. Nursing internships involve an educational experience that provides a transition from student to practitioner. Internships are primarily offered by employing agencies and may last from 2 weeks to a year. The internship provides classroom experience, often in the area of nursing management as well as clinical practice. Internships may be used as a recruitment tool for health care agencies, which benefit from having well-oriented and well-prepared staff nurses who are likely to remain at the agency for an extended period of time.

Preceptorships. Preceptorships are specially designed relationships matching a novice with an expert to facilitate individualized acquisition of skills, knowledge, values, and orientation to the work environment. Like internships, preceptorships bridge the gap between education and nursing service.[29,71] Although preceptorships are primarily offered by an employing agency, they may also be incorporated into senior courses in nursing curriculum. Here preceptors are matched with a senior student to facilitate the transition from student to staff nurse. When preceptorships were integrated into a senior practicum in a baccalaureate nursing program, students who had a preceptor experience demonstrated significantly different professional socialization and were better able to make the transition from student to staff nurse.[18] Preceptorships are not limited to generic undergraduate students but have also been designed for R.N. mobility and graduate nursing students.[71]

Work-Study. Work-study programs combine employment and education. The study and work may be alternated; that is, students may engage in a period of study followed by a period of employment. The classroom experiences provide the theory base, and the employment period provides time for application and testing of theory. Work-study arrangements may also be designed so that employment and study take place concurrently. Various mechanisms are used to grant credit for the employment experience, which may range from full to additional credit or partial credit. The advantages of work-study accrue to the employer and the student and include self-paced education, recruitment and retention opportunities, and financial benefits.

Access to Nursing Education: Distance Education and Virtual Schools of Nursing

As nursing students who live and work at a distance from schools of nursing seek access to basic, advanced, and continuing education, distance education provides alternatives for pursuing nursing course work and degrees. *Distance education* refers to the use of technology (instructional delivery systems) to provide instruction for students who are separated from teachers by time and space. Courses and programs or parts of courses and programs can be delivered by print media such as self-directed learning modules or correspondence courses; television (video conferencing), such as courses offered on satellite, cable, or dedicated phone lines; and on the Internet, such as academic and continuing education courses on the World Wide Web (WWW). Opportunities for distance learning are increasing as information technology becomes available at colleges and universities, health care agencies, and in the home. Recent research about distance education in nursing indicates that learning outcomes of course achievement, student satisfaction, and course progress completion are comparable when distance education delivery is compared with instruction in the traditional classroom.*

*References 6, 11, 16, 17, 36, 38, 42, 64.

Self-Directed Learning

In self-directed learning, or independent study, students and faculty advisors design a personal learning plan. The plan includes the course content, how the content will be learned, the time period, and the criteria for evaluation of outcomes.[17] The content is comparable to courses in the curriculum and carries equivalent course credit. Self-directed learning courses encourage flexibility and independence in meeting course objectives and foster responsibility for self-learning. Self-directed learning is particularly useful as instructional delivery system in mobility programs and to meet elective requirements.[14] Increasingly, self-directed learning opportunities will be offered on the Internet.

Video-Teleconference

Video-teleconferencing uses television to broadcast courses to students at distant sites.[7,11] The course is broadcast from a studio classroom and received at one or more reception sites. The same class that is offered on campus is thus available to students at other reception sites throughout the city or state, or in other parts of the world. Video conferences can use *one-way* video technology, in which students at reception site(s) see and hear the students and faculty at the origination site but the origination site cannot see the reception site(s), or *two-way* video, where all site(s) can see other connected site(s). With current computer technologies it is also possible to use computers with cameras to establish video connections between faculty and students.

The Internet and the World Wide Web

The personal computer has opened new channels for delivering instruction to students through an electronic communications network (the Internet) used to provide interactive instruction to students worldwide. The World Wide Web establishes linkages with multiple users. Increasingly, schools of nursing will be offering academic courses and continuing education to students who can enroll and complete the courses using computers in their homes or work sites.[13] Emerging technologies promise the capability of bringing Internet access through telephone lines to home television sets. Nursing students, nurses, and their clients will have the potential to establish a variety of virtual learning communities to promote lifelong learning and access to health education and health care.

Off-Campus Programs

Another approach to serving distant students is to bring the academic program to a geographically convenient site, often referred to as an *outreach site.*[47,75] This may involve developing nursing programs in an existing system campus, developing a local school site, or having faculty commute to the site. The curriculum offered on the parent campus is thereby offered at a time and place convenient to students who might otherwise be unable to attend the program.

■ ISSUES FACING NURSING EDUCATION

Nursing education is embedded in a dynamic social, educational, legislative, economic, and professional context. Although currently several types of nursing education programs prepare nurses for a variety of nursing practice roles, multiple opportunities for educational mobility, and flexible curriculum plans, the nursing profession must continue to examine the issues affecting curriculum and instruction. Input into these issues must be sought from nurses in the education and practice settings and from consumers. The following issues are raised to stimulate discussion about the future of nursing education.

Students

Who will be the nursing students of the future? Nursing students of the future will be older, more culturally diverse, and are likely to be married and have children. Many will be employed, have previous educational degrees and experience,[3] and live at a distance from an institution of higher education. Costs in terms of time and money influence decisions about the educational options. Will the cost of a nursing education deter future students? How can students knowledgeably choose the type of nursing programs that will enable them to most effectively achieve their career goals? Where will funding to recruit and educate students be found? What support services will be necessary to retain students in nursing programs? Furthermore, other desirable employment options for both men and women outside the profession of nursing will continue to be available. What incentives will attract qualified future nurses to the profession?

Currently there is strong support for educational mobility within the nursing profession. How can educational mobility for students continue to be enhanced among the multiple pathways that exist in nursing education? How can students economically and conveniently access nursing education? How will instructional delivery systems that support distance education and take advantage of educational technology be developed and funded for undergraduate and graduate outreach programs? What shifts in responsibility for learning are required in distance education?

Nurse Educators

Nurse educators have stated that significant curriculum revision is necessary to adequately prepare nurses to practice in today's complex health care system. Fundamental assumptions about learning, teaching, and curriculum are being challenged. How are nursing programs responding to the need for change? How will curricula need to be revised to most effectively prepare nurses to practice in a community-based health care delivery system? What does nursing education research reveal about effective and efficient teaching-learning strategies that promote the development of critical thinking and decision-making skills? What implications do these curricular changes have for student-faculty relationships? What can nurse educators do to promote collaborative, congenial relationships among faculty, students, and nursing staff? How will student and program outcomes be evaluated? Do current accreditation models serve the needs of students, educators, and clients?

Nurse educators are the leaders and developers of nursing programs of the future. The changing health care environment and the increasingly-diverse student population entering nursing have led to the need for changes in nursing curricula. Nurse educators must be prepared to teach in the information age of education and health care. What will be the qualifications for nurse educators? How can nurse educators prepare for the challenges of teaching in future educational systems? How will nurse educators be prepared to fulfill the role of educator in a community-based health care system that emphasizes health promotion and health prevention? Who will support funding for nursing education research and the development of high-technology teaching systems of the future?

Linking Nursing Education and Nursing Practice

If nursing is to influence health care and health policy, nursing education and practice must establish a common base of scholarly nursing practice. New models of collaboration for both nursing education and practice are evolving. What types of collaborative models between nursing practice and nursing education will be needed to disseminate knowledge throughout the nursing profession? How can up-to-date nursing curricula and clinical practice be maintained in this age of rapidly changing technology and information? What technical and professional mix of nursing graduates will most likely meet the health care needs of society? Will graduates of varied programs and curricula be employed in settings that effectively use the differences rather than the similarities of the outcomes of nursing education?

The issues facing nursing education pose challenges for students, educators, and the health care system. To meet the challenges of health care reform, it is likely that significant changes will have to occur in nursing education. Open dialogue between nursing education and nursing practice is essential to the development of nursing education programs that will meet the needs of all the stakeholders.

■ SUMMARY

Rapid and continuing changes in society's health care delivery system have compelled corresponding changes in the way nursing professionals function. As a result, institutions that educate nurses must be responsive to these developments. A large part of the challenge is that nursing educators and practitioners alike must be sensitive to the current health needs of people while anticipating future trends that will affect their profession. On the one hand, quality of care is a major concern to the recipients of nursing and health care. On the other hand, quality control challenges the institutions and educators preparing nurses for practice. State and federal governments must respond more quickly than ever before to provide necessary funding as well as mechanisms for licensing and credentialing. All of these aspects must be coordinated to ensure that the profession serves the people who are the reason for its existence.

The profession has developed numerous types of education programs to address the need for increased nursing manpower and also to allow a variety of channels for obtaining a nursing education. Numerous educationally innovative approaches to nursing education have resulted. Education mobility programs are an example. The challenge is to keep up with the ever-changing demand for nurses. The resulting variety of functional nursing levels, as well as the corresponding degrees and credentials, has become complex. Material presented elsewhere in this text describes some of the complexities and assists with placing the multidimensional dynamics in perspective.

CRITICAL THINKING *Activities*

1. What is meant by technical and professional nursing? What educational programs prepare students for these two levels?
2. What is your ultimate educational goal in nursing? How might you achieve it, based on discussion in this chapter?
3. How do nursing programs fit in a college or university setting? Can you see ways to improve that fit?
4. What do you think it will take to establish nursing on an equal basis with other health professions?
5. What is meant by the statement, "The common base of nursing education and practice must be scholarly nursing practice"?
6. What is distance education? What nursing courses (credit and noncredit) are offered on the Internet? Conduct an Internet search to answer this question.

References

1. American Association of Colleges of Nursing: *Integrity in college curriculum: a report to academic community,* Washington, D.C., 1985, AACN.
2. American Association of Colleges of Nursing: *Position statement for addressing nursing education's agenda for the 21st century,* Washington, D.C., 1993, AACN.
3. American Association of Colleges of Nursing: *The baccalaureate degree in nursing as minimal preparation for professional practice,* Washington, D.C., 1996, AACN.
4. American Nurses Association, Board of Directors: *Scope of nursing practice* (Report: DA-87), Kansas City, MO, 1987, ANA.
5. Andreoli KG: Specialization and graduate curricula: finding the fit, *Nurs Health Care* 8(2):65-69, 1987.
6. Billings D, Bachmeier B: Teaching and learning a distance: a review of the nursing literature. In Allen L, ed: *Review of research in nursing education,* New York, 1994, National League for Nursing.
7. Billings DM and others: Videoteleconferencing: solving mobility and recruitment problems, *Nurs Educ* 14(2): 12-16, 1989.
8. Billings D, Jeffries P, Kammer C: *R.N. to B.S.N.: review and challenge for R.N. mobility,* Philadelphia, 1989, Lippincott.
9. Bloom A: *The closing of the American mind,* New York, 1987, Simon & Schuster.
10. Bowles JG, Lowry L, Turkeltaub M: Backgrounds and trends related to nursing articulation in the United States. In Rapson MF, ed: *Collaboration for articulation: R.N. to B.S.N.,* New York, 1987, National League for Nursing.
11. Boyd N, Baker CM: Using television to teach, *Nurs Health Care* 8(9): 523-527, 1987.
12. Brower HT, Tappen RM, Wever MT: Missing links in nurse practitioner education, *Nurs Health Care* 9(1): 33-36, 1988.
13. Brown JS, Dugid P: Universities in the digital age, *Change* 28(4): 11-19, 1996.
14. Carroll TL, Artman S: Fitting R.N. students into a traditional program: secrets for success, *Nurs Health Care* 9(2): 88-91, 1988.

15. CBHDP acts on wide range of issues at annual meeting, *Nurs Health Care* 10(1): 37-40, 1989.
16. Clark CE: Telecourses for nursing staff development, *J Nurs Staff Dev* 5(3): 107-110, 1989.
17. Clarke LM, Cohen JA: Distance learning: new partnerships for nursing in rural areas, *Rural Health Nurs* 359-388, 1992.
18. Clayton G, Broome M, Ellis L: Relationship between a preceptorship experience and socialization of graduate nurses, *J Nurs Ed* 28(2): 72-75, 1989.
19. Clinton HR: Nurses in the front lines, *Nurs Health Care* 14(6): 286-288, 1993.
20. Coleman E: On redefining the baccalaureate degree, *Nurs Health Care* 7(4): 193-196, 1986.
21. De Back V: Competencies of associate and professional nurses. In *Looking beyond the entry issue: implications for education and service,* New York, 1986, National League for Nursing.
22. DeTornyay R: Nursing education—staying on track, *Nurs Health Care* 14(6): 302-306, 1993.
23. Diekleman N: Curriculum revolution: a theoretical and philosophical mandate for change. In *Curriculum revolution: mandate for change,* New York, 1988, National League for Nursing.
24. Diploma programs in nursing accredited by the NLN, 1996-97, *Nurs Health Care* 17(5): 268-269, 1996.
25. Downs FS: Doctoral education: our claim to the future, *Nurs Outlook* 36(1): 18-20, 1988.
26. Duffey ME: Innovation as a survival strategy. In *Patterns in nursing: strategic planning for nursing education,* New York, 1987, National League for Nursing.
27. Eden GE, Labadic GC: Opinions about the professional doctorate in nursing, *Nurs Outlook* 35(3): 136-140, 1987.
28. Edge S: Appendix B: State positions on tutoring and licensure. In *Looking beyond the entry issue: implications for education and service,* New York, 1986, National League for Nursing.
29. Ellis LA, Clayton GM: Preceptorship. In Fuzard B, ed: *Innovative teaching strategies in nursing,* Rockville, MD, 1989, Aspen.
30. *Essentials of college and university education for professional nursing,* Washington, D.C., 1985, American Association of Colleges of Nursing.
31. Fagin CM, Lynaugh JE: Reaping the rewards of radical change: a new agenda for nursing education, *Nurs Outlook* 40(5): 213-220, 1992.
32. Farley VM: Strategic planning: an organizing framework for nursing education. In *Patterns in nursing: strategic planning for nursing education,* New York, 1987, National League for Nursing.
33. Fields WA: The Ph.D.: the ultimate nursing doctorate, *Nurs Outlook* 36(4): 188-189, 1988.
34. Forni PR: Nursing's diverse master's programs: the state of the art, *Nurs Health Care* 8(2): 71-75, 1987.
35. Forni PR, Welch MJ: The professional versus the academic model: a dilemma for nursing education, *J Prof Nurs* 3(5): 291-297, 1987.

36. Fulmer J and others: Distance learning: an innovative approach to nursing education, *J Prof Nurs* 8(5): 289-294, 1992.
37. George S, Young W: Baccalaureate entry into practice: an example of political innovation and diffusion, *J Nurs Educ* 29(8): 341-345, 1990.
38. Henry P: Distance learning through audio-conferencing, *Nurs Educ* 18(2): 23-26, 1993.
39. Hickey MR: *Competence statements for differentiated practice in critical care,* Newport Beach, CA, 1989, American Association of Critical Care Nurses.
40. Deleted in proofs.
41. Keating SB: Baccalaureate to M.S.N.: an accelerated pathway for second degree students, *Nurs Educ* 14(1): 35-36, 1989.
42. Keck JF: Comparison of learning outcomes between graduate students in telecourses and those in traditional classrooms, *J Nurs Educ* 31(5): 229-234, 1992.
43. Keith N: Assessing educational goals: the national movement to outcomes evaluation. In Garbin M, ed: *Assessing educational outcomes,* New York, 1991, National League for Nursing.
44. Lambeth SO, Volden CM, Oechsle LH: Portfolios: they work for R.N.s, *J Nurs Educ* 28(1): 42-44, 1989.
45. Lenburg CB: Assessing the goals of nursing education: issues and approaches to evaluation outcomes. In Garbin M, ed: *Assessing educational outcomes,* New York, 1991, National League for Nursing.
46. Lenburg CB: Preparation for professionalism through regents' external degrees, *Nurs Health Care* 5(6): 319-325, 1984.
47. Lethbridge DJ: Independent study: a strategy for providing baccalaureate education for R.N.s in rural settings, *J Nurs Educ* 27(4): 183, 1988.
48. Linderman CA: Curriculum revolution: reconceptualizing clinical nursing education, *Nurs Health Care* 10(1): 23-28, 1989.
49. Lut EM, Schlotfeldt RM: Pioneering a new approach to professional education, *Nurs Outlook* 33(3): 139-143, 1985.
50. Meleis AI: Doctoral education in nursing: its present and its future, *J Prof Nurs* 4(6): 436-446, 1988.
51. Miller C: Transforming the patterns of nursing education. In *Looking beyond the entry issue: implications for education and service,* New York, 1986, National League for Nursing.
52. Mitchell CA: Future view: nontraditional education as a norm. In *Pattern in nursing: strategic planning for nursing education,* New York, 1987, National League for Nursing.
53. Montag ML: *Community college education for nursing,* New York, 1959, McGraw-Hill.
54. National Commission on Nursing Implementation Project: *An introduction to timeline for transition into the future nursing education system for two categories of nurse and characteristics of professional and technical nurses of the future and their educational programs,* Milwaukee, WI, 1987, NCNIP.
55. National commission on Nursing Implementation Project: *Overview of the project,* Milwaukee, WI, 1987, NCNIP.
56. National League for Nursing: *A vision for nursing education,* New York, 1993, National League for Nursing.
57. National League for Nursing: *Characteristics of baccalaureate education in nursing,* New York, 1987, National League for Nursing.

58. National League for Nursing: *Characteristics of master's education in nursing,* New York, 1987, National League for Nursing.

59. National League for Nursing: *Educational outcomes of associate degree nursing programs: roles and competencies,* New York, 1990, National League for Nursing.

60. National League for Nursing: *1995 nursing data review,* New York, 1995, Division of Research, National League for Nursing.

61. National League for Nursing: *Roles and competencies of graduates of diploma programs in nursing,* ed 2, New York, 1989, National League for Nursing, Council of Diploma Programs.

62. Oesterle M, O'Callaghan D: The changing health care environment: impact on curriculum and faculty, *N&HC: Perspectives on Community* (17)2: 78-81, 1996.

63. Parietti ES: The development of doctoral education in nursing. In Allen JC, ed: *Consumer's guide to doctoral degree programs in nursing,* New York, 1990, National League for Nursing.

64. Parkinson CF, Parkinson SB: a comparative study between interactive television and traditional lecture course offerings for nursing students, *Nurs Health Care* 10(9): 499-502, 1989.

65. Pender NJ and others: Health promotion and disease prevention: toward excellence in nursing practice and education, *Nurs Outlook* 40(3): 106-112, 1992.

66. Peterson JM, Duda S: System theory facilitates student practice in self-directed learning courses, *Nurs Educ* 11(5): 12-15, 1986.

67. Rapson MF, ed: *Collaboration for articulation: R.N. to B.S.N.,* New York, 1987, National League for Nursing.

68. Redman BK, Dassells TM, Jackson SS: Generic baccalaureate nursing programs: survey of enrollment, administrative structure/funding, faculty teaching/practice role, and selected curriculum trends, *J Prof Nurs* 1: 369-380, 1985.

69. Reed SB, Hoffman SE: The enigma of graduate nursing education: advanced generalist? or specialist? *Nurs Health Care* 7(1): 43-49, 1986.

70. Reilly DE: *Graduate professional education through outreach: a nursing case study,* New York, 1990, National League for Nursing.

71. Rosenlieb CO: A profile of preceptorships in baccalaureate-degree nursing programs for registered nurses. In Diekelman N, Rather M, eds: *Transforming RN education: dialogue and debate,* New York, 1993, National League for Nursing.

72. Simmons J: *Prospectives—celebrating 40 years of associate-degree nursing education,* New York, 1993, National League for Nursing.

73. Stull MK: Entry skills for B.S.N.s, *Nurs Outlook* 34(3): 138, 153, 1986.

74. Tanner C: Curriculum revolution: the practice mandate, *Nurs Health Care* 9(8): 427-430, 1989.

75. VanHoff A: An off-campus second-step B.S.N. program, *Focus on critical care* 10(3): 50-53, 1983.

76. Williams C, Gallimore K: Educational mobility in nursing, *Nurs Educ* 12(4): 18-21, 1987.

77. Woodman E and others: Assessment of effective outcomes in R.N./B.S.N. programs: advancing toward professionalism. In Garbin M, ed: *Assessing educational outcomes,* New York, 1991, National League for Nursing.

LAWS RELATING TO
THE MINNESOTA BOARD OF NURSING
NURSE PRACTICE ACT

Extract from Minnesota Statutes 1996

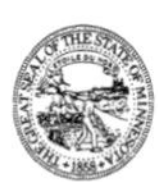

The Minnesota Board of Nursing
2829 University Ave. W., Suite 500
Mpls.,MN 55414-3253

Text Provided By
The Office of Revisor of Statutes
7th Floor, State Office Building, St. Paul, MN 55155

Prepared By
Minnesota's Bookstore
117 University Avenue (Ford Bldg.) St. Paul, MN 55155
Metro: 612-297-3000, MN Toll Free: 1-800-657-3757
TTY (Telecommunications Device for the Deaf)
Metro: 612-282-5077, MN Toll Free: 1-800-657-3706

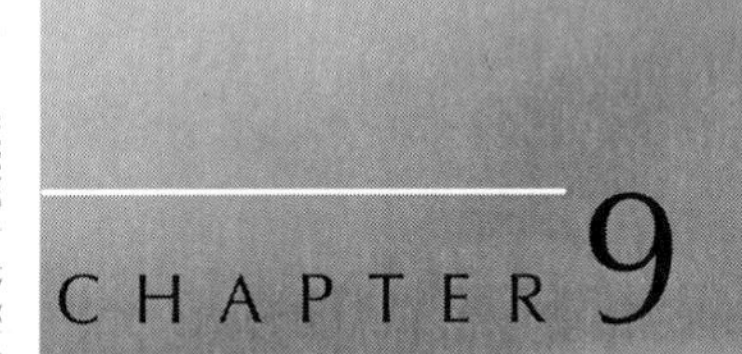

Licensure and Related Issues in Nursing

Linda Seppanen

OBJECTIVES After completing this chapter the reader should be able to:

- **Understand the historical perspective of licensure for nurses and its purposes**
- **Describe state regulatory systems for nursing, including boards of nursing and how they function**
- **Explain the federal role in occupational regulation**
- **Describe the national focus of nursing regulation and collaboration among the jurisdictions**
- **Discuss issues and trends in nursing regulation**

From the beginning of organized nursing, the establishment of standards was closely linked to societal needs. The goal that the ideals of the nursing profession would be practiced by every nurse strengthened efforts in mandating requirements. Nurses influenced legislation to provide safe and effective nursing care for the citizens of their respective states. Coupled with this altruistic goal was an acute awareness of society's needs and the contributions nurse could make in meeting those needs. With core principles, nursing regulation is in a dynamic relationship with nursing practice and thus changes as nursing as a profession grows (Box 9-1).

■ HISTORICAL PERSPECTIVE OF NURSING REGULATION

Initiating the Regulation Process

The regulation of nursing by legal entities arose from a quest for reform. Many who presented themselves as "nurses" had never received any training as nurses. There was no legal constraint against implying or indicating to the public that one was a

Box 9-1 Nursing Regulation

Exists to protect and benefit the health, safety, and welfare of the public.
Requires adherence to ethical, professional, and legal standards.
Is administered in a fair, ethical, and impartial manner.
Requires anyone practicing nursing to be accountable for obeying all laws governing practice.
Is based on sound reason as opposed to being arbitrary or capricious.
Is administered in a cost-effective and cost-conscious manner.
Encompasses the enforcement of laws governing practice.
Is at the least restrictive level needed to ensure public safety.
Ensures the licensed nurse has demonstrated the knowledge, skills, and abilities to provide safe and effective nursing care.
Provides for protection of the public by dissemination of information about disciplinary action within the jurisdiction.
Includes provision of information about disciplinary activity across jurisdictional boundaries.
Includes participation in the development of regulatory policy at the state and national level.
Includes setting and monitoring of standards for nursing education.
Ensures consumer participation in the regulatory process.
Is based upon research findings, experience, and collaboration with others.
Includes provisions that ensure protection of due process for all parties.
Provides for costs to be born by those regulated.
Provides for remediation of nurses within the boundaries of the laws governing nurses.[24]

From National Council of State Boards of Nursing: Delegation: concepts and decision-making process, Chicago, 1995, NCSBN.

fully trained graduate. It was from the need to protect the health and welfare of the public and to have professional identification that legislation and organized state associations evolved. The drive for regulation began in England where, as early as 1867, Dr. Henry Wentworth Ecland sought credentialing of nurses. Ethel Gordon Bedford Fenwick continued this effort in 1887 with the founding of the British Nurses' Association. They worked to obtain a royal charter for the testing and registering of nurses. This group met substantial opposition, including that of Florence Nightingale, who believed that the focus should be on social and moral standards of the nurse rather than abilities of nurses. Several countries instituted nurse registration to separate the trained from untrained nurses at about the same time: South Africa in 1891, New Zealand in 1901, and Great Britain in 1902. In the United States this kind of legislation would come through the state rather than the federal level.

The first public statement on nurse licensure in the United States came in a consumer group in 1898. Sophia Palmer read a paper before the New York State Federation of Women's Clubs. In 1900 Philadelphia nurses reacted to the announcement by the Medical Society and College of Physicians that they were starting a program that prepared nurses in 10 weeks. At the same time several correspondence schools advertised home study courses lasting a few weeks. In September 1901 the International Council of Nurses met in Buffalo. The several hundred nurses in attendance left motivated to procure state registration of nurses.

The companion activity at the time was formation of state nurses' associations that spearheaded the drive for passage of legislation. In 1897 the Association Alumnae of Trained Nurses of the United States and Canada (now the American Nurses Association [ANA]) was founded. One of its fundamental goals was to establish uniform standards for nursing education. From 1898 to 1902 the Association Alumnae established state nurses' associations.

The first state to enact a registration law was North Carolina in early 1903, with 27 states following by 1910. Within 20 years of the first legislation all 48 states, Hawaii, and the District of Columbia enacted laws regulating nursing training. These early laws were weakened as a result of opposition from medical societies and hospital administrators. The most progressive legislation was that of New York, where nurses had to be graduates from training schools approved by the regents of the State University and those already in practice but trained out of state had to meet requirements to continue their in-state practice. The education requirements set out the minimum amount of practice and theory instruction in subjects deemed essential. The result was schools both in and out of state expanding their courses to meet these requirements. In addition, the nurse examining board in New York was composed entirely of nurses.

These early laws shared some basic provisions: (1) use of the title "registered nurse" denied to untrained nurses; (2) completion of an educational program that met standards set by the board of nursing; (3) mechanism for examining training school graduates through an examination and/or performance; (4) mechanism to recognize individuals already practicing as nurses (grandmothering provision); and (5) evaluation of moral and character fitness appropriate for a nurse. In contrast to current laws, these first laws had neither a definition of the practice of nursing nor a limitation of the practice of nursing to those who qualified. Nursing was viewed as mainly custodial. It is a tribute to these early nurses' use of the political process that they were able to influence the enactment laws designed to protect both the regulated personnel and the public from unqualified, unethical practitioners.

Definitions of Nursing

Early regulation of nursing established a registration process that protected the registered nurse (R.N.) title of those who met a minimum set of criteria for registration. These initial laws were permissive; that is, they did not mandate licensure to practice the profession but only to use the title. Consequently, nursing organizations directed efforts at protecting the public and profession from individuals who were not nursing qualified. To accomplish this objective it was necessary to define the scope of nursing practice. Again New York state was progressive, with the first law in 1938 defining the scope of nursing practice, differentiating between the licensed registered nurse and the licensed practical nurse, and adopting a compulsory law. This mandatory licensure law (establishing a precise definition of a licensed nurse and barring all unauthorized persons from nursing practice) met both resistance and support in the various states. Thus further passage was slow, with only 10 states having legislated definitions of nursing by 1946. Nurse employers objected because of fear of loss of practicing unlicensed nurses resulting in shortages and higher costs. Even in those states where licensure was mandatory, the practice acts were filled with exemptions from licensure requirements, such as gratuitous services, recent graduates, federal employees, and emergency care. In addition, World War II delayed implementation of mandatory licensure because of the acute nursing shortage. This shortage hastened the full recognition of the licensed practical or vocational nurse so that by the 1950s they were included in nurse practice acts. Other movements influenced changing licensure laws. The publishing of a standard curriculum guide for schools of nursing in 1937 and the establishment of a national examination in the 1940s were significant influences. ANA adopted a model definition in 1955 that eventually was included in legal definitions by the mid-1960s.[3,16]

This model definition from ANA excluded nurses from diagnosis or prescription of therapeutic or corrective measures. These efforts attempted to distinguish nursing from medicine, but they unfortunately failed to clarify the difference in focus. These definitions did enable nurses to progress from a dependent role to varying levels of independence in increasingly technologic and complex care. In 1973 the work of the New York State Nurses' Association led to passage of a revised nurse practice act that recognized nursing as an autonomous profession. This act distinguished between medical and nursing practice, described nurses' independent functions, and defined nursing as "diagnosing and treating human responses to actual or potential health problems through such means as case finding, health teaching, and counseling." Numerous jurisdictions attempted to accommodate the expanding role of nursing in health care by including in their definitions the authorization of nursing acts of diagnosis and treatments and by including language that made the individual accountable for educational preparation and experience in rendering nursing care.

Changing state law is not easy because so many other groups, particularly hospitals and physicians, have an interest in how nurses practice. Consequently, provisions in other related state statutes or provisions were introduced that affected the definitions of nursing practice; for example, blanket prohibitions against medical diagnosis and treatment, including prescription and dispensing of medications. These provisions unfortunately hindered nursing efforts to be recognized for reimbursement for services and to implement the full scope of nursing practice in contemporary settings. Even so, mandatory licensure has helped nursing become a recognized entity in the health care delivery arena. All jurisdictions in the United States require mandatory licensure now. Numerous health occupations continue to seek recognition by licensure to gain legal recognition that benefits the public and at times nursing; at other times such recognition erodes nursing's role.

One of the recurring arguments against licensure is the cost of mandatory regulations. Nurses bear the cost through the fees as licensees. These self-supporting regulations focused attention to costs and resulted in promulgation of "sunset laws" in the 1970s. These laws reexamined the concept of licensure and the inherent regulatory costs by using state-developed criteria to determine continuation or discontinuation of all kinds of licenses. Even though these review processes tended to be very expensive, they did result in continuation decisions and, in many states, recognition for the effectiveness and efficiency of boards of nursing.

Change is possible when nurses work together. However, the regulation of nurses in the United States has been troubled with internal conflict and controversy. The multiple organizations of nursing have not accepted a universal professional definition of nursing. There were serious concerns about control when the National Council of State Boards of Nursing (NCSBN) was formed as a freestanding organization in 1978. Before that time boards of nursing were organized under a Council of State Boards of Nursing housed with ANA. Faced with the challenges of potential conflict with government groups, the ANA Council separated. Disagreement heightened with NCSBN's intent to develop a model nursing practice act and its imbedded definition of nursing. Activity directed at establishing a model nursing practice act had been the sole prerogative of ANA to this point, despite the establishment of many other specialty nursing organizations and the omission of the licensed practical or vocational nurse.

Model Nursing Practice Act

The Nursing Practice and Standards Committee of the NCSBN began to develop a model nursing practice act shortly after NCSBN was organized. The first task was to establish a definition of nursing, which they based on the 1977 definition of licensure by the U.S. Department of Health, Education, and Welfare. *Licensure* is the process by which an agency of government grants permission to an individual to engage in a given occupation upon finding that the applicant has obtained the minimal degree of competency necessary to ensure that the public health, safety, and welfare will be reasonably well protected.

As an organized profession, nursing has a responsibility to define nursing so that its nature and components are adequately described. For nursing this is done in interaction with the public to meet the health needs of the public. A professional definition originates from professional peers and evolves with the practice as needed. A legal definition is influenced by case law, interpretation within the context of the existing nursing practice act, and determination of whether certain actions fall within the bounds of the legal definition as well as the professional definition. A legal definition is limited to what is necessary or indispensable. It determines the basis for licensure, sets essential standards of nursing education and practice, and prohibits or removes unqualified and incompetent persons from the nursing practice. In its statement *The Scope of Nursing Practice,* published in 1987,[3] ANA states that there are parallel relationships of the component parts of professional and legal regulations of nursing practice.

The 1994 Model Nursing Practice Act by the NCSBN[27] can be used in combination with suggested models from professional associations and demonstrates how far nursing has come. In it "the practice of nursing means assisting individuals or groups to maintain or attain optimal health, implementing a strategy of care to accomplish defined goals, and evaluating responses to care and treatment." This practice includes, but is not limited to, initiating and maintaining comfort measures, promoting and supporting human functions and responses, establishing an environment conducive to well-being, providing health counseling and teaching, and collaborating on certain aspects of the health regimen. This practice is based on understanding the human condition across the lifespan and the relationship of the individual within the environment. This definition is sufficiently broad to include all levels of practice, including that of registered nurse, licensed practical/vocational nurse, and advanced practice registered nurse. This model act further articulates the responsibilities and scopes of practice for each of these levels of nursing, something that was missing in the infancy of nursing regulation.

Evolution of Advanced Practice Nursing

Even though advanced practice nursing is thought of as a recent expansion of nursing practice, around 1900 the nebulous concept of postgraduate training was in place. The term *postgraduate* was used indiscriminantly for many clinical courses, which were available to diploma nurses as substitutes for advanced nursing education. Most of these postgraduate courses were characterized by service with a tremendous lack of uniformity. Again the fledgling profession of nursing began reforming itself. Through the efforts of the American Society of Superintendents of Training Schools for Nurses, in 1899 Teachers College, Columbia University, added courses for the purpose of preparing graduate nurses to become teachers in training schools and superintendents of nursing in hospitals. The goal was to attain uniformity in training school methods; then nurses graduating from a school that was part of a general hospital would have similar training.

The development of nursing theory and more precise definition of the scope of nursing practice began in the late 1950s and 1960s. During this time educational preparation of nurses at the baccalaureate levels flourished. Preparation at the master's and doctoral levels progressed similarly but at a much slower pace. Nurses applied such terms as *nursing diagnosis* and *nursing process* to practice, and they demonstrated expanding skills. In fact, the concept of the expanded role for the nurse was not completely new. Some public health nurses have always engaged in many practices that only belatedly became recognized as nursing. Especially in many rural areas, nurses had functioned in a relatively independent manner in collaboration with the local physician. For example, since 1926 nurses in the Frontier Nursing Service in Kentucky had functioned in areas commonly considered part of the physician's domain.

The momentum to expand the traditional nursing role increased in the early 1970s with the report *Extending the Scope of Nursing Practice* from the U.S. Department of Health, Education, and Welfare.[36] The report acknowledged that the implementation of expanded roles would require careful legal evaluation. However, the report noted that orderly transfer of responsibilities from medicine to nursing had been occurring anyway, so there was no reason to assume that this process would be impeded. The title *nurse practitioner* was first used in a demonstration project funded by the Commonwealth Foundation at the University of Colorado in 1965. This demonstration prepared professional nurses to give comprehensive well-child care in ambulatory settings. The accompanying study by the Bureau of Sociological Research at the University confirmed the value of the new role. In the 1970s several approaches were being used by states to extend the functions that qualified nurses might perform. There were "non-amended statutes," where the wording of the statute was interpreted broadly or where words were substituted to accommodate more autonomous functions. Some states used amended new authorization statutes, where clauses or completely redefined nurse practice were added to include the expanded role. Several states used new administrative regulations, promulgated by the board of nursing and/or board of medicine. In addition to redefining nursing, most states mandated additional requirements necessary to function in the expanded role, such as formal education, pharmacology courses, a master's degree, and professional certification.

Critical elements in the regulation of nursing persisted and interfered with expansion of the scope of nursing practice. These critical elements, which were carefully guarded by the medical profession and later by the pharmacy profession, involved diagnosis, prescription and dispensation of drugs, and treatment. These groups maintained that their practice laws exclusively reserved these activities to licensed physicians and pharmacists. These groups proposed the creation of still other health care provider categories such as physician assistants, registered care technologists, pharmacy technicians, and clinical pharmacists. Many nurse practitioners felt that physicians expected them to perform many more independent functions than the physicians were willing to legally support in the nursing practice act.

In the interest of maintaining high standards of practice and moving to some uniformity, both the ANA and the NLN passed resolutions in 1993 favoring a graduate degree as the minimal educational requirement for advanced practice nurses. At this time the certifying bodies giving professional recognition to advanced practice nurses did not uniformly require a master's degree for certification. Boards of nursing did not have such uniform requirements either; in fact, such consistency has yet to be attained. According to the NCSBN, specific elements related to the regulation of advanced practice registered nurses (A.P.R.N.) vary greatly from jurisdiction to jurisdiction.[21] They include such things as prescriptive authority or lack thereof; the scope of practice authorized for an A.P.R.N. category; whether physician supervision, collaboration, and/or back-up is required; the criteria for national certification used in the regulatory process; and requirements for maintaining continued competence.

Determination of Competence

Traditionally, boards have met their responsibility to protect the public by licensing qualified individuals to practice nursing, denying licenses to the unqualified, and disciplining those individuals who are incompetent, negligent, or in violation of the nursing practice act. The usual qualifications for licensure are educational preparation in an approved program and passing the licensure examination. In the 1960s and 1970s the consumer movement raised the issue of the continued competence of licensees, which contributed to the passage of Sunset legislation. As previously discussed, such legislation challenged regulatory bodies to demonstrate their cost effectiveness. As an outcome of the Sunset review process, many professional and occupational boards, including nursing, were mandated to establish mechanisms for assuring the continued competence of their licensees. The most common measure adopted was continuing education. This makes logical sense, but the effectiveness of continuing education in practice has not been documented. Several other approaches were discussed then and continue to be considered now, such as peer review, self-evaluation, employer-directed evaluation, and reexamination. In 1985 the NCSBN published a position paper on continued competence. In 1993 they presented a new paradigm.[22] Licensees, not the regulatory body, are primarily responsible for their own competence. The board shifted from being assurer to collaborator with licensees and employers. The licensee is responsible for self-assessment and self-limitation. A model for nursing competence is continuing in discussion and review. The increasingly complex health care environment, rapid advances in health care sciences, and growing public sophistication create an expectation that boards of nursing provide assurance that the licensed nurse is competent.

Disciplinary action against licensees was rare until the 1970s.[25] Before that time other societal influences or employer action removed unfit or incompetent individuals from practice. In the area of misappropriation or abuse of drugs, there has been a drastic change in the processing of disciplinary cases in reporting and action taken by boards. The trend in disciplinary action parallels the increased use and abuse of chemical substances in society today. Nursing practice acts and other state statutes have been revised to include mandatory reporting of licensees suspected of violating the law, such as for substance abuse, failing to provide child support or pay taxes, abusing relations with clients, abusing vulnerable adults, and termination of employment at agency.

▪ LEGAL AUTHORITY AND THE REGULATION OF NURSING

As granted by the U.S. Constitution and state constitutional parameters, each state has jurisdiction over its own affairs. It is the obligation of state legislatures to protect their citizens. One way this is done is through enactment of laws that govern any occupations that meet criteria set by the state and the regulatory requirements. Bearing this in mind, Toni M. Massaro, in response to an inquiry from the NCSBN, cited the following three principles of occupational law that provide guidance in setting such requirements.[19]

The more restrictive a regulatory scheme is on the right to practice nursing, the more vulnerable that regulatory scheme becomes to legal challenges on constitutional grounds and to resistance from the profession. As such, the objective basis for increased regulation should be clear and documented.

The more subjective the regulatory requirements are (peer review rather than an objective written examination), the more vulnerable the requirements are to charges of unlawful arbitrariness, discrimination, or unreasonableness. In correlation, subjective requirements must be accompanied by greater procedural mechanisms to protect against unfairness or discrimination. These procedures, which may include evidentiary hearings, involve time and money. Increased regulation of the profession may have anti-competitive effects. Special licensure, relicensure, certification, or other restrictions on the right to practice nursing will create a special group of nurses who have met the qualifications or have been "grandfathered." This group may charge higher rates for their special services, or may enjoy advantages in the job market in general. Increased regulation may also extend the time necessary for individuals to enter the new field and reduce access to the field. These anti-competitive effects may violate the federal antitrust laws. The state cannot safely delegate general authority to the state board members to adopt regulations with anti-competitive effects; nor can the board cede its regulatory authority to private entities. In either situation a court may conclude that the regulatory scheme violated the antitrust laws and enjoin enforcement of the regulations or award money damages.[19]

Further, Massaro stated that the United States Constitution limits the states' authority to regulate the professions in two ways: (1) the regulatory scheme must bear a rational relationship to a valid state purpose, and (2) the regulatory scheme must provide a person who is denied the right to practice the profession or specialty within this profession certain procedural rights, such as notice and an opportunity to be heard about the denial.[19]

Regulation as a Rational Relationship

The "rational relationship" test is satisfied when two conditions are met: (1) the intent of regulatory law is to protect the public from licensees who are incompetent or unfit to practice an occupation, and (2) regulation is deemed to be a reasonable means of accomplishing the goal of public protection. When the state empowers a board of nursing to set new requirements for the licensing of the nursing occupation, additionally imposed regulation on current licensees must be an accurate measure of relevant, job-related skills, and thus rationally related to a legitimate state goal.[19]

Boards of nursing exercise caution when new regulations are being promulgated so that they have solid rationales. They look for any adverse impact on minorities and those protected in the Americans with Disabilities Act. Because members of boards of nursing are predominantly licensed nurses, any regulation that decreases competition can lead to accusations that new regulations are for the benefit of the profession versus the public good and that they may increase costs. The recent moves to further regulate advanced practice nurses have met the requirement of the rational relationship test by looking at the possibility of a separate examination, by working with the certifying bodies on entry level, by establishing legally defensible criteria, and by completing studies of functional abilities essential for nursing practice. NCSBN provides position statements and model rules and regulations as guidelines to assist boards. New regulations not expressly authorized by statute have the potential for closer scrutiny by the judiciary system. Challenges to licensure examinations have not been successful, and most regulation of the nursing occupation by boards of nursing has widespread acceptance.

Due Process in Regulation

States are obligated by the U.S. Constitution to develop procedures that ensure due process in enforcement of requirements imposed on applicants or licensees. Such procedural rights provide the framework for making decisions that are unbiased, sound, and fair, even though the public at times views these as self-serving for the profession. Notice and opportunity to be heard are two basic requirements of due process; they also extend the time required to remove the incompetent and negligent nurse from practice. An individual licensee's right to notice involves notification and time to meet requirements or time for defense in a disciplinary action. Consequently, boards of nursing develop internal administrative procedures to handle complaints against licensees in a timely, efficient, legal manner.

Many states also have uniform administrative procedure acts and elaborate review in promulgation of new regulations by boards of nursing and other agencies. Even though costly, these protect agencies and provide for input before regulations become effective. The former detail procedures that protect agencies when taking disciplinary actions or when denying licensure to applicants. Regardless of the type of regulatory processes adopted by a board of nursing, active state supervision is a critical feature. A board of nursing may not delegate the responsibility for enforcement of requirements to private entities nor accept the administration of the requirements by bodies outside itself without active participation. This has come to the fore in the regulation of advanced practice nursing and the role of national certifying organizations in that process.

Regardless of the previous discussion of states' authority to regulate activities that affect the health, safety, and welfare of their citizens, the federal government can preempt any state regulation. The Medicare and Medicaid programs do so now. The advent of telehealth raises this issue again. Telehealth, or telemedicine, offers the potential to provide health services across vast distance to underserved areas. Even though telehealth knows no boundaries, health professionals must be licensed and regulated at the state level. Although there is strong presumption against state preemption, the Supremacy Clause of the Constitution mandates that even state regulation designed to protect vital state interests gives way to paramount federal legislation. Should Congress decide to regulate telemedicine or telehealth licensure, it could do so.[35] States would be able to continue their own licensing systems in the absence of complete preemption. Thus the ultimate question of preemption will lie with the intent of Congress.

Licensure and Alternative Methods of Regulation

Although licensure is a predominant mode for regulation of the nursing profession, other modes of occupational regulation are used. The criteria that are considered when selecting an appropriate level of regulation include the risk of harm to the consumer; the specialized knowledge, skills, and abilities required for professional practice; the education needed; the level of autonomy; the scope of practice; economic impact; alternatives to regulation; and a determination of the least restrictive regulation consistent with the public safety.[7]

The least restrictive and first mode of regulation corresponds to designation/recognition. Through statutes or rules, or both, this mode can establish restrictions on the practice of an occupation and may establish inspections, enforcement mechanisms, and penalties. It does not require any assessment of the practitioner's credentials or competency.

The second mode of regulation is registration, where a state agency can require persons in an occupation to register and supply certain information. Registration is not exclusionary, but it does grant some limited protection to the public with the listing.

Certification is a third mode of regulation and may be thought of as title protection. Through regulation an occupation member can be required to meet certain standards; only those who meet these predetermined qualifications may legally use the designated title of the occupation. This mode entails standards, testing, codes of practice, possible inspections, and enforcement. Certification may come through a government body or a private organization.

Licensure, the fourth mode of regulation, is the most restrictive form of occupational regulation, providing for both title control and an exclusive area of practice. It requires standards of practice, education, knowledge or minimum competency, and inspection and enforcement with civil and criminal penalties.

The complexity of nursing regulation is better understood when these modes are applied to the current regulation of nursing and health care. An example of designation/recognition is the requirements that health facilities must meet for Medicare/Medicaid reimbursement. They must be listed but are not evaluated according to standards. Registration can be applied to certain states that use a minimal practice standard for recognition of advanced practice nurses. Federal reimbursement mechanisms for agency providers of health care also use this type of process and require minimum standards to be met by registrants. Another example is the recent requirements of the federal government for employment of nurse aides in nursing homes and in home health care for Medicare/Medicaid reimbursement. The early regulation of nursing fell into this category, since standards were minimal; thus the title "registered" nurse.

Certification is applicable to the regulation of advanced practice nurses. There is title control and also the requirement to meet certain standards such as additional educational preparation and clinical experience. There is recognition of certification processes conducted by nongovernment groups with the standards set by the state and a mechanism for enforcement (loss of one's certification). Certifying organizations evaluate members who wish to enter, continue, or advance in a nursing specialty through a certification process that results in the issuance of credentials to those nurses who meet the required qualifications and level of competence. Such certifying bodies assist in providing credentials for public information and, to the extent that the standards mean anything, contribute to the public protection. Certification in nursing has been voluntary, and there are programs for L.P.N./L.V.N.s, R.N.s, and advanced practice nurses. As an example of multiplicity of private certifications, nurse practitioners, nurse anesthetists, nurse-midwives, and clinical nurse specialists are certified by the American Nurses Credentialing Center (ANCC); the Council on Certification of Nurse Anesthetists (CCNA); the National Certification Board of Pediatric Nurse Practitioners and Nurses (NCBPNP/N); the National Certification Corporation for the Obstetric, Gynecologic and Neonatal Nursing Specialties (NCC); and the American College of Nurse Midwifery (ACNM) Certification Council, Inc.

Finally, licensure limits the practice of nursing only to registered nurses and licensed practical/vocational nurses with limitations. Licensees have completed approved nursing education programs, passed the licensure examination, show continuing competence with no disciplinary actions against them, and may use the respective title. Those who have not completed these requirements may not use the title and will have action against them if practicing nursing. Enforcement is the job of the board of nursing. The minimum standards of practice provide for public protection.

State Government Organization and Regulation of Nursing

The administration of the nursing practice acts in 61 jurisdictions of the United States is vested in agencies of the executive branch of state and territorial governments. The 61 jurisdictions are the 50 states; five states with separate boards for practical/vocational nurse licensure (California, Georgia, Louisiana, Texas, and West Virginia); the District of Columbia; and the territories of Guam, the Virgin

Box 9-2 Boards of Nursing Responsibilities

Licensure
Registration renewal
Establishing practice standards
Making definitive practice decisions or giving guidelines for practice
Regulating advanced practice
Establishing fees
Imposing fines
Investigating complaints against licensees
Conducting formal disciplinary hearings
Approving education programs
Reviewing licensure examinations/items for currency and legal scope
Promulgating rules that regulate nursing
Overall enforcement of the provisions of the statutes related to nursing practice

Islands, American Samoa, the Northern Mariana Islands, and Puerto Rico. The statutes or nurse practice acts authorize the agency, which is usually the board of nursing, to promulgate rules and regulations that are necessary for implementation of the statute.

Boards are appointed and structured in a variety of ways. Nurse board members are appointed by the governor in 31 jurisdictions, with another 20 requiring confirmation by the state Senate. Thirty boards are independent or quasiindependent agencies, and 21 are part of an umbrella agency. Boards size range from 7 to 25, with 9 to 13 the norm. All boards that regulate both R.N. and L.P.N./L.V.N. practice include both categories of nurses on the board. Those boards that regulate just R.N. practice do not include L.P.N./L.V.N. board members. All but 5 of the 61 jurisdictions have public members. Michigan, which has the largest board, has the most public members, numbering eight. Seven boards continue to have physicians as board members.

Responsibilities of Boards of Nursing

The powers and duties of nearly all of the boards fall into several categories. See Box 9-2 for the responsibilities of the board.

Some boards have additional responsibility in regulating other groups; 17 do so, the majority with unlicensed assistive personnel or nursing assistants. These responsibilities are carried out directly by board members with the assistance of staff within a separate nursing agency or under a centralized agency. For example, some states have an umbrella agency that handles the administrative procedures for occupational relicensure for all licensees in the state. Implicit in these responsibilities is the mission of public protection and thus rule-making authority, quasijudicial authority, and administrative authority. Rule-making authority provides for setting of standards, as well as for due process requirements. Quasijudicial authority provides for enforcement standards and outlines procedures for adjudication of contested matters. Administrative authority provides for elements needed to enforce standards, such as agency budget, personnel, and office management. Boards of nursing maintain control of professional licensing issues and matters dealing with disciplinary action, which are examples of rule-making and quasijudicial authority. The greatest variety of structures in the jurisdictions is found in the area of administrative authority where state government bureaucracies have attempted to be more innovative, cost effective, and responsive.

NCSBN has developed two resources for states as they consider changes in their statutes and administrative rules: Model Nursing Practice Act and Model Nursing Administrative Rules.[26,27] As states and territories have attempted to respond to the many changes in nursing practice evolving over the years, significant differences have resulted in the manner in which the same subject matter has come to be statutorily and administratively regulated. Since states have the right to enact legislation that best meets the needs of its citizens, there will always be some variation. However, the national need exists for some uniformity so that there is a common understanding of what constitutes a legally recognized profession and facilitation of the geographic mobility of nurses to meet national health needs and personal interests. Most boards of nursing are authorized by the jurisdiction's Nursing Practice Act to develop administrative rules that are used to clarify or make more specific the statutes. Administrative rules must be consistent with the Nursing Practice Act, cannot go beyond the law, and once in place have the force and effect of law. The Model Nursing Administrative Rules provide a blueprint for regulation with important elements developed in the language of the rules, but not every aspect that might be possibly codified. These models must be considered in the context of the law in the particular jurisdiction. To those outside of the regulatory community, these models give a national overview of what to expect in laws and rules and a way to better understand the concepts through the comments and explanations within the documents.

Board of Nursing Processes

A license is granted when an applicant meets the requirements set by state law and that board of nursing or another administrative agency. Such requirements include graduation from an approved nursing program. The criteria for such program approval vary from jurisdiction to jurisdiction. In 35 jurisdictions, for the program to retain approval its graduates must have a certain passing rate on the NCLEX examination for those taking it for the first time, with 75% to 80% passing as the norm. In a few jurisdictions the board establishes a minimum number of credit hours in theory courses and in clinical experiences for program approval. In about half the jurisdictions student-faculty ratios are prescribed, use of clinical preceptors are regulated by the board, and clinical education facilities used by programs are approved by the board. Most boards require English-language proficiency of applicants. In all states felony convictions of applicants are reviewed for their relationship to nursing practice. In about one third of the states the applicant must demonstrate good moral character and good mental and physical health. The applicant must successfully complete the licensure examination (NCLEX-RN or NCLEX-PN), which will be further discussed later. All jurisdictions accept the same passing standard. A license is valid during the life of the holder unless revoked or suspended for some reason. Licensure by endorsement refers to mutual acceptance by another state of a previously issued and unencumbered state license. The licensure decision is based on verification of licensure in the original state of licensure and meeting all licensure requirements, just as those seeking initial licensure in the state. About half the states issue temporary permits to practice to U.S.-educated candidates while awaiting completion of the total process. Forty-nine states issue interim permits to endorsement candidates. Very few states renew permits.

Not only does the nurse need to be licensed, but she or he also needs to also have current registration in the jurisdiction where she or he is practicing nursing. *Registration* refers to listing the license with the state or jurisdiction for a fee, also called license renewal. There is some variation in requirements for renewal, including continuing education and active practice hours. Disciplinary action can be taken against the licensee for practicing without current registration.

The first step in the process of becoming licensed is completing the application form for the state where one wishes to be licensed. This form typically has questions related to that state's licensing requirements. These forms are obtained from the specific state board of nursing. For the new graduate the application, licensure and test fees, documentation of graduation, and application to sit for the National Council Licensure Examination (NCLEX-RN or NCLEX-PN) are submitted; this process can be initiated even before graduation. Licensure by endorsement will have a similar but obviously different process. Nurses should allow sufficient time for this process, so it is advisable to contact the new state board as soon as a possible relocation becomes known. It is important in any correspondence to have complete name and address on all materials to expedite the process. The application process is fairly standard in all states. Addresses and phone numbers for boards of nursing are widely available and can be also accessed through NCSBN by mail, phone, and computer.

Licensure Examination

The successful completion of an examination before licensure has widespread acceptance in nursing, as it has in other professions. If the state specifically mandates the examination requirements and actively supervises its implementation, the state protects itself against challenges of anticompetitiveness. Consequently the examination development must clearly include measures showing job relationship. The purpose of the licensing examination is to determine whether a licensure candidate possesses the minimum knowledge, skills, and abilities to provide minimally safe and effective nursing care.

NCSBN is responsible to its member boards for the preparation of psychometrically sound and legally defensible licensure examinations and for the administration of those examinations. All states and jurisdictions use the National Council Licensure Examination (NCLEX). The test plan serves as a guide for both examination development and candidate preparation. The test plan for NCLEX-RN uses the framework of the nursing process and client needs across the lifespan with the categories of safe, effective care environment; health promotion and maintenance; psychosocial integrity; and physiologic integrity. The test plan for NCLEX-PN has the same categories but focuses on the knowledge, skills, and abilities to meet the needs of clients with commonly occurring health problems having predictable outcomes while using parts of the nursing process. Both are regularly updated. Copies of the current test plans are available from NCSBN and boards of nursing. The periodic performance of job analysis studies of newly licensed R.N. or L.P.N. practice assists in evaluating the validity of the test plans that guide content distribution of the licensure examination. Because of changes that have been occurring in practice, job analysis studies are conducted on a 3-year cycle. In addition, a longitudinal cohort study was implemented to identify trends in the employment settings and work environments of newly licensed R.N.s and L.P.N./L.V.N.s. The identification of these trends further assists in test item construction to maintain currency of the licensing examinations and to inform internal and external groups interested in the educational preparation and employment of newly licensed nurses. Among a variety of considerations, the National Council monitors adverse effects on minority groups. The actual test items are written by practicing nurses and nursing educators, reviewed by nurses and psychometricians, and tested before being used for actual scoring.[15]

On April 1, 1994, the National Council replaced the written examination of all candidates in all jurisdictions with computerized adaptive testing (CAT) for the NCLEX-RN and NCLEX-PN examinations. With CAT, candidates are administered items appropriate for their current estimated competence level until a confident pass or fail decision can be made, the maximum number of items are answered, or they run out of time. This methodology for administering tests uses today's computer technology and measurement theory. With CAT each candidate's test is assembled interactively as the individual is tested. As the candidate answers each question, the computer calculates a competence estimate based on how previous questions were answered and selects the next question from the large item pool. Since the practice of nursing requires application of knowledge, skills, and abilities, the majority of questions in the examination are written at the application and/or analysis level of cognitive ability. The test bank of questions is classified according to the test plan and level of difficulty. This test plan reflects the totality of entry-level nursing practice, based on the job analysis studies and professional judgments. Since targeted questions are given to each candidate, the amount of measurement information in each response is maximized. Items that are neither too easy nor too hard for a candidate contribute the most measurement information. Thus tests do not need to be as long as the paper-pencil forms. Pass or fail reports result. These are sent to the respective boards of nursing, where they are used along with other requirements to make the actual licensure decision. Consequently, a candidate can pass NCLEX but not be licensed. In 1996, 90.5% of U.S.-educated candidates taking the NCLEX-PN for the first time passed the examination. For the same year, 88% of U.S.-educated candidates taking the NCLEX-RN for the first time passed the examination.[4,15]

The licensure examination's purpose is to provide a determination of those who are or are not competent according to a minimum requirement, not how far above or below competence they are. In general candidates can progress through CAT at their own pace; however, there is a 5-hour time limit. A minimum number of questions do need to be answered to adequately sample competence throughout the whole test plan. NCSBN contracts with a testing service and testing centers for the actual administration of NCLEX, with the results reported to the respective boards of nursing for their licensure decisions. Candidates schedule their own appointments with their preferred testing center once they are deemed eligible to test. A candidate need not test in the state or jurisdiction in which she or he plans to be licensed. The NCLEX is administered in each of the 50 states, the District of Columbia, Guam, the Virgin Islands, Puerto Rico, American Samoa, and the Commonwealth of Northern Mariana Islands. National Council's current policy limits retesting to a maximum of four times per year, based on psychometric research. However, an individual board policy may limit such retesting less frequently.

Disciplinary Processes

The primary responsibility of boards of nursing is the protection of the public health, safety, and welfare through the regulation of nursing practice. Incompetent nursing practice places the client at risk of harm. Investigating, disciplining, and monitoring nurses who practice incompetently is becoming increasingly complex. In most jurisdictions board of nursing members and staff must devote the majority of their time and efforts for the board with disciplinary matters. Statutory language differs from state to state, but grounds for discipline typically include unprofessional conduct, incompetent practice, unethical practice, and criminal convictions. Sources of nursing standards include the American Nurses Association (ANA), other nursing associations, the jurisdiction's rules/regulations, National Council models and papers, Agency for Health Care Policy and Research (AHCPR) guidelines, Health Care Financing Administration (HCFA), and other federal agency regulations, as well as nursing textbooks and other nursing literature.

To carry out their disciplinary functions, licensing boards depend on receiving timely information about allegations of substandard practice. One source of information, and for some boards the only source of information, is consumer complaints. Even though very important, consumer complaints by themselves do not keep a board fully informed about incompetent practice. Those who receive substandard care may not be aware of the fact, may not wish to make a complaint, may not know where to send the complaint, or may decide that a malpractice suit is the right recourse. Consequently, some states have enacted laws that give boards access to information from other sources, such as insurers, practitioners, facilities, and the courts. The Citizen Advocacy Center's study "Enforcement of Mandatory Reporting Laws by State Boards of Medicine and Nursing"[32] looked at how well hospitals and individual licensees are reporting in those jurisdictions where such reporting is required. The majority of the 41 responding boards of nursing believed that useful "leads" came from mandatory reports, that hospitals were complying with mandatory reporting laws, and that mandatory reporting laws were effective as currently written. The majority held similar views regarding reporting by licensees under "tattle-tale" laws. Of those boards that sent information on the number of reports received from mandatory reporting sources, the numbers of such reports were low and the number of enforcement actions for failure to comply were low. This could indicate a gap between perception and performance. The overall numbers in this study were low, so results must be carefully weighed.

Although jurisdictions may vary on the disciplinary processes, a general generic process is followed. The Disciplinary Case Analysis Focus Group of NCSBN described this process.[25]

- *Complaint Receipt and Review.* Staff of the board of nursing receives and reviews complaints initially in most jurisdictions; complaints typically need to be in writing. The complaint would be dismissed if there would not be grounds for discipline (no violation) or when the board does not have jurisdiction. Some states require a board member to review each complaint before dismissal. If there is no jurisdiction, the complaint may be referred to another agency that does have jurisdiction. If the facts alleged are true and there would be grounds for disciplinary action, then an investigation is conducted. In many states a priority ranking is assigned to the case according to the seriousness of the allegation.
- *Investigation.* Investigations can include requesting additional documents from a complainant, phone calls to clarify information, interviewing the licensee identified in a complaint and other witnesses, investigating the site of the alleged incident(s), and checking the Disciplinary Data Bank (DDB). NCSBN maintains the DDB for across-jurisdiction sharing of disciplinary actions taken by boards of nursing. The DDB was established in 1980, has since been computerized, is open to electronic access and reporting of information by boards, and has data fields congruent with the National Practitioner Data Bank. This investigatory process varies from state to state, but the objective is gathering evidence so that the board can resolve complaints.
- *Evaluation of Complaint and Investigatory Findings.* The determination of whether to proceed with a disciplinary case is a crucial point in this process. At this decision point the question is probable cause: Is there reasonable belief in the existence of facts warranting administrative or board action? If so, charges are filed. If not, the case is dismissed.
- *Formal and Informal Disciplinary Proceedings.* The disciplinary process takes time, so most jurisdictions provide procedures to act quickly in cases where an emergency situation exists that is a grave risk of harm to the public. Boards may also seek a court injunction requiring a nurse to cease and desist from practice. Standards and procedures for emergency actions are strict because of due process considerations. The format and drafting of official documents and the procedures and conduct of hearings are state specific. Whether through formal or informal administrative proceedings, the goal is to determine findings of fact, whether the proven facts constitute a violation of the grounds for discipline, and what remedy should result.
- *Selection of Appropriate Remedies.* The choice of disciplinary remedies is tailored to the grounds violated. Factors considered include (1) a lack of knowledge, skills, and abilities, (2) poor judgment, and (3) intentional acts. Cases in the first category involving incompetence often result from inadequate understanding of concepts and procedures. Inexperience may contribute to the situations. Cases of poor judgment, the second category, may result from problems with assessment, analysis, and decision making. Personal problems may also affect a nurse's judgment and result in cases before the board. Cases involving intentional acts, the third category, reflect a knowing or willful commission or omission of actions. The board may identify factors of fraud, misrepresentation, or dishonesty that result in cases before the board.

- *Board Action.* The board's determination of the need for disciplinary action results in a legal document specific to that state. These documents reflect the findings of fact, the grounds for discipline, what the remedy is, and the mechanism for reinstatement. Contrary to the misperceptions of many nurses, boards of nursing do not capriciously "take away licenses," but rather carefully follow due process. By the same token, sometimes the public sees this as unduly protecting the profession. Consequently, board members take their responsibilities very seriously in balancing both interests. They must hold themselves separate from workplace, friendships, and professional vested interest. Likewise, all nurses have a responsibility to their clients to help their colleagues practice competently and reduce the load on the disciplinary process.

Federal Government Involvement in Occupational Regulation

Federal agencies have increasingly become involved in scrutinizing effectiveness and operations of state licensure and disciplinary practices. As the largest purchaser of health care in the United States, the federal government examines and implements ways to ensure that only services provided by competent licensees and their unlicensed assistants are reimbursed. Some of the federal initiatives currently in effect give the appearance of developing "federal credentials." The provisions of the Omnibus Budget and Reconciliation Act of 1987 (PL 100-203) include mandates for training, competency evaluation, and registration of nurse aides and home health aides. Medicare- and Medicaid-approved agencies must meet the requirements or risk losing their funding. The National Practitioner Data Bank, enacted by federal legislation (PL 99-660), is a key federal initiative that mandates reporting and releasing information on members of the health professions. Physicians and dentists were the first groups included. Nurses and other health professions have since been added. The implementation is moving slowly as administrative procedures are being worked out. The purpose of the databank is laudable: to track licensees who have been found to be incompetent, disciplined by a licensing board, involved in malpractice suits, and subject to adverse actions taken against them by their professional society or in regard to clinical privileges. The Health Insurance Portability and Accountability Act (PL 104-191), in its Title II: Preventing Health Care Fraud and Abuse, mandates reporting by state and federal agencies. Included are agencies that license or certify health care providers, practitioners, or suppliers.

Interstate commerce issues are a federal role. The Federal Trade Commission (FTC) has not directed major effects toward nursing, but it continues to review and evaluate rules to ensure that trade restrictions are not occurring by the promulgation of licensure requirements. Most of the focus is on advertising. The North American Free Trade Agreement (NAFTA) has an effect on nursing regulation with its goal of objective, transparent, and competency-based requirements for licensure of professionals in the U.S.A., Canada, and Mexico. The Comprehensive Telehealth Act (S. 385) would put a range of health care services within reach of people living in small and rural communities through telecommunication. Its author has a commerce focus.

The Health Services and Resources Administration is currently funding a project with the National Council of State Boards of Nursing that is designed to create a common lexicon of disciplinary grounds and sanctions used by boards of nursing. Ultimately this will assist in creating common reporting formats for the disciplinary databank. The Omnibus Consolidated Appropriations for Fiscal Year 1997 Act requires that foreign-educated health care workers, including nurses, complete a screening program to meet requirements for certain occupational visas. The Commission on Graduates of Foreign Nursing Schools (CGFNS) is identified as an agency qualified to do this screening. This processing has implications for state licensing processes. The Health Care Financing Administration has proposed new rules for home health participation that have a fundamental shift in regulatory approach. They attempt to promote an interdisciplinary view of client care.

Partnerships with other groups are advocated by the federal government via its support of the Clearinghouse on Licensure, Enforcement, and Regulation of the Council of State Government and the National Commission for Health Certifying Agencies. The latter serves as a primary source for dissemination of information on state regulatory agencies, whereas the former sets standards for organizations that certify allied health personnel.

■ A NATIONAL ORGANIZATION OF NURSING BOARDS

With the regulation of nursing a function of the states, there is a need for a national perspective and coordination of regulation but no desire for a federal agency. NCSBN grew from that need. For many years representatives of state boards of nursing met as a council within the American Nurses Association (ANA). Various ANA committees and councils examined the regulatory needs of the nursing profession. Because of concern about potential conflicts of interest, as well as often-heard criticisms that professional boards primarily serve the interests of the profession they are to regulate, the NCSBN was created as a separate entity in 1978. NCSBN is organized as a not-for-profit organization whose purpose is to provide an organization through which boards of nursing act and counsel together on matters of common interest and concern affecting the public health, safety, and welfare, including the development of licensing examinations in nursing. It is composed of 61 member organizations, consisting of boards of nursing or agencies that regulate nursing in the 50 states, the District of Columbia, and five U.S. territories; five states have two boards of nursing. Adopted by the 1996 Delegate Assembly, the mission of NCSBN is to advance the safe and effective practice of nursing in the interest of protecting the public's health and welfare. This mission is reflected in the organization's goals: (1) provide member boards with examinations and standards for licensure and credentials; (2) provide information, analyses, and standards regarding the regulation of nursing practice and nursing education; (3) promote the exchange of information and serve as a clearinghouse for matters related to nursing regulation; and (4) foster an organizational environment that enhances leadership and facilitates decision making in the nursing regulatory community.

The structure of NCSBN includes a delegate assembly, board of directors, committees, and staff. The policy-making body is the Delegate Assembly, composed of two representatives from each member board. The elected Board of Directors is charged with overseeing implementation of policy and directing activities of National Council. Most of the National Council's objectives are accomplished through the committee process. Composition of committees reflects representation regionally, staff and board members, R.N.s and L.P.N./L.V.N.s, and consumers. A professional staff provides expertise in support of all National Council activities, projects, and programs. Consistency in regulation is an overarching motive in its services and products, whether in testing, research, public policy, or communications.

■ ISSUES AND TRENDS IN NURSING REGULATION

Challenge to Regulation by Pew Commission

There have been many criticisms of the health care workforce and the regulation of these professions in this time of rapidly changing health care delivery system in the United States. The Pew Health Professions Commission has spurred on national discussions. This Commission is funded through the grantmaking of the Pew Charitable Trusts, a national and international philanthropy. The Trusts seek to encourage individual development and personal achievement, cross-disciplinary problem solving, and innovative, practical approaches to meet the changing needs of society.

The Commission issued its first report in 1991, *Healthy America: Practitioners for 2005,*[31] in which they set out 17 competencies describing the skills and attitudes required of health care providers of the twenty-first century. In 1993 the Commission published *Health Professions Education for the Future: Schools in Service to the Nation,*[30] which offered specific strategies for reform of each of the health professions at the time that a national consensus seemed imminent for federal reorganization of health care. The Commission's third report, *Critical Challenges: Revitalizing the Health Professions for the Twenty-First Century,*[29] is intended as a guide to health professionals, their schools, and their governing and policy bodies for surviving the transformation and for thriving in the emerging health care culture. Another major impetus for discussion is the *Report of the Taskforce on Health Care Workforce Regulation.*[12] Their work set out to identify and explore how regulation protects the public's health. They then studied the current regulatory system and determined that it does not fit the current needs and expectations of public protection. The regulatory system contributes to increasing costs in health care, restricting managerial and professional flexibility, limiting access to care, having an equivocal relationship to quality, and failing to be accountable to the public through its boards. The Taskforce proposed new approaches to health care workforce regulation to better serve their view of the public's interest.

The Pew Commission's recommendations for the preparation of all health professions are far reaching. Schools must enlarge the scientific bases of their educational programs. Interdisciplinary education is necessary along with partnerships and alliances with new entities such as managed care, computer and software companies, and state governments. Future clinicians will be required to use the sophisticated information and communication technology, to promote health and prevent disease, to be more customer- or client-focused, and to take on new roles that require equitably balancing resources and needs. Cultural sensitivity and commitment to diversity must continue. Future professionals must be prepared to practice in settings that are more intensively managed and integrated. Specific recommendations for nursing were included. Nursing should recognize the value of the multiple points of entry into professional practice at the associate degree, baccalaureate degree, and master's degree levels. At the same time nursing should consolidate nomenclature so that there is a single title for each level of nursing preparation and service and differentiation of practice responsibilities. The associate degree preparation focuses practice on entry-level hospital and nursing home settings; the baccalaureate on the hospital-based management and community practice; and the master's on specialty practice in the hospital and independent practice as a primary care provider. The career ladder programs should be strengthened to facilitate movement through these levels. In conjunction with better focusing education, the size and number of associate and diploma degree programs should be reduced by about 10% to 20%, taking into account regional supply issues in the transition. Master's level nurse practitioner training programs should expand. New models of integration between education and managed and integrated systems of care need to be developed so that appropriate training and clinical practice opportunities are available. In addition, the clinical management role of nursing must be recovered and strengthened at all levels.

Many of these recommendations fit what educational programs have articulated as their values for many years; however, the actual implementation of interdisciplinary efforts were not essential until the delivery system reformed. Just as health care delivery has transformed itself in recent years, we can expect to see higher education in the United States going through transformations. The specific recommendations for nursing have raised the greatest opposition in the educational sector of associate degree and diploma programs who wish to have neither their size nor number reduced. There is less opposition to the nomenclature of single titles for every level in nursing if that of registered nurse remains with the associate degree preparation. Implementation of these recommendations would have far-reaching effects on nursing education and regulation. No school or faculty wishes to lose students. Curricula change anyway; the process just would be more rapid. Public and private funds supporting education will be reallocated, never an easy process. Nursing practice acts across the country will need to be revised to reflect the nomenclature and scope of practice changes. The health care system will need to adjust to these proposed levels more formally.

Reforming Health Care Workforce Regulation: Policy Considerations for the 21st Century has focused attention on the fundamental transformation of the health care delivery and its financing and the impact on regulation. Its authors based their work, which addresses more than just nursing, on a set of principles for a health care workforce regulatory system. Regulation best serves the public's interest by promoting effective health outcomes and protecting the public from harm; by holding regulatory boards accountable to the public; by respecting consumers' rights to choose their health care providers from a range of safe options; by encouraging a flexible, rational, and cost-effective health care system that allows effective working relationships among health care providers; and by facilitating professional and geographic mobility of competent providers. See Box 9-3 for 10 specific recommendations.

The NCSBN response to the Pew Taskforce for Health Care Workforce Regulation[14] supports the articulated principles as desirable and laudable. However, the principles go far beyond what the regulatory boards have as authority and resources

Box 9-3 10 Recommendations to Reform Health Care Workforce Regulation

Recommendation 1: States should use standardized and understandable language for health profession regulation and its functions to clearly describe them for consumers, provider organizations, businesses, and the professions.

Recommendation 2: States should standardize entry-to-practice requirements and limit them to competence assessments for health professions to facilitate the physical and professional mobility of the health professions.

Recommendation 3: States should base practice acts on demonstrated initial and continuing competence. This process must allow and expect different professions to share overlapping scopes of practice. States should explore pathways to allow all professionals to provide services to the full extent of their current knowledge, training, experience, and skills.

Recommendation 4: States should redesign health professional boards and their functions to reflect the interdisciplinary and public accountability demands of the changing health care delivery system.

Recommendation 5: Boards should educate consumers to assist them in obtaining the information necessary to make decisions about practitioners and to improve the board's public accountability.

Recommendation 6: Boards should cooperate with other public and private organizations in collecting data on regulated health professions to support effective workforce planning.

Recommendation 7: States should require each board to develop, implement, and evaluate continuing competency requirements to assure the continuing competence of regulated health care professionals.

Recommendation 8: States should maintain a fair, cost-effective, and uniform disciplinary process to exclude incompetent practitioners to protect and promote the public's interest.

Recommendation 9: States should develop evaluation tools that assess the objectives, successes, and shortcomings of their regulatory systems and bodies to best protect and promote the public's health.

Recommendation 10: States should understand the links, overlaps, and conflicts between their health care workforce regulatory systems and other systems that affect the education, regulation, and practice of health care practitioners and work to develop partnerships to streamline regulatory structures and processes. Each recommendation has policy options for state consideration. The Commission's intent is to stimulate extensive debate and discussion with a call for responses. A revision for further discussion and debate will then come.

to do. The National Council recommends a validated consensus regarding appropriate regulatory outcomes before seeking to design the workforce regulation for the twenty-first century. The past should not be allowed to thwart evolution of regulation, but diversity, historical roots, and legal precedents must be considered. Competence is best assessed from multiple sources with periodic demonstration to ensure reliability and validity. In addition, competence most benefits the consumer when it is focused on ensuring knowledge and skills in the current area of practice so that safe and competent care is continually enhanced. A more effective approach to ensuring continuing competence of licensed professionals assesses random groups or selected groups of licensees based on "triggers" that identify a particular need for competence demonstration rather than performing superficial sweeps of all licensees.

National Council points out that health professions overlap in both knowledge base and clinical application. Thus scopes of practice should delineate the boundaries necessary for the appropriate education and experience but not define exclusive territory for one group. Licensing boards need consistent and easy access to data sources, including disciplinary data, malpractice payments, and criminal records. Crimes that have potential impact on the nurse's ability to practice safely or predict how he or she might treat vulnerable clients should be considered as part of a licensure or credentialing decision. Informal processes provide cost-effective and expeditious means of resolving disciplinary matters; such processes enable boards to deal with cases in a more timely manner while still taking action as stringent as needed to protect the public.

Any additional oversight boards with the authority to amend or reject decisions of professional boards just add another layer of bureaucracy to the system. Boards can bring together diverse viewpoints by having both public members who articulate viewpoints and needs of consumer and professional members who provide professional expertise and judgment. Coordination and collaboration of regulatory agencies can be accomplished through existing boards. Enhanced communication among the multiple licensing agencies, the federal, state, and local authorities, and private entities is imperative. In addition, adequate funding and staffing are necessary to ensure that any policy implementation is successful since many boards are currently underfunded, understaffed, and underdeveloped on technology. Standardization of regulatory terms and language requires the major stakeholders who are affected by the language to be involved; one group cannot unilaterally do this. Any such body must include the public, regulated health providers, providers and payers of health care, regulators, and legislators. Boards of nursing are willing and committed to pursue needed regulatory reform.

The ANA response declared that any effort to reform health care workforce regulation must be based on a commitment to ensuring a stronger, more effective system that places primary emphasis on protection of the health and safety of the public. ANA opposes attempts to weaken the functioning and enforcement abilities of the regulatory system. Regulatory terms should be standardized so that consumers and health care professionals can better understand qualifications and abilities of different categories of personnel. Boards should be utilized to increase collection of workforce data and to make more relevant information available to the public. Concerns are raised about some of the recommendations or policy options because they seem to provide opportunity to weaken regulatory mechanisms at a time when the safety and quality of health care services are threatened by attempts to cut costs inappropriately. ANA is opposed to any effort to increase institutional control of professional nursing practice, to flexible scopes of practice, and to consolidation of medical and nursing boards. Clear and consistent educational standards for nursing practice are necessary with the full range of competencies taken into account in regulations.[17]

ANA differs with the Pew recommendation about involvement of health professions in their regulation. ANA wants a continued, visible role for nursing in its regulation through setting and refining standards for clinical practice and ethical behavior, through accreditation, and by close collaboration and participation on regulatory boards. Neither regulation nor discipline can be administered effectively or appropriately without utilizing nursing's professional standards for practice and ethical behavior. ANA endorses the goal of ensuring that all health care professionals remain able to practice safely and competently; however, they want ways that take into account the broad range of roles, specialty areas, and settings in which nurses practice.

In her presentation *Viewpoints on Vision for the Regulatory System,* Joyce Schowalter[33] asks some challenging questions about regulation and its future. What amount of regulation of nurses is desired or needed by the public? How can this be determined? Because the practice of nursing is currently so intertwined with the practice of medicine and pharmacy and, increasingly, with social work, what regulatory reforms can nursing make unilaterally? How can regulators of nurses develop an effective public constituency and yet receive the necessary technical information from the profession? How can national change come through state actions? Can the system accept multiple experiments before agreeing on the best changes? How can we accomplish recommended change in our ever-changing political environment?

The Pew Commission sought to stimulate national discussion of the regulation of health care providers. Some of their recommendations do not stem from the situation in nursing per se. Even so, the points are useful, have generated much self-examination, and reinforced on-going evolution of regulatory mechanisms that accommodate changes in health care. The subsequent discussion of issues and trends reflects this.[29-31]

Entry into Practice Requirements

Pressure to increase educational requirements for entry into various professions persists. Nursing has been discussing the appropriate educational level for registered nurse practice for the past 30 years, with numerous position statements recommending that it should be at the baccalaureate degree level. Resistance has come from employers, from associate degree educators, from legislators who are reluctant to overregulate or go against powerful stakeholders, and physicians and other related professionals. An overriding question is whether the additional education requirement would make any difference in client care. North Dakota is the only state that requires the baccalaureate degree for R.N. licensure and the associate degree for L.P.N. licensure. Maine has the enabling legislation to do so. Much time and energy goes into differentiating practice levels in nursing, which can be seen as counterproductive to the larger issues nursing faces in demonstrating positive client outcomes as a result of nursing care. A similar discussion is unfolding in relationship to advanced nursing practice, especially that of the nurse practitioner. The evolution of the nurse practitioner role has resulted in varying levels of education. Now the consensus is shifting to requiring master's degree preparation.

Ensuring Continuing Competence

As we have rapid technological and scientific development in nursing and health care, one of the great challenges for health care professionals is the attainment, maintenance, and advancement of professional competence. Licensing boards have a role in assuring the public of the competence of licensees; the focus has been at entry level but the need is also throughout their careers. The issue is the inherent change in practice from the new graduate, entry-level generalist level to a focused-practice competence level. Nursing careers take widely divergent paths in terms of settings, types of clients, disease conditions, therapeutic modalities, and level of health care delivery. What is the standard that shows continuing competence:—the current entry-level competency for nursing?—the generalist core competency of nursing?—the competency needed for safe and effective practice in the focused area of practice or specialty in nursing? To benefit the consumer it makes the most sense to focus on competence related to daily practice.[9]

A regulatory model for competence may facilitate the board of nursing efforts in meeting its public accountability. The foundation for a model for competence assurance requires (1) articulating a definition of competence; (2) setting standards of competence to compare and evaluate the practice of individual nurses; (3) identifying behaviors that demonstrate competence; and (4) implementing a system to discipline individuals who fail to meet the standards for safe and effective practice.[22,23]

The model is useful in giving general direction, but work is still required to give specificity to what are considered areas of practice, or specialties. In addition, the system to identify those who are not competent must meet the standard of timeliness, cost-effectiveness, and openness. Much work for boards and licensees would be required depending on the mechanisms utilized—peer review, professional portfolio, professional certification, testing, retesting. A system of "triggers" could reduce that workload and better target those at high risk for less-than-competent practice. Promotion of professional competence requires a collaborative approach with the board of nursing, individual nurses, employers, and educators rather than an adversarial process between board and nurse. It incorporates professional accountability on all levels.

The most-used mechanisms to indicate continued competence are continuing education, refresher courses, and minimum practice requirements. Currently approximately 30 states require continuing education for renewal of licenses for R.N.s, L.P.N./L.V.N.s, and/or A.P.R.N.s. This makes logical sense, but the effectiveness of continuing education in practice has not been documented and is in much debate.

As a new measure for competency, the NCSBN is developing Computer Clinical Simulation Testing (CST). CST is an uncued, dynamic, interactive test that permits examinees to realistically simulate clinical decision-making activities used in the nursing management of client needs. A brief introduction to a client is presented and the desired nursing actions are then specified by the examinee through free-text entry. The client's condition changes over time in response to the action or inaction of the examinee, as well as the natural course of the health problem. In spring 1998, the National Council will conduct a nationwide investigation to determine whether CST meets the stringent criteria for high-stakes testing as the NCLEX does. Some of its uses may be at entry-level in conjunction with NCLEX, in renewal for everyone or those who may trigger an examination of competence, and/or for reinstatement after discipline. It is not anticipated that any official use would occur before 2001 once all criteria have been successfully met.

Functional Abilities Essential to Nursing Practice

The initial and continued competence of persons with disabilities to practice nursing has been debated for many years. In fact, several boards of nursing have a mechanism whereby a limited license may be issued to individuals whose ability to practice is affected by the presence of a disability. A board's responsibility to protect the public and the issue of competence was heightened with the passage of the Americans with Disabilities Act (ADA). Questions are raised about the types of the *functional abilities,* those activities and attributes that are not domain specific but that a nurse must have to practice safely and effectively. Also, questions are raised about what compensatory accommodations can be used by nurses to practice competently. Historically, boards of nursing have relied on two major domain-specific sources of information to evaluate the competence of licensure applicants: that is, nursing-specific knowledge, and skills and abilities. These information sources include documentation from nursing education programs that graduates have demonstrated satisfactory levels of competence and performance on standardized objective tests such as the NCLEX examination.

To address issues of essential functional abilities, NCSBN undertook a study to obtain validation of the essential non–domain-specific functional abilities that a nurse must possess to perform nursing activities in a safe and effective manner. Examples of functional abilities range from the ability to pick up objects with hands to tell time to use of long-term memory to reading and understanding printed documents to transferring knowledge from one situation to another. The greatest proportion of reported disabilities involved neuromusculoskeletal system problems and, in this group, the majority were back-related problems. The predominant accommodations for participants identifying the presence of a disability were workload and work schedule adjustments, the provision of assistance by other staff, or a change in employment status or location. For example, the primary accommodation for those with a hearing impairment was the use of a hearing aid or other amplification devices. Depending on its severity and effect on the ability to function, the reported disability may or may not be covered under the ADA and, therefore, may or may not trigger a legal requirement for an accommodation. A core of 27 essential activities/attributes was identified for L.P.N./L.V.N.s providing direct client care, and a core of 17 was identified for R.N.s providing direct and indirect client care. For the R.N.s all but two of the activities/attributes represent psychosocial skills and higher cognitive functioning abilities.[38-41]

The possession of functional abilities necessary for nursing is a concern for those entering the field, educators, employers, boards of nursing, and consumers. Prospective nursing students, along with the educators who help them decide about their education, need to be aware of their abilities in such things as fine motor skills, physical endurance, mobility, hearing, vision, reading, arithmetic, emotional stability, analytic thinking, interpersonal skills, and communication skills, and how they accommodate any limitations in these areas. Employers typically are not under the domain of the board of nursing; instead they are usually acutely aware of legal requirements related to ADA. Boards of nursing have a legislative mandate to protect the public from incompetent providers of care. To the extent that a nurse with a disability cannot give competent care with reasonable accommodation, that nurse is subject to the board's nondisciplinary and disciplinary processes. By the same token, boards do not want to evaluate nurses with disabilities so stringently as to exclude many who could function safely and effectively in selected employment settings/environments and positions. Consumers can legitimately expect the nurse with a disability to withdraw herself or himself from practice when there is threatened or actual harm as a result of the nurses' status. It is not just the employers' responsibility to make such arrangements.

Alternatives to the Disciplinary Process

An ongoing concern for boards of nursing is the need to identify strategies for the prevention of common nursing practice deficiencies and ways to help keep competent nurses in practice. A majority of board members' and staff time is devoted to the disciplinary process of handling complaints, investigating, holding hearings, and taking final legal action. This is a costly process usually borne by licensees' fees and a diversion of professional resources that could be used in improving the health care of all. One approach for reducing deficiencies is promoting professional accountability among nursing students, applicants, and licensed nurses. The Nursing Practice and Education Committee of NCSBN studied the application of an accountability framework in reviewing a sample of discipline cases. The cases were analyzed to determine the presence or absence of essential elements of professional accountability. The critical elements used in the framework were: (1) the nurse is responsible for actions, practice, and decisions; (2) the nurse demonstrates honesty and integrity; (3) the nurse maintains continued competence; and (4) the nurse is self-reflective, critically reviewing actions, practice, and decisions. The committee determined that there is initial support for using the above indicators to evaluate licensees for the responsibility element of professional accountability. A way to look at professional accountability is proposed for further discussion. Professional accountability represents the process of balancing the various components of practice between nurses' rights to practice and nurses' duties to do so for public safety and protection. The accountable nurse fits together knowledge, skills, and abilities; competence in role; functional abilities; professional conduct/behavior; accommodations for any disability; and self-limitations. When these are not put together in adequate balance, the nurse would be subject to disciplinary review. A mistake does not necessarily reflect incompetence, since some mistakes are trivial. It is when a pattern of behavior represents a consistent imbalance of practice components, or when a single very serious mistake occurs, that efforts are needed to reeducate, to rehabilitate, and to work to restore balance.

Chemical substance abuse is a major contributor to nursing incompetence and to nurses' practice being restricted through discipline. The chemically impaired licensee's practice does not exemplify accepted standards, and recipients of nursing care are exposed to threatened or actual harm. Over the past 10 years it has been argued that a nondisciplinary approach can protect the public from unsafe practitioners while promoting treatment and rehabilitation of impaired licensees. A nondisciplinary program (often termed diversion program) offers a confidential, voluntary alternative to license discipline for nurses with a substance abuse or dependency problem. The nurse may also have accompanying psychiatric and/or physical conditions. Objectives of such programs are to ensure public health and safety through a program that provides close monitoring of nurses who are impaired as a result of chemicals, and to decrease the time between the nurse's acknowledgment of a problem and the time she or he enters a recovery program. Early help will allow the nurse to practice in a manner that will not endanger public health and safety and will redirect the nurse's energies to the provision of client care much sooner. Proponents of this approach contend that it is more cost effective and successful. However, little conclusive data is available for boards of nursing and other policy makers in their evaluation of policies and procedures established to protect the public while still promoting the recovery/rehabilitation of licensed nursing personnel.

NCSBN conducted a study of two regulatory approaches to the management of chemically impaired nurses in 1996. Participants who volunteered for the study were 39 L.P.N./L.V.N.s and 158 R.N.s, including A.P.R.N.s. The most frequently abused prescription and street/recreational drugs were amphetamines, barbiturates, tranquilizers, alcohol, and marijuana. The results of the study demonstrate that the outcomes of both disciplinary and nondisciplinary approaches are equivalent in regard to continued use or abuse of alcohol and drugs by nurses (including those who returned to the workforce), in deterring recidivism, in keeping impaired nurses from practice, and in returning/retaining abstinent nurses in the workforce.

Boards of nursing take seriously their mandate to protect the public and to uphold due process rights for nurses. Consequently they seek validated outcomes in developing policies. Research is still needed to identify factors that contribute to abstinence and recidivism and to identify facilitators and barriers to nurse rehabilitation and recovery. This is all in the context of professional accountability, which all nurses have a stake in ensuring.

Utilization of Unlicensed Individuals in Nursing Care

As the demand for accessible, cost-effective client care services escalates, optimal use of registered nurses' time is an important strategy in maintaining the delivery of high-quality care. Optimal use of R.N. time involves allocating resources based on client needs, providing adequate personnel levels, and establishing efficient support systems for individual clients and their families. In 1988 the Department of Health, Education and Welfare Secretary's Commission on Nursing recommended that health care delivery organizations should preserve the time of the nurse for the direct care of clients and families by providing adequate staffing levels for clinical and nonclinical support services. The Institute of Medicine's Committee on the Adequacy of Nursing Staffing[13] rejected the idea of mandatory minimum nurse staffing levels in hospitals. Reporting in 1996, the Committee concluded that there was insufficient quality outcome evidence to support the imposition of mandated nurse staffing ratios.

Nurses, who are uniquely qualified to promote the health of the whole person by virtue of their education and experience, are in the position to coordinate and supervise the delivery of nursing care, including the delegation of nursing tasks to others. Delegating selected activities usually performed by nurses does not mean delegating nursing. Nursing is a knowledge-based and process-oriented practice profession, not a task-oriented profession, but it is also a profession that needs to adjust to the reformed health care system. The two most frequent reasons cited for malpractice claims against nurses and hospitals are failure to communicate and failure to intervene in a timely fashion. Both require knowledge and judgment. Health care organizations are responding to pressures to reduce costs by management restructuring, clinical integration, care and case management, customer service, outsourcing, and continuous quality improvement. Reengineering and redesigning initiatives have also taken hold in health care, primarily to maintain market share.[5]

Delegation is transferring to a competent individual the authority to perform a selected nursing task in a selected situation. The nurse retains accountability for the delegation, that is, being responsible and answerable for actions or inaction of self or others in the context of delegation. One major problem in this area is the lack of understanding about delegation by nurses themselves, whether in direct client care or in managerial positions. In addition, they do not always recognize or act in situations of inappropriate direction from employers to delegate when, in the nurse's professional judgment, delegation is unsafe and not in the client's best interest. The nurse should assess the following five factors before deciding to delegate: (1) potential for harm; (2) complexity of task; (3) problem solving and innovation required; (4) unpredictability of outcome; and (5) level of client interaction. Since delegation is usually done in the context of an institutional setting, certain institutional requirements should be in place before delegation of selected nursing activities can be considered.[1,6,10]

The NCSBN produced conceptual and historical papers on delegation in recent years, 1987, 1990, and 1995, an example of the continuing difficulties. They serve as a resource for boards of nursing, health policy makers, and health care providers on delegation and the roles of licensed and unlicensed health care workers. There is no reason to expect any decrease in the use of unlicensed persons for the delivery of nursing care, given the dynamics of the delivery system and lack of widespread documentation of any detrimental effect of such unlicensed assistive personnel in client outcomes. In addition, there is a projected shortage of R.N.s by 2020 according to the Division of Nursing, U.S. Department of Health and Human Services, 1996, which will contribute to the push to replace R.N. responsibilities with other levels of personnel. These are hard times in health care with the cessation of unquestioned payments. Boards of nursing base their activities in terms of maintaining consumer safety rather than professional job interests.

One of the concerns at issue today is whether we have reached the point where legislatively set standards are too wide of the reasonable mark for public protection. This leads to the argument that titles should be protected but that scopes of practice be eliminated. Such a practice gives greatest flexibility and improves workforce utilization but dilutes regulatory control. To be proactive in protecting the public, boards of nursing will be part of developing public health policy. They will maintain ongoing collaboration with consumers, other regulatory agencies, and health care providers to increase access and delivery of quality care. In addition, they will regulate the utilization of any unlicensed person, regardless of title, to whom nursing tasks are delegated.

Regulation of Advanced Nursing Practice

There is an old adage: "History repeats itself." In the regulation of the new specialty usually referred to as advanced practice nursing, this adage appears to be true. With the growth of specialty or advanced preparation nurses, controversy within nursing persists over whether this new group of nurses should be regulated by legal entity or by self-regulation through an evolutionary and professional process. This controversy is similar to the one that existed at the beginning of the regulatory movement in nursing.

NCSBN produced position papers, concept documents, and studies on advanced nursing practice in recent years, 1986, 1993,[28] and 1995, an example of the continuing difficulties in this area. "There is no doubt about it: lack of uniform regulation between states and strict guidelines for reimbursement, prescriptive authority, and physician supervision can be harmful both to the public who demands access to cost effective primary health care and to the practitioners who wish to provide it."[37] Wilken's statement reflects the concerns of boards of nursing that led to the study of advanced nursing practice mobility and credentialing. This study looked at regulation of certified registered nurse anesthetists (C.R.N.A.s), certified nurse midwives (C.N.M.s), and Nurse Practitioners (N.P.s) and found variation from jurisdiction to jurisdiction. Thirty-five boards answered questions on prescriptive authority or lack thereof; the scope of practice authorized; whether physician supervision, collaboration or back-up is required; the criteria for national certification used in the regulatory process; and requirements for continued competence maintenance. The majority has minimum education requirements for a postbasic program. Most recognize the requirements established by the national certification body. Half the boards require that the certifying body meet specified board of nursing requirements. Different educational and credential requirements, titles, authority, scope of practice, formularies, protocols, and practice agreements create a mixed bag of regulatory approaches. Such diversity creates confusion for the consumer and difficulty for A.P.R.N.s when state lines are crossed. The term *advanced practice* implies to the public that these nurses are prepared in every way clearly beyond the R.N. level in education and standards.

The NCSBN went through a shift in recommending licensure as the preferred method of regulation for advanced nursing practice from a recognition/designation method between the 1986 and 1993 papers. The evolution of advanced practice registered nursing has produced an expanded scope of practice and a high level of autonomy based on advanced knowledge, skills, and abilities. As mentioned, these roles are clinical nurse specialist, nurse anesthetist, nurse-midwife, and nurse practitioner. As the health care delivery continues to change, other A.P.R.N. roles may emerge to meet future needs. While the scope of practice of each of these is distinguishable from the others, an overlapping of knowledge and skills exists within these roles. ANA sees certification by the profession as recognition of excellence and continued competency of the A.P.R.N. by professional nursing organizations and the preferred way to ensure competence.[2] No other profession requires multiple licenses to practice a profession that has the same academic base. Safe, competent practice requires licensure, the highest level of regulation, to best protect the public from fraud and malpractice. Although not the regulatory concern, licensure would foster the A.P.R.N.'s legitimacy to diagnose and treat health problems, ensure prescriptive authority, give title protection, and, most importantly, provide the foundation for direct supervision of nursing services. There is legitimate concern about the costs of professional licensure, and these must be weighed against the value of the service and the potential risks in not regulating the profession. At this point most boards and licensees are experiencing such costs anyway in the patchwork regulation of advanced nursing practice. Unlike physicians, scopes of practice for nurses are not generally expansive enough to include all aspects of advance practice nursing; thus additional legal authority must be secured through nursing statute or rules. ANA argues that advocating additional licensing requirements sends the wrong message—that nurses need the state to police their practice to ensure public safety. In addition, second licensure would put nurses in an uphill battle with medical and pharmacy boards at a time when nursing needs to be focused on health care reform.[2,8]

The question is not *whether* boards of nursing regulate advanced nursing practice but *how* boards regulate. There does seem to be general agreement that the appropriate regulation for A.P.R.N.s includes predetermined qualifications, evaluation of applicants, title protection, a defined scope of practice, and authority to take disciplinary action. The National Council position advocates that regulatory jurisdiction for advanced practice registered nurses (A.P.R.N.) be solely under boards of nursing, a master's degree be required as minimum educational preparation, and prescriptive authority be granted as appropriate to the practice area. Appropriate considerations for transition periods, such as "grandmothering," are described in model administrative rule language. As of January 1997 all states regulate advanced practice nurses in some manner. Eighteen license nurse practitioners. Thirty-two additional jurisdictions grant authority to practice through certificates, recognition, registration, or similar means. Thirty-eight currently rely on national certification programs.[21]

As part of an effort to assist member boards in moving to more uniformity in 1994, National Council performed two studies, one to identify core competencies of nurse practitioners and another to explore the regulatory, fiscal, and political implications of developing a core competency examination for nurse practitioners. The Council really found out the political implications with the resulting very strong negative reaction and misunderstanding of certification bodies. The collaboration process to demonstrate regulatory sufficiency in nurse practitioner certification examinations has and will continue.

There has been activity the last few years to monitor the status of clinical nurse specialists, another category of advanced nursing practice. Clinical nurse specialists (C.N.S.s) are experiencing restructuring of their role since they have traditionally practiced in the acute-care setting and care is shifting to community-based care. The core role components of the C.N.S. consist of expert clinician, consultant, researcher, and educator. NCSBN looked at the regulatory status of the C.N.S. across the country in 1996.[20] As previously mentioned, the scope of C.N.S. practice is changing so the C.N.S. has an opportunity for increased responsibility in the medical management of clients. There is a proliferation of very subspecialized practice, as well as an increase in numbers of C.N.S.s seeking prescriptive authority. The question becomes how well does the educational preparation match the current C.N.S. scope of practice, given that fact that it is at the graduate level. Not all boards grant C.N.S.s authority to practice beyond the basic nurse practice act. From the 1996 survey, 62.5% of the 40 boards of nursing responding indicated that they regulate C.N.S.s as A.P.R.N.s in their state. Of those who regulate, 36%

do so by licensure, 12% by certification, 24% by letter of recognition, and 28% by means not specified. Sixty percent of this group indicated that recognition gives use of the title, and 56% gives a scope of practice. Of those who regulate C.N.S.s, 78% require a master's degree in nursing or other field. Of the 40 boards, 23% indicated that the educational standards for the N.P. and C.N.S. were the same. Fifteen percent were considering rule changes that would require the same criteria for C.N.S. and N.P. recognition.

The regulatory mechanisms in place for C.N.S.s are working adequately for what the designed role was, but with the possibility of C.N.S. diagnosis, treatment, and prescription and a scope of practice similar to medicine, the design is different and needs different regulation. In addition, there appears to be an informal merging of the C.N.S. and N.P. roles. If so, the standards need to be congruent. Schools with clinical practice graduate programs must create a consistent product. With interstate mobility and onset of telecommunication technology, similar regulatory requirements need to be in place to ensure consistent protection for the citizens of the United States. The legal entanglements of trying to include C.N.S.s in existing advanced practice legislation and titling issues are certainly correctable since they are already part of the patchwork regulatory process.

A principle to keep in mind when regulating a given occupation is that of the public's right and need to know. A historic statement published by the ANA, titled *Nursing, a Social Policy Statement,* emphasizes the obligation and responsibility of a professional group to the society it serves. To that end, the adoption of uniform standards on a national scope is urgently needed so that the public will be better served and the talents and skills of nurses who have excelled in specialty or advanced practice will be recognized.

Reimbursement Issues in Nursing

With advanced practice prescription privileges, there is increased activity regarding legislative actions on payment mechanisms for reimbursement of nursing services. States that enact reimbursement legislation usually exclude payment for nursing services in hospitals, nursing homes, and physician's offices. Another area of concern is that of malpractice insurance for nurses. Premium rates have increased much faster than salaries. The premiums for specialty groups such as anesthetists and midwives have not been justified by the numbers of lawsuits and monetary damages awarded. Although the costs to nurses are not a primary concern of regulation, they still must be taken into consideration to get competent care to the public. For example, if it is economically impractical for a nurse practitioner to be in practice, then her or his potential clients are deprived of access to that level of very competent care provider. Since nurses are unique providers and not interchangeable with other professionals, the public suffers from lack of nursing care and nursing perspective in the health care team. As we see the "graying" of the American population, a growing age group is in need of the holistic approach nursing offers. The nursing workforce is economically or job driven, just as any other occupational group in this country. If there is not adequate compensation, the numbers of nurses entering the field will decrease and, along with the aging of the current nursing workforce, shortages can occur. When qualified personnel are not available in a geographic area, less-prepared individuals must function out of need. Since the profession is dynamic and changing, licensure requirements will change as they also reflect the professional standards and scope of practice that are dominant in the care settings.

Regulation of Nursing Education

There is currently much flux and concern about accreditation, approval, and recognition of educational programs. The accreditation process at all levels is under intense scrutiny.[34] Essential values of the voluntary, peer-review nature of accreditation are being debated from the perspectives of the federal government, faculty, students, institutions, state government and regulatory agencies. At issue in nursing regulation is the appropriate role between accreditation and approval of nursing education programs. Boards of nursing currently vary in their approaches to approval of nursing education programs. According to *Member Board Profiles 1996*, 56 state boards of nursing approve basic education programs; of these, 17 boards also approve R.N. baccalaureate completion programs. Nondegree programs are approved for A.P.R.N.s by 15 jurisdictions. Graduate programs for nursing are approved in 12 jurisdictions. The approval of R.N. baccalaureate completion programs has been consistently questioned since these students are already licensed and the board of nursing does not separately regulate baccalaureate-level nursing practice. A second approach used by 11 boards of nursing in approval is granting initial approval to new programs and then utilizing specialized accreditation for renewal of approval. A third approach is that of nursing recognition as an accrediting agency by the U.S. Department of Education; these include Maryland, Missouri, Montana, New Hampshire, Vermont, and Iowa. A final approach to approval exists in jurisdictions where a state agency other than the board of nursing approves educational programs; these include New York, Mississippi, and Puerto Rico.

Colleges and universities hold regional accreditation for the institution. In the United States such has been the primary vehicle for standardization and quality improvement, whereas in other countries similar functions were within a government entity. Typically professions, including nursing, have specialty accreditation of their programs. The National League for Nursing (NLN) is the accrediting body for all levels of nursing education programs through master's degree level. Some boards of nursing call their approval processes accreditation, and some boards are recognized as accrediting agencies by the Department of Education, further complicating the scene. Standards for board of nursing approval address minimum or essential competencies as laid out in the nursing practice act and rules. Standards for accreditation address quality issues in professional education and go beyond the minimum standards. Approval is basically required for a school "to be in business" since it is necessary for their graduates to take NCLEX, the licensure examination. Accreditation is voluntary and market driven to the extent those accreditation criteria are important to the public. Accredited nursing programs have complained of duplicative paperwork in documenting board of nursing requirements and accreditation self-study.

The face of nursing accreditation may change radically in the near future. The National League for Nursing Accrediting Commission, now an autonomous arm of NLN, received recognition from the Department of Education in June 1997. In

June 1996 the National Advisory Committee on Institutional Quality and Integrity had recommended withdrawal of recognition based on review. NLN appealed that recommendation and made many necessary changes in structure and function. NLNAC plans to continue accrediting practical nursing programs, associate degree nursing programs, diploma programs, and baccalaureate and higher degree programs. The American Association of Colleges of Nursing (AACN) has begun an accreditation initiative through its Steering Committee for the Establishment of an Accreditation Alliance. The Commission on Collegiate Nursing Education (CCNE) will be an autonomous arm of AACN and will develop accreditation criteria and processes for baccalaureate and graduate nursing education programs. They further propose a formation of an alliance of nursing organizations concerned with credentialing and accreditation to look at effectiveness of program review and accreditation processes. Schools offering baccalaureate and graduate degrees will have a choice in accreditation bodies if NLNAC is recognized. If NLNAC is not recognized by DOE, programs at the practical nursing, associate degree, and diploma levels will be without a specialty accreditation resource. Those that are in institutions of higher education will still be part of regional accreditation; however, those outside of academia, especially diploma programs, will not have a recognized accreditation organization. Such accreditation controls the flow of federal dollars to students for loans and schools. Boards of nursing will need to review the CCNE criteria for comparability to their standards and adjust their language, which is usually in rules, that currently only recognizes NLN as the accrediting body. New approaches to approval and accreditation merit investigation. Research is certainly needed in the effectiveness and outcomes of various approaches in approval and accreditation of nursing education.

Telenursing and Regulation of Multistate Nursing Practice

As competition among service and academic organizations increases and consumers increasingly desire and use information for their own health care, telecommunications offers programming and health care advice to an audience well beyond the local area and beyond state and national borders. Telenursing is nursing practice that occurs through the utilization of telecommunications and includes the use of nursing knowledge, skills and abilities; the application of critical thinking and nursing judgment; and/or the provision of nursing direction or care in specific client situations. The key question for determining whether an electronic interaction is the practice of nursing is whether the interaction would be considered the practice of nursing if it occurred in a face-to-face interaction rather than electronically.[18]

Telenursing, telemedicine, or telehealth care, whatever the terminology, is part of the delivery system now, not a future concept. Nurses are part of the system of teleservices, triage, algorithm-driven care guidelines, and provider services databases. Called *demand management,* decision and self-management support systems are used to mobilize consumers and help them decide how, where, when, and why to use health care services, a major goal of all client advocacy in nursing. The technology has the capability to function in a wide variety of ways to facilitate health care via phone, Internet, high-resolution video, or satellite transmission.

A number of legal issues are raised in considering telehealth/telenursing and multistate practice. These fall into the following categories: jurisdictional issues, confidentiality of information/privacy issues, telehealth/telenursing terminology, federal legislation/preemption, equal protection issues, and discipline and implementation concerns. Individual boards of nursing have the authority to regulate nursing practice, but interpretations and implementation of that authority vary somewhat from state to state. Plus the decision of which board has jurisdiction is difficult when the nurse is in one state and the client is in another. States also vary greatly on how data collection and privacy issues are reflected in their laws and rules. Again, this particularly comes into play for dealing with incompetent and unethical behavior in telenursing and multistate practice. The terminology in statutes and rules was created when the world was a much smaller place and may not clearly reflect the different types of care now. Given the introduction of federal bills on telehealth, where it is characterized as interstate commerce, and the political attention that telehealth is receiving nationally and at state levels, a confrontation between federal powers and states' rights appears to be a real possibility.[35] Some of the possible regulatory approaches seem to put boards of nursing that chose more stringent licensure requirements in the position of requiring their citizens to meet a higher standard than noncitizen nurses originally licensed in other states, thus appearing to have a double standard. The board of nursing's disciplinary activities are a crucial regulatory responsibility. The prospect of dealing with multiple boards, investigations, actions, and monitoring over even greater distances seems insurmountable. What state would be responsible for taking discipline in a multistate practice situation: the state issuing the license, which would likely have the clearest authority, or the state where the harm was done, which would likely have the best access to information about the complaint? Identifying all the possible legal issues is difficult. Creative regulatory approaches are possible but must be legally defensible, economically affordable, professionally acceptable, and publicly credible. Boards of nursing through the NCSBN are exploring a system that would provide for multistate licensure, beyond simply an expedited endorsement process within the existing structures. The features of such a system may include state-based authority with licenses linked to the state of residence, a central database of licensees, core standards for licensure across all states, revenue neutral with the current system, and expedited processing of licensure applications. The goal is to retain a state-based system with permeable boundaries for the competent nurse.

■ SUMMARY

Now is an exciting time for nursing and health care, with the advent of sophisticated telecommunications and information technology, redesigned and reengineered health care organizations, expanded nursing science, consumer interests in self-care, many new roles for nurses, and an overall system focus on health rather than just illness. Nurses have almost an unlimited array of new and creative ways to serve clients' needs. Likewise, nursing regulation has the opportunity to redefine and restructure its activities to avoid regulatory barriers to the innovations of the profession while still meeting their mandate to protect the public. The boards of nursing in the future may not look like those of the past, but neither will health care itself.

CRITICAL THINKING *Activities*

1. Discuss the reasons for initial legislation for regulating nursing and the process for obtaining it.
2. Describe the relationship between professional associations and boards of nursing from their start to today.
3. Identify what nursing regulation is and how it is accomplished in the United States.
4. Differentiate the roles of the state government, the federal government, and the national organization of boards of nursing in the regulation of nursing.
5. Discuss trends in regulating the various levels of nursing: A.P.R.N.s, R.N.s, and L.P.N./L.V.N.s, and unlicensed assistive personnel.
6. Analyze the major challenges in nursing practice today and how they affect boards of nursing and vice versa.

References

1. American Nurses Association: *Policy series: regulation of unlicensed assistive personnel,* Washington, D.C., 1996, American Nurses Association.
2. American Nurses Association: *Scope and standards of advanced practice registered nursing,* Washington, D.C., 1996, American Nurses Publishing.
3. American Nurses Association: *The scope of nursing practice,* Kansas City, MO, 1987, American Nurses Association.
4. Brown V, Yocom C, White E: *1995-1996 licensure and examination statistics,* Chicago, 1997, NCSBN.
5. Buerhaus PI: What is the harm in imposing mandatory hospital nurse staffing regulations? *Nurs Econ* 15 2:66-72, 1997.
6. Canavan K: Combatting dangerous delegation, *Am J Nurs* 97:5, 57-58, 1997.
7. Commonwealth of Virginia Policy Review: *The regulation of the health profession,* Richmond, VA, 1983, Department of Regulatory Boards.
8. Cronenwett LR: Molding the future of advanced practice nursing, *Nurs Outlook* 43 3:112-118, 1995.
9. Curtin LL: Your license and mine, *Nurs Manag* 26 12:7-8, 1995.
10. Delegation: a tool for success in the changing workplace, Aliso Viejo, CA, 1995, American Association of Critical Care Nurses.
11. Dower C: Regulating health professionals through titles and scopes of practice, *State Health Workforce Reforms,* 1995.
12. Finocchio LJ and others: *Reforming health care workforce regulation: policy considerations for the 21st century,* San Francisco, CA, 1995, Pew Health Professions Commission.
13. Institute of Medicine: *Nursing staff in hospitals and nursing homes: is it adequate?* Washington, D.C., 1996, National Academy Press.
14. *Issues,* Chicago, National Council of State Boards of Nursing, 18:1, 1997.
15. *Issues: special edition on computerized adaptive testing,* Chicago, 1993, National Council of State Boards of Nursing.

16. Kalish P, Kalish B: *The advance of American nursing,* ed 2, Boston, 1986, Little, Brown.
17. Keepnews D: Emerging issues in licensure and regulation, *Am J Nurs* 96:10, 70-72, 1996.
18. Kjervik DK: Telenursing-licensure and communication challenges, *J Pro Nurs* 13:2, 65.
19. Massaro TM: Legal opinion on advanced practice, unpublished, 1984.
20. National Council of State Boards of Nursing: *Clinical nurse specialists: a regulatory profile,* Chicago, 1997, NCSBN.
21. National Council of State Boards of Nursing: *Profiles of member boards, 1996,* Chicago, 1997, NCSBN.
22. National Council of State Boards of Nursing: *Assuring competence: a regulatory responsibility,* Chicago, 1996, NCSBN.
23. National Council of State Boards of Nursing: *Professional accountability: allowing holistic integration of the many components of nursing practice,* Chicago, 1996, NCSBN.
24. National Council of State Boards of Nursing: *Delegation: concepts and decision-making process,* Chicago, 1995, NCSBN.
25. National Council of State Boards of Nursing: *Disciplinary case analysis report,* Chicago, 1994, NCSBN.
26. National Council of State Boards of Nursing: *Model nursing administrative rules,* Chicago, 1994, NCSBN.
27. National Council of State Boards of Nursing: *Model nursing practice act,* Chicago, 1994, NCSBN.
28. National Council of State Boards of Nursing: *Position paper on the regulation of advanced nursing practice,* Chicago, 1993, NCSBN.
29. Pew Health Professions Commission: *Critical challenges: revitalizing the health professions for the twenty-first century,* San Francisco, CA, 1995, UCSF Center for the Health Professions.
30. Pew Health Professions Commission: *Health professions education for the future: schools in service to the nation,* San Francisco, CA, 1993, UCSF Center for the Health Professions.
31. Pew Health Professions Commission: *Healthy America: practitioners for 2005,* San Francisco, CA, 1991, UCSF Center for the Health Professions.
32. *Preview of endorsement of mandatory reporting laws by state boards of medicine and nursing,* Washington, D.C., 1996, Citizen Advocacy Center.
33. Schowalter J: Viewpoint on vision for the regulatory system, *The Proceedings: Crafting Public Protection for the 21st Century: the Role of Nursing Regulation,* Chicago, 1995, NCSBN.
34. Seppanen L: Accreditation: differentiation from regulation, *Issues* 16:2, 3-5, 1995.
35. U.S. Department of Commerce: *Telemedicine report to Congress,* Washington, D.C., 1997, Government Documents.
36. U.S. Department of Health, Education, and Welfare, Secretary's Committee to Study Extended Roles for Nurses: *Extending the scope of nursing practice: a report of the secretary's committee,* Washington, D.C., 1972, Government Printing Office.
37. Wilken M: Non-physician providers: how regulation affects availability and access to care, *Nurs Policy Forum* 1(2): 28-37.
38. Yocum CJ: *Employment and work environment trends in newly licensed nurses,* Chicago, 1997, National Council of State Boards of Nursing.

39. Yocum CJ: *Job analysis: newly licensed registered nurses, 1996,* Chicago, 1997, National Council of State Boards of Nursing.
40. Yocum CJ, Haack MR: *Interim report: a comparison of two regulatory approaches to the management of chemically impaired nurses,* Chicago, 1996, National Council of State Boards of Nursing.
41. Yocum CJ: *Validation study: functional abilities essential for nursing practice,* Chicago, 1996, National Council of State Boards of Nursing.

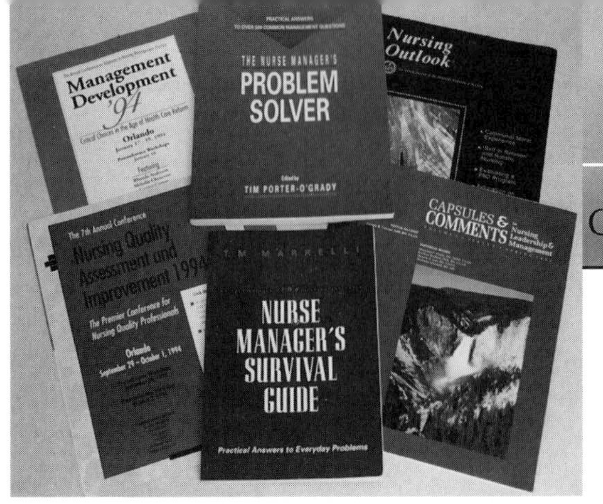

CHAPTER 10

Continuing Education for Relicensure

Gloria Y. York

OBJECTIVES After completing this chapter the reader should be able to:

- **Identify the reasons continuing education is necessary for nurses**
- **Specify the individual credited with being the first nurse to recognize the need for continuing education**
- **Recognize the role professional nursing organizations played in the development of continuing education for nurses**
- **Indicate the role that university schools of nursing took in the development of continuing education for nurses**
- **Recognize ways in which the federal government was supportive in the development of mandatory continuing education for nurses and other health professionals**
- **Specify the challenges that face groups, organizations, and institutions offering continuing education for nurses**
- **Identify some of the problems that could be addressed by boards of nursing as they relate to the multiplicity of continuing education providers, course offerings, and needs of nurses**

One of nursing's early founders, Florence Nightingale, identified the need for nurses of her day to continue learning after their training.[7] Today's need is more intense because nurses are required to keep current in a field that is exploding with new information. Technical and scientific advances in medicine, increasing consumer demand for high-quality health care, and the extraordinary transformation of health care in the last few years have increased the need for continuing education for nurses.[21]

Today continuing education (CE) includes programs developed in many diverse content areas and in many different media. At any one time, the type and number of courses and content of programs offered to nurses across the country are dependent on numerous factors, including client care requirements, types of health care organizations, infrastructures of the organizations, the marketplace (which courses sell best), and economic conditions of the organizations that provide the CE.

Health care reform has had varied effects on the education provided by health care institutions. According to predictions made by the American Nurses Association (ANA), the work nurses are doing will change as much as the health care delivery systems they are working within.[1] These changes and the rapid advancement in medical science, even in specialized areas, can be handled by nurses taking an active, responsible role in their own continued growth and learning. Many nurses find this challenge exciting and seek out CE courses in their specialty area. These nurses are fulfilling the idea of continuing education as many of nursing's founders envisioned it.

■ HISTORY OF CONTINUING EDUCATION IN NURSING

Most nursing CE literature identifies postgraduate courses as the earliest sources of CE for nurses. These courses were prevalent in the early 1900s and for many years were almost the only source of CE for nurses. Most of the postgraduate courses were offered by hospitals and provided training in selected clinical areas. Because there was no educational requirements for the courses, they often became a means for hospitals to obtain free help from the course participants.[7]

In the 1920s ANA and the National League of Nursing Education sponsored institutes for nurses, and universities became involved in CE. Lecture courses became more popular by the 1940s as nurses began to obtain college preparation for their profession. In-service education and refresher courses were available by the early 1930s, and the Social Security Act provided the first federal funds for CE in 1935.[5]

By 1941 New York had developed the first statewide refresher program for inactive nurses. Federal legislation supporting refresher courses came in 1941 with Public Law 146 (77th Congress), and federal funds were allocated the following year. The Manpower Development and Training Act of 1962 made provisions for many of the refresher courses for the years that followed.[7]

In 1955 the University of Wisconsin department of nursing created an extension division to provide CE for nurses throughout the state. This started the trend for university schools of nursing to accept responsibility for nursing CE courses.[7]

In 1968, 34 national organizations developed a standard measurement of educational activity other than collegiate credit. As a result the continuing education unit (CEU) was developed.[11]

By 1970 the Carnegie Commission report on *Higher Education and the Nation's Health* stated that, "In view of the rapid rate of progress of medical and dental knowledge and the associated problem of educational obsolescence of practicing physicians and dentists, the Commission recommends the development of national requirements for periodic reexamination and recertification of physicians and dentists."[13] These reports, and others with similar recommendations, lead many states to develop a system for monitoring and requiring CE for registration renewal of physicians and nurses. In 1971 California became the first state to pass a law requiring CE for nursing relicensure.[8]

In 1974 the Office of Prevention, Control, and Education of the National Heart, Lung, and Blood Institute initiated a review of continuing medical education. The report from this review states, "Conceivably, the issue of malpractice insurance may become linked to either recertification or relicensure as a means of reducing risk. Should that occur, effective continuing education would become essential to every physician as a means of ensuring his livelihood."[25]

Health care organizations and regulatory bodies also began to recognize the value of organized staff development, in-service training, and continuing education. In 1976 ANA published a pamphlet titled *Guidelines for Staff Development,* and in 1978 the Joint Commission on Accreditation of Healthcare Organizations (JCAHO) required that a position be established for overseeing staff development activities such as orientation, in-service education, and continuing education.[16]

Once states began to require continuing education for relicensure, provider groups spread from colleges and universities to include nursing organizations, health care employers, proprietary businesses, and other nonprofit and specialty organizations. Since states required providers of nursing CE to become accredited by national, regional, state or professional associations, CE programs had to conform to guidelines and standards established by these regulating bodies.[2] All this led to the beginning of the boom of continuing education in the early 1970s and the proliferation of organizations creating or accrediting nursing CE.

■ CONTINUING EDUCATION TODAY

ANA defines CE in nursing as "planned educational activities intended to build upon the educational and experiential bases of the professional nurse for the enhancement of practice, education, administration, research, or theory development to the end of improving the health of the public."[3]

The process of planning and developing a nursing CE offering involves consideration of many factors. The factors CE providers appraise are results of needs assessment, content of the program, cost effectiveness of the offering, the appropriate levels of materials, method of presentation, media to use for the presentation, evaluation methods for the program, and continuing education hours to be awarded for the offering. Each of these factors is significant to the success or failure of the CE offering.

Needs Assessment

What do nurses need to know? Health care agencies, educational institutions, state boards, accrediting agencies, and independent providers all have difficulty finding the answer to this question. Part of the difficulty in assessing learner needs is that nurses are such a heterogeneous group. They are diverse in their:

1. Educational preparation
2. Areas of expertise and specialization
3. Work setting
4. Job descriptions within each work setting

Health care organizations have access to data that provide excellent opportunities to conduct valid needs assessments. In health care organizations data can be collected in the following ways:

1. Interviews with supervisors and head nurses
2. Data collected from nursing care audits of client records
3. Reports from quality assurance committees

4. Recommendations from JCAHO
5. Needs assessment surveys of staff[4]

Health care organizations have access to data about performance problems nurses have on the job. Nursing care audits and quality assurance reports, when used in conjunction with other needs assessment tools, can provide needs analyses that differentiate perceived learning needs from actual performance needs.

If needs assessments lead to the design and implementation of CE courses, these same data can be used to evaluate the success or failure of the programs. Decreased incident reports, better client care, and decreased nursing turnover are ways in which health care organizations can measure the success of CE.

Cost Effectiveness of Continuing Education

For health care institutions that employ nurses, if CE programs lead to changes in behaviors that result in fewer costs (or risks of liability), the CE offerings are determined to be cost effective. However, cost effectiveness is often difficult to measure since continuing education is designed "to enhance the professional knowledge base; to facilitate practice toward higher levels of practice, and to improve health care delivery."[16] Increased knowledge does increase overall performance, but the specific financial gain for CE offerings is difficult to measure. Even when measured, the costs of needs assessments, developing, implementing, and evaluating programs may outweigh the financial gains to the health care institutions. This is considered conventional wisdom by many health care institutions, but they continue to offer CE to their nurses. Health care institutions continue to provide CE courses for several reasons, even when they are not found to be cost effective. Providing continuing education is:

- Consistent with many institutions' mission and philosophy of nursing staff development[16]
- An attractive employment benefit that will attract and retain staff when it is provided at the institution's expense
- Compatible with the education standards listed for hospital accreditation by JCAHO[14]

Many health care organizations offer their programs to nurses outside their employment and collect fees to increase attendance and make CE more cost effective to provide. As the wave of cost control continues in the future, education departments will be required to become increasingly effective to justify their existence.[1] This trend will most likely motivate more health care institutions to create self-sustaining for-profit education departments, or education departments that at least generate enough outside income to reimburse more of the costs of providing CE programs.

Independent providers and some educational institutions are also required to show a profit, or at least break even, to continue to provide CE courses. In some cases providers become more concerned with making a profit than with filling the learning needs of particular target groups. Many providers send mailers to all nurses in states where they have provider numbers 3 to 6 months before nurses' license renewal dates. These providers rely on the fact that most nurses procrastinate when obtaining their CE and often select courses out of interest, convenience, and low price rather than real learning needs. Providers who market in this way get better responses than those providers who mail to groups targeted because of their learning needs.

Cutting the costs of program development is another method used by providers to stay in business. This problem has caused some states to develop stricter guidelines for providers to curtail this problem.

CE providers need to be careful to take the responsibility for needs assessment and pragmatic analysis of the demographics of the nurses in their target audiences before developing CE programs. If their courses are on-site or seminar-type presentations, the needs of nurses in their cities and states need to be researched, as well as how far nurses are willing to travel for particular offerings. Reports from state boards, state nurses' associations, state affiliations of national professional specialty organizations, and data about nurses in local health care settings need to be collected so CE providers can offer courses that will be well attended.[4]

Methods and Media

The first courses in CE for nurses were formal classroom programs and clinical practicums. Today advanced technology not only influences how quickly our fields of practice change, it also influences the methods used to educate us about those changes. CE programs are offered via the media of print, video tapes, computers, interactive videodisc systems, teleconferencing systems, and live presentations. Nurses have the choice of obtaining CE credit offered in the following formats:

1. Seminars
2. Institutes
3. Conferences
4. Symposia
5. Workshops
6. Home study
7. Teleconferences
8. Clinical practicums
9. Self-directed learning projects

Seminars, institutes, conferences, symposia, workshops, and teleconferences are all popular group presentations that are frequently provided for large groups of nurses and marketed to large geographic areas. These large-group programs may be sponsored by health care organizations, professional nursing organizations, university schools of nursing, university departments of CE, national or state health care organizations, or private CE businesses. Home-study courses are also developed by these organizations in addition to nursing journal publishers and book publishers. Home-study courses are marketed to large geographic cross sections of nurses. Courses prepared for nurses within health care organizations use multiple formats and are provided for the employees of the organization and sometimes other nurses in the community. These courses may or may not be marketed to the nurses in the local or state community.

Self-directed learning is a process in which learners assume the initiative for identifying, developing, and evaluating their own learning activities. ANA has published guidelines for nurses wishing to use this as an alternative to learning programs designed by others.[8] At present, not all states that have mandated CE allow nurses to use self-directed programs as an option for relicensure requirements. The criteria for approval in many states is basically the same as those a provider has to develop for acquiring a provider number. The individual must submit a proposal before starting the learning experience. Although nurses using this alternative are on the increase, the process can be lengthy and limit the growth of self-directed learning as a viable alternative for many nurses.[10]

Live presentations such as seminars, conferences, institutes, and symposia may use two or three types of media, e.g., oral presentations, written materials, and films or slides. Some home study courses combine video or audio tapes and written materials. Appropriate media selections for a course's content help sustain learner attention and thus increase learning. If instruction is systematically designed, the media in which subjects are presented should be determined by the subject matters and learner assessments. Ideally, analyses of the subjects, learners, and learning environments should be done before the selection of a medium for a CE offering. However, many times the criteria for media selection is based on the equipment or facilities in which the provider has already invested, rather than the appropriate media for the subject. Providers of CE are involved in some of the following businesses:

1. Seminars
2. Journals
3. Home-study courses
4. Computer programs
5. Interactive videos
6. Teleconferencing

CE course developers who are not confined to producing programs in a particular medium can best develop CE programs that are appropriate for their learners and subjects. As the field of instructional design becomes more well known, and health care organizations, nursing schools, specialty nursing organizations, and private providers become more aware of the increased learning that takes place when media selection is a result of front-end analyses and needs assessment, professional help from this field will be used more often.

Content of Continuing Education

ANA describes the content of CE programs as consisting of concepts, principles, research findings, or theories related to nursing that build on the nurse's previously acquired knowledge, attitude, and skills.[14] Many states have adopted similar specifications for subject matter that is considered appropriate for CE. California's content statement is a good example:

> The content of all courses of continuing education must be relevant to the practice of nursing and must: (a) be related to the scientific knowledge and/or technical skills required for the practice of nursing, or (b) be related to direct and/or indirect patient/client care. (c) Learning experiences are expected to enhance the knowledge of the Registered Nurse at a level above that required for licensure. Courses related to the scientific knowledge for the practice of nursing include basic and advanced courses in the physical, social, and behavioral

> sciences, as well as advanced nursing in general or specialty areas. Content which includes the application of scientific knowledge to patient care in addition to advanced nursing courses may include courses in related areas. . . . Courses in nursing administration, management, education, research, or other functional areas of nursing relating to indirect patient/client care would be acceptable. Courses which deal with self-improvement, changes in attitude, financial gain, and those courses designed for lay people are not acceptable for meeting requirements for license renewal.[20]

Educational Level of Courses

At what academic entry level should CE courses be designed? The academic level of the CE course's content is left up to the CE provider, depending on the target audience and learner needs assessments. Many accrediting bodies contend that the level of all CE courses should be at a level above that required for licensure. California's regulations state that "Learning experiences are expected to enhance the knowledge of the Registered Nurse at a level above that required for licensure."[20] According to this statement and similar guidelines in other states, many courses that nurses need would be inappropriate for CE. However, courses such as cardiopulmonary resuscitation (CPR) are considered acceptable in some states and can be used for relicensure in every renewal period.

Some providers analyze and note the level of the course in their advertising so nurses may take courses at the appropriate education level for them. However, most boards leave the decision of what courses nurses should take up to the nurses themselves. The rationale for this is that nurses are the only ones who know what knowledge is useful to them. This permits providers to develop courses and allow both R.N.s and L.V.N.s to attend the same offerings.

If the goal of continuing education is to provide nurses with "content related to the development and maintenance of current competency in the delivery of nursing care,"[20] it is unrealistic to expect all CE courses to be developed above the participants' level of schooling. CE should be based on the awareness that individuals all have different learning needs, no matter what their educational background. The common phrase "use it or lose it" is important to consider when attempting to meeting the learning needs of nurses. Continued learning should include learning new information, reviewing previously learned but forgotten information, and revising new schemas to fit the pieces of information together.

Continuing Education Hours

California and most states define an hour of CE as "at least fifty (50) minutes of participation in an organized learning experience."[20] California's Board of Nursing accepts CE on the following basis:

1. Each hour of theory shall be accepted as one hour of Continuing education.
2. Each three hours in course-related clinical practice will be accepted as one hour of continuing education.
3. Courses less than one (1) hour in duration will not be approved.
4. One (1) CEU (Continuing education unit) is equal to ten (10) continuing education contact hours.

5. One (1) academic quarter unit is equal to ten (10) continuing education hours.
6. One (1) academic semester unit is equal to fifteen (15) continuing education hours.[20]

In 1968, 34 national organizations developed a standard measurement of educational activity other than collegiate credit. As a result the continuing education unit (CEU) was developed.[11] The CEU is defined as "Ten contact hours of participation in an organized CE experience under responsible sponsorship, capable direction, and qualified instruction."[9] A contact hour is 50 minutes long; 1 contact hour = 0.1 CEU. CEUs are awarded by providers of CE courses. If providers award CEUs to participants of the courses they are confirming that the courses meet the criteria set up by the Council on the Continuing Education Unit.[9] Fortunately this system for measuring credit has been accepted by all nursing boards as the standard that will be used for measuring CE. Each state sets up its own standard for a number of CEUs needed for relicensure in a license renewal period. Most states' requirements fall somewhere in the 1.5 to 4.5 CEU range per renewal period.

No national organization authorizes providers to grant CEUs. The responsibility of awarding CEUs rests with the provider of the CE courses. Providers who grant CEUs to course participants are affirming that their program meets the criteria set up by the Council on Continuing Education Unit.[11]

In the past few years the concern with solely using contact hours as a measure of achievement has come into focus because of the acceptance of nontraditional learning modalities in CE. *Nontraditional* courses are those courses that are not grouped or monitored meetings. For example, seminars are traditional classroom situations, and contact hours are measured by the time participants are actually present at seminars "under responsible sponsorship, capable direction, and qualified instruction."[9] In home study, however, the amount of actual time spent is individual, depending on how long it takes learners to read materials and whether they simply look up answers to posttests or study materials until they can answer the questions with the book closed. (Participants may pass the posttest without following directions and spending time to study the course.)

In past nontraditional learning the number of hours was assigned by providers estimating the length of time participants would need to complete the programs. Before 1988 most state boards did not require that providers use a systematic approach to estimate the number of hours assigned to each course nor did they require documentation that courses actually took the amount of time assigned to them. Florida was the first state to address this problem by organizing a task force of continuing educators to develop more specific guidelines for nontraditional learning modalities. Recommendations were made that providers retain documentation of summative evaluations that prove that average learner times are the same as the number of hours providers assign to courses.

Video and audio tapes, computer programs, and interactive video instruction (IVI) are also a part of nontraditional learning. Contact hours for linear video and audio tapes are considered easy to measure because the length of tapes' playing times and average testing times will vary only slightly among participants. In computer and interactive video programs, however, nurses may do several reviews,

Box 10-1 Typical Questions on a Program Evaluation Form

Did the offering meet your educational needs?
How would you rate the quality of the program?
Did the program meet the stated objectives?
Was the program well presented?
Will you use your new knowledge in your workplace?
What suggestions do you have for improvement of the program?
What other topics would you like to have offered?

practice exercises, or select different submenus that contain expanded information on the subject. In other words, the content of the program and amount of detail presented to learners is learner controlled. With interactive video and computer programs, average participant completion times are not valid measurement tools for contact hours. If participants are not monitored, providers of these types of programs have to be able to justify learner self-reporting. Because self-reporting is not accepted for written material, providers of written materials want to know why should it be acceptable for computer and interactive video programs. The solution to this problem is for providers of IVI and computer programs to offer these programs in such a way that actual contact hours can be verified.

Home study providers also maintain that although seminar and group presentations frequently do not require participants to be doing anything but passively sit, courses that are based on reading or responding (such as computer or interactive video programs) require much more participation on the part of learners. Participants may be learning much more from these types of home study programs and receiving less credit because they are not monitored.

Predetermining credit based on averages of contact hours brings up many problems for both learners and CE providers. This system, which is the basic system used for all our formal education, is internationally recognized. Many students probably believe that the four-credit college chemistry course they struggled through would have given them eight semester credits if the college system could actually measure the amount of time they put into the course.

Evaluation of Continuing Education

Evaluation is the means of gathering, analyzing, and interpreting indications of how well an instructional product or system performs.[12] ANA states, "Evaluation is an integral, ongoing, and systematic quality assurance process of the continuing education provider unit and each program. Evaluation includes measuring the impact on the learner, and where possible, on the organization and on health care."[3]

In 1988 both California and Florida enacted requirements for CE programs to have participant *program* evaluations as a part of the offerings. These evaluations for program questionnaires presented to participants to rate the offerings are commonly used for all types of CE offerings (Box 10-1).

Although these evaluations provide valuable information for providers about improving their programs, they do not measure what participants have learned or the effectiveness of programs. Most unmonitored nontraditional programs develop posttests to ascertain whether participants have actually taken the course. The posttests measure learning as a result of the CE offerings.

Many state boards do not require that providers give posttests or that providers who do give posttests require participants to achieve minimum passing scores. The lack of regulations for all providers to measure learning, and the lack of specifying standards for passing scores on posttests has been explained in the following way: There has been no large-scale documentation indicating that CE has an actual impact on client care. Nurses who are taking CE for relicensure and have actual evidence of participation (e.g., monitored attendance or their attempt at completing a posttest) are entitled to CE credits. If the state boards were to specify that participants must show evidence of learning (e.g., an acceptable posttest score), and participants took courses and failed posttests, those nurses could be denied renewal of their licenses and suspended from work until completion of their CE requirements. Some state boards feel they cannot defend the refusal of nurses' licenses on the basis of failed posttests. They feel that nurses could challenge the assumption that the courses have a bearing on their ability to practice competently. Until more data exist to prove impact, some state boards are hesitant to require that participants pass posttests.

■ CHALLENGES FACING CONTINUING EDUCATION

Nursing CE has seen many changes since 1971, when California first mandated CE for nurses. One of the most positive changes is a trend toward increased support. In California the mandate stimulated more courses to be developed, and nurses reported a higher quality and quantity of courses than in Michigan, a state that has not yet mandated CE.[22] According to the 1996 Annual CE Survey conducted by *The Journal of Continuing Education in Nursing,* 25 states had continuing education requirements for license renewal. These requirements were either for all their nurses or, in some states, for those who worked in specialized fields.[15]

Past studies have shown a growing satisfaction with mandated CE among nurses and state board administrators who have been using a mandated system. This does not mean that the states implementing the systems do not have problems. The task of setting up workable and equitable systems for providers, nurses, and consumers is tremendous. There are bound to be problems in any regulatory system, and mandated CE is no exception. State nursing boards and accrediting agencies have problems setting up equitable regulations, setting up sufficient recording systems, and maintaining systems that make sure nurses and providers of CE conform to regulations. State boards have found that getting nurses to comply with the mandate has not been as difficult as ensuring that providers of CE are observing standards that assure the development of quality courses.

CE for relicensure has not been welcomed by all. Some of the arguments against CE are listed as follows:

1. Participation in educational opportunities is no guarantee of learning.
2. Education cannot be equated with competence and accountability.
3. The mandate causes programs to be geared toward the median needs of all nurses, which are inferior learning opportunities for some nurses.

4. It violates the principles of adult education to make education mandatory.
5. There is no proof that what is taught in courses affects job performance.[23]

These arguments stimulated studies on motivational factors affecting attendance of CE offerings. Many studies conclude that most nurses are motivated to attend CE opportunities because of their desire for job improvement and advancement, and indicate that more educated nurses are most motivated to attend.[24] Studies in some midwestern states show 24% to 28% of nurses would not attend CE on a voluntary basis.[9,10] In one of these studies the typical profile of nonparticipants in states that do not mandate CE was documented as nurses who (1) worked part-time in single-nurse or chronic care settings, (2) had relatively low-level positions, and (3) had no education beyond professional training. Apparently, the nurses least likely to voluntarily attend CE offerings are the ones who might need them the most.[23] However, the extra cost to the family may be a significant factor in these findings. One educator found that because the large majority of nurses are women, the mandate helps to release the restrictions they place on themselves. The fact that CE is the law serves to release some nurses from feelings of guilt regarding spending additional time away from home and spending money on CE.[6]

Another positive effect of increased availability and quality of courses in states where CE is mandatory might be contrasted with the problems caused by so many providers trying to compete for nurse participants. Although competition keeps prices lower and increases the availability of courses, it also causes problems for accrediting agencies that are obligated to monitor providers who cut the quality of courses to offer their programs at competitive prices.

Low correlation of nursing impact is another problem that afflicts CE. CE impact studies, conducted by some health care and educational institutions, result in cost-benefit analyses to health care agencies or research studies by universities. Nursing audits have been used to determine effect of CE on client care. Although some studies show a positive correlation between CE and impact on client care, the results of most studies are mixed and portray a difficulty in any CE correlation.[27]

Nursing audits may measure the impact of CE courses on client care, but other variables that cannot be controlled may be the reason for low impact scores. Some factors that influence client care and interfere with positive correlations between education and increased job performance include the following:

1. Staffing patterns
2. Workload
3. Fluctuations in client census
4. Variations in hospital and administrative support
5. Role modeling and motivational factors[18]

Nurses in one impact study conducted at Marquette University, however, had an increased probability of practice change if the participants perceived the program as being applicable to their current nursing practice.[26]

These findings present challenges for educators interested in developing high-quality courses for CE. How can accrediting agencies and providers meet the challenges? By determining appropriate audiences, subject matters, education levels, contact hours, media, evaluation techniques, and costs for CE offerings. Additionally, all accrediting agencies could develop stricter guidelines for providers to prevent cutting quality instead of using careful planning to maintain cost effectiveness.

▪ RECOMMENDED PROVIDER GUIDELINES

With all the problems that exist, what is the future of CE in nursing? If the problems are analyzed, it appears that solutions to many of them will take time to resolve but are nonetheless attainable. Accrediting agencies may be able to solve some of these problems by increasing provider regulations. I suggest changing regulations in the following areas:

1. Requirements that advertising specify the education level the course was developed for so that participants may choose courses that are appropriate for their education and learning needs
2. Requirements that providers furnish a statement to nurses informing them they should notify the board if the quality of the course is poor
3. Requirements that all courses develop both posttests to measure learning and course evaluations to collect data on quality of courses and actual time spent completing the courses; these should be kept as records for audits and studies by accrediting agencies
4. Requirements that providers use the expertise of credential educators and develop needs assessments for at least 25% of their offerings, and that providers of significant size should measure and report at least one impact study per year
5. Requirements that providers help reduce board workloads by participating in peer review at least once a year
6. Requirements that all nurses take certain CE courses that have been identified by the state as being a large-scale learning need, and requirements that nurses update their education in areas that have been added to nursing school curricula
7. Revisions in the definition of CE to include review courses and courses that encompass all nursing learning needs

Besides these regulatory changes, state boards might also conduct large-scale studies to help establish general needs assessments and impact of CE on nursing practice. Because large-scale studies could be used to justify CE for all licensed professions, funds from all the Departments of Consumer Affairs could be used for the studies. States with large nursing populations could pool resources and obtain funds from the Federal Department of Education. Biennial large-scale needs assessments could be conducted. Providers could be required to offer at least one of the topics that were identified in these studies.

These studies and regulations would increase the accountability of providers and nurses and would lead to improved CE systems. If states are to continue mandating CE for relicensure, they may find they need to mandate higher standards. Many nursing educators are eager to meet the challenges of nurses' learning needs. As professionals they want to offer nurses the best possible CE system.

▪ CONTINUING EDUCATION IN THE TWENTY-FIRST CENTURY

The nurses of today trek into the frontier of the twenty-first century confronted with an era of monumental transitions in professional nursing and the continual restructuring of health care. Entering into this challenging age, nurses are discovering that computer technology, medical and scientific advances, increased consumer demand for high-quality health care, and the new roles and responsibilities under managed care systems have all escalated the need for continuing education and professional metamorphosis in their careers.

Like all health care providers, nurses have professionally dealt with the medical information explosion and demand for expertise by becoming specialists in narrower fields of practice. Nursing specializations help provide a way of dealing with the overwhelming body of knowledge in medicine, but nurses also face rapid change in their specialized areas. Medical advancements and greater responsibilities for managing and directing unlicensed assistive personnel in acute-care and community-care settings create a need for a new direction for continuing education in nursing.[17]

In the twenty-first century the new map for continuing education will be charted by the persistent technology explosion and health care restructuring. Most organizations will redesign their staff into self-directed work teams. Nurses will become more empowered and have greater accountability for their jobs. In the next few years nurses will need to direct their attention to continuing their education in leadership skills, computer skills, and learning to work well in culturally diverse environments. These skills, along with learning to become masters of change and giving up traditional ways of thinking, will help nurses face the challenges of the health care age they are entering.[19]

CRITICAL THINKING *Activities*

1. **What was the first state to require continuing education (CE) as mandatory for relicensure?**
2. **Describe the development of CE for nurses, beginning with the early 1900s to the present.**
3. **What are some of the arguments pro and con regarding the issue of mandatory CE for relicensure?**
4. **Does the state in which you reside or plan to practice nursing have mandatory CE for relicensure?**

References

1. Abruzzese RS: *Nursing staff development: strategies for success,* St. Louis, 1996, Mosby.
2. Alspach JG: *The educational process in nursing staff development,* St. Louis, 1995, Mosby.
3. American Nurses Association: *Standards for continuing education in nursing,* Kansas City, MO, 1984, American Nurses Association.
4. Bell EA: Needs assessment in continuing education: designing a system that works, *J Contin Educ Nurs* 17(4):112, 1986.
5. Bowser MR: *Selected factors related to participation in continuing education of dental hygienists, nurses, and physical therapists,* Doctoral thesis, 1979, University of Pittsburgh.
6. Brooks CM: In defense of mandate, *J Contin Educ Nurs* 19(3):129, 1988.

7. Cooper SS, Hornback MS: *Continuing nursing education,* New York, 1973, McGraw-Hill.
8. Cooper SS, Neal MC, eds: *Perspectives on continuing education in nursing,* Pacific Palisades, CA, 1980, NURSCO.
9. Council on the Continuing Education Unit: *Criteria and guidelines for use of the continuing education unit,* Silver Springs, MD, 1979, Council on the Continuing Education Unit.
10. DeSilets L: Self-directed learning in voluntary and mandatory continuing education programs, *J Contin Educ Nurs* 17(3):81, 1986.
11. Dolphin P, Holtzclaw BJ: *Continuing education in nursing,* Englewood Cliffs, NJ, 1983, Reston.
12. Gagne RM, Briggs LJ: *Principles of instructional design,* New York, 1979, Holt, Rinehart, Winston.
13. Hennelly M and others, eds: *Higher education and the nation's health, a digest of the Carnegie Commission on Higher Education,* Berkley, CA, 1974, McGraw-Hill.
14. Joint Commission on Accreditation of Healthcare Organizations: *Accreditation manual for hospitals,* Oakbrook Terrace, IL, 1994, JCAHO.
15. Journal of Continuing Education in Nursing: Annual CE survey, *J Contin Educ Nurs* 27(1):3, 1996.
16. Kelly KJ: *Nursing staff development current competence, future focus,* Philadelphia, 1992, Lippincott.
17. Krapohol GL, Larson E: The impact of unlicensed assistive personnel on nursing care delivery, *Nurs Econ* 14(2):99, 1996.
18. Meservy D, Monsond MA: Impact of continuing education on nursing practice and quality of patient care, *J Contin Educ Nurs* 18(6):214, 1987.
19. Nowicki CR: 21 predictions for the future of hospital staff development, *J Contin Educ Nurs* 27(6):262, 1996.
20. *Nurse practice act with rules and regulations,* section 1456, pg 58, Sacramento, 1994, California Board of Registered Nursing.
21. O'Conner AB: *Nursing staff development and continuing education,* Boston, 1986, Little, Brown.
22. Pituch MJ: *Perceptions of nurses toward mandatory CE,* doctoral dissertation, University of Michigan, Ann Arbor, MI, 1979, University Microfilms International.
23. Puetz BE: Providing an empirical basis: legislating a CE requirement for licensure renewal, *J Contin Educ Nurs* (14)5:5, 1983.
24. Urbano M and others: What really motivates nurses to participate in mandatory professional continuing education? *J Contin Educ Nurs* 19(1):38, 1988.
25. U.S. Department of Health, Education and Welfare: *Competence in the medical professions: a strategy,* Hyattsville, MD, 1974, U.S. Department of Health, Education and Welfare.
26. Wake M: Effective instruction in continuing education, *J Contin Educ Nurs* 18(6):188, 1987.
27. Warmuth J: In search of impact of continuing education, *J Contin Educ Nurs* 18(1):4, 1987.

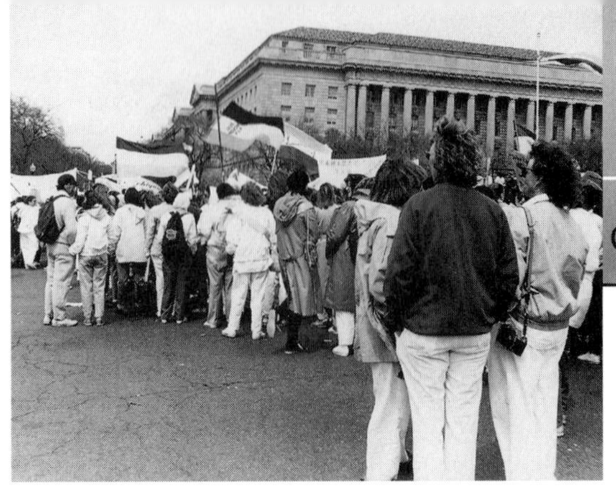

CHAPTER 11

Political Awareness in Nursing

Mary Jane Zusy

■ NURSING'S GROWING POLITICAL INVOLVEMENT

The past two decades have brought a virtual revolution in the delivery of health care in America that has affected every aspect of nursing, as well as client care. Increasingly nurses have realized that government policy and programs significantly influence their day-to-day practices—how they are educated, where they practice, and how they are reimbursed. As major providers of health care, nurses have come to realize that they must play an active role in the development of public policy in that field through politics.

Politics has been described as "the art of the possible." Whenever a few people gather together to effect change, politics is there. Someone has an idea, facts are gathered, a decision is made as to what to do, persuasion is used, alliances are formed, positions are taken, and members of the group go out and persuade others. This is politics at its most basic, and every one of us have experienced it in our private, public, and professional lives.

Although organized nursing's emergence on the political scene seems recent, modern professional nursing owes its beginning to Florence Nightingale's political skills, as well as her vision, intelligence, education, and position in society. Probably the towering figure of her era, Nightingale was a persuasive and tireless crusader for her causes, a voluminous writer, a statistician, and a consummate politician. Since her time, a growing number of nurses have used politics in the public arena to attain greater professionalism for nursing and improved access to health care for everyone.

Near the turn of the century, Lillian Wald was determined to change for the better the deplorable conditions of the immigrants housed in the tenements of the New York City's Lower East Side. From her Henry Street Settlement House, in 1893 she organized the first community nursing services and is credited with subsequently establishing its branches—public health, rural nursing, and school nursing. She was a committed nurse who wrote engagingly, used statistics to make her points, and enlisted the help of politicians, government officials, and philanthropists to address the problems she saw. She repeatedly looked to legislative solutions to social and health problems. "I was in politics," she wrote.[2]

Another nurse who had a larger vision was Lavinia Dock, an active suffragette who was convinced that the way for women to attain equality with men was through the right to vote. She also believed nurses, not doctors, should control nursing, and that nurses should organize to promote professional goals. Her goals were licensing to control nursing practice and the establishment of standards for nursing education. In 1893 she was one of the founders of the organization that was to become the National League for Nursing (NLN).

The struggle for nurse licensure was long and difficult, since the fight for enabling legislation had to be won in every state. New York, North Carolina, New Jersey, and Virginia passed licensure legislation in 1903, but it was almost 20 years before every state had such laws in place. As is often the case, legislation passed in one state served as a model for others. The effort did much to strengthen and unite nursing and represented organized nursing's first experience in the achievement of professional goals through legislation.[3]

The American Nurses Association (ANA) formed a legislative committee in 1923 and continued to speak for nursing through the depression years and World War II, but it was not until the early 1980s that ANA became markedly more assertive on health policy.[5]

The consciousness raising of the women's movement in the 1970s and 1980s had a great impact on nursing, since it remains a predominantly female profession. Many nurses became interested in political involvement and saw opportunities to both professionalize nursing and improve the public health through political action. Realizing that in numbers there is strength, nurses became aware of their potential power. ANA coined the slogan "One in 44"—one in every 44 women voters is a nurse.

Nursing organizations proliferated. In addition to the early ones, ANA and NLN, nurses from almost every specialty organized. There are now more than 100 national nursing organizations, and the larger ones have legislative programs.[9]

■ THE PACs

In the early 1970s a change in the federal election laws governing the financing of political campaigns by capping the size of individual campaign contributions opened the door for political actions committees (PACs). An organization's PAC raises money for political campaigns of candidates for elective office—ones endorsed on the basis of the candidate's sympathy with the parent organization's agenda. As the costs of campaigns have escalated, PACs have become a major source of funding.

Though far from a perfect system, PACs have broadened the base of people contributing to campaigns. Someone has quipped that giving money, in addition to helping one's cause, is a little like betting on a horse race. One's bet increases one's interest in the race.

At its convention in June 1974 ANA announced the formation of its nonpartisan political action unit, Nurses' Coalition for Action in Politics (N-CAP). In 1986 the name N-CAP was changed to ANA/PAC to facilitate easier identification with its parent organization.

PACs do no direct lobbying. By law their only function is to raise money and provide financial and other support for candidates of their choice. They solicit voluntary contributions from the members of their parent organizations. Their governing boards then distribute the money to the political campaigns of candidates friendly to the parent organizations' positions and whom they believe they may be able to influence if they are elected. PAC dollars do not actually buy influence, but they do facilitate access to elected officials who have received them.

In 1984, for the first time, ANA/PAC, in addition to congressional candidates, endorsed the candidates for President and Vice President—Democrats Walter Mondale and Geraldine Ferraro. In each presidential campaign subsequently it has endorsed candidates at the top of the ticket believed to be friendly or potentially friendly to nursing.

Although controversial, the practice has paid off in getting for nurses access to people in high places. President Bill Clinton, having received ANA/PAC support in 1992, returned the favor by keynoting the 1996 ANA convention in Washington, D.C. The Secretary of Health and Human Services, Donna Shalala, addressed a nurses' luncheon at the 1996 Democratic convention in August. Being able to get these high-level people to speak at their events gives nurses reason to feel their voices will be heard and their opinions valued.

In addition to a Board of Directors, ANA/PAC set up a Congressional District Coordinator (CDC) network. The goal is to have a CDC (a nurse) in every one of the 435 Congressional districts to serve as a liaison between the PAC board and the field. The effort also develops grass-roots support among nurses and promotes nursing's visibility with candidates.

In 1996 ANA/PAC raised more than a million dollars and distributed nearly that amount to its 270 endorsed Congressional candidates (both Democratic and Republican)—77% of whom won.[8]

ANA/PAC, replicated on the state level, contributes dollars, mailing lists, and volunteer support to candidates for state office. This has greatly increased nursing's visibility in the state as well as in the national political arena.

■ ISSUES

In 1992 some 70 health care groups, most of which were national nursing organizations, networked, collaborated, and came together to form the Nursing Organizations Liaison Forum. It developed a "nursing agenda for health care reform." The leadership believed nursing was strong enough to have a place at the table when the debate began.

It is not, perhaps, surprising then that several nurses were asked to serve on First Lady Hillary Rodham Clinton's Health Care Task Force. Its mission was to find ways to broaden the availability of health care to underserved populations and at the same time cut costs. After months of closed hearings and study, the Task Force came up with a rather complicated legislative proposal. After spirited debate, Congress rejected the package as a whole. Some valuable goals were accomplished, however. One was the education of the public about the scope of the problems and some of the possibilities for meeting them. Out of that momentum some beneficial legislation was passed, such as the bipartisan Kassebaum-Kennedy bill, which made health insurance portable from one job to another.

In the mid-1990s ANA, concerned that cost cutting, hospital downsizing, and the substitution of unlicensed personnel for R.N.s threatened client safety and welfare, promoted relevant federal legislation. It was aimed at ensuring safe quality nursing care in hospitals and other health care institutions and the protection of nurses who speak out on client care issues. The bill, The Patient Safety Act of 1996, was introduced by Rep. Maurice Hinchey (D-NY) on the eve of National Nurses' Week at an attention-getting press conference on the Capitol steps. A prominently displayed ANA banner declared, "Nurses: the heart of health care."[7]

During the same period, among other initiatives on its agenda, ANA lent its influence to orchestrate the "Every Patient Deserves a Nurse" campaign and to support the "Every Child by Two" immunization program. It also took positions on issues of national debate. One such position was a firm stand against assisted suicide, while at the same time supporting the delivery of dignified and humane end-of-life care.[10]

■ HOW CAN INDIVIDUAL NURSES MAKE A DIFFERENCE?

With the growing awareness that many professional nursing and health care issues are driven by legislation or the regulations implementing it, it is not surprising that nurses are now becoming involved in politics in the public arena at every level. So let's look at some of the keys to political effectiveness.

The Basics

Every citizen 18 years or older has a basic privilege and responsibility to register to vote, become informed on the issues, and to vote his or her conscience.

The first step is to register to vote. Most states make opportunities to do this very conveniently during a designated period preceding both primary and general elections. Tables may be set up in supermarkets, libraries, or other public places where you can fill out a voter registration form, or you can request one from the local board of elections.

The registration form will ask for a party alignment (Democrat, Republican, or other), although you can designate "Independent." Although many people like to think of themselves as independent voters, registering as an Independent means you lose the opportunity to take part in the early part of the election process—the primary.

Party affiliation gives you a voice in choosing the party's candidates. But, in fact, you are completely free to vote for the candidates of your choice (regardless of party) in the general election in November, and party designation can be changed.

The majority of states hold direct primary elections in the spring before a general election. At that time party members go to the polls to vote for the candidates who will make up their slate in November. In a few states there are "open primaries" in which voters can choose to vote in the primary of either major party.

In others, however, parties select their candidates through party caucuses (e.g., Iowa) or conventions (e.g., Virginia). In these, party members meet in designated places around the state and select their candidates. Regardless of the procedure in your state, to participate in this phase of the election process when parties are choosing their slates of candidates, you must have a party affiliation. To learn whether your state has primaries, caucuses, or conventions, call the League of Women Voters or your local board of elections.

Study the Issues

Every citizen has a responsibility to study the issues and the candidates in preparation for casting a thoughtful vote. Newspapers that cover the news and feature a variety of editorial opinion are probably the most important sources of information. There are also news magazines, television, and citizen's forums. In some communities the League of Women Voters publishes a Voter's Guide. These are nonpartisan and provide profiles of all the candidates who wish to be represented in the guide.

For nurses, our organizations and their news organizations should be the very best sources of information on nursing and health care issues. Joining a nursing organization, then reading its publications and newsletters and attending its meetings, are important ways to stay informed. When nursing organizations have members on important city-, county-, or state-wide committees or commissions having to do with health, it gives them a direct pipeline to developments and an active role in decision making.

ANA, with its state constituents, is the largest and most influential nursing organization and is accepted as the general spokesperson for the profession. It also works through coalitions and networks with many other nursing organizations. In that each one of these represent a certain constituency of nurses, each is important. The more they pool resources and work together, the stronger they are.

Once informed, every citizen's responsibility is to go to the polls on election day and cast a thoughtful vote. It is the most basic act of citizenship. Democracy depends on the participation of its citizens. Our founding fathers assumed that having been given the vote, people would exercise their will for the benefit of all.

Through the years efforts have been made to expand the voting pool, such as lowering the voting age from 21 to 18, although participation in that age group has been disappointingly low. The National Voter Registration Act (NVRA), also known as the "motor voter" act, was passed in 1993. It was an effort to make registration easier by offering citizens the opportunity to register to vote or update their voter registration at driver's license agencies, unemployment offices, libraries, and public assistance agencies. It is believed to have produced the largest 2-year increase in voter registration in American history.[4] Nevertheless, despite the increase in registration, the voter turnout in the 1996 presidential election was very disappointing. Less than half of our country's eligible voters exercised their franchises. The downward trend in voter turnout begun in 1960 continued.[4]

Although many pundits blamed the lackluster campaign and blurred definition of issues, persons who did not vote may have failed to consider that even if you do not vote it makes a difference. Unless there is broad participation in the election process, the small number of persons who do vote exercise unfair power. Their candidates and positions on issues may not represent the will of the majority, but they will prevail if the majority of persons fails to vote.

Beyond the Basics

Beyond turning out to vote, what can we as nurses do politically to further nursing and its agenda?

It is accepted as axiomatic that "all politics is local." Getting involved in the local politics in your own community is the perfect place to start. One way is to work in a campaign of a candidate in whom you believe. To be most effective as a nurse, choose a candidate endorsed by one of the nursing PACs—a Congressperson endorsed by ANA/PAC, or a candidate for your state and county government endorsed by your state nurse association's PAC—a nurse candidate, if possible.

Literally dozens of jobs need to be done in any campaign. As an individual, call the candidate or her campaign manager and ask how you can help. You may be asked to work in the campaign headquarters. Most candidates in local elections rely on "shoe leather," which means going door to door to introduce themselves to voters, to talk with them, and to distribute campaign literature. You may be asked to distribute literature either with the candidate or on your own, perhaps in a shopping center on a busy day or in your neighborhood, and on election days just outside a polling place.

You and other nurses may work in a telephone bank calling voters to remind them to vote for your candidate. Or you and your colleagues may organize a fundraiser for your candidate—a coffee, a tea, or a reception, in which a fee is charged, the food is donated, and all of the proceeds go to the campaign.

Finally, you may be asked to work in the inner circle of a campaign, keeping track of the candidate's appointment schedule or helping develop strategy.

■ THE NURSE LEGISLATOR ADVANTAGE

Nothing is perhaps more advantageous to nursing than having nurses in elective office. Nurses were delighted when Eddie Bernice Johnson, M.P.A., R.N., was elected Congresswoman from her Texas district in 1992—the first nurse to sit in Congress.

Although it seems that the first nurse in Congress has been a long time in coming, nurse politicians have been remarkably successful on the state level. By 1997 approximately 75 nurses were sitting in 34 state legislatures across the country. In New Hampshire alone there were eight in its House of Representatives. In Maryland, where nurses have had a history of political activism, one was in the state Senate and four were in the House of Delegates (the lower house).[1]

Nurse legislators, with their understanding of health care, become mentors on that subject for their colleagues in their legislative bodies. Nurses who have an agenda for legislation directly related to nursing find their familiarity with their issues invaluable. As an example, in the late 1970s nurses in advanced practice in Maryland brought a proposal to Delegate Marilyn Goldwater, R.N. They wanted legislation that required insurance companies to compensate them directly for the professional work they were licensed to perform. They worked with Goldwater in drafting the legislation, preparing testimony on behalf of it, and organizing lobbying efforts. They were rewarded when Maryland passed pioneering legislation making third-party reimbursement for nurses in advanced practice mandatory—first for nurse-midwives in 1978, then for nurse practitioners in 1979. The legislation served as a model for other states. If Maryland nurses had taken this proposal to a legislator who was not a nurse, it is doubtful whether the issue would have been understood or championed.[5]

Maryland nursing organizations learned early the value of political action and continue to educate nurses about the issues and to mentor them in political skills such as how to analyze proposed legislation, take positions, and lobby effectively.

Every other year, near the beginning of the Maryland legislative session, nursing organizations sponsor an all-day legislative workshop in Annapolis, the state capitol. It is scheduled on the day of the nurses' legislative reception. Workshop participants attend the reception and can immediately put new skills and information to work.

The reception, "Nurses' Night in Annapolis," is now sponsored by the Maryland Nurses Association and as many as 15 cosponsoring nursing organizations. Every January it brings together as many as 300 nurses and legislators, who use the opportunity to get acquainted and talk about the issues to be tackled in the upcoming session. This is a very convivial form of lobbying.

Nurses, prepared on their issues, are also at the state House every other Monday evening during the session when legislators set aside time for more serious talk with constituents about bills under consideration.

Maryland's example is only one of several that might be explored. Nursing organizations in other states, including California, Illinois, New York, New Mexico, and Mississippi, have strong programs to educate and mentor their members on how to be effective politically.

■ ON THE NATIONAL SCENE

Our nation's capitol, Washington, D.C., has been a magnet in recent years for nurses interested in influencing health care policy.

Nurses have been given high-level and very visible positions. One was Carolyne K. Davis, Ph.D., R.N., F.A.A.N., who was appointed administrator of the Health Care Financing Administration (HCFA), U.S. Department of Health and Human Services, by President Ronald Reagan in 1981. She became the first woman to hold that top health policy–making position in the federal government.[5]

Another was Sheila Burke, M.P.A., R.N., F.A.A.N., who for many years was a valued staffer of Senator Robert Dole (R-Kansas). She won her spurs politically as the president of the National Student Nurses' Association, and started out as a legislative assistant in Senator Dole's office in 1977. In 1982 she became deputy staff director of the U.S. Senate Committee on Finance, on which he served. In that role she was the staff's chief contact on such programs as Social Security, disability insurance, Medicare, Medicaid, maternal and child health, and peer review organizations. In 1986 Burke became Senator Dole's chief of staff, and was seen at his side from that time through his 1996 campaign for President. She subsequently became an Associate Dean at the Kennedy School at Harvard University.

Still another was Mary Wakefield, Ph.D., R.N., F.A.A.N., who was administrative assistant to Senator Quentin Burdick (D-ND) from 1989 to 1993, and chief of staff for his successor Senator Conrad Kent (D-ND) from 1993 to 1996. She later became Director of the Center for Health Policy at George Mason University College of Nursing and Health Science in Fairfax, Virginia.

By the mid-1990s many nursing organizations recognized the practicality of being near the seat of power and had located their national headquarters in Washington, D.C. Among those were ANA; the American Association of Colleges of Nursing; the American College of Nurse Midwives; the American College of Nurse Practitioners; the Association for Professionals in Infection Control and Epidemiology; the Association of Women's Health, Obstetric, and Neonatal Nurses; and the Nurses' Organization of Veterans Affairs, to name a few. Many more had Washington legislative offices. All were organized to bring their issues to Capitol Hill and to collaborate with each other on many of them.

In 1997 ANA had a director of federal government relations and four paid lobbyists on Capitol Hill, each assigned to work on specific issues. There were in total approximately 40 lobbyists (some volunteer and some paid) at that time making the rounds in Congress for their nursing organizations.[9]

During the 7 years between 1985 and 1992, when nursing was coming of age politically, Nancy J. Sharp, M.S.N., R.N., Executive Vice President of the American College of Nurse Practitioners, developed and ran a week-long political education workshop, the "Nurse in Washington Internship" (NIWI)—some years twice. Her goal was to plant the seeds of political awareness in nurses around the country and give them the tools to be politically effective. Over those years some 750 nurses came from all parts of the United States to participate in these workshops. They included education on nursing and health care issues and actual hands-on experiences, such as attending Congressional hearings and visiting their Congresspersons.[9] Since 1992 the National Federation of Specialty Organizations has offered a shortened version of the NIWI program annually.

During roughly the same period, nurses in the nation's capitol interested in health policy organized the Nurse in Washington Roundtable, which brought together health policy makers and interested nurses on a bimonthly basis for dinner, talks by high-level speakers, questions and answers, and networking. Its success ultimately became its undoing. The numbers of nurses interested in attending became so great, and the cost so high, that the event became too unwieldy to manage on such a frequent basis. It is now held once a year at the time of the NIWI conference.[9]

■ SUMMARY

The late 1990s are challenging times for nursing. In a sense the field is in the eye of a hurricane, with forces committed to changing the health care delivery system swirling around it.

Several issues that affect nursing directly are being debated all across the country. They include:

- How to contain costs, particularly of the major government health care programs—Medicare for the elderly, and Medicaid for the federal/state partnership for the care of the indigent
- How to provide access to care for the 37 million people without health insurance, either private or government
- How much profit-making by some of the health maintenance organizations (HMOs) and the insurance companies is reasonable and fair
- How we can provide quality client care both during shortened stays in hospitals and after clients return home

- How professional nurses will be utilized and what responsibilities for client care can be delegated to less qualified personnel
- How advanced practice nurses can best be utilized

Every one of these issues directly affects us. Nurses, 1.2 million strong, constitute by far the largest numbers of health care providers, and we must be involved in finding solutions to these very complicated problems.

Increasingly, health policy is being made by government—by elected and appointed officials who are not really knowledgeable about health care or about nursing. It is up to us to educate them and the public about both. We must do it through political involvement.

For every nurse there are limits of time and talent. There should be no limit on commitment. Each of us should do what she can: join a nursing organization; study the issues; vote; educate friends, neighbors, and particularly political officials and candidates about the realities of health care delivery and nursing's role; support candidates friendly to us; and, finally, support the nurses who are willing to provide leadership in this field, particularly those who are willing to run for office.

It is critical that nurses play an active part in resolving the health care delivery problems presently facing the country. Nurses have unique experience and insights concerning these issues. Their full participation in working out solutions to these difficult problems is absolutely essential.

CRITICAL THINKING *Activities*

1. **Describe what the political process is.**
2. **How has nursing officially influenced public policy, political decisions, and elections?**
3. **Name nurses who have been politically active and changed the course of conditions and events.**
4. **What are some top priority issues of this decade?**

References

1. ANA/PAC list, Nurse state legislators, Washington, D.C., January 1997.
2. Chinn PL, ed: Nursing history, *Adv Nurs Sci* 7(2):10, 1985.
3. Donahue MP: *Nursing: the finest art,* St Louis, 1985, Mosby.
4. Duskin M: Who voted and why, Washington, D.C., *National Voter* 46(2):5, 1997.
5. Goldwater M, Zusy MJL: *Prescription for nurses: effective political action,* St. Louis, 1990, Mosby.
6. Deleted in proofs.
7. Helmlinger C: ANA's landmark patient safety legislation debuts on Capitol Hill, Washington, D.C., *Am Nurse* 28:4, p. 1.
8. Schumacher K, ANA/PAC coordinator: Washington, D.C., personal communication, January 1997.
9. Sharp NJ: Personal communication, Washington, D.C., January 1997.
10. *Am Nurse,* Washington, D.C., June 1996, pp. 5, 9, 11.

PART THREE

Nursing Practice

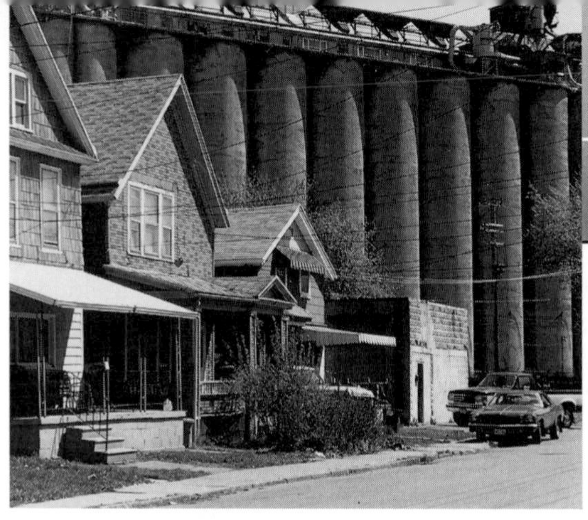

CHAPTER 12

Urban Health Care Problems

Iris R. Shannon

OBJECTIVES After completing this chapter the reader should be able to:

- **Describe the particular characteristics of urban communities that influence health**
- **Identify selected environmental, social, and health issues that affect urban populations**
- **Understand the role of government public health in the reduction of population health risks, including the delivery of public health nursing services**

Urban communities represent an array of attractions: employment and other economic opportunities; education, cultural, and recreation diversity; government and private sector resources; commercial, technical, and industrial advances; and extensive levels of religious, social service, and health resources. As a result of these and other attractions, cities are challenged by large and concentrated populations and by diverse groups that often have conflicting goals. The growth of cities has always been influenced by powerful forces. For example, cities are seen as a resource for an increasing world population that reached 1 billion by 1830, 5 billion by 1987, and is expected to reach 8 billion by 2022.[23,36] In 1995 George Silver[26] wrote that "given present estimates, the world will double its present population in about 50 years and will have surpassed its space and resources for the accommodation of such a multitude." Cities are viewed as important attributes in coping with the increasing number of persons living in poverty.

Nationally, significant numbers of city dwellers are at high risk of illness, disability, and premature death because of their compromised socioeconomic, environmental, physiologic, and other conditions. For example, the 1992 U.S. Department of Commerce estimate of the persons living below the poverty level was 36.9 million (14.5% of the nation's population), of which 42.4% lived in central cities.[35] Poverty has long been established as a causative factor in illness.

In addition to poverty, density, and poor health outcomes, the increased vulnerability of inner-city populations is partly explained by the disproportionate representation of minorities, increased numbers of homeless persons, high crime rates, drug use, violence, environmental pollution, substandard housing, unemployment, undereducation, and other social problems with health consequences. Collectively, this myriad of issues affects urban health problems, resources, and needs.

■ PUBLIC HEALTH AND PUBLIC HEALTH NURSING

A public health perspective was selected for the exploration of issues that affect urban health. This perspective provides a holistic approach to problem solving and is population based and community focused. Fundamental to public health practice is the science of epidemiology, which describes and explains health problems among populations and provides a basis for appropriate interventions.[25] Although public health involves public and private resources, this chapter will focus on government public health. Government public health's functions are concerned with issues of the public good and include assessment, assurance, and policy development. Public health functions are aimed at the identification of populations at risk and at optimizing the health of the community.[13]

Members of the Public Health Nursing Section of the American Public Health Association submitted an updated definition and role statement at the Association's 1996 Annual Meeting. *Public health nursing* was defined as "the practice of promoting and protecting the health of populations using knowledge from nursing, social, and public health science." The definition is congruent with the functions of public health and a practice in which prevention and health promotion are dominant.

This chapter will proceed by providing an urban framework followed by brief discussions of environmental, social, and medical concerns. References will be made in these discussions to selected findings from a 1993 study completed by the author involving public health nurses from seven city health departments: Baltimore, Chicago, Los Angeles, Memphis, New York, San Francisco, and Washington, D.C.*

■ AN URBAN FRAMEWORK

Great cultures are said to be city-born. Estimating that by the year 2000 more than half of the world's population will live in cities, Schiffer and Cooke[23] identify the need and challenge for cities to absorb "an exploding population into a limited infrastructure of jobs and homes."

Doxiadis[14] is credited with describing an evolutional progression of cities. His conceptualization considers the sequence of time matched to a sequence of scale as

---

*Appreciation is expressed to the Loewenberg School of Nursing, Memphis State University, for their support of this research. Findings were reported by the author in a presentation given at the American Public Health Association's 132nd Annual Meeting, Washington, D.C., November 1, 1994.

they relate to human spaces. The sequence of his "system of settlement" for human living space included room, dwelling, group of dwellings or neighborhood, small town, city metropolis, conurbation, megalopolis, urban region, urbanized continent, and ecumenopolis. Each is an extension of the preceding smaller unit. Jones[14] characterized *ecumenopolis* as an extension of a megalopolis, an extrapolation of Western tendencies and more of what we already have. The point was made by Jones that technology ensures communication even when populations are dispersed, and he suggested that it is no longer necessary to live in a city to be a part of an urban civilization. His position is vindicated by the current explosion of technology associated with cyberspace. As a further extension of this taxonomy and of an awareness of current and developing scientific and technical advancement, the concept of *planetopolis* (space cities in the galaxy) has emerged.[23]

Although the most frequently used measures of *urban* are demographic (e.g., trait lists based on size, density, and heterogeneity), the common view of large cities is that they collectively represent social illness. This is partially true because crime statistics are easier to obtain and more widely disseminated by the popular media than positive measures of urban life involving culture, the arts, or community achievements. This places additional responsibility on public health nurses and other workers to include in their assessments and planning the strengths of the individuals, families, and communities.

Cities are economic, geographic, cultural, educational, and ecologic units. They go beyond their charters and formal organization and represent dynamic, varied, and complicated cultures. In 1991 an estimated 196 million Americans lived in metropolitan areas (76 million in central cities and 120 million outside of central cities).[35] Estimates about cities in the next millennium suggest continued growth. For example, by the year 2000 some 25 cities worldwide are expected to have populations of 10 million or more, including the American megacities of New York (15.8 million) and Los Angeles (11.0 million).[17,23]

Varied economic and sociologic factors affect U.S. megacities, such as high taxes, racial tensions, violence, and decreasing social and health resources for the disadvantaged. The environmental impact of megapopulations on the supply, safety, and quality of water, food, and air varies as a function of technologic and other available resources.

Based on studies that included New York City, the Wallaces[39] suggested that urban afflictions such as homelessness, addiction, mental illness, AIDS, and crime and violence are not separate and disparate problems. The researchers attribute these and other health and social problems to "an interwoven pattern of urban ecological collapse."

The 1990 U.S. census confirmed distributional changes in the population. For example, the new emerging majority is people of color.[15] The greatest growing minority populations are represented by Hispanic and Asian groups.

In 1992, 36.9 million Americans had incomes below the poverty level.* Almost 60% (12.7 million) of those in poverty lived in central cities. Poor Americans are essentially concentrated in metropolitan areas: 92.0% of poor Hispanics, 81.8% of poor African Americans, and 71.9% of poor whites. Central cities have even greater

*Poverty thresholds are updated every year to reflect changes in the Consumer Price Index.

concentrations of the poor: 73.5% of poor African Americans, 64.8% of the poor Hispanics, and 49.1% of poor whites.[35] Given the growth in population diversity and its concentration in urban communities, nurses must be prepared to deliver culturally competent and sensitive care.

Another example of changing demographics that will greatly influence urban health and resources is referred to as the "aging of America." Schiffer and Cooke[23] provide this account of projected changes in New York City's population:

> The people of New York are getting older . . . By the year 2000, the ratio will be higher . . . especially the number of "old old" past eighty-five, and New York will then be another of the twenty-first century's cities of the aged. (p. 178)

The U.S. Congress oversees the status of the nation's urban areas. In a hearing of the Senate Banking, Housing and Urban Affairs, chaired by Donald Riegle (D-Michigan) on September 17, 1992,[34] testimony and comments from an array of experts raised many complex issues:

- In our cities, 40% of children drop out of school, 30% of children are in poverty, 25% of babies born in city hospitals are drug addicted, and African American teen pregnancy has not dropped since the mid-1970s
- Disinvestment in many cities is evident from levels of unemployment, scarce educational resources, high crime rates, and "heavy" infrastructure problems related to water, energy, and transportation, including roads and bridges
- Urban problems cannot be solved by philanthropic organizations and must be considered with national macroeconomic policy
- The May 1992 Los Angeles riots were symptoms of the problem—society is divided by racism and classism, and government and the public must develop partnerships for the resolution of urban problems
- Building equity in individuals and communities is necessary, beginning with children and the availability of proper health care
- The antecedents of poor health include poverty, unemployment, AIDS, violence, crime, and tuberculosis
- At a time of increased demand for services, public health infrastructures in urban communities have experienced significant decreases, including public health nursing positions

The preceding comments are not inclusive of the extensive testimony given and the discussion that took place during the hearing. However, to achieve improvement in the quality of life, the need to resolve issues around the organization, delivery, and cost of health care emerged as a paramount consideration resolving urban problems.

Adequate resources to support large population centers are always a challenge. Funding, particularly from various levels of government, is of great concern to urban areas given the magnitude of services that must be maintained. Therefore analysts, policy makers, and critics of the complex federal budget maintain a constant vigil as budget bills are presented to Congress. For example, in the U.S. Conference of Mayors (USCM) report of the administration's Budget, Fiscal Year 1996, [32] concern was raised regarding funding for health care.[31] One concern focused on the proposed consolidation of categorical grants such as those previously sent directly to cities for STDs, HIV prevention, HIV surveillance, tuberculosis, and immunization programs. This gives states great latitude in the use of federal health dollars within certain broad categories. The impact of this approach on cities will require careful assessment.

Social change and social dislocation, characteristics of inner cities, influence the health and well-being of their residents. (Random House defines an *inner city* as the older part of a city, densely populated and usually deteriorating, inhabited mainly by the poor who disproportionately represent minority groups.) These characteristics have been explored and analyzed in books written or edited by Wilson,[40] Braithwaite and Taylor,[2] Conrad and Kern,[5] Hacker,[10] and Dula and Goering.[6] Wilson describes the social problems of urban life in the United States as "problems of racial inequality." He further posits that in recent years the uneven racial distribution of these problems is demonstrated by the overrepresentation of minorities in crime rates, drug addiction, out-of-wedlock births, female-headed families, and welfare dependency.

For a variety of reasons, minorities are among the at-risk groups identified in national health goals for the year 2000 as "special populations" needing targeted preventive efforts.[37] Existing health disparities, especially between minority and nonminority population groups, are important factors in defining special populations. Poverty and near-poverty are posited by the U.S. Department of Health and Human Services (DHHS) as underlying "elements" for many of the health problems experienced by African American, Hispanic, Asian and Pacific Islander, Native American, and Alaskan Native groups. Successful outcomes from interventions targeted at the reduction of health risks among special populations depend on understanding the differences in health disparities in and among population groups and on understanding their epidemiologic bases.

Effective nursing care must reflect population differences and the cultural context in which care is given. Therefore, along with negotiating the visible aspects of the city, nurses working in urban areas should become familiar with such intangible characteristics as prevailing value systems, behaviors, relationships, and institutions. These understandings contribute to a more accurate assessment of a community's health needs. Abraham[1] describes the health experiences of an inner-city Chicago family and concludes that inner-city emergency rooms are where "the hospital collides hardest with the neighborhood around it, where the products of a broken-down inner-city come to be put back together again" (p. 94). It is apparent that the issues that affect health in urban communities are complex, requiring public and private resources and multifaceted effort and disciplines.

■ URBAN HEALTH ISSUES

Given the complexities of urban communities, nurses working with such populations encounter a host of environmental, medical, and social problems. These problems may not be uncommon in their practice but appear more frequently in densely populated communities.

Environmental Health

Saucier[22] considers the environment as possibly the "single most important determinant of health in the near future" (p. 173). Chapter 11 of *Healthy People 2000 National Health Promotion and Disease Prevention Objectives*[37] includes 16 objectives related to environmental health problems such as asthma, waterborne diseases, lead poisoning, air pollution, radon testing, solid waste disposal, safe water, hazardous waste, and others. In addition, an objective related to establishing and monitoring sentinel environmental diseases is included for the surveillance of lead and other metals, pesticides and carbon monoxide poisonings, heatstroke, hypothermia, and respiratory diseases. There are few limits on the opportunities for nurses to contribute to the reduction of environmental risks through education, advocacy, and treatment. The impact on health of non–disease-causing agents, as well as disease-causing agents, must be considered.

Although cause and effect relationships are difficult to establish, an increasing number of studies have reported that environmental hazards in the air, water, and soil are barriers to good health. Nurses must understand the effect of the environment on disease and disability including risk factors associated with age, location, occupation, and other socioeconomic determinants. Leptospirosis, asthma, lead poisoning, and heat-related deaths are offered as examples of the impact of urban environmental conditions on health.

Leptospirosis

The reemergence of the disease leptospirosis (a flu-like disease that is usually mild but can become life threatening) was recently reported in *The Nation's Health*[28] as an environmental problem. Among the populations at risk are inner-city residents, particularly children, because of their exposure to rat urine when they play in vacant lots and alleys. The disease is transmitted through breaks in the skin or through the linings of the eyes, nose, and throat. Although the disease is also transmitted by dogs and livestock, these animals can be vaccinated. Flood victims, farmers, sanitation and sewer workers, campers, and freshwater swimmers are also at risk for the disease. Rodent control measures in cities, in addition to community education that includes identification of environmental risks, safe play areas, and disease symptoms are important public health nursing interventions.

Asthma

The prevalence of asthma is increasing among all ages, races, and sexes but particularly among children. According to the Department of Health and Human Services, increases are attributed to environmental factors such as ozone and other air pollutants.[37] DHHS reports that African Americans die at three times the rate of whites and attributes their excessive deaths to residence in urban areas where air pollution may be more prevalent.

Consistent findings were reported by Targonski and others,[27] who studied asthma mortality in Chicago among African Americans and whites age 5 through 34. The researchers found that African Americans experienced consistently higher asthma mortality throughout the study period. They also identified a shift in deaths from inpatient to noninpatient settings (e.g., emergency room and outpatient facilities). Findings were inversely correlated with measures of income in the Chicago study group, as well as in a similar New York City study group. According to the researchers, "Lack of access to health care has been proposed as a contributor to the increase in mortality from asthma," as well as an increased exposure to environmental allergens and irritants (pp. 1832–1833). They conclude that death from asthma continues to be preventable but is interrelated with social, cultural, and economic factors, including access to health care. Therefore a multidimensional public health approach is appropriate to assess the problem, ensure services are available, and formulate needed policy for risk reduction among high-prevalence population groups.

Lead Poisoning

The estimate given by Glotzer and others[9] in addressing the issue of lead testing procedures was that one of every six children in the United States has an elevated lead level ($\geq$ 0.72 μmol/L [15 μg/dL]) associated with "adverse effects." Another estimate of the problem among children is that 12 million American children under the age of 7 may be at risk of elevated lead levels, and 3 to 4 million American children under the age of 6 may have toxicity levels above 10 μg/dL. Low-level lead exposure in children is associated with disturbances in cognition, behavior, and attention disorders. Although sources of lead are found in air, water, food, and soil, paint remains the most important source for children. The most devastating form of lead poisoning is found in inner cities where old, dilapidated housing containing chipped and peeling paint is responsible for poisoning thousands of children. Peeling paint with a lead base forms colorful, sweet-tasting chips that are attractive to young children. Lead abatement is an expensive process, and the Residential Lead-Based Paint Hazard Reduction Act of 1992 specifically provides grants to assist state and local governments to reduce lead-based paint hazards in low-income private housing.

According to Needleman,[19] "Over 50% of Black children in poverty enter the first grade with elevated blood lead levels considered neurotoxic." He offers this explanation for why so little prevention has been implemented and why the condition continues to prevail:

> First, is the enduring belief that this is a problem only for poor inner city black children. Related to this is the assertion that the mother's inferior care is responsible for the child's lead exposure and poor learning ability. Society has always been myopic about the problems of poor minorities, and once the mother has been blamed for the problem, official consciences can rest. (p. 686)

However, he identifies the more "intractable" problems to be the beliefs held by many that the problem is too big to handle, too expensive, and that society would never be willing to pay the cost. The national health objectives for the year 2000 regarding lead are aimed at eliminating elevated blood lead levels in the United States by the year 2010.

Public health and other community-oriented nurses have the opportunity to reduce health risks associated with lead poisoning. They can educate the public about the danger that peeling paint in older houses represents to young children and about existing or needed community resources for lead testing and treatment.

Heat-Related Deaths

Chicago experienced a record-setting heat wave in July of 1995, resulting in over 700 excess deaths. Temperatures ranged from 93°F to 119°F between July 12 and 16, peaking at 119°F on July 13. The risk of heat-related death was found to increase in persons with known medical problems who were confined to bed, for persons who did not leave home each day, for those who lived alone, and for those who lived on top floors of buildings. Researchers studying the heat wave concluded that those at greatest risk of dying from the heat were persons with medical illnesses who were socially isolated and did not have access to air conditioning.[24]

Stimulated by the heat-related crisis, city government initiated policies and procedures (based on meteorologic data) that included public health warnings when conditions warranted. In addition, agents of the city visited and checked persons at risk who lived alone; additional cooling centers were made available; electric fans were issued when needed; and a public campaign was initiated to encourage family members, friends, and neighbors to monitor those at risk. Although transportation was made available to cooling centers, some persons were too fearful to leave their homes. Among population groups where strong family relationships prevailed, fewer deaths occurred. This natural environmental disaster had complex social, political, and health implications. Community-based nursing, working with other disciplines, assisted in the planning and implementation of services needed by individuals, families, and communities to cope with the heat.

Other Disasters

Another example of public health nursing's response to environmental challenges is contained in the following recommendation for the Lillian Wald Service Award, Public Health Nursing Section, American Public Health Association, which I submitted in 1994:

> In the past year, the challenges to the resources and ingenuity of the Los Angeles County Department of Health Services have received national attention because of their unusual and calamitous nature. Repeated catastrophes (riots, fires, mud slides, earthquakes and windstorms) occurred throughout the year that required the Department's public health nurses to reorganize and provide services to existing and resulting vulnerable populations. These skills required knowledge of County and community resources, the ability to negotiate and use such resources efficiently and effectively and the ability to work in high stress situations. In spite of the impact of events on their personal lives, public health nurses, in the tradition of Lillian Wald, demonstrated extraordinary dedication in responding to the community health needs created by repeated crises. The Department's decisions and planning were influenced by public health nurses' first-hand knowledge of community resources, by their resourcefulness and their ability to assess population needs. Nursing's presence in devastated communities not only represented help, but hope, order and reassurance to frightened, disoriented and displaced persons.

Recognition was given to the Los Angeles public health nursing staff regarding their response to repeated environmental challenges at the 1995 Annual Meeting of the American Public Health Association.

Environmental health has enormous dimensions; this discussion is not intended to be inclusive. The reader is advised to consult environmental texts and journal

TABLE 12-1

Selected Mortality Rates per 100,000 Population in Seven American Cities, 1992

City	Homicide	Lung Cancer	Heart Disease	HIV/AIDS	Infants**
UNITED STATES	10.5	41.0	144.2	12.6	8.5
Baltimore	47.0	55.7	207.9	76.2	13.8
Chicago	34.6	43.7	199.7	34.7	13.7
Los Angeles (County)	22.3	38.2 (1991)	148.6	25.0	7.3*
Memphis (Shelby County)	24.7	45.6	181.9	13.6	13.4
New York City	28.0	32.7*	196.8	79.8	10.2
San Francisco	15.9	31.0*	130.1*	180.8	7.6*
Washington, D.C.	64.1	57.8	301.2	87.7	18.3

*Not in excess of U.S. rate

**Per 1000 live births

From: Chicago Department of Health: *Big cities health inventory,* Chicago, 1994, CDOH; Chicago Department of Public Health: *Big cities health inventory,* Chicago, 1995, CDPH.

reports for a more inclusive consideration of the subject. Social issues also have significant implications for urban settings as evidenced by their impact on health.

■ SOCIAL ISSUES

The "new urban health crisis" is described as a complex catastrophe generally involving those located in low-income minority communities and having as its core the interrelated conditions of HIV and other infections, homelessness, violence, drug use, and mental illness.[11] It is important to realize that the mix of residents in urban communities is not the same as it was 23 years ago. Population distributions for the seven cities included in my study of public health nurses shown in Table 12-1 demonstrate some of these changes over time. Extensive disaggregated racial and ethnic distributions were only available after the last census.

Los Angeles (L.A.) serves as an example of increased diversity. As a megacity, its racial and ethnic composition has changed dramatically over recent years.[18] The greatest percentage increase in population groups since 1980 have been Asian/Pacific Islanders (110% increase representing 20 different nationalities) and Latinos (70% increase). Latinos now constitute the largest ethnic group in L.A. Over 100 languages are spoken in L.A., and 45% of its residents speak a primary language other than English. Health care providers must be sensitive to socioeconomic and diverse lifestyle factors shaping health behaviors. Disparate health needs differ among L.A.'s population groups (African Americans, Native Americans, Anglos, Asian/Pacific Islanders, and Latinos). The number of persons in L.A. with incomes below the poverty level had increased in the 1990 census and is expected to reach 1.6 million by the year 2000. In addition to poverty in this community, other factors identified associated with poor health outcomes included unhealthy living conditions, inadequate diet, violence, lack of transportation, and lack of access to health care.

Kotlowitz,[16] an investigative journalist, presents an exploration of poverty in Chicago. He provides insight into the multiple government and nongovernment systems influencing the health and the well-being of an inner-city Chicago family living in a public housing high rise.

Hunger and Homelessness

The United States Conference of Mayors (USCM) has followed hunger and homelessness in American cities for 12 years, completing their most recent assessment in 1996.[29] Among the 29 major cities participating in the USCM study, three were cities also included in my study of public health nursing: Los Angeles, Chicago, and San Francisco. The 1996 findings related to hunger in these cities were based on changes in the status of hunger since 1995:

- An average increase of 11% in requests for emergency food, with 83% of the 29 cities participating registering an increase
- An average of 18% of the requests for emergency food assistance was estimated to have gone unmet
- Sixty-two percent of those requesting emergency food assistance were members of families
- Thirty-seven percent of the adults were employed
- In 26 cities, emergency food assistance was relied on by families and individuals in emergencies and as a steady source of long-term food

Local food assistance efforts in the 29 cities were supported by a variety of sources: locally generated revenues, federal funds, and state grants. Causes cited for hunger included unemployment and other employment-related problems, high housing costs, poverty (lack of income), low-wage jobs, and inadequate public assistance benefit levels and welfare cuts.

Health department nurses, with others, assist in the assessment of hunger in the populations they serve through the delivery of direct services, observations, and involvement with community groups. Assessment includes the adequacy and accessibility of government and private resources to meet the community's needs. In addition, through referral systems and working with others, public health nurses can ensure that persons needing food assistance are aware of available community resources.

In the same manner, homelessness in 1996 compared to 1995 was reported in the 29 cities:

- Cities experienced an average increase of 5% in the number of requests for emergency shelter
- An average of 20% of homeless individuals' and 24% of homeless families' requests for shelter were unmet
- The average length of time that persons remained homeless was 6 months
- In over half of the cities (56%) families may have to be separated to have shelter or leave the shelter they were staying at during the day

The population included in the survey was on average 45% male, 14% single females and unaccompanied minors, 38% families with children (children represented 27% of the total population and the fastest-growing subpopulation among the homeless), 57% African American, 30% white, 10% Hispanic, 2% Native American, and 1% Asian. Eighteen percent of the homeless were employed, and 19% were veterans. An average of 24% of the homeless in the survey were considered mentally ill, 43% were substance abusers, and 8% had AIDS or

HIV-related illness. All homeless shelters participating in the survey reported receiving government funds to support their services. The reasons given for homelessness by city officials included lack of affordable housing, substance abuse, lack of "needed" services, mental illness, unemployment, domestic violence, poverty, and family crises or other family problems.

The Committee on Health Care for Homeless People, Institute of Medicine, National Academy of Sciences[12] reported that the homeless are a special challenge to health agencies because of their mobility and because they are at high risk of disease, disability, and premature death. Nurses, including nurse practitioners, are major providers and organizers of health care for the homeless and participate in a variety of public and private community-based programs providing care to this population. Homeless persons with comorbidity (multiple health problems) are very problematic since treatment facilities for homeless persons with secondary and tertiary diagnoses are very limited. Homelessness is recognized as a cause of illness, and illness is recognized as a cause of homelessness. Many health departments and voluntary agencies have designed special programs that provide essential health and medical care to this group.* In June of 1997 the annual conference on health care for the homeless convened in Washington, D.C. Health care providers, policy makers, and advocates discussed the clinical and administrative challenges associated with providing health care to the homeless.

According to the USCM report, city officials paint a bleak picture of the effect that welfare reform, food stamp cuts, and immigrant benefit cuts will have on hunger and homelessness during 1997. Recent changes in public policy are expected to increase the numbers experiencing hunger and homelessness.

Violence

Many consider violence as one of the most critical problems affecting our cities today. It affects all aspects of urban life and is considered a major and difficult public health problem. Violence has many forms; among them are homicide, suicide, abuse, assault, and civil unrest.

Civil unrest erupted in L.A. in 1992. The public health significance of this unrest was described by Evans[7] and included 53 deaths, 2325 reported injuries, and the destruction by fire of 600 buildings. Evans reported that the city of L.A. suffered 76% of the damages at an estimated cost of $735 million. Health department services were disrupted by the unrest. Because of the extensive destruction, new Women, Infants and Children (WIC) food distribution points were needed, as well as relocation of methadone and alcohol program services. Alternative arrangements were necessary to continue pharmacy and medical services. Health department nurses were identified among the many staff who provided care and assistance to affected residents. About 25,000 residents lost their jobs, adding to the 2.7 million persons then uninsured in Los Angeles County. Environmental problems included polluted water from the runoff used to fight fires in buildings containing hazardous

---

*In 1993, Chicago's Interfaith House was established. It describes itself as a respite, assessment, and supportive living center for the homeless and targets its services to those "too sick for the streets, but not sick enough for the hospital." This organization estimates that Chicago has a homeless population of 50,000 during the span of a year.

materials and fires involving gas stations. Resulting air pollution from the disaster was a concern for persons with chronic upper respiratory problems. The L.A. racial riots of 1992 and 1965 were examples of the characterization given to megacities as places of racial conflict. The collective costs of such violence to any community include potential years of life lost; cost of treatment, rehabilitation, and long-term care resulting from accidental and intentional injuries; and an array of social costs.

According to a report from the Chicago Department of Health:

> Violence has also had a social and psychological impact in Chicago's communities. A recent Police Department study has found that while overall crime has not increased significantly in recent years, the fear of crime within communities has. Indeed, senior citizens are often afraid to seek health care in the afternoon, preferring early morning appointments in order to avoid encounters with gang members. (p. 58)

The issue of community-level violence in the delivery of public nursing services emerged in my study. Some nurses attributed heightened levels of violence in their communities to drug use and, because of the perceived danger, made visits in pairs. Other nurses felt that their partnership with the community represented a safety factor and were less fearful about their personal safety. In this regard, district nursing assignments were considered by some to enhance the public health nurse's ability to function effectively in communities where health and social risks were high.

Among the societal conditions contributing to violence are lack of access to care, issues of unemployment, discrimination, poverty, neglect, and lack of police presence. Violence is described as being in "epidemic proportions in America's cities." Multiple resources are being targeted to the problem and its prevention.[31] Health departments around the nation are in collaboration with others to define the problem; disseminate information to policymakers, media, and the public; develop content for the education of children; and develop, implement, and evaluate prevention programs. Public health, school, and other community-oriented nurses are participants in these programs. Urban health departments report that their efforts to reduce violence are inclusive and involve other government agencies, existing networks and coalitions, and collaboration with community groups. In the USCM report on violence prevention for youth, profiles of 13 urban health department violence prevention programs are presented, including five of the city health departments in my study of public health nurses: Baltimore, Chicago, Los Angeles, New York City, and San Francisco.

Poverty is a strongly associated causation for many social problems with health consequences, including hunger, unemployment, homelessness, violence, teen pregnancy, undereducation, and others. Some would add to this list such medical problems as tuberculosis, HIV/AIDS, infant mortality, and substance abuse. These are among the multiple medical problems associated with concentrations of disadvantaged populations characteristic of urban communities.

Other Health Issues

Health problems in cities mirror the health problems of the nation. Nationally the leading causes of death in order of magnitude are heart disease, cancer, stroke, injuries, chronic lung disease, pneumonia/influenza, diabetes, suicide, liver disease, and atherosclerosis. However, when age, gender, race/ethnicity, residence, and income are statistically controlled, differences emerge in the causes of death. Epidemiologic data supporting national public health objectives and goals have been presented by controlling for these various factors and appear in *Healthy People 2000.*[35] Therefore variation in morbidity and mortality rates within and among urban populations is dependent on multiple statistical factors. For example, in almost all of the seven cities included in the study of public health nursing, infant mortality rates were in excess of the 1992 national rate of 8.5/1000 live births. The rate for African American infants was more than twice the rate for white babies. Deaths are associated with low birth weight (considered the greatest single hazard), congenital anomalies, sudden infant death syndrome, and respiratory distress syndrome. Health indicators related to specific urban areas are usually available from local or state health departments.

"Fulfilling Society's Interest"

In a report of a national study on public health by the Institute of Medicine, National Academy of Sciences,[13] public health is defined as "fulfilling society's interest in assuring conditions in which people can be healthy" (p. 140). The public concerns addressed by this specialty are community and population focused and related to the prevention of disease, health promotion, and "encompassing physical, mental, and environmental health." The Institute further explained that:

> Many distinct and diverse professional disciplines are necessary in this effort, such as nursing, medicine, social work, environmental sciences, dentistry, nutrition and health education. These professions are unified within public health by dedication to its value system, by the public interest in health, and by its core science, epidemiology—the study of health problems in populations and the factors that affect them. (p. 140)

To carry out public health's mission requires an organized community effort that includes private organizations and individuals. Governmental public health's role is to see that the mission is adequately addressed. Although population-focused prevention and health promotion activities have distinguished public health practice, urban health departments also provide personal health services, including general medical and primary health care for the uninsured (currently estimated at 40 million) and the poor. For many, health departments are the providers of last resort. At the delivery level, nurses represent the largest group of care providers in urban health departments. As shown in Table 12-2, public health nursing services within core government functions are envisioned on three levels: community, family, and individual.[21]

The 75 public health nurses respondents from seven urban health departments in my study reported changes in the organization of their services over a 20-year time frame (1970 to 1990). These changes included health departments' emphasis on primary care services driven by the availability of Medicaid reimbursement with the subsequent conversion of public health nurse positions to nurse practitioner positions and with the introduction and use of lay workers to perform nursing

TABLE 12-2

Public Health Nursing within Core Public Health Functions Levels of Public Health Nursing Service*

Core Function	Community	Family	Individual
Assessment	Participate in data collection Conduct surveys or observe populations at risk	Comprehensive assessment of physical, social, and mental health needs Evaluate environment	Identify individuals in need of services Develop nursing care plans
Assurance	Service to target population groups Maintain safe levels of communicable disease surveillance and outbreak control Provide expert public health nursing consultation in the community	Provide services to a cluster of families. Services may include physical assessment, health education and counseling, and developmental screening	Provide nursing services across the lifespan Consult with other health care providers Prioritize individual's needs Participate on quality assurance teams
Policy Development	Provide leadership in convening and facilitating community groups to evaluate health concerns and planning Raise awareness of key policy makers about health matters Act as an advocate for target populations	Recommend programs to meet specific family needs Identify and work with families toward the support of specific policies	Develop standards for individual client care Participate in the development of job descriptions and role clarification for the various members on the team

*Selected activities

From Public Health Directors of Washington: *Public health nursing within core public health functions,* July 1993.

functions. Another significant change over the 20-year period was the reduction in public health nursing staff in all but one of the urban health departments visited. Reductions were attributed to changes in federal funding from general to categorical programs, the impact of Medicaid and Medicare reimbursement on agency priorities, and the change from community prevention to primary care.

Support for these observations has been reported by others. In the June 1993 issue of *Governing,* Brenda Wilson observed that before the 1978 passage of Proposition 13 in California there were over 100 public health nurses in the county and "today, there are 50" (p. 30). Gerzoff and others[8] analyzed changes in local health department spending in 1989 and 1992. They concluded that although the demand for public health services increased as a result of increased numbers of

TABLE 12-3

Employment Settings of Registered Nurses, 1972, 1979, and 1992

Selected Employment Settings	Total Number of Registered Nurses and Estimated Percentage of Total					
	1972		1979		1992	
Type	Number	Percentage	Number	Percentage	Number	Percentage
All	778,470 (1974)	100	1,272,851 (1980)	100	1,853,024	100
Hospital	449,594	64.2	823,321 (1980)	64.6	1,232,717	66.5
Board of Education	19,798	2.5	21,626	1.7	36,776	2.0
Local Health Departments	18,093	2.3	26,598	2.1	25,765	1.4
Visiting Nurse Service	5,830	0.07	9,936	0.07	34,350	1.8
Home Health	1,859	0.02	10,224	0.08	58,088	3.1

From U.S. Department of Health, Education and Welfare: *First report to Congress, February 1, 1977, Nurse Training Act of 1975,* Hyattsville, MD, DHEW; U.S. Department of Health and Human Services: *Nurse supply, distribution and requirements, 3rd report to the Congress, February 17, 1982, Nurse Training Act of 1975,* Hyattsville, MD, DHHS; U.S. Department of Health and Human Services: *Fifth report to the President & Congress on the status of health personnel in the United States, March 1986,* Springfield, VA, Dept. of Commerce; U.S. Department of Health and Human Services: *The registered nurse population: findings from the national sample survey of registered nurses, March 1992,* Washington, D.C., 1992, GPO.

uninsured, Medicaid-eligible clients and other factors, there was virtually no increase in local health department budgets. Levels and sources of funding have profound influence on public health nursing staffing patterns (Table 12-3).

The 1992 national survey of registered nurses[38] also supports decreasing percentages of local health department nurses. However, fifteen other subcategories of employment for community/public health nurses represent a diversity of competing opportunities for nurses interested in community and public health (Box 12-1).

The need for and commitment to community-oriented preventive efforts prevailed among the public health nurse respondents. Health indicators for the seven cities as measured by mortality data are shown in Table 12-4. For these health department nurses, interventions must be congruent with public health functions with emphasis on prevention at the individual, family, and community levels (Table 12-2).

Many urban residents experience the coexistence of multiple medical and social problems. This intensifies their need for human services and creates special challenges for community resources. Problem identification is done not only to target populations in need but also to efficiently and effectively use the scarce resources available.

A correlation matrix was developed to show the relationships among the incidence of syphilis, gonorrhea, tuberculosis, and AIDS.[3] Two correlations were statistically significant: gonorrhea and syphilis (r = 0.79), and tuberculosis and AIDS (r = 0.50). The problems associated with tuberculosis and HIV as infectious and life-threatening illnesses are of paramount concern to the health of the public.

Box 12-1 Employment Settings of 180,132 Registered Nurses Working in Community/Public Health, 1992

Employment Setting	Total	Percentage of Total
Other home health agency (non–hospital based)	58,088	32.2
Visiting Nurse Service	34,350	19.1
City/County health departments	25,765	14.3
State health department	17,570	10.0
Neighborhood health centers	8,527	5.0
Hospice	7,634	4.0
Community mental health services	7,218	4.0
Other settings	5,920	3.3
Totals	165,072	92.0

Note: Settings reporting less than 5000 registered nurses included state mental health department, Planned Parenthood/family planning, rural health care center, day care center, retirement community center, and substance abuse outpatient facility.
From: U.S. Department of Health and Human Services: *The registered nurse population: findings from the national sample survey of registered nurses, March 1992,* Washington, D.C., 1992, GPO, p. 46.

Tuberculosis and HIV

Tuberculosis is described in uncomplicated cases as curable with 6 months' treatment if that treatment is correctly prescribed and taken. If treatment is inadequate, the possibility of developing drug-resistant tuberculosis exists. This form of tuberculosis is resistant to the two drugs of choice (isoniazid and rifampin) and is known as multidrug-resistant tuberculosis (MDRTB). The problems associated with this form of tuberculosis include that it is more expensive to treat and that the failure rate for treatment is higher. The prevention of MDRTB requires a strong public health control program that ensures that every case of tuberculosis is treated appropriately and that contacts are found quickly and adequately assessed and managed. Public health departments have established programs of Directly Observed Therapy (DOT) where public health nurses and other health department workers directly observe on site the ingestion of medications. In cities, outbreaks of MDRTB have been reported in hospitals, prisons, methadone centers, and other sites frequented by drug abusers, the homeless, or mentally ill persons. Outbreaks in New York and Miami in the 1990s occurred in AIDS clients, resulting in high mortality rates and cases and deaths among health workers.[20]

The 26 cities surveyed in 1991 by USCM[33] accounted for 56.1% (94,134) of the nation's known AIDS cases (167,803). Five of the cities were also included in my study of urban public health nursing: Baltimore, Chicago, Los Angeles County, New York City, and San Francisco. These five areas represented 62.2% (58,627) of the AIDS cases reported. Chicago, in 1994, reported that the incidence of AIDS continued to increase among all risk groups, including women and minorities. Table 12-4 indicates the changing characteristics of AIDS cases in Chicago comparing data from 1990 and 1993.

Holistically, HIV and TB are evolving into diseases of poverty because of their impact on the homeless and drug abusers. Therefore some persons advocate that the approach should include stable housing, medical care, and drug treatment. In

TABLE 12-4

Characteristics of 1990 and 1993 AIDS Cases, Chicago, Illinois

Characteristics	1990	1993
Total Cases	1068	1578
African American	45%	57%
Hispanic	14%	13%
White	40%	29%
Homosexual contact	66%	49%
Injecting drug use	20%	32%
Heterosexual contact	4.5%	12%
AIDS with TB	7.6% (1989)	15%

From: Chicago Department of Public Health: *Chicago IPLAN community health needs assessment and public health plan,* 1994, p. 27.

fact, in November of 1993 the integration of tuberculosis services with drug and alcohol treatment programs, the expansion of public education, and the adoption of infection-control measures by health care facilities and prisons were included in the guidelines developed by the Advisory Council for the Elimination of Tuberculosis. Consistent with government police power and responsibility to protect the public, clients who are unable or unwilling to comply with their treatment can be committed to an institution as a last resort until they are no longer infectious.[30]

■ SUMMARY

Urban health problems are multidimensional and complex. Given the array of societal resources that urban areas represent and given the concentrations of diverse populations they also represent, efforts to reduce health and social risks for the good of the community seem an appropriate use of available resources. Government public health has responsibility to provide leadership in urban areas based on their functions of assessment, assurance, and policy development. As agents of local departments of health, public health nurses work with diverse populations and provide care to individuals, families, and communities that consider needs and strengths. Public health nursing participation and staffing levels are significantly influenced by funding sources and levels. But in urban areas their practice is also influenced by an array of social problems with health outcomes such as poverty, undereducation, abuse, unemployment, violence, racism, and drug addiction. These problems necessitate that nurses, working with others, have responsibility to advocate for social and health care reform that create environments in which citizens can maximize their full potential. The concentration of populations in urban areas at risk of disease, disability, and premature death challenges cities to develop effective prevention and health promotion programs. To maximize effort and achieve reductions in health risks, health care must be provided in culturally appropriate and sensitive environments. Given their commitment to population-based nursing, public health nurses, in partnership with the community, have a long and distinguished history of successfully contributing to the quality of life of urban residents.

CRITICAL THINKING *Activities*

1. **Given that the resources of urban health departments are limited and given the need to provide preventive and health promotion services to concentrations of populations at risk of poor health outcomes, how would you determine who should receive services?**
2. **As a public health nurse working in an inner-city community, you have been given an opportunity to organize a community advisory committee focused on reducing infant mortality. What representation would you seek on the committee?**
3. **Do nurses have any responsibility to work and advocate for the reduction of social problems?**

References

1. Abraham LK: *Mama might be better off dead: the failure of health care in urban America,* Chicago, 1993, The University of Chicago Press.
2. Braithwaite RL: Taylor SE, eds: *Health issues in the black community,* San Francisco, 1992, Jossey-Bass.
3. Chicago Department of Public Health: *Big cities health inventory, 1995,* Chicago, 1995, Chicago Department of Public Health.
4. Chicago Department of Public Health: *Chicago IPLAN community health needs assessment and public health plan,* Chicago, 1994, Department of Health.
5. Conrad P, Kern R, eds: *The sociology of health & illness,* New York, 1990, St. Martin's Press.
6. Dula A, Goering S, eds: *"It just ain't fair": the ethics of health care for African Americans,* Westport, CT, 1994, Praeger.
7. Evans CA: Public health impact of the 1992 Los Angeles civil unrest, *Public Health Rep* 108(3): 265-272, 1993.
8. Gerzoff RB and others: Recent changes in local health department spending, *J Public Health Policy* 17(2): 170-180, 1996.
9. Glotzer DE and others: Screening for childhood lead poisoning: a cost-minimization analysis. *Am J Public Health* 84(1): 110-112, 1994.
10. Hacker A: *Two nations black and white, separate, hostile, unequal,* New York, 1992, Scribner's.
11. *Health/PAC Bulletin,* Activism in the new urban health crisis, Winter 1991, 3.
12. Institute of Medicine, National Academy of Sciences: *Homelessness, health and human needs,* Washington, D.C., 1988, National Academy Press.
13. Institute of Medicine, National Academy of Sciences: *The future of public health,* Washington D.C., 1988, National Academy Press.
14. Jones E: *Metropolis,* New York, 1990, Oxford University Press.
15. Johnson T: Changing demographics in minority populations of the United States. Caring for the emerging majority: Creating a new diversity in nurse leadership, proceedings of an invitational congress sponsored by the Division of Nursing and Office of Minority Health, USDHHS, January 8-10, 1992, Bethesda, MD.
16. Kotlowitz A: *There are no children here: the story of two boys growing up in the other America.* New York, 1991, Doubleday.
17. Linden E: Megacities, *Time,* January 11, 1993, 28.

18. Los Angeles County Task Force for Health Care Access: *Closing the gap,* report to the Los Angeles County Board of Supervisors, November 4, 1992.
19. Needleman HL: Editorial: Childhood lead poisoning: a disease for history texts, *Am J Public Health* 81(6): 685, 1991.
20. Paul W: Update on multidrug-resistant tuberculosis: a presentation to the Chicago Board of Health, September 20, 1995.
21. Public Health Directors of Washington: *Public health nursing within core public health functions,* July 1993.
22. Saucier KA: *Perspectives in family and community health,* St. Louis, 1991, Mosby.
23. Schiffer RL, Cooke J: *The exploding city,* New York, 1989, St. Martin's.
24. Semenza JC and others: Heat-related deaths during the July 1995 heat wave in Chicago, *N Engl J Med* 335(2): 84-90, 1996.
25. Shannon IR: Epidemiology and the public policy process. In Oleske DM, ed: *Epidemiology and the delivery of health care services,* New York, 1995, Plenum Press.
26. Silver G: Editorial: beyond population statistics, *Am J Public Health* 85(10): 1345-1346, 1995.
27. Targonski PV and others: Trends in asthma morality among African Americans and whites in Chicago, 1968 through 1991, *Am J Public Health* 84(11): 1830-1833, 1994.
28. *The Nation's Health, American Public Health Association:* Inner-city residents found at risk for rat-borne bacterial disease, 27(1):6, 1997.
29. United States Conference of Mayors: *A status report on hunger and homelessness in America's cities: 1996.* Washington, D.C., 1996, United States Conf. of Mayors.
30. United States Conference of Mayors: *AIDS information exchange: TB and HIV—tuberculosis adds to the challenge of the HIV epidemic,* Washington, D.C., 1994, United States Conf. of Mayors.
31. United States Conference of Mayors: *Local health departments and violence prevention for youth,* Washington, D.C., 1995, U.S. Conf. of Mayors.
32. United States Conference of Mayors: *The federal budget and the cities,* Washington, D.C., 1995, United States Conf. of Mayors.
33. United States Conference of Mayors: *The impact of AIDS on America's cities,* Washington, D.C., 1991, United States Conf. of Mayors.
34. U.S. Congress. Senate. Senate Banking, Housing and Urban Affairs Committee, 102nd Cong. 2nd Sess., 9 September 1992.
35. U.S. Department of Commerce, Bureau of the Census: *Poverty in the United States: 1992,* Washington, D.C., 1993, Government Printing Office.
36. U.S. Department of Commerce, Bureau of the Census: *World population profile: 1991,* Washington, D.C., 1991, Government Printing Office.
37. U.S. Department of Health and Human Services: *Healthy people 2000—national health promotion and disease prevention objectives,* Washington, D.C., 1991, Government Printing Office.
38. U.S. Department of Health and Human Services: *The registered nurse population: findings from the national survey of registered nurses,* Washington, D.C., 1992, Government Printing Office.
39. Wallace R, Wallace D: Contagious urban decay and the collapse of public health, *Health/PAC Bulletin* Summer 1991, 13.
40. Wilson WJ: *The truly disadvantaged—the inner city, the underclass and public policy,* Chicago, 1987, University of Chicago Press.

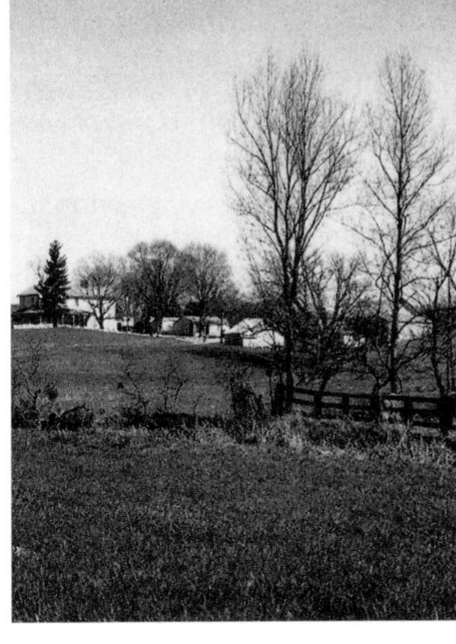

CHAPTER 13

Rural Nursing

Barbara Hulsmeyer

This chapter addresses the trends and issues related to rural nursing and health care services for vulnerable populations in rural areas. The history of nursing in rural areas, characteristics and major health problems of persons living in rural communities, health care delivery to such persons, and potential ways to improve the health status of rural populations are considered.

Rurality is defined in several ways. The U.S. Census Bureau describes *rural* as a community of less than 2500 people. Another designation by the Office of Management and Budget is that of *nonmetropolitan,* based on Standard Metropolitan Statistical Area (SMSA)—a city of at least 50,000. A rural area would be from 40 to 75 miles from a major urban area and located in a county with no population of 50,000 or more people.[31] The U.S. Department of Health and Human Services developed the category *frontier* as a description for very rural and remote areas. Frontier is used to indicate an area with a population density of less than six persons per square mile, 25 hospital beds or less or no hospital, a driving time of 1 hour to the nearest health care facility, or severe geographic limitations.[6] Geographic and population factors are generally used to designate rurality, but there are also subjective elements, such as having no cable television or living on a farm.[8]

Although the American health care system is the most costly in the world, it has inequities, and in some areas health care is limited. For rural populations health care has historically been inadequate and often inaccessible.

■ HISTORY OF RURAL NURSING

The Frontier Nursing Service (FNS), located in Hyden, Kentucky, was founded in 1925 by Mary Breckinridge, a member of a prominent Kentucky family, who decided to devote her life to the health care of women and children after her own two children died in early childhood (Figure 13-1). After graduating from St. Luke's Hospital School of Nursing in New York in 1910, she traveled to France during World War I to work with the American committee for Devastated France where she met a British nurse and midwife; this led Mary Breckinridge to study nurse-midwifery at the British Hospital for Mothers and Babies in London, and that motivated her to think about alternative options for women (Figure 13-2).

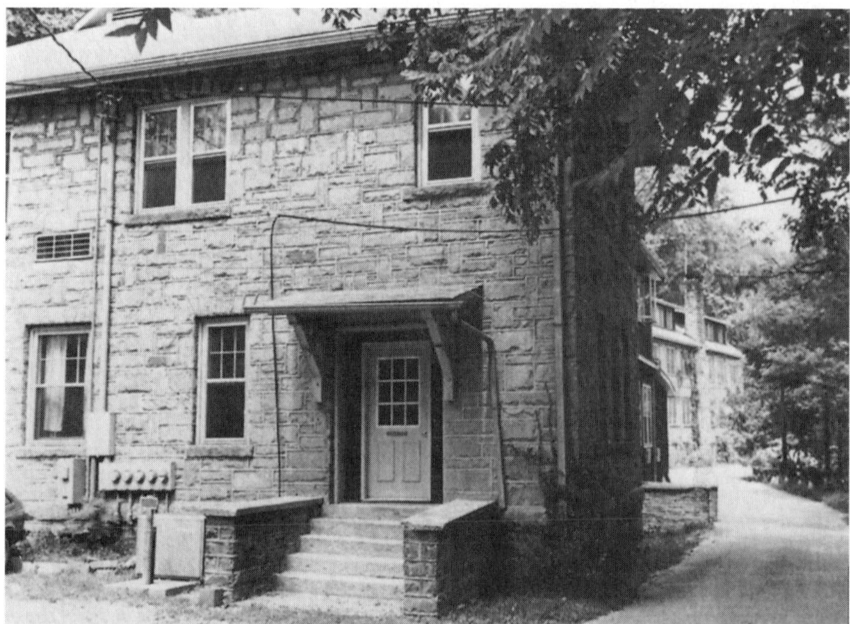

FIG. 13-1 The Morton Gill Building, originally the Hyden Hospital, now home of the Frontier School of Midwifery and Family Nursing.

> In France midwives were not nurses. In America nurses were not midwives. In England trained women were both nurses and midwives. After I had met British nurse-midwives, first in France and then on my visits to London, it grew upon me that nurse-midwifery was the logical response to the needs of the young child in rural America. In America much had been done for city children, whereas remotely rural children had been neglected. My work would be for them.[5]

After completing her work in France, Mary Breckinridge returned to the United States to supplement her education by taking a year of courses in public health nursing at Teachers College, Columbia University, after which she began her work in Leslie County, Kentucky, then one of the country's poorest and most inaccessible areas.

This initial work involved conducting a survey of Leslie, Knott, and Owsley counties. Traveling alone and spending nights in residents' cabins, she covered nearly 700 miles on horseback. She learned from the people their greatest needs and how they might be met. At the time there were no roads within 60 miles, and not one licensed physician in the area. She believed that if her efforts and plans were successful in such an inaccessible area, they could be successful anywhere.

After assessing the people and their needs, Mary Breckinridge returned to London where she studied nurse-midwifery. After completing this program, she went to Scotland where she observed the work of the Highlands and Islands Medical and Nursing Service, which provided the kind of decentralized care that became the model for the FNS.

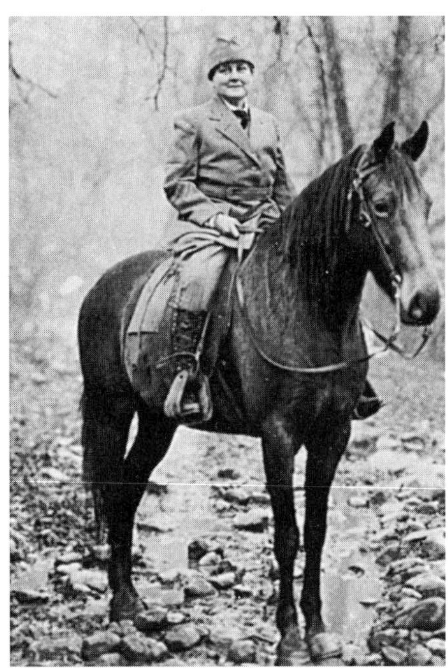

FIG. 13-2 Mary Breckinridge on horseback in 1930.

In 1928 the Hyden Hospital and Health Center was established. Six outpost nursing centers were built between 1927 and 1930. The nurse-midwives provided bedside nursing, midwifery, and public health nursing and education to nearly 10,000 people in eastern Kentucky. Until her death in 1965, Mary Breckinridge continued her life's work of caring for women and families.

The FNS is currently organized as a parent holding company for Mary Breckinridge Healthcare, Inc., home health agency, four outpost clinics, one primary care clinic in the hospital, Kate Ireland Women's Healthcare Clinic, and the Frontier School of Midwifery and Family Nursing— the largest midwifery program in the United States.[37]

■ LEGISLATION AND RURAL HEALTH CARE

In 1921 the Sheppard-Tower Act strengthened rural county health departments by providing federal grants to states for the support of maternal and child health stations, but funding was terminated in 1929 under the conservative administration of Herbert Hoover. The year 1929 marked the beginning of the Great Depression, which essentially halted all health programs.

By the early 1930s one fifth of the rural counties in the United States had a full-time public health service, though fewer than 50 of them were adequately staffed and budgeted. It was not until 1935, with the passage of the Social Security Act, that efforts to improve the public's health resumed in both rural and urban areas. This was the only major federal program for the provision of maternal and child health until the passage of Medicaid in 1965.

Another program of the 1930s was the Voluntary Prepaid Health Plan, set up by the U.S. Farm Security Administration in 1935. This federal program was specifically directed to low-income farm families and implemented to deal with rural health problems. This program was designed to furnish and improve the delivery of medical services (including general practitioner care, dental services, and hospitalization and surgical services) to dependent farm families through the concept of voluntary group action.[36]

Another program of the 1930s was the Voluntary Prepaid Health Plan, set up by the U.S. Farm Security Administration in 1935. This was an example of a federal program that was specifically directed to low-income farm families and implemented to deal with rural health problems. This program was designed to furnish and improve the delivery of medical services, including general practitioner care dental services and hospitalization and surgical services, to dependent farm families through the concept of voluntary group action.

At its peak in 1942, over 600,000 persons in 1100 rural counties were enrolled in the program. By the mid-1940s, however, the program declined because there were not enough enrollees to make it viable. To be successful, it should have been available to all rural farmers, not just those who were borrowers from the Farm Security Administration. After World War II and subsequent withdrawal of federal funds, the program was discontinued.

By 1940 the shortage of rural health practitioners became acute, with only 18.6% located in rural areas; a highly disproportionate number, given the fact that 43.55% of the total population lived in rural areas. World War II brought a lack of financial resources that, combined with a lack of human resources, attributed to the period of decline in rural health care facilities and the delivery of health care.[36]

Congress passed the Hill-Burton Act in 1946. This act provided federal funds for construction and renovation of nonfederal health care facilities. Nearly 40% of the projects funded were in communities of less than 10,000 people.[25] Although this legislation was intended to alleviate the physician shortage in rural areas, recruitment and retention were, and still remain, problematic.

One significant rural program of the 1950s was the United Mine Workers of America Welfare and Retirement Fund, which provided a full range of health benefits for miners and their families. This rural program is claimed to have had a major impact on the medical care delivery system in Southern Appalachia. But the recession of the coal industry in the early 1960s resulted in financial difficulties for the Fund and, like many other attempts to boost services and accessibility of health care in rural areas, this one became ineffective.[20]

Further expansion of the federal government's rural health programs occurred when the Indian Health Service was transferred from the Department of the Interior to the U.S. Public Health Service (USPHS) in 1955. Although the Indian Health Service has been a major combative force in social and medical problems, Native Americans as a group are still the most unhealthy population in the United States. Native Americans have a shorter life expectancy, with higher- than-national-average mortality from tuberculosis, influenza and pneumonia, renal disease, and diabetes.[19] Currently 1.5 million Native Americans are living on or near reservations in 28 states.[6] These reservations are generally located in isolated rural areas. Poverty, alcoholism, the travel distance to health care providers, and a tendency toward obesity further exacerbate overwhelming health care problems. Passage of the 1975 Indian Self-Determination and Education Assistance Act empowered Native Americans to participate in choosing essential health care services.[19]

In 1957 the Sears Roebuck Foundation introduced its Community Medical Assistance Program (CMAP) to assist rural communities in building medical clinics. As with the Hill-Burton Act, this effort was based on the assumption that modern new facilities would enhance physician recruitment in rural areas.[20]

During the existence of this program, from 1958 to 1970, a total of 625 communities completed its survey, and 253 were accepted into the program by the foundation. The CMAP provided design, fund-raising, and planning assistance for 165 physicians' offices in rural areas. However, the turnover was high, with approximately 30% of the recruited physicians leaving after 1 year or less. Although this attempt demonstrated that a new facility could induce a physician into a rural area, it had a short-term effect and failed to anticipate or deal with the problem of retention.

Many health care programs developed in the 1960s were also characterized by inequities with regard to rural populations. The Medicaid and Medicare programs were initiated in 1965 as amendments to the Social Security Act of 1935, with a major goal of improving access to health care for the disadvantaged. As a result of this legislation poor, elderly, and disabled persons have greater access to health care, but reimbursement for health care services to providers has been less in rural communities than in urban areas. This has resulted in less incentive for health care providers to practice in rural areas.

In the 1960s and early 1970s concern over the rural physician shortage became acute. Although the number of physicians had increased from 119 per 100,000 in 1950 to 137 per 100,000 in 1970, the urban versus rural disparity was apparent, with 41 physicians per 100,000 practicing in rural areas compared with 192 physicians per 100,000 in urban areas.[2] The federal government initiated programs to encourage physicians to practice in rural areas. Between 1970 and 1980 millions of dollars in grant funding were provided for the following efforts:

- Regional Medical Programs
- National Health Service Corps
- Health in Underserved Rural Areas
- Area Health Education Centers program
- Rural Health Initiative
- Community Health Centers Program
- Migrant Health Program
- Rural Health Clinic Services Act
- Farmer's Home Administration Rural Health Facility Loan Program

One of the earliest congressional attempts to improve access and availability of health care services to rural areas resulted in the development of the Regional Medical Programs (RMP), initiated in the mid-1960s and established through the United States. The inception of this program was largely in response to widespread public and professional concern regarding the need to institute effective and efficient mechanisms for providing education, research opportunities, and health resources to rural areas, thereby improving the physical, mental, and social well-being of many underserved populations. This effort to stimulate initiative and innovation at the regional level through planning, coordinating, and sharing limited health care resources and facilities was thought to be the most effective way of providing and maximizing the quality and quantity of care and services to populations of many rural regions.

The Regional Medical Programs became particularly instrumental in improving the care of clients with heart disease, cancer, and stroke, but also focused on the following issues:

1. Biochemical screening (Missouri)
2. Development of a comprehensive utilization and client information statistical system (Connecticut)
3. Provision of optimum clinical lab services for 3 million people (Connecticut)
4. A multimedia approach to the learning of health science personnel (Colorado and Wyoming)
5. A telephone network for continuing education (central New York)
6. Continuing education for physicians (West Virginia and the District of Columbia)
7. Guest resident programs (Maine)
8. Studies to determine whether comprehensive, family-oriented health care in a neighborhood health center, coordinated with an automated multiphase screening laboratory could result in improved mortality, morbidity, health services use, and health attitudes (Tennessee—mid-South)

By the end of 1967, 54 such programs were established throughout the United States, and they continued into the 1979s until dwindling federal funding and support led to their demise. As Milton Roemer said, "Except for the recent major cutbacks in federal Regional Medical Program funds, this program was helping to extend the qualitative influence of the urban medical center to rural locations."[44]

The National Health Service Corps (NHSC) was the first federal effort designed to directly place physicians and other health professionals in rural areas. Through the NHSC medical students could receive loan forgiveness in exchange for serving in designated health care shortage areas. As the NHSC increased in size, it shifted from the development of self-sufficient rural practices to become the staffing mechanism for other federal rural health programs.[36] After the cutbacks of the 1980s, this program became a viable option for placing health care professionals in medical shortage areas. Interestingly, increased funding also helped place nurse practitioners, nurse midwives, and physician assistants in these shortage areas.

The Area Health Education Centers (AHEC) program was established to provide medical education linkage between academic settings and rural practice sites. These centers provide opportunities for health care students to gain first-hand experience in medicine, health care, and the lifestyle of rural communities. Their impact on rural physician recruitment and retention has been difficult to assess. Presently 33 states have AHEC programs.[2]

Health in Underserved Rural Areas (HURA) was established in 1974 to develop comprehensive health care systems for underserved populations in rural areas. These programs include primary care, radiology, dentistry, pharmacy services, and other specialized programs in an area-wide network of health services.[38] Many of the programs demonstrated the effect of nurse practitioners and physician assistants in enhancing the health of rural populations.

All four of the preceding efforts—RMP, NHSC, HURA, and AHEC—implemented represented joint ventures between federal government and local communities. Whereas HURA emphasized research and evaluation of existing models of health care delivery, RHI was an effort to efficiently direct federal resources toward the development of comprehensive primary care in rural areas.

The Community Health Centers Program, combining three independent programs—the Neighborhood Health Centers (NHC), Family Health Centers (FHC), and the Community Health Networks (CHN)—was established to support ambulatory health care projects in areas with scarce or nonexistent health services. With the ever-shrinking federal dollar, a 1987 survey of 183 community health centers showed a 60% federal funding cut with a 27% cutback on nonrequired services and 12.6% cutback on required services.[21]

In 1977 the Rural Health Clinic Services Act amended Titles XVIII and XIX of the Social Security Act to permit cost-related Medicare reimbursement for nurse practitioner and physician assistant services provided at health care centers in rural, federally designated, medically underserved areas. Implementation of this law was gradual, with only a small portion of the clinics participating and many states unwilling to promote the program. The number of rural health clinics is currently greater than 1100. This program offers hospitals that sponsor clinics increased revenue and opportunities for expansion of services.[42]

Unfortunately, the majority of efforts to improve health services in rural areas in the 1970s were too often characterized by fragmentation, duplication, ineffectiveness, and, finally, lack of longevity, thus perpetuating a critical situation in our country. In fact, Rosenblatt and Moscovice[36] refer to it as a "rural health care crisis," claiming "the study of rural health care shows that the government tends to go from crisis to crisis, rather than coming to grips with the true, underlying problems of rural health care." They argue that rural programs have consistently been developed without sufficient thought regarding concurrent technologic processes and concern about the consequences for rural residents.

In 1987 the Office of Rural Health Policy (ORHP) was established within the Health Resources and Services Administration of the DHHS. Moscovice believes that policy makers are recommitted to ensuring a viable rural health care system.[49] Its main responsibility is to work with other agencies to seek solutions to health care problems in rural communities. In particular, this office:

- Advises the Secretary of State on the effects that the Medicare and Medicaid programs have on access to health care by rural populations
- Coordinates rural health research within the DHHS and administers a grant program that supports the activities of the Rural Health Research Centers
- Provides staff support to the National Advisory Committee on Rural Health. This committee focuses on the issues and unique problems related to providing and financing health care services in rural areas
- Articulates the views of rural constituencies with the federal establishment
- Supports a national clearinghouse for collection and dissemination of rural health information[30]

The Omnibus Reconciliation Act (OBRA) of 1989 called for the DHHS to establish an Essential Access Community Hospital (EACH) Program providing grants in up to seven states for the purpose of developing rural health care plans.[13]

The plans designate EACHs and Rural Primary Care Hospitals (RPCHs). The RPCH facilities provide 24-hour emergency care, with no more than six inpatient beds to provide temporary care for periods up to 72 hours for clients requiring stabilization or transfer. These facilities can be staffed by physicians, nurse practitioners, or physician assistants. An EACH is a facility with 75 or more beds that will accept transfers and provide emergency and medical backup services to RPCHs. As more providers are dealing with managed care, the limited services offered by rural hospitals are a basic factor in the development of health care networks to serve rural citizens.[42] These innovative models of health care will continue to be assessed as a possible means of providing accessible and affordable quality care to rural populations.

Up to this point, primary emphasis has been placed on government attempts to improve health care services in rural areas. Less well known are the efforts by school nurses and school-based clinics to provide health promotion, disease prevention, and health maintenance services to children in rural areas. School health services started in the 1900s, when it was necessary to identify and exclude students with contagious diseases from the classroom. The role of the school nurse has expanded to deal with the needs of single families, working mothers, and exceptional children in the school system.

Because of these societal trends, several demonstration projects have helped to change the way health care is delivered in schools. In 1978 the Robert Wood Johnson Foundation, a private foundation, funded a school-based clinic demonstration project in four states using 18 school districts. The results showed that nurse practitioners can successfully diagnose and treat health problems in these settings.[9] Since then the Robert Wood Johnson Foundation has funded other school health demonstration projects for adolescents and high-risk youth. Presently teen pregnancy, school truancy, substance abuse, and mental illness are just a few of the problems that are encountered in the over 150 school-based clinics located in both rural and urban areas.[23] With one fifth of our nation's children living in poverty,[27] these clinics provide primary care services to a number of them. School-based clinics may be one of the best-kept secrets when it comes to providing primary health care to rural children.

▪ ISSUES

Characteristics of Rural Populations

About 27% of the U.S. population lives in rural areas.[23] Persons living in sparsely populated regions tend to develop independence and to rely on family and neighbors in time of need rather than on social service agencies, which may not be accessible. Rural residents learn to differentiate between health problems that will interfere with functioning if untreated and those that can be tolerated for a while.[27] Rural persons' views of health and illness are affected by their lower average incomes, less access to Medicaid coverage, and significant numbers of people who are medically uninsured or underinsured as compared with urban residents.[48] This helps to explain the tendency for rural people to use health services less frequently than urban inhabitants.

Although rural occupations of farming, mining, lumbering, and fishing are still important, a growing population of persons work in urban areas and live in the country. There are seven times as many nonfarming rural residents as those involved in agriculture.[27] In addition to diversity of occupations, the rural population differs in ethnicity. Lifestyles are influenced by both culture and environment. For example, there are the rural poor in the South, Hispanics in the Southwest, farmers in the Midwest, and small groups of Amish in Pennsylvania, Indiana, and Kentucky.

Rural populations share some characteristics. There tends to be more emphasis on traditional gender roles among rural people, compared with urban populations.[7] Rural residents are more likely to be white and married than persons living in urban areas. Although one study indicated few differences between rural and urban adults, rural elders are in significantly poorer physical and mental health.[28]

Health Issues of Rural Populations

Research suggests a variety of health problems face rural populations. A study of pregnant women receiving prenatal care in health department clinics indicated that rural women were younger, had poorer nutrition, and had more low birth weight infants than urban women. The rural group was also more like to have delivered infants by cesarean section than the urban group. This could be a result of limited access to obstetric practitioners in the isolated rural area.[1]

In a review of occupational health problems related to farming, mining, and logging in rural areas, ailments were specific to the occupation. Farm workers were affected primarily by psychologic problems, injuries, skin disease, and toxicity of agrichemicals. Farmers had a high suicide rate and job-related fatality rate. Miners and loggers performed dangerous work and experienced trauma, respiratory illnesses, cardiovascular problems, and malignancy.[34] South Dakota, where 60% of the country is considered frontier, has the highest rate of lost working years of life compared with rural and urban areas.[3] This suggests the possibility that in addition to occupation, environment is a factor in health and illness.

Over a 43-month period, 2089 farm injuries occurred in nine Kentucky counties; 17% were injured children. Farm machinery, usually a farm tractor, was associated with 22% of the injuries, followed by farm animals (19%) and falls (17%) for all age groups.[41] Children of any age can participate in farm work on their parents' farm; children age 12 and older may work on other farms with parental consent according to federal law. Risks involved with farming, rural isolation, and incomplete training in rescue strategies result in excessive injuries and deaths associated with farming.[23]

In comparison with urban populations, rural people have higher infant and maternal morbidity rates; higher rates of chronic illness such as hypertension and cardiovascular problems; occupation-specific problems, such as machinery accidents, skin cancer, and respiratory difficulties resulting from exposure to agrichemicals; and mental health problems. In addition, rural adults are less likely to participate in preventive health care.[8]

A study of the relationships among health risk factors and physical findings in well rural Appalachian women indicated that the most prevalent risk factors were cigarette smoking, hypertension, high cholesterol levels, physical inactivity, obesity, and older ages. The mean age of the women, however, was 49 years.[15] Poverty, lack of access, cost of health care, and rural persons' tendency to delay seeking health care secondary to needs of other family members are associated with the failure to seek or follow through with health care directives.

In a study of rural people in Pennsylvania to test two different methods of covering health promotion services—paying for services on a fee-for-service basis through physicians' offices or by establishing centers that would operate like an HMO—health screening and disease risk factor interventions were offered at no cost. The rural elderly preferred treatment at a physician's office rather than at a clinic located in the local hospital. Persons were more likely to use services that required little involvement on their part, such as health screening and immunization, instead of services involving behavior modification, such as smoking cessation and nutrition. The main problems identified were obesity, smoking, and high cholesterol levels in this elderly population. Study findings indicate that rural residents would use health promotion services if encouraged to do so by their physicians.[26]

In a study of factors that influence health care perceptions of rural persons in Georgia, Horner and others[25] found that before seeking care, people tend to wait because of financial concerns, having undergone health care, or seeking advice from family and friends. Many rural residents could not afford insurance, especially the elderly, and Medicare/Medicaid did not cover all health care expenses. Participants would follow health care providers' advice if they could afford to do so and if their problems improved as a result of treatment.

In a comparison of health service use patterns in a sample of elderly persons in Pennsylvania, cognitively impaired individuals were more likely to have been hospitalized and to have received home health care, social services, and mental health services than those without cognitive impairments. Social services, however, consisted of Meals on Wheels from informal service providers. This suggests that health care professionals and informal service providers should be informed about the warning signs of dementia and be given information that would enable them to refer clients and their families appropriately.[18]

Another issue in rural nursing is the increasing homeless population, especially homeless families.[33] In a study of homeless persons from five rural counties in Ohio, there were 76 homeless families with 125 children under 12 years of age. Although the women (18 to 40 years old) were relatively healthy, 41% complained of gynecologic disorders. Risk factors included illegal drug use (37%), alcohol use on a regular basis (49%), and cigarette smoking (74%). Only 41 (48%) of children under 6 years of age passed the Denver Developmental Screening Test; 52% needed additional screening to determine the presence of a developmental lag.[46] Social services and housing are inadequate in rural areas to meet the needs of this vulnerable population.

Barriers to Health Care

Problems that have historically plagued rural residents are still present: limited access to health care, cost of health care, inequities in reimbursement for providers, inadequate political influence, and insufficient numbers of health care providers. Health promotion and disease prevention programs are needed in rural areas. A study of indigent, rural Appalachian clients showed that most had seen a physician during the previous year, but 85% of 188 patients were lacking at least one applicable preventive measure. More than 605 were lacking mammography, diphtheria-tetanus immunization, and cholesterol testing. Clients' reasons for not receiving care were lack of knowledge about prevention, cost, lack of location to obtain screening, and transportation problems.[16] Clients expressed willingness to obtain preventive care if barriers were removed. Other barriers identified by elderly persons in rural areas included lack of awareness of existing services and long distances to obtain services.[35] Health care providers may be viewed as "outsiders" and, therefore, not trusted. Mental health care, in particular, can be jeopardized if provided by persons new to the area or just located there for a short time.[27]

It is an altogether different problem when nurses providing care in rural areas also reside in the community. Clients may be reticent to confide in nurses who also may be neighbors and friends.[10,11] This situation may also be a positive factor, in that rural people may feel safer discussing health matters with an "insider." The social and cultural dynamics of nurse/client relationships differ significantly between urban and rural settings.

Another barrier for home health nursing services in remote areas is the long travel times for home visits. Time involved in visits, in addition to Medicare's reimbursement ceilings for sparsely populated rural areas, make provision of home health services costly for agencies.[10]

The combination of poverty, inadequate health care resources, lack of awareness of available services, costs, and rural persons' propensity toward self-reliance make the health status of rural populations an ongoing concern. There are, however, promising signs for improvements.

■ TRENDS

Health promotion and disease prevention efforts have gained emphasis because of the national directive *Healthy People 2000*,[43] and the health insurance movement toward managed care that started in the private sector and is gaining popularity as a vehicle for Medicaid and Medicare management. As nurses become increasingly involved in health teaching with rural populations, success can be enhanced by careful planning and working with people in target communities. In planning health screening services and educational offerings, rural work schedules, weather conditions, and availability of transportation are important factors that will affect client participation.[27] Recognition of local health experts, such as a county extension agent, minister, or pharmacist, may be an avenue for establishing trust with residents. Dewar[12] found that rural women's groups were the major source of health education rather than health professionals. Veterinarians and farm suppliers trained in farm health and safety education might be effective in teaching rural men.[12] Farm hazard recognition and injury prevention should be community based and incorporated into the grade school safety program.[41] Another important consideration for nurses and other health care planners is recognition of the lower educational level of some rural populations compared with urban groups. Educational programs and reading materials should be modified to match literacy levels as well as cultural differences of clients.[1]

Health Care Delivery

A collaborative model for health care in which practitioners and clients work together to determine communities' needs, set priorities, and develop strategies to make the most of scarce resources is most acceptable to residents. In working with community residents, professionals can gain cultural sensitivity and devise holistic care for the target population.[7] In rural Arizona, empowerment was the key to health promotion efforts of community health nurses working with lay health workers, called *protomoras.* The largely Mexican-American population became involved in decision making and implementation of health teaching activities as a result of door-to-door surveys and interviews with key informants to determine community health goals.[29]

Nursing education has a responsibility to introduce students to rural locations as clinical sites. During a summer course, student nurses in South Carolina practiced in a rural community, developed their sensitivity to barriers that may affect their efforts to care for rural clients, and gained insight into clients' lifestyles. They also learned that success of health education and care depend on cooperation with key informants in the target community.[17] Nurses can establish nurse-managed centers, network with existing agencies, and provide outreach programs to underserved rural populations.[45]

Although rural nurses have not seen the numbers of clients with HIV/AIDS that are now familiar to nurses practicing in urban areas, there is a growing need for nurses in rural areas who have the expertise to care for this vulnerable population. Nurses' attitudes are relatively favorable about working with HIV-positive clients, but rural nurses expressed concerns about the opinions of significant others and a need for training in sexuality counseling.[22] In an effort to address continuing education needs of rural nurses in Georgia, a program was developed to teach nurse practitioners, public health nurses, and home health nurses to be primary care providers for persons with HIV/AIDS.[39] There is no shortage of nurses in urban areas; however, large portions of the country are designated as shortage areas, specifically, the Mountain, West North Central, and East South Central regions. About 92% of the federally designated nurse-shortage areas are in nonmetropolitan counties.[40] Educating more nurses is not as likely to solve the problem as changing the way health professionals are educated. A survey of nurses indicated that the main reasons for choosing a rural practice setting were home town, or near home; spouse's employment; and enjoyed rural life.[14]

Although many rural hospitals are at risk for closure, a greater concern is developing systems of care that are appropriate, that are responsive to the health status of the community's residents, that facilitate the capabilities of nurses and other health professionals, and that use new technologies that are transforming some aspects of health care delivery.[47] For example, two or more small rural hospitals could develop a consortium to share the cost of a clinical nurse specialist.[24] Home health agencies are also more likely to succeed by affiliating with hospitals or adult day care centers, senior housing, and community social service organizations.[11]

As managed care programs increase in prevalence, the special needs of rural populations for affordable access must be considered.[15] For the past 20 years, nursing care has been increasingly delivered in nurse-managed centers. The emphasis on nurse-managed care is an impetus for the growing numbers of nurse practitioner programs at the graduate level in response to the shift from acute care to community-based health care delivery.

In every state, with the exception of Illinois, nurse practitioners have prescriptive authority. The scope of practice and extent of prescriptive authority vary among states. The board of nursing in 26 states is sole authority in scope of practice with no requirement for physician collaboration or supervision.[32] Nurse practitioners (79.2%) practice in community-based settings. Forty-nine percent of nurse practitioners are baccalaureate prepared, and the remaining 51% hold at least a master's degree; about 16% of physician assistants have associate degrees or diplomas, 72% have baccalaureate degrees, and 13% hold a master's degree or higher.[33] Nurse practitioners are employed in Rural Health Clinics to meet the requirement for midlevel practitioners to provide at least 60% of service hours in the clinic.[42] Physician assistants work under the supervision of physicians, and nurse practitioners are relatively independent. Most nurse practitioners (61.7%), however, have a physician available much of the time, and more than 29% practice under written protocols.[33]

Rural nurses must become more active in developing health policy at all levels of government.[10] Nurses should be involved in professional organizations, such as the National Rural Health Association; American Public Health Association, Rural Health Section; and their state nurses' association. Such organizations lobby for adequate funding for health services and forming coalitions can increase nurses' power to improve health care delivery and access to care for rural populations.

Communications Technology

Advances in communications technology can provide educational support and information about health policy for nurses in rural areas. In 1990 Congress authorized the State Office of Rural Health grants program, which provides matching grants to states to establish and maintain offices of rural health.[48] These state offices serve as clearinghouses for information and create an ongoing database of rural health information. They also are likely to have home pages on the Internet available to health care providers in rural areas. Most offices of rural health are located in state health departments, but others are affiliated with universities. At the national level, the Office of Rural Health and the Rural Health Association are resources with home pages on the Internet. Linkages are possible for online computer searches, databases, and current nursing information. Another use for computer technology is contracts with third-party payers that require information systems to monitor services and charges. It will be necessary to access Medicare/HMO working files to establish eligibility and obtain prior authorization for client services.[11]

▪ SUMMARY

The history of rural health care services is marked by numerous attempts to address the needs of people with a wide range of risk factors as a result of their cultural diversity, environment, and socioeconomic conditions. Disparities between the health status of rural and urban residents indicate that rural populations are more vulnerable, have less access to health promotion initiatives, and need more health care providers and resources. A variety of government-initiated and community-based programs have been established over the years, and innovative efforts of concerned individuals and professionals continue to seek ways to improve health care delivery to vulnerable populations in rural areas.

CRITICAL THINKING *Activities*

1. **Discuss legislation enacted to improve the health of rural populations.**
2. **Explain health problems that affect rural residents.**
3. **Describe innovative ways to meet health care needs of rural populations.**

References

1. Alexy B and others: Prenatal factors and birth outcomes in the public health service: a rural/urban comparison, *Res Nurs Health* 20:61-70, 1997.
2. Berstein JD, Hege EP, Farran CC: *Rural health centers in the United States,* Rural Health Center Development Series, no. 1. Cambridge, MA, 1979, Ballinger Publishing.
3. Bigbee JL: Frontier areas: opportunities for NP's primary care services, *Nurse Pract* 17(9):47, 1992.
4. Deleted in proofs.
5. Breckinridge M: *Wide neighborhoods: the story of the Frontier Nursing Service,* Lexington, KY, 1952, The University Press of Kentucky.
6. Buehler J: Nursing in rural Native American communities, *Nurs Clin North Am* 28(1):211, 1993.
7. Bushy A: Rural women: lifestyles and health status, *Nurs Clin North Am* 28(1):187, 1993.
8. Bushy A: Women in rural environments: considerations for holistic nurses, *Holistic Nurs Pract* 8(4):67-73, 1994.
9. Children's Defense Fund: *A call for action to make our nation safe for children: a briefing book on the status of American children in 1988,* Washington, D.C., 1988, The Fund.
10. Congdon JG, Magilvy JK: The changing spirit of rural community nursing: documentation burden, *Public Health Nurs* 12(1):18-24, 1995.
11. Dansky KH: The impact of health care reform on the rural home health agencies, *J Nurs Admin* 25(3):27-33, 1995.
12. Dewar DM: Farm health and safety issues: do men and women differ in their perceptions? *Am Ass Occup Health Nurs J* 44(8):391-401, 1996.
13. Dryfoos JG: School-based health clinics: three years of experience, *Fam Plann Perspect* 20(4):193-200, 1988.
14. Dunkin JW and others: Why rural practice? *Nurs Manag* 27(12):26-28, 1996.
15. Edwards JB and others: Relationships among health risk factors and objective physical findings in well Appalachian women, *Family Comm Health,* 67-80, 1996.
16. Elnicki DM and others: Patient-perceived barriers to preventive health care among indigent, rural Appalachian patients, *Arch Int Med* 155:421-424, 1995.
17. Erkel EA and others: Intensive immersion of nursing students in rural interdisciplinary care, *J Nurs Ed* 34(8):359-365, 1995.
18. Ganguli M and others: Cognitive impairment and the use of health services in an elderly rural population: the MOVIES project, *J Am Geriatr Soc* 41(10):1065-1070, 1993.
19. Gessler W, Ricketts T, eds: *Health in rural North America—the geography of health care service and delivery,* New Brunswick, NJ, 1992, Rutgers University Press.
20. Greeley C: Health status of Native Americans, *JAMA* 265(17):2272, 1991.

21. Hassinger EW: *Rural health organization: social networks and regionalization,* Ames, IA, 1982, Iowa State University Press.
22. Highriter ME and others: HIV-related concerns and educational needs of public health nurses in a rural state, *Public Health Nurs* 12(5):324-334, 1995.
23. Hill DE: FARMEDIC: a systematic approach to train rural EMS, fire, and rescue personnel at the grassroots level, *J Agromed* 1(4):57-64, 1994.
24. Hjelm JS: The rural health care setting: is there need for a CNS? *Clin Nurse Special* 9(2):112-115, 1995.
25. Horner SD and others: Traveling for care: factors influencing health care access for rural dwellers, *Public Health Nurs* 11(3):145-149, 1994.
26. Lave JR, Ives DG: Participation in health promotion programs by the rural elderly, *Am J Prevent Med* 11(1):46-53, 1995.
27. Long KA: The concept of health: rural perspectives, *Nurs Clin North Am* 28(1):123, 1993.
28. Mainous AG, Kohrs FP: A comparison of health status between rural and urban adults, *J Comm Health* 20(5):423-431, 1995.
29. May KM and others: Community empowerment in rural health care, *Public Health Nurs* 12(1):25-30, 1995.
30. Oda D et al: Nurse practitioners and primary care in schools, *MCN* 10(2):127-131, 1985.
31. Office of Technology Assessment: *Health care in rural America,* Washington, D.C., 1990, U.S. Government Printing Office.
32. Pan S and others: A comparative analysis of primary care nurse practitioners and physician assistants, *Nurse Pract* 32(4):14, 16-17, 1997.
33. Pearson LJ: Annual update of how each state stands on legislative issues affecting advanced nursing practice, *Nurse Pract* 22(1):18-86, 1997.
34. Pratt D: Occupational health and the rural worker: agriculture, mining and logging, *J Rural Health* 6:399-417, 1990.
35. Roemer MI: *Rural health care,* St. Louis, 1976, Mosby.
36. Rosenblatt RA, Moscovice IS: *Rural health care,* New York, 1982, Wiley.
37. Severance D: The Frontier Nursing Service, *Frontier Nursing Service Q Bull* 72(3):1, 1997.
38. Shride SE: Strategies for the nurse executive to keep the rural hospitals open, *Nurs Admin Q* 21(2):40, 1997.
39. Sowell RL, Opava WD: The Georgia rural-based nurse model: primary care for persons with HIV/AIDS, *Public Health Nurs* 12(4):228-234, 1995.
40. Stratton TD and others: Redefining the nursing shortage: a rural perspective, *Nurs Outlook* 43(2):71-77, 1995.
41. Stuttmann T: Farm injury surveillance in Kentucky—what have we learned? *Kentucky Epidemiolog Notes Reports* 31(10):1-4, 1996.
42. U.S. Bureau of the Census: *Statistical abstract of the United States: 1984,* ed 10, Washington, D.C., 1985, U.S. Government Printing Office.
43. U.S. Department of Health and Human Services: *Healthy people 2000: national health promotion and disease prevention objectives, full report, and commentary,* Washington, D.C., 1991, U.S. Government Printing Office.

44. U.S. Department of Health and Human Services: *On the move: innovation in rural health care delivery,* 1991, National Rural Health Association.

45. Vrabec NJ: Implications of U.S. health care reform for the rural elderly, *Nurs Outlook* 43(6): 260-265, 1995.

46. Wagner JD and others: What is known about the health of rural homeless families? *Public Health Nurs* 12(6):400-408, 1995.

47. Weinert C: Rural nursing: legacy, science, trajectory, *Communicating Nursing Research* 27:63-77, 1994.

48. Weinert C, Burman ME: Rural health and health-seeking behaviors, *Ann Rev Nurs Research* 12:65-92, 1994.

49. Wysocki S: Rural health care: a challenge and opportunity for nurse practitioners, *Nurse Pract Forum* 1(2):68, 1990.

CHAPTER 14

International Nursing

Edwina A. McConnell

OBJECTIVES After completing this chapter the reader should be able to:

- **Explain the effect of at least four factors on international nursing**
- **Discuss the impact of international trends in nursing education on primary health care**
- **Compare the purpose of at least three international nursing organizations**
- **Contrast the mission, purpose, and function of the World Health Organization with those of the International Council of Nurses**
- **Describe ways in which international nursing research can affect nursing and health care worldwide**
- **Design a plan for becoming involved in international nursing**

■ FACTORS AFFECTING NURSING INTERNATIONALLY

As the profile of world health continues to change, the role of nursing personnel continues to evolve to meet the changing health needs.[43] Health care and nursing do not exist in a vacuum. They are shaped by the environment in which they take place, and this environment is affected by several factors, including culture. Culture provides the context of socially transmitted assumptions that are shared among a country's people and the understanding those people have about the nature of the physical and social world, the goals of life, and the appropriate means of achieving those goals.[33] Other factors influencing the context of health care and nursing are a country's size, demography and epidemiology, social structure, political factors, economic resources, level of scientific knowledge and technology, and history.[3,4,43] Furthermore, nursing is directly affected by education, leadership and management, working conditions, legislation and regulation, and research.[43]

Country Size, Demography, and Epidemiology

A country's size and demography (that is, the size, structure, and distribution of its population) affect nursing. Health care and nursing needs of large, sparsely populated countries differ from those of small, densely populated countries, and differ as well from those of large countries with great diversity in terms of population density, climate, and topography. Due to access, a densely populated small country may find it easier to organize health services than a large, sparsely populated country. Fewer nurses may be available in areas that are isolated, are remote, have difficult terrain, are climatically unpleasant, and have poor cultural and educational resources.[4,43]

The structure of a country's population in terms of age affects health care needs and nursing practice as well as nursing education. Populations with high birth rates and moderate-to-low death rates will be relatively young. A median age in the late teens in developing nations contrasts sharply with a median age in the thirties in industrialized countries. Furthermore, disease distribution is strongly related to the age distribution of certain populations.[3]

Developing countries with 50% of the population under the age of 21 years require nursing care directed toward maternal-child health more than toward the care of persons with chronic diseases. In Europe, North America, and Australia an ever-increasing proportion of the population is elderly. In fact, in many industrialized countries the 80-plus age group, or the "oldest old,"[12] is the largest-growing segment of the population. This increase, in large measure a result of improved nutrition, sanitation, and immunization programs, has come at a time in some countries when traditional family support systems are in transition. More women are working outside the home, and immigration to the cities is massive.

Disease patterns in industrialized countries tend to be associated with lifestyle. Increased incidences of cancer are partly a consequence of smoking but also result from pollution, which increases with industrialization. Certain cancers develop in older people, and consequently as people age, their risk of these cancers increases. Sedentary lifestyles, increased alcohol consumption, and obesity—all of which are common in wealthy industrial nations—contribute to the development of chronic disease and disability.[4,43]

In nearly every country populations tend to clump. "The proportion of people living in urban areas is increasing at a rate faster than the underlying population growth."[3] Cities worldwide are becoming larger rather than more intensely populated; the average population density in major cities is declining.

Urbanization is the result of many factors, including near-to-impossible survival in some rural areas, war, revolution, political agitation, ethnic or religious persecution, boredom, social ferment, weakening of traditions, and natural disaster.[3] Additionally, the attractions of city life, such as a stable wage structure, public services, shopping, schools, and educational opportunities, are appealing.

Migration to cities can result in numerous health problems both for individuals and for communities. Such problems include psychologic and emotional stress, the breakdown of extended family life, and a physical environment that may be unhealthy. For example, housing may be inadequate, sanitation poor, and water unsafe, all of which contribute to disease.

Demographic changes are not isolated. Each change in a population's size, structure, or distribution affects other facets and, ultimately, the relationships of individuals, families, and communities. The resulting social and economic challenges present nurses internationally with numerous opportunities to design models of care that would be both economic and humane.[19]

Just as a country's size and demography affect the need for health services and nursing care, so also do environmental factors, as previously suggested. For example, the increase in nuclear waste and other hazardous materials influences the health of the world's population, as do increases in air and water pollution. Furthermore, industrial injuries and poisonings from pesticides are not uncommon.

Problems related to environmental factors occur to a greater or lesser degree in both developing and industrialized countries. Their incidence depends, in part, on the lack of an organized approach to environmental issues and implementation of appropriate programs.

Social Structure

Key factors in a country's social structure are religion, language, the political system, and economic resources. These factors, their interrelationship, and their effect on nursing and health care emphasize that health cannot be discussed in isolation. Health is embedded in the socio-cultural-economic factors of a country and is only minimally affected by activities in the health sector.[3,43]

Religions are a major source of values. Different religions extol varying views about the value of an individual life, the role of women, the correct approach to life and death, the extent of social compassion appropriate under conditions of discomfort and suffering, the ideology of stoicism or verbalization of complaint, and whether one accepts one's fate or fights to the last breath.[4] Religious beliefs influence people's thoughts about health and illness, as well as the role of nurses.

A country's social structure also determines societal norms, including the role of men and women in society. This, of course, extends to the role of nurses, as well as the way in which nursing and nurses are perceived. The low status of nursing, a predominantly female profession, reflects the low status of women in general.[19,43]

Political Factors

Health is a political issue integral to a country's development. Furthermore, health must be part of socioeconomic plans developed at the national level.[43]

The interplay of health and politics is evident in matters such as national health insurance, drug control, long-term care for the elderly and chronically ill, and public funding for AIDS research. Nurses are directly influenced by these matters. Recruitment, retention, education, and practice of nurses are affected by the demand for services, reimbursement systems, prevalent health care problems, and research findings.[43]

Government structure and political systems influence the distribution of wealth and power, as well as the definition of health care policy and resource allocation. Political systems vary—from democracy to pseudodemocracy to control by a powerful leader, either civilian or military. The government in most countries establishes health policies and is the principal employing agency. The existence of a Chief Nursing Officer (CNO), particularly in a line position, implies recognition of nursing.

Ultimately, political forces influence the demand for health care. War and political unrest, either overt or covert, can increase refugee populations, which in turn increase the need for nursing services. Furthermore, nurses working in countries where imprisonment for political and religious reasons is common are confronted with the dilemma of being required to participate in the torture of prisoners.

Political factors influence legislated regulations about who may practice nursing, as well as the working conditions and education of nurses. For example, in countries where administration of nursing services and nursing education is centralized, a few officials at the national level determine the content of nursing education programs, the number of nurses to be educated and employed, their places of employment, and their salaries. Conversely, in the United States each nursing school has its own unique curriculum, and the majority of nurses practice in nongovernment institutions.[32,43]

The status of a country's professional nursing organization, especially its degree of independence from both the government and the medical establishment, is an indication of nursing autonomy. The functions of this professional organization reflect the levels of nursing education and the licensing or registration system.

Economic Resources

A country's economic resources are part of its social structure, and a country's economic status can be determined by looking at its level of development. Economic development is closely aligned with the state of both individual and public health. Consequently, health programs are a part of a country's economic strategy, both at the microeconomic and macroeconomic levels.[3,43]

At the microeconomic level each human life has a certain monetary value. Briefly, for example, costs associated with pregnancy and childbirth include loss of productivity and earnings, special foods, and the cost of prenatal care and delivery. In developed countries these costs may be very high, whereas in developing countries little cash may be invested in pregnancy. However, other costs, including decreased attention to other children and loss of productive time, may be substantial. Death of a child represents the loss of these investments, as well as time that could have been otherwise used. In countries with very low economic bases, and where at least half of all deaths occur by 5 years of age, infant and child mortality are a great financial burden and an unproductive investment. A person's economic value can also be addressed in terms of present and future earning power.[3]

At the individual level, health is an investment, and illness has two aspects of cost. The first is loss of working time and decreased effectiveness or productivity. The second is money spent to alleviate the condition; for example, money spent on medical and nursing care, medications, special foods, or devices. If the individual is not covered by a social welfare scheme, these costs must be borne privately.

At the macroeconomic level is the recognition that all resources—whether human, financial, material, or informational—are finite. Competition is severe. Public and private expenditures for health purposes compete not only with other sectors within health and welfare but also with all other sectors, including defense.[3]

The resources available and allocated for health care services, including nursing, depend on a country's economic status. Poorer countries, although expending a larger percentage of their gross national product (GNP), may still be spending relatively small amounts for health. Wealthier countries may spend more on health while expending a lesser portion of their GNPs. (GNP is defined as the income generated within a country and assets owned overseas.) In recent years, with an increasing percentage of many governments' budgets being used for defense and debt reduction, the financial resources for health have diminished worldwide.[5,39]

The economic forces influencing nursing extend beyond the availability of resources to their distribution. The widening gap between the rich and the poor is a global concern.[5,39] Those who can afford health care receive it. Those who cannot are left without health services. Additionally, they may not have the resources to obtain nutritious food, safe water, and education. Clearly economic forces influence the health needs of people and how nurses meet these needs.[13]

Economics is concerned not only with income and wealth, but also with using resources to achieve significant ends such as the prevention of disease and the promotion of health.[13] Thus the economic success of any country, developed or developing, can be judged not only by the end product of its resource utilization but also by the health of its citizens.[35]

The ability of poorer countries to achieve improvement in health care and life expectancy that may rival those of more affluent nations has tremendous policy implications. Education and health care are both labor intensive, but these services cost less in a cheap-labor economy than they do in wealthier countries.

The role of public policy in extending life expectancy has worldwide implications. Public intervention in health, education, and nutrition has historically been integral in increased longevity in the West and in Japan. The decades of World War I and World War II in England and Wales were

> characterized by the most significant increase in life expectancy found in any decade in this country. War efforts and rationing led to a more equitable distribution of food, and the government paid more attention to health care—even the National Health Service was set up in the 1940s. In fact, these two decades had the slowest growth of gross domestic product per capita; indeed, between 1911 and 1921, growth of GDP was negative. Public effort rather than personal income was the key to increasing life expectancy during those decades.[35]

Although related to economic development, improved health is the result of a multiplicity of factors, including education. The one most important indicator of improved health status has been education, particularly education of women.

Scientific Knowledge and Technology

A country's level of scientific knowledge and technology affects all aspects of nursing, including where nurses practice, how they practice, and indeed how they and their publics define professional nursing practice. Furthermore, scientific knowledge and technology affect not only the basic and advanced education of nurses but also educational strategies. For example, advances in communication technology make it possible to learn via computer-assisted instruction and to participate in distance education programs.

Nurses must be competent, regardless of their work setting and the level of available health care technology. Technology, particularly in Western cultures, has an aura of power that may exceed the technology's proven capabilities.[6] The introduction of sophisticated health care technology does not guarantee quality client care, nor can all technology be simply transferred to all countries.[14,30] Essential to quality health and nursing care in any country is nurse use of appropriate technology, defined by the World Health Organization (WHO) as methods, procedures, techniques, and equipment that are scientifically valid, adapted to local needs, and acceptable to those for whom they are used, maintained, and utilized with resources the community or the country can afford.[46] Inappropriate use of health care technologies is associated with a high cost of health care and, equally important, with high personal, ethical, and psychologic costs to clients, families, nurses, and society.[6,28,34]

Acquisition and use of appropriate technologies can be facilitated by applying the process of technology assessment. Technology assessment can be used to evaluate emerging as well as existing technologies and to identify problems needing solutions, thus improving the quality of care while decreasing or containing costs.

Technology assessment is defined by the Swedish Council of Technology Assessment in Health Care as

> the complete, scientifically based assessment of a technology's benefits, safety, and social, ethical, and economic consequences. Assessments should even include organizational aspects and educational issues. Assessment cannot rely on any one methodology, but rather on a process which synthesizes several scientific works concerning the overall value of a given technology.[9]

A comprehensive technology assessment is a five-step process. Although each step can be considered individually, all aspects of a technology assessment are interrelated, and short- and long-term consequences can both be considered.[41]

The first step in a comprehensive assessment considers need. *Need* refers not only to the health problem to be treated but also to its dimensions, including urgency, severity, or scope. Furthermore, a needs analysis also considers existing alternative technologies and potential effects of substitution.[15]

The second step addresses safety. This is "a judgment of the acceptability of risk in a specified situation."[2] A technology's safety is measured in terms of its risk-to-benefit ratio, which is a relative term.

Evaluating those aspects pertaining to conditions of use, effectiveness, and efficacy constitute the third step. Concerned with the benefits of using a technology in a defined population, effectiveness and efficacy also consider the environmental and operational factors inherent in a technology's application. Specifically, are infrastructure facilities such as water, storage, and power supplies adequate? How will staff be educated to use the technology and at what cost? Are maintenance staff, facilities, and equipment readily accessible and available to keep the technology working?[14,40]

Economic appraisal, the fourth step in a comprehensive technology assessment, compares estimated costs of providing a technology with projected returns in anticipated benefits. Cost analysis also considers costs from other vantage points, such as opportunity cost. Opportunity cost explores the value of alternatives or activities that could be undertaken with the same resources.[25] Specifically, if foreign exchange is spent on a specific technology, what *cannot* be purchased?

The fifth step addresses social impact. Nursing and health care are culturally defined and must be culturally congruent to be acceptable. Therefore social issues, such as the legal, ethical, cultural, environmental, and political impact of a technology, are explored.

The political impact of a technology can have local, regional, national, and international consequences. Technology is frequently transferred from one country to another. However, moving a specific technology from one situation to another requires changes in the technology, the context to which it is moved, or both.[7] From a global perspective, the transfer of technology from one country to another can lead to technologic dependence, which is "the difficulty that governments face in trying to use science and technology to attain social, economic, and political goals."[11]

The main purpose of health care technology is to improve human health.[2] The involvement of nurses in technology assessment empowers them and can positively affect the nature and quality of health care, from the individual level through and including national health policy.[30]

History

A country's history determines its system of government, the values of its communities, and the development of its institutions. Typically, the current pattern "of provision (of health care) reflects the priorities and solutions of the past rather than reflecting present needs, or even present philosophies."[4]

Societal needs change as populations change, whether these changes result from war, aging, or immigration. The number of cultural groups and the extent of their acculturation affect the kind of health and welfare services needed, as well as the role of the nurse.

■ PRIMARY HEALTH CARE

In 1977 the Thirtieth World Health Assembly passed a resolution (WHO 30.43) stating that "the main social target of governments and WHO in the coming decades should be the attainment by all the citizens of the world by the year 2000 of a level of health that will permit them to lead a socially and economically productive life."[3] This goal is commonly known as *Health for All by the Year 2000,* or *HFA2000.*

A series of preliminary conferences laid the groundwork for HFA2000 and culminated in the International Conference on Primary Health Care (PHC), held September 6 to 12, 1978, in Alma-Ata, capital of Kazakhstan, then a Soviet republic in central Asia. A landmark in international health, this conference was the largest single-theme conference ever held. Representatives of 143 countries and 57 organizations, including United Nations agencies and nongovernment organizations, attended this meeting, which was cosponsored by WHO and the United Nations Children's Fund (UNICEF). On September 12, 1978 the attendees adopted the Declaration of Alma-Ata, which identified primary health care as the key to attaining HFA2000. This conference was a "concerted international effort to

Box 14-1 The Essential Components of Primary Health Care

1. Health education
2. Environmental sanitation, especially of food and water
3. The employment of community or village health workers
4. Maternal and child health programs, including immunization and family planning
5. Prevention of local endemic diseases
6. Appropriate treatment of common diseases and injuries
7. Provision of essential drugs
8. Promotion of nutrition
9. Traditional medicine

From World Health Organization: *Alma-Ata 1978: Primary Health Care* (Health for All Series no. 1), Geneva, Switzerland, 1978, WHO.

expand and redirect health programs in countries throughout the world. Its goal was to make substantial, rapid, and inexpensive improvements in the delivery of preventive and curative services at the community level, primarily in rural areas."[3]

Primary health care is defined in conference documents as:

> Essential health care based on practical, scientifically sound and socially acceptable methods and technology made universally accessible to individuals and families in the community through their full participation and at a cost that the community and country can afford to maintain at every stage of their development in the spirit of self-reliance and self-determination. It forms an integral part of both the country's health system, of which it is the central function and main focus, and of the overall social and economic development of the community. It is the first level of contact of individuals, the family and the community with the national health system bringing health care as close as possible to where people live and work, and constitutes the first element of a continuing health care process. (Alma-Ata Conference Documents).[45]

The essential components of primary health care are shown in Box 14-1. Although implementation differs among countries, depending on local conditions and customs, the basic theory represents an integration of PHC with socioeconomic development so that each supports the other in a context of equity and social justice.[3]

Primary health care is considered the ideal standard for health care,[42] and nursing and midwifery, as the largest sector of the workforce, have a pivotal role to play in it.[18] In 1978 Dr. Halfdan Mahler, then Director-General of WHO, acknowledged the involvement of nurses in PHC and presented them with the following challenge:

> If the needs of communities are to be met, the ranks of health workers, including nursing and medical personnel, will need to consist predominantly of people who genuinely care about the health and welfare of impoverished communities, who want to help such communities, who are willing to learn what has to be done, and who cannot only do it, but do it without dependence on sophisticated and costly technology. [The world's population] needs nurses who can diagnose commu-

> nity health problems and institute measures to protect, advance, and monitor the health of populations as a whole, nurses who can care for the sick or the disabled, nurses who can teach people to care for themselves.[26]

In the years since 1978 every country member state of WHO has accomplished something toward attaining HFA2000. However, the level of achievement tends to be very unbalanced, and the WHO periodic updates on HFA2000 have become increasingly cautionary in tone.[24] In a May 1991 address to the executive board and World Health Assembly, Dr. Hiroshi Nakajima, Director-General of WHO, said:

> [T]he monitoring of progress toward the goal of health for all has shown that at best it has been slow . . . it is becoming clear that we need to improve our understanding of the close relationship between health, the economy and development.[24]

As the year 2000 approaches, the goal of health for all is clearly unattainable in many countries. Thus WHO is renewing its health for all strategy. WHO has asked member states and has called on a variety of personnel, including national decision makers, technical experts, and representatives, to assess the current health situation and trends and identify the major health issues for their countries. Nurses, too, are being asked to reflect on their role in PHC and to identify ways to collaborate in the renewal effort.[37]

■ INTERNATIONAL NURSING ORGANIZATIONS

International nursing organizations facilitate the exchange of knowledge and information while affording nurses opportunities for networking and collaboration. These organizations provide mechanisms for nurses to develop standards of care and codes of ethics, to cooperate in improving the socioeconomic and working conditions for nurses worldwide, to stimulate research and theory development, and to develop creative solutions to common problems. Such organizations include the International Council of Nurses, WHO, Pan American Health Organization, Sigma Theta Tau International, and Nurses' Christian Fellowship International.

International Council of Nurses

The International Council of Nurses (ICN) is the oldest international organization for professionals in the health care field. An idea among nursing leaders at the Columbia Exposition in 1893, ICN was established in 1899 at a meeting of the International Council of Women in London. The constitution was adopted the next year, with English, American, Canadian, New Zealand, Australian, and Danish nurses as founding members.[16] One of the major attractions at the 1999 centennial celebration conference in London will be the special ICN Centennial History Project.[8,21]

For nearly a century ICN has served as the authoritative voice of the nursing profession worldwide.[23] Its structure is a nongovernment federation of national nurses associations from 118 countries,* representing nurses who are members of

---

*As of October 1997.

constituent organizations. ICN was one of the first organizations to adopt a policy of nondiscrimination based on nationality, race, creed, color, politics, gender, or social status.

Run by nurses for nurses, ICN provides a medium through which the interests, needs, and concerns of member nurses associations can be addressed, to the advantage of both the public and nurses. The stated purposes of ICN are to:

> (1) promote the development of strong national nurses associations, (2) assist national nurses associations to improve standards of nursing and competence of nurses, (3) assist national nurses associations to improve the status of nurses within each country, and (4) serve as the authoritative international voice for nurses and nursing.[16]

Activities of ICN reflect its purposes as well as the diverse interests and needs of its international membership. These interests include education, nursing practice and service, the economics and welfare of nurses, research, legislation, and cooperation with other health professions. At any one time ICN is involved in 30 to 40 projects such as regulating nursing practice, revising and updating the ethical code, offering legislative seminars for member associations, and issuing policy statements about health and social issues such as equal pay for equal work and the role of nurses in caring for prisoners and detainees. Four of ICN's major contributions to nursing are (1) an internationally accepted definition of nursing, (2) a code of ethics, (3) the document on conditions of work and life of nursing personnel, which was adopted by the International Labor Organization, and (4) work on an international classification for nursing practice (ICNP).[10,20,36]

Information is disseminated through seminars, meetings, and publications. Quadrennial congresses are conducted in various countries and provide unique and stimulating experiences. All nurses worldwide are invited to attend, although only those belonging to national nurses associations may present papers. *The International Nursing Review,* published bimonthly, is the official journal of ICN. Other publications, such as *Guidelines for National Nurses' Associations and Others—Preparation of Nurse Managers and Nurses in General Health Management, Guidelines for Public Policy Development Related to Health, Guidelines for Nursing Research Development,* and *Guidelines for Nurses Applying for Senior Positions,* provide direction for advancing the nursing profession. The *Caring for the Carers* series was developed to help nurses deal with a variety of work situations.

ICN supports education through the Florence Nightingale International Foundation, an endowed trust established to advance nursing education. ICN also administers the ICN/3M Nursing Fellowship program, which awards three fellowships annually for advanced study.

Originally located in London, ICN relocated in 1966 to Geneva, Switzerland, headquarters of many international health care organizations. This move not only increased ICN's power base but also facilitated communication and networking with other humanitarian organizations. ICN maintains an official relationship with such international organizations as WHO, United Nations Education, Scientific, and Cultural Organization (UNESCO), International Labour Organization (ILO), UNICEF, Economic and Social Council (ECOSOC), and the International Committee of the Red Cross (ICRC).

TABLE 14-1

Regional Headquarters of WHO

Region	Headquarters City
Europe	Copenhagen, Denmark
Eastern Mediterranean	Alexandria, Egypt
Africa	Brazzaville, Congo
Southeast Asia	New Delhi, India
Western Pacific	Manila, Philippines
The Americas	Washington, D.C.

World Health Organization

WHO has its origins in the United Nations charter, which was signed and came into being in 1945. The U.N. Charter provided for the creation of a specialized health agency with wide powers. Constituted in 1946, the new General Assembly adopted a resolution "to call an international conference to consider the scope of, and the appropriate machinery for, international action in the field of public health and proposals for the establishment of a single international health organization of the United Nations."[3] The Conference met in New York and, together with other accomplishments, produced the Constitution of the World Health Organization. Signed in 1946, the constitution was sent to member states for ratification. Final ratification occurred on April 7, 1948, a date known as World Health Day.[3]

The work of WHO is carried out in Geneva, Switzerland, at the six regional headquarters, at offices in numerous countries, and in many projects in the field. Both WHO, with its 193 (as of June 1997) members, and ICN are divided into the same six regions (Table 14-1), but only WHO has offices in each region.

Policy is set at the parliament-like World Health Assemblies, which are held in Geneva in May of each year. Delegates of all member governments and observers from affiliated organizations and other agencies attend.

The mission of WHO, which is contained in Article 1 of its Constitution, is "the attainment by all people of the highest possible level of health."[3] The Preamble to the Constitution is shown in Box 14-2, and the specific functions of WHO as listed in Article 2 are identified in Box 14-3.

The two major categories of WHO's work are central technical services and services to governments. The central services include epidemiologic intelligence; work toward international agreements relative to health aspects of travel and commerce; international standardization of vaccines and pharmaceuticals; and the dissemination of knowledge through meetings and the publication of technical and other literature about world health problems. Headquarters in Geneva also coordinates the work of WHO Collaborating Centres, as well as several hundred laboratories and institutes throughout the world that offer expert consultation and services in many areas. WHO's fellowship program, which has enabled thousands of persons to participate in brief study tours abroad in nursing, public health, maternal and child health, and other health services, is administered through regional offices.[3]

Box 14-2 Preamble to the Constitution of the World Health Organization

The States Parties to this Constitution declare, in conformity with the Charter of the United Nations, that the following principles are basic to the happiness, harmonious relations and security of all peoples:

Health is a state of complete physical, mental and social well-being and not merely the absence of disease or infirmity.

The enjoyment of the highest attainable standard of health is one of the fundamental rights of every human being without distinction of race, religion, political belief, economic or social condition.

The health of all peoples is fundamental to the attainment of peace and security and is dependent upon the fullest co-operation of individuals and States. The achievement of any State in the promotion and protection of health is of value to all.

Unequal development in different countries in the promotion of health and control of disease, especially communicable disease, is a common danger.

Healthy development of the child is of basic importance; the ability to live harmoniously in a changing total environment is essential to such development.

The extension to all peoples of the benefits of medical, psychological and related knowledge is essential to the fullest attainment of health.

Informed opinion and active co-operation on the part of the public are of the utmost importance in the improvement of the health of the people.

Governments have a responsibility for the health of their peoples which can be fulfilled only by the provision of adequate health and social measures.

Accepting these principles, and for the purpose of co-operation among themselves and with others to promote and protect the health of all people, the Contracting Parties agree to the present Constitution and hereby establish the World Health Organization as a specialized agency within the terms of Article 57 of the Charter of the United Nations.

Services to governments are provided at the request of member countries, typically in the form of discrete projects established through the appropriate regional office. However, some larger cooperative programs are established on an interregional basis; for example, a working group about the role of nursing and midwifery in maternal and child health care in Latin America. The heart of WHO services is in the thousands of individual country projects. Although many of these are for training, especially in health manpower development and strengthening of health services, a great many others focus on primary care or specific disease control programs.

WHO has two nurses in the chief nurse's office in Geneva; the Chief Scientist for Nursing and a nurse scientist. Other nurses work in parallel programs or come to Geneva from around the world to serve as consultants. Additionally, every region has a nurse advisor who is responsible for all nursing activities in that region. Furthermore, there are approximately 20 collaborating centers for nursing around the world. The nurses work with many other health and health-related personnel to identify health problems and strategies for coping with them. An international approach is needed because health and disease know no boundaries. Both WHO and ICN remain committed to HFA2000.

Despite differences in size, structure, and political affiliation, remarkable and productive collaboration occurs between ICN and WHO. This relationship has

Box 14-3 Specific Functions of WHO as Listed in Article 2[3]

(1) To act as the directing and co-ordinating authority on international health work;
(b) to establish and maintain effective collaboration with the United Nations, specialized agencies, governmental health administrations, professional groups and such other organizations as may be deemed appropriate;
(c) to assist Governments, upon request, in strengthening health services;
(d) to furnish appropriate technical assistance and, in emergencies, necessary aid upon the request or acceptance of Governments;
(e) to provide or assist in providing, upon the request of the United Nations, health services and facilities to special groups, such as the peoples of trust territories;
(f) to establish and maintain such administrative and technical services as may be required, including epidemiological and statistical services;
(g) to stimulate and advance work to eradicate epidemic, endemic and other diseases;
(h) to promote, in co-operation with other specialized agencies where necessary, the prevention of accidental injuries;
(i) to promote, in co-operation with other specialized agencies where necessary, the improvement of nutrition, housing, sanitation, recreation, economic or working conditions and other aspects of environmental hygiene;
(j) to promote co-operation among scientific and professional groups which contribute to the advancement of health;
(k) to propose conventions, agreements and regulations, and make recommendations with respect to international health matters and to perform such duties as may be assigned thereby to the Organization and are consistent with its objective;
(l) to promote maternal and child health and welfare and to foster the ability to live harmoniously in a changing total environment;
(m) to foster activities in the field of mental health, especially those affecting the harmony of human relations;
(n) to promote and conduct research in the field of health;
(o) to promote improved standards of teaching and training in the health, medical and related professions;
(p) to study and report on, in co-operation with other specialized agencies where necessary, administrative and social techniques affecting public health and medical care from preventive and curative points of view, including hospital services and social security;
(q) to provide information, counsel and assistance in the field of health;
(r) to assist in developing an informed public opinion among all peoples on matters of health;
(s) to establish and revise as necessary international nomenclatures of diseases, of causes of death and of public health practices;
(t) to standardize diagnostic procedures as necessary;
(u) to develop, establish and promote international standards with respect to food, biological, pharmaceutical and similar products;
(v) generally to take all necessary action to attain the objective of the Organization.

resulted in advancement of the nursing profession and the health of the world's population.

Pan American Health Organization

The Pan American Health Organization (PAHO) is an autonomous organization closely affiliated with WHO. Composed of 35 member governments in the Americas and three European governments with Western Hemisphere interests,

PAHO serves member countries in meeting the health needs of their populations. Nurses from the United States benefit from collaborating with nurses in other countries in North, Central, and South America through PAHO. One of the PAHO programs of interest to many nurses is the Women in Health and Development Program, which focuses on women's special health needs and enhances women's role in providing health services.

Sigma Theta Tau International

Sigma Theta Tau, from its founding in 1922 until 1985, was confined to recognizing superior scholarship and leadership of nurses in the United States. In 1985 this honor society for nursing expanded its constitution to become the International Honor Society of Nursing. As evidence of the organization's commitment to excellence in nursing globally, eight international chapters have been chartered since 1989. The chapters are in Taiwan, Korea, Canada (5), and Australia. Members are active in 73 countries and territories worldwide.

The commitment of Sigma Theta Tau to excellence in nursing worldwide extends beyond membership. Such commitment is evidenced in the establishment of the International Nursing Library, the promotion of research internationally, and the publication of articles in *IMAGE: Journal of Nursing Scholarship* by nurses from countries other than the United States.

Nurses' Christian Fellowship International

Nurses are drawn together around the globe by religious organizations such as Nurses' Christian Fellowship International (NCFI). NCFI is an interdenominational organization for nurses who hold essential Christian beliefs. Its purposes include the development and maintenance of Christian beliefs among nurses worldwide and the promotion of Christian principles in professional life. The journal of NCFI, *Christian Nurse International,* includes articles pertaining to issues of concern to nurses, such as ethics, cross-cultural communication and practice, standards of practice, management problems, and the spiritual care of clients and their families.

■ INTERNATIONAL TRENDS IN NURSING EDUCATION

Three interrelated patterns of nursing education have affected the development of nursing education systems around the world: the French, the British, and the American. Colonization of countries by France or Britain led to the perpetuation of the colonizing country's model of nursing education.[32,43]

The French system is the most medically oriented and consists of a hospital-based apprenticeship, typically 28 months. Similarly, the British system involves a 3-year hospital-based apprenticeship. Graduates qualify for nursing in general, sick children, or psychiatric areas. However, the British system, unlike the French, includes public health nursing and midwifery. After completing a basic education program, a nurse can continue in specialty certificate programs. The American model began as the British model, but quickly moved from hospitals to institutions of higher education and is based in academia.

The nursing education models are losing their distinctiveness with the worldwide trend toward moving nursing education into institutions of higher learning.

This shift is slow but consistent. If the university pattern of nursing education is viewed as the American pattern, then many countries have begun to introduce the American pattern into their systems of basic and graduate nursing education.[32]

Baccalaureate programs of nursing are not unique to developed countries. However, while colleges and universities are the sites of nursing education in the United States, this is not yet so in most other countries. Furthermore, many countries' baccalaureate programs in nursing were instituted to prepare students for teaching positions in schools of nursing. These programs have been seen, therefore, as teacher education programs, unlike U.S. nursing programs, which prepare beginning-level practitioners.[20,32]

Advanced nursing education programs in many countries other than the United States include "graduate programs" in nursing that confer academic degrees and other programs of study for graduate nurses. However, relatively few graduate programs in countries other than the United States lead to master's and doctoral degrees in nursing. Some countries offering the baccalaureate in nursing have also implemented programs leading to higher degrees in nursing. However, the vast majority of these advanced nursing studies are generally referred to as *postbasic* programs. They are offered in areas such as nursing education, nursing administration, or a clinical nursing area such as critical care. These programs, which are of 1 or 2 years' duration, confer a diploma or certificate in the area of specialization. Even though they may be offered from a university setting, they do not culminate in a degree.[32]

These programs, while excellent in some countries, exist where nursing does not have entry into the university. Developed to meet a country's health care needs, these programs are the prime resource for preparation in nursing leadership roles. These programs have had a critical place in the educational systems of many countries.[32]

In most countries nursing education has occurred primarily in hospital settings. In the past most nursing schools were established and functioned under the auspices of the nation's ministry of health, rather than the ministry of education. However, the establishment of baccalaureate, master's, and doctoral programs in nursing has led to placement of these programs within the ministry of education. Although it facilitates standard settings for curriculum development, this system can limit individuality, creativity, and experimentation.[32]

Traditionally, nursing education programs of developed, as well as developing, nations have focused on skill training and preparing students to care for persons within the acute care setting. In many countries around the world physicians outnumber professional nurses and thus have primary responsibility not only to teach the theoretic content of the nursing curriculum but also to determine it. Nursing faculty monitor the students in their clinical work on the wards.[32]

Nursing curricula in most countries must be radically altered to prepare nurses to meet the health needs of the greatest number of people in the community. Government and nongovernment international health agencies have identified the need for curriculum changes in both basic and advanced programs of nursing education as one of the most significant changes facing nursing as it participates in achieving HFA2000.[32] Additionally, national nurse associations (NNAs) responding to ICN's 1993-1994 biennial worldwide survey of nursing issues, priorities, and activities ranked nursing education a top priority. "With the trend toward health sector restructuring, nursing curricula must coincide with changes in health systems and be geared to preparing nurses in community-oriented care and to respond to such pressing health problems as HIV/AIDS, mental health issues, and 'life-style diseases.' "[22]

International Nursing Research

The importance of nursing research was emphasized when the Forty-Second World Health Assembly encouraged member states and asked the Director-General of WHO to promote and support the education of nurses, including education in research methodology. The crying need is for research that reorients nursing practice, education, and administration to ensure the participation of nurses in health research programs, in the development of national health care strategies, and in strengthening the provision of primary health care and care at all levels.[44] Similarly, the Forty-Ninth World Health Assembly supported the training of nursing/midwifery personnel in research methodology.[38]

Research must address all the factors that affect nursing practice in whatever situation it is carried out.[43] "[D]evelopments in the nature and scope of nursing practice must be supported by research so that the effectiveness of nursing can be evaluated and practice can be supported by research findings."[43]

Analysis of the most significant health care needs is a first step in designing and implementing practical, educative, and administrative interventions in the communities where the problems exist. The results of such endeavors can then be compared with findings in other communities and countries.[17,46,47]

International nursing research has great potential to significantly affect the health of all people. Therefore Henry and Nagelkerk reviewed international nursing research, defined as: "(a) scientific work conducted worldwide, (b) addressing problems in clinical nursing, nursing education, or nursing administration, and (c) using the methodologies of description, hypothesis-testing, program evaluation, policy research, or diffusion of knowledge."[17] The review was limited to studies reported in English-language nursing journals between 1985 and 1989 and conducted in countries other than the United States. Nearly 400 research studies were chosen from the following journals: *Australian Journal of Advanced Nursing* ($n = 45$), *Canadian Journal of Nursing Research* ($n = 71$), *International Nursing Review* ($n = 11$), *IMAGE: Journal of Nursing Scholarship* ($n = 5$), *Journal of Advanced Nursing* ($n = 192$), *Nursing Research* ($n = 2$), *Scandinavian Journal of Caring Sciences* ($n = 53$), and *Western Journal of Nursing Research* ($n = 8$). Furthermore, to broaden the analysis, studies in the 1980, 1984, 1985, and 1989 proceedings of the Workgroup of European Nurse Researchers were included, bringing the total to 549 research reports.[17]

Research problems identified in the studies were analyzed. Approximately 50% of the identified problems focused on clinical practice, 25% on nursing education, and 15% on nursing administration, with an additional 10% on the nursing profession. Of the studies, 75% were descriptive, approximately 14% were hypothesis-testing, 6% were program evaluations, and the remaining few were analyses of diffusion or policy research. Three fourths of the studies were cross-sectional, and a nurse was first author in 75% of the articles.

Study findings led to suggestions for future international nursing research. For example, more clinical research studies are needed that examine safe environments and lifestyles. Such studies would facilitate the understanding of the most appropriate interventions, especially those aimed at decreasing the prevalence of communicable diseases in many countries. Additionally, more research is needed that focuses on the costs and benefits of care particularly for the aged, on safe motherhood interventions, on damaging lifestyles, and on care and services for people with infectious disease, including AIDS.[17]

Comparative international research is needed to describe educational programs both in developing and in industrialized countries. Programs of education and research can enhance nurses' leadership in organizing, managing, and evaluating health care services. Additional studies should also focus on the planning, organization, management, and evaluation of effective health care services. Other areas that could be explored include alternative organizational designs, nurse managers' work technology, on-the-job management training, and nurse migration.[17]

Scientific research comprises three major stages, each of which is meritorious in its own right. In the first stage, a problem is perceived and new phenomena are sought. Systematic analysis to understand cause and effect characterize the second stage of scientific research. In the third stage theories and models are developed and tested.[17] Nursing research in most countries is primarily first-stage science, as exemplified by the fact that most studies are explorative-descriptive projects undertaken to identify problems, develop concepts, and generate hypotheses.[17] The potential for second-stage science is high, as understanding of health and illness and the accompanying care requirements escalates.

International nursing research is essential for the discovery of knowledge and new approaches to cost-effective care.[17] Though the underlying causes of health problems/illness may be universal, their efficient and effective eradication depends on adequate funding. Resources are limited, and competition is keen for them in all countries. Therefore programs with the best-documented need and return for monies spent are more likely to be supported. Such documentation requires research at the international level.

Although important, international nursing research has not flourished for several reasons. One reason has been the heavy workloads of international advisors. Another reason has been the reticence of the countries involved. Some have been concerned that results would be used to promote the researcher's interest and not those of the host country.[31] Additionally, in some countries research is considered an elite and inappropriate activity for nurses.[43]

Even when research is conducted, a number of factors make it difficult for nurses to share results with their international colleagues. Problems relate to language difficulties, data compilation and analysis, and preparation of a manuscript in a format acceptable for publication.[48] One solution to these problems is international collaborative projects. International nursing consultants can provide the research expertise, and nurses from the host country can provide entry into the health system and intimate knowledge of the culture.[31] However, to have a positive impact, research results must be published.

A survey undertaken by McConnell focused on English-language nursing publications originating in countries other than the United States.[29] Publications included journals, in-house journals, journals published by state or provincial nurses' associations, newsletters, and abstract review publications. Questionnaires were mailed to editors of 102 publications. Of these, 32 questionnaires were not returned, 2 were returned undeliverable, 5 were returned not completed, 10 were ineligible, and an additional 11 publications did not grant permission to publish their data.

The questionnaire had 40 open- and closed-ended questions pertaining to four areas: (1) journal characteristics, (2) readership characteristics, (3) review process characteristics, and (4) journal staff characteristics. Twenty-seven of the available 42 journals (64.3%) had been founded since 1970, including 4 since 1990. The journals represented 14 countries, with Australia, Canada, and England accounting for 69% of the publications.

Each publication available in 1991 (n = 40) was placed into one of five categories: administration (2 publications), education (2), general practice (24), research (2), and specialty practice (10). Editors of 28 journals provided information about the work focus of their readers. Direct care was the focus for at least half the readers for 67.9% of these publications. Nearly all publications included some research articles. The two most frequent reasons cited for manuscript rejection were "poorly written" and "idea poorly developed."

The results of this study identify the international publishing opportunities for nurses. International collaboration facilitates international nursing research as well as "breaking into print."

Participating in International Nursing

Nurses are part of a worldwide community, and outcomes of participating in international nursing are an increased awareness of the world as a global village and of the universality of nursing. Worldwide, nurses and nursing are more similar than dissimilar. Differences are a matter of degree.[21]

All the various ways of participating in international nursing begin with an attitude. This attitude values the differences inherent in a global perspective and readily acknowledges that nurses have much to learn from and about each other. Nurses can participate in international nursing by reading the *International Nursing Review* (the official journal of ICN); reading about nursing and health care in countries other than one's own; attending international conferences such as ICN's Quadrennial Congress; participating in a nursing cultural exchange across countries; conducting or participating in international collaborative research; and working in an international setting.

Nurses work in international settings in a variety of positions. Some work as teachers, others as supervisors or consultants. A few work as clinicians giving direct client care. Employers are as varied as the roles nurses fulfill. For example, some employers are private multinational corporations, whereas others are the United States government or national governments abroad. Nongovernment volunteer agencies such as CARE and Project HOPE and religiously affiliated organizations also hire nurses for international employment. Furthermore, universities promote international nursing through faculty and student exchange programs.

International nurses constitute a minority. Much information about their work comes from personal experiences shared through presentations or anecdotes in the nursing literature. The few research studies providing an organized description of nurses working internationally were conducted in the late 1970s and mid-1980s.[1]

Working in international settings is challenging, rewarding, and exciting. However, nurses undertaking international work must be flexible and prepared to appreciate and accept cultural differences. Nurses involved in international nursing are cautioned to help local people do what is culturally congruent for their country, today and tomorrow.[21] Nurses considering international work benefit both from general and specific preparation. Knowledge and understanding of the following enhance their effectiveness:

1. International health and health issues
2. Health, nursing roles, and nursing systems in other countries
3. Health needs and priorities in other countries
4. The influence of politics on health services and nursing

Additionally, skills in cross-cultural communication, problem solving, and decision making are beneficial, as are adaptability and proficiency in a language other than one's own.[27]

■ CHALLENGES CONFRONTING INTERNATIONAL NURSING

In today's global society the nursing profession may be viewed as a unified worldwide group.[32] Nursing has the ability, as well as the responsibility, to help redirect the focus of health care worldwide. Achievement of this goal necessitates changes in the practice of nursing and the preparation of nurses. Five strategies for change will help ensure nursing's success:

1. Develop a corps of nurse leaders in each country who are informed about primary health care and ready to expedite necessary changes in the nursing system
2. Include nursing personnel in policy making and administration at all levels of health care services
3. Institute basic changes at all levels of nursing education (basic, postbasic, and continuing) to ensure that students are prepared to meet priority needs of populations
4. Involve nurses in the initiation or extention of primary health care
5. Conduct research about nursing administration, practice, and education both to demonstrate the need for nursing's contribution to primary health care and to evaluate the results of such contributions.[32]

■ SUMMARY

Nursing in a country is affected by that country's culture. To know the size and demography of a country, its social structure, political factors, economic resources, level of scientific knowledge and technology, and history is to begin to understand nursing and health care in that country. To have knowledge about primary health care, international nursing organizations, international trends in nursing education, and the status of nursing research internationally is to begin to understand nursing from a worldwide perspective.

International nursing is challenging and exciting, and nurses who participate in international nursing have the opportunity to make a difference in the health of people nationally and internationally. At its best, international nursing reminds us that nursing and health care are culturally defined. To be accepted, they must be culturally congruent.

CRITICAL THINKING *Activities*

1. Explain the influence of factors that affect nursing and health care internationally.
2. Describe the role of the nurse in primary health care.
3. Compare at least three international nursing organizations.
4. Explain the role of nurses in fulfilling the mission of WHO.
5. Categorize articles about international nursing that have been published in the last 12 issues of *IMAGE: Journal of Nursing Scholarship* in terms of focus (that is, clinical practice, administration, education, or research).
6. Compare the requirements for international nursing positions as advertised in two current nursing journals.
7. Evaluate the adequacy of an undergraduate nursing curriculum in preparing nurses to work in primary health care.

Addresses of Organizations

International Council of Nurses
3, place Jean-Marteau
CH-1201
Geneva, Switzerland
Telephone: (41-22) 908 01 00

World Health Organization
CH-1211
Geneva, Switzerland
Telephone: (41-22) 791 21 11

Pan American Health Organization
525 23rd St. NW
Washington, DC 20037-2895
Telephone: 202-974-3000

Sigma Theta Tau International
550 West North
Indianapolis, IN 46202
Telephone: 317-634-8171

Nurses' Christian Fellowship International (NCFI)
American Office
PO Box 7895
Madison, WI 53703-7895
Telephone: 608-274-9001
International Office
18 Buckland Road
Maidstone, Kent
ME16 OSL
England

References

1. Andrews MM: U.S. nurse consultants in the international marketplace, *Int Nurs Rev* 33(2):50-55, 1986.
2. Banta HD, Behney CJ: Policy formulation and technology assessment, *Milbank Memorial Fund Quarterly/Health and Society* 59:445-479, 1981.
3. Basch PF: *Textbook of international health,* New York, 1990, Oxford University Press.
4. Bates E, Lapsley H: *The health machine: the impact of medical technology,* Victoria, Australia, 1985, Penguin Books Australia.
5. Bergstrom S, Mocumbi P: Health for all by the year 2000? *BMJ* 313(7053):316, 1996.
6. Brans YW: Biomedical technology: to use or not to use, *Clin Perinatol* 18:389-401, 1991.
7. Brown JN, Jr, Wooten FT, Fischer WA: Technology transfer in medicine, *CRC Critical Reviews in Bioengineering* 4(1):45-79, 1979.
8. Brush BL, Stuart M: Unity amidst difference: the ICN project and writing international nursing history, *Nurs History Rev* 2:191-203, 1994.
9. Castaneda ME, Breivis J: Technology assessment, *Healthc Forum J* 33(6):100-105, 1990.
10. Clark J: How nurses can participate in the development of an ICNP, *Int Nurs Rev* 43:171-174, 1996.
11. Coe GA, Banta D: Health care technology transfer in Latin America and the Caribbean, *Int J Technol Assess Health Care* 8:255-267, 1992.
12. Crossette B: As population ages, demographers foresee business accommodating over-80 crowd, *Fort-Worth Star-Telegram,* December 22, 1996, p. A24.
13. Curtin LL: Keepers of the keys: economics, ethics, and nursing administrators, *Nurs Admin Q* 17(4):1-10, 1993.
14. Erinosho OA: Health care and medical technology in Nigeria, *Int J Technol Assess Health Care* 7:545-552, 1991.
15. Glasser JH, Chrzanowski RS: Medical technology assessment: adequate questions, appropriate methods, valuable answers, *Health Pol* 9:267-276, 1988.
16. Hamilton PM: *Realities of contemporary nursing,* Menlo Park, CA, 1992, Addison-Wesley.
17. Henry BM, Nagelkerk JM: International nursing research, *Ann Rev Nurs Res* 10:207-230, 1992.
18. Hirschfield MJ: Challenges from the World Health Organization, *Nurs Admin Q* 16(2):1-2, 1992.
19. Hirschfield MJ: Nursing research and community nursing-the work of family care, *Proc 12th Workgroup Meeting and International Nursing Research Conference, Workgroup of European Nurse Researchers,* Frankfurt, Germany, 1989, German Nursing Association.
20. Holleran CA: Perspective of the International Council of Nurses, *Nurs Admin Q* 16(2):2-3, 1992.
21. Holleran CA: The many labors of the International Council of Nurses, *Nurs Health Care* 14(4):206-207, 1993.
22. International Council of Nurses: Worldwide survey of nursing issues, *Int Nurs Rev* 42:125-127, 1995.
23. Kim M: Overview: the International Council of Nurses: the past, present and future, *Imprint* 40(3):57-60, 1993.
24. Little C: Health for all by the year 2000: where is it now? *Nurs Health Care* 13(4):198-201, 1992.

25. Luce BR, Elixhauser A: Estimating costs in the economic evaluation of medical technologies, *Int J Technol Assess Health Care* 6:57-75, 1990.
26. Mahler H: Action for change in nursing, *World Health* 12:1, 1978.
27. Masson V: *International nursing,* New York, 1981, Springer.
28. McConnell EA: Complexity in selecting health care technology in diverse settings, *Holistic Nurs Prac* 9(2):1-8, 1995.
29. McConnell EA: Journal and publishing characteristics for 42 nursing publications outside the United States, *IMAGE: J Nurs Scholar* 27(3):225-229, 1995.
30. McConnell EA, Murphy EK: Nurses' use of technology: an international concern, *Int Nurs Rev* 37:331-334, 1990.
31. Meleis AI: International nursing: a force for knowledge development, *Nurs Outlook* 33(3):138-142, 1985.
32. Ohlson VM, Franklin M: An international perspective on nursing practice, *Issues Prof Nurs Prac,* Kansas City, MO, 1985, American Nurses Association.
33. Paul BD: *Health culture and community: case studies of public reactions to health programs,* New York, 1955, Russell Sage Foundation.
34. Quivey M: Advanced medical technology: finding the answers, *Int Nurs Rev* 37:329-330, 1990.
35. Sen A: The economics of life and death, *Scientific American* 268(5):18-25, 1993.
36. Staff: Introducing ICN's International Classification for Nursing Practice (ICNP): a unifying framework, *Int Nurs Rev* 43:169-170, 1996.
37. Staff: Nurses asked to renew Health-for-All strategy, *Int Nurs Rev* 43:42, 1996.
38. Staff: Nursing received overwhelming support at World Health Assembly, *Int Nurs Rev* 43:97-98, 1996.
39. Subramanian M: The World Health Report 1995: bridging the gaps, *World Health* 48(2):4-5, 1995.
40. Tan-Torres T: Technology assessment in developing countries, *World Health Forum* 16:74-76, 1995.
41. U.S. Office of Technology Assessment (OTA): *Strategies for medical technology assessment,* Washington, D.C., 1982, U.S. Government Printing Office.
42. Vatre NJ: Global issues for nurses and nursing, *J Prof Nurs* 8(5):259, 1992.
43. WHO Expert Committee: *Nursing practice,* Technical Report Series No. 860, Geneva, Switzerland, 1996, WHO.
44. World Health Assembly Resolution 42.27: *Strengthening nursing midwifery in support of strategies for health for all,* Geneva, Switzerland, 1989, WHO.
45. World Health Organization: *Alma-Ata 1978: Primary health care* (Health for All Series No. 1), Geneva, Switzerland, 1978, WHO.
46. World Health Organization: *Education and training of nurse teachers and managers with special regard to primary care,* Geneva, Switzerland, 1984, WHO.
47. World Health Organization: *Evaluation of the strategy for Health For All by the Year 2000,* Geneva, Switzerland, 1987, WHO.
48. Zanotti R: Overcoming national and cultural differences within collaborative international nursing research, *Western J Nurs Res* 18(1):6-11, 1996.

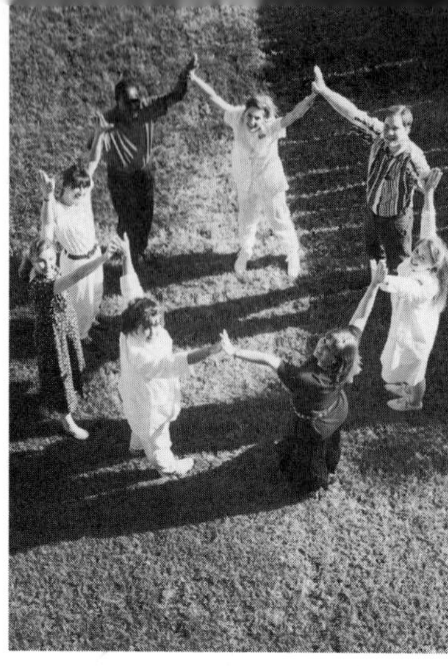

CHAPTER 15

Image of Nursing

Carmen Germaine Warner,

Vicki L. Black, Pat C. Parent

OBJECTIVES After completing this chapter the reader should be able to:

- **Describe the current broad public perception of the nursing profession and some of the sources of this image**
- **Describe ways in which the media have influenced public perception of nurses and nursing**
- **Discuss how gender issues, past and present, affect the nursing profession**
- **Suggest ways in which nurses individually and collectively can improve the status of their profession**
- **Discuss the ramifications of the increasing number of male nurses**

■ HISTORICAL DEVELOPMENT OF NURSING'S IMAGE

Credit is given to Florence Nightingale for the written history and development of modern nursing. The image of nursing may also have its roots in the Victorian Age during which she lived.[39] At that time men were the laborers and the breadwinners, and almost all women were socialized into becoming wives, mothers, and housekeepers. Nursing was perceived as "women's work"—a natural extension of all of the altruistic qualities valued in women.[45]

Women were expected to lovingly devote themselves to the health and well-being of other people, and they were also expected to do this without any thoughts of autonomy at the bedside or in their identified professional activities. In the hospital setting nurses were recognized as physician extenders. Unlike today, physicians by the late 1800s were exclusively male and nurses were female. The expectations of nurses were altruism, sacrifice, and submission. These expectations were not just encouraged but demanded. Obligation and love, rather than having to earn a living, were required to bind the nurse to her client. In a society thus oriented, it was natural that women viewed nursing as a means of manifesting their love to others; such a noble characteristic was attractive to many women and drew them into nursing. This thought process became a part of a girl's upbringing, and nursing skills were integrated into the teachings passed from mother to daughter.

The usual image of Florence Nightingale is of a self-sacrificing young woman with no desire or need for money, rest, or recognition. Even today, the image of Florence Nightingale as the "lady with the lamp" remains perhaps the most popular public image of the founder of modern nursing. Actually, she was a courageous, liberated, independent woman who may be credited with leading the nursing profession into a new era.[37] Ms. Nightingale had strong convictions about what nursing should be, and she fought hard to see that certain clinical and educational standards were maintained.[40]

Florence Nightingale also had a strong sense of spirituality, which she viewed as intrinsic to human nature, accompanying our most potent grounding for healing. Ms. Nightingale also perceived nursing as a means of searching for truth and discovering God's laws of healing, with their appropriate and relevant application.[32]

■ LINKAGE BETWEEN MASS MEDIA AND NURSING IMAGE

Extensive research on the image of the nursing profession has been done by Kalisch and Kalisch.[23-27] Although somewhat harsh at times, these authors make some worthwhile statements that can assist the nursing profession to view itself more objectively. They identify six periods during which distinct corresponding images of the nursing profession can be seen. These periods will be reviewed here next. Because of its pervading influence, emphasis will be placed on the effect that mass media had on the image of nursing during these periods.

Period 1: Angel of Mercy (1854-1919)

In the pioneer days of nursing there were two prominent images of nurses. One image, in a novel by Charles Dickens, was Sairy Gamp, the poorly educated alcoholic nurse who worked in primitive conditions primarily performing domestic chores. The second prevailing image was Florence Nightingale, the original "Angel of Mercy."

In the early 1900s nurses were viewed as honorable, moral, spiritual, self-sacrificing, and ritualistic. World War I media representations continued the "Angel of Mercy" image, idealizing nurses and making them a totem of exemplary moral purity.

This time period corresponded with the silent era of the film industry. In these films the function the nurse served was more symbolic than useful. Neither the role of the nurse nor her educational preparation was well presented. The nurses' role in films was influenced by a moral code from the Victorian era. Just as in society in general at that time, the image of women in films was defined primarily by their economic and marital status. A female nurse was almost always depicted in relation to a male. A familiar theme in the motion pictures was that of the male client falling in love with his nurse. Amusement was frequently derived through the antics resulting from a nurse being pursued by an ardent admirer.

During the "Angel of Mercy" era, nurses appeared in a substantial number of literary endeavors. Nurse heroines were characterized as being involved in a dual search: (1) success and meaning through nursing and (2) happiness and fulfillment through love and marriage. This dichotomous representation often resulted in a mixed image. Conflict within the nurse herself often ensued because success as a nurse demanded intelligence, expertise, perseverance, and leadership, whereas success at love and marriage still required the stereotypical feminine qualities of compliance and obedience. The seeming dichotomy was as confusing for the nurse as it was for the public.

From 1916 to 1918 the nursing profession received its greatest attention in the propaganda films of World War I. Nurses were consistently cast as Red Cross nurses and represented an idealized and almost mythical womanhood. The extent to which nursing activities were illustrated was largely limited to gentle, maternal concern for the client's comfort. Films generated from Hollywood emphasized nursing as it was during the war. The war provided an improvement of the professions' image in novels. Although skilled nursing activities and knowledge were seemingly deemphasized, the nurse was portrayed as an autonomous and intelligent health care provider.

Period 2: Girl Friday (1920-1929)

With the passage of the Women's Suffrage Reform in 1919, women entered a new domain of professional endeavors and activities. World War I and the 1918 influenza epidemic created a vast need for nurses to decrease human suffering on many fronts. The invention and use of aircraft in war, as well as chemical warfare, resulted in new problems in the health field. The influenza epidemic also increased the importance of instructing nurses in the area of home nursing. In addition, this was a time when the Red Cross was active and publicly visible; it expanded rapidly and created a high demand for nurses. As a result of all these factors, efforts toward increased regulation of nursing education were hampered.

Nursing students were exploited as cheap labor, literally staffing entire hospitals. Nurses were described as faithful, dependent, cooperative, long-suffering, and subservient. Their careers culminated in marriage, which represented a woman's only legitimate destiny. This attitude was conveyed in the enterprises of Hollywood in which nursing was depicted as a conscientious and admirable job choice, but acceptable only until time for marriage. In films of this era nurse heroines were not cast as career nurses. Nursing was simply a means to an end.

In novels written after World War I, nurses diminished in importance. They were depicted as remedies for the emotional turmoil that active soldiers suffered and endured, and the nurse's duty was that of instilling hope into the lives of wounded soldiers.

Period 3: Heroine (1930-1945)

For the next 15 years, nursing was acknowledged as a worthy and important profession that enabled women to earn an honorable living. Nurses were identified as educated and owning certain abilities. Adjectives such as courageous, chivalrous, fearless, reasonable, clear-headed, humanitarian, and magnanimous were used to illustrate and portray nurses.

The only feature-length films ever produced that focused entirely on the nursing profession— seven in number—were released in the 1930s. These films stressed the education and work of professional nurses. Attractive young women were portrayed as putting the demands of their profession before personal ambitions. One of the most popular films, nominated for the 1934 Academy Award for best picture, was *The White Parade.* Loretta Young provided audiences with a realistic portrayal of the challenges and problems encountered in becoming a nurse in a large hospital school. The plot stressed that not every woman was destined to become a nurse, but those who were could expect a life of hard work, minimal monetary reimbursement, and immense personal satisfaction. The heroine of the film rejected a millionaire's offer of marriage to continue her career as a nurse.

In the Depression years of the 1930s, such devotion and selflessness meant a great deal. The viewing public understood that the nursing profession maintained high standards and insisted on rigorous self-restraint among its practitioners and students. Hollywood ceased to present nursing as a short-lived humanitarian hobby for rich girls before their more permanent status as wife and mother.

During World War II the perceived worth of professional nurses by American society intensified tremendously. This was magnified on the screen as nursing assumed a loyalist and activist character never before or since matched in feature films. In 1943, at the zenith of the war, the studios produced their greatest accolade to the profession: *So Proudly We Hail* (1943), a Paramount release based on the experiences of nurses on Bataan and Corregidor when the war began in the Philippines, was one of the biggest successes of the year. Its image of nursing was very positive.

Period 4: Mother (1946-1965)

It may have been a natural development after World War II that a major goal for many American women was to stay home and care for children. Nurses during this period were chronicled as maternal, compassionate, unassertive, submissive, and domestic. Postwar society would not support independent and autonomous women. Their place was typically perceived as being in the home raising children.

During the 1950s television programs usually portrayed nurses as worthy of respect and appreciated for their skills. They were depicted in roles subordinate to physicians and employed in positions that they would easily surrender for marriage or children. Work as a nurse was often seen as a means to obtain amenities such as vacations or luxuries for the home and family.

The American public was captivated by the medical world in the figures of Ben Casey and Dr. Kildare in the 1960s. Although the nurse was positively portrayed in these films as intelligent, altruistic, perceptive, and energetic, there was a subtle erosion of the nurse's image.

Period 5: Sex Object (1966-1982)

After 1966 the mother image of the nurse, which was popular in the mid-1940s, changed to the sex object image. Nurses were increasingly depicted as being sexually promiscuous, self- indulgent, superficial, and unreliable. Nurses became "sexual mascots" for health care teams and were seen in X-rated movies. They were often depicted as more interested in linen closet trips than in professional growth and development. Eventually, nurses were portrayed as cold, uncaring, power-hungry, and unmotivated persons, and the once-honored and virtuous film image of the nurse was a thing of the past.

Television censorship standards were lax in the early 1970s. Nurses who were portrayed in appropriately or provocatively dressed were no longer censored.

During this decade nurse figures were cast primarily in series that accentuated the medical model and made physicians seem almost superhuman. In films of these years, nurses were undervalued and poorly represented. Their contributions to health care were not addressed. For example, Major Margaret Houlihan on *MASH* was technically competent but had little effect on client welfare. As a surgical nurse she was supportive of the surgeons, but they were clearly the heroes. The scene was further skewed by the fact that the client received little emotional support or physical comfort from the nurse and was rarely seen by Major Houlihan.

The television show closely associated with scientific endeavors was the portrayal of the nurse in *Doctors' Private Lives.* In her off-duty hours the nurse served as an assistant to a physician-researcher. The nurse was often chastised, insulted, and sexually manipulated by the physician.

The 1970s represent the lowest point in film history for the nursing profession. Certainly, nurses were not portrayed as altruistic, intelligent, and virtuous. Instead, a new nurse characterization appeared—that of the malevolent and sadistic personality. For example, the highly acclaimed *One Flew Over the Cuckoos' Nest* (1975) depicted Nurse Ratched as a soul-destroying, castrating mother figure. She abused her position as a psychiatric nurse to arrange cruel punishments. In one scene she has a client, McMurphy, lobotomized to demonstrate her ultimate power over the clients. In another box office hit, *Coma* (1978), a nurse plays a key role in a murderous conspiracy to sell needed transplantable organs to unethical and ruthless surgeons.

The mass media of the 1980s did not improve the image of the profession. Movies such as *Terms of Endearment* endorse the image of the cold-hearted, punitive, sadistic nurse who derives pleasure from client suffering.[9,10]

Bumper stickers and T-shirts claiming "Nurses Call the Shots" and greeting cards that depict nurses who derive pleasure from the discomfort of clients may, on the surface, appear fairly innocent and cute, but they relay a subtle message to those who interpret them in various ways. Television shows during the 1980s declined to promote a positive professional image of nursing. Shows such as *St. Elsewhere, Trapper John, M.D.,* and daytime dramas depicted nursing in an unfavorable and unprofessional light. Perhaps the television show that most blatantly demoralized and insulted nurses was *Nightingales.* In this show, student nurses— five single females—were cast as brainless male-chasing dummies who wore skimpy underclothing or bath towels. They demonstrated no clinical competence or expertise but exhibited playful sexual escapades in the linen closet.[1] As Dickson notes, media images are important because they have an impact on clients' and their families' perceptions and expectations of what nursing is about.[11] The image may also deter some persons from becoming nurses.

Period 6: Careerist (1983-Present)

The careerist has become the new image for the mid-1980s and 1990s, portraying nurses as intelligent, logical, progressive, sophisticated, empathetic, and assertive. Men and women in the nursing profession are dedicated to providing the highest standards of health care and the greatest expanse of excellence to the consumer.[29]

Recognizing that the previous period identified nurses as sex objects, it has become increasingly more important for nurses to endeavor to share, spread, and practice the new image of the careerist. Each one of us holds the responsibility and the privilege of making this image the commonplace awareness in every household.

Kalisch and Kalisch[26,27] clearly showed that the negative image of nursing precipitated a problem where both the quantity and the quality of persons who choose nursing as an occupation are affected.

One positive advance in reversing the negative image has been the TV program *China Beach.* In this series nurses were portrayed in a positive light, depicting nursing during the Vietnam War in a realistic and sensitive manner. *Nursing Approach,* an international production of a television series, has helped nurses connect with other nurses, using the media to assist in improving care.

Nurses of America (NOA) was organized for the purpose of monitoring the media for health-related issues and for projecting the best image of nursing along with the role that nurses play in the health care system. Their newsletter publication *Media Watch* has been established for the purpose of disseminating a positive, realistic image.

Another factor contributing to the enhanced image of nursing in the careerist period is the collaborative practice that has encouraged nurses and physicians to practice in tandem for the quality care of all, with nurses being recognized as the pivotal provider for entry into the health care system.

It has become the responsibility of each nurse to expand out of the paradigm, depicting nursing as an integrated way of living, seeking, and achieving wholeness beyond the institution and extending into all walks of life. The ultimate image of nursing, as we approach the millennium, is for nursing to:

- Touch the hearts of the homeless and abandoned by working for change in the policy of local health agencies
- Enhance the minimum level of education for all nurses by involving them in collaboration with community business and political and social endeavors
- Expand the involvement of political integration by visualizing total health care as the responsibility of the entire community
- Enlighten the public through all forms of media of the positive dynamics of nursing by showcasing personal stories as shared by clients
- Affect the escalating trend in violence, drug influence, and family disruptions by incorporating the compassionate and hopeful heart of our heritage through involvement in the health care within areas such as prisons, community agencies, shelters, and clinics

Our greatest advocate is the client. As we reach out to care for them heart to heart, they will reach out to work with us hand in hand.

■ NURSING'S IMAGE OF ITSELF

Nurses may sometimes feel that it is not important how they perceive nursing—their 8-, 10-, or 12-hour days should speak for them. However, individual attitudes, feelings, and perceptions are reflected in one's appearance, behavior, and outcomes of interactions with others, including clients, peers, and the public. Collectively, these individual nurses' attitudes, behaviors, and interactions constitute nursing's self-image. The image of nursing held by nurses is cited as perhaps the most damaging influence affecting the profession's image.[6,52,56,57] Until the profession changes its lack of occupational prestige, it is unlikely to persuade the public to do so.[8] Nurses who verbalize comments such as "I'm only a staff nurse" or "I was just following the physician's order" are not improving the image of nursing. It is the challenge for each nurse to extend the best image possible and offer the utmost by substantiating the value of that service.[21]

Self-Image Psychology

In addition to her contribution to nursing theory, the late Martha Rogers (1914-1994) made a major contribution to nursing through her presentation of principles regarding self-image psychology. These principles focus on the self-concept of the individual nurse.[53] Tracy explored specific principles of the self-concept model and studied how these principles actually determine individual achievement.[54] Tracy describes two basic principles that Strasen believes have significant implications for improving the image of the nursing profession.

The law of belief. This major principle of the model declares that whatever an individual strongly believes is actualized. This principle is commonly known as the *self-fulfilling prophecy.*[53] Everything an individual subconsciously believes becomes reality.[49] Only information consistent with internal beliefs is allowed to pass through to the conscious mind. Therefore self-concept affects one's image of self and thus one's professional image. Actualized feelings are reflected on others. The key, Strasen emphasizes, is to focus one's energy on oneself and not on external factors over which one has no control.

The responsibility/achievement relationship. This model states that an individual experiences a confident self-concept, the attitude of being in control, and achievement in equal proportions to the willingness and ability of that individual to take responsibility for her or his own life without blaming external factors. Applied to the nursing profession, the concept implies that until nurses internalize feelings of control and professionalism, they will collectively continue to act as if they are powerless and not in control of their own destiny. Nurses must believe that they are meritorious professionals willing to accept accountability for their lives and practices no matter what external factors are present. Strasen suggests that full professional potential for nursing will not be attained until these beliefs are internalized and incorporated into each nurse's daily professional practice.

Professional Pride

Nurses frequently become trapped in one particular image. They may believe that to be a "real" nurse one must work in a hospital providing direct client care and that when one moves away from the bedside or the hospital setting, status as a "real" nurse is lost. Nurses must begin to educate members of the profession, the public, and nursing students that "real" nurses are involved in a variety of interesting and valuable professional activities in many diverse settings. The belief that it is acceptable not to be at the bedside must be generated, discussed, encouraged, and disseminated. Real nurses engage in research, deliver babies in hospitals and in homes, consult, participate in ministry, administer anesthesia, provide psychotherapy, care for individuals with complex disabilities in the home, collaborate with administration, and teach. Real nurses also work in jails, homes, clinics, hospice settings, colleges, industries, private businesses, reservations, and in rural and urban areas. Nurses participate in all areas of life.

There is a dearth of research in the United States on the perception of nurses as a group. Also, virtually no research exists on the self-image of nurses as compared to their "ideal self-image." Zalar and Suter developed the Nursing Image Survey and completed a study that included 486 working nurses and nursing students in Northern California.[57] The survey indicated a difference between nurses' self-image and ideal self-image, specifically in the areas of professionalism and stress. The actual self-image tends to be less positive. To strengthen the nursing profession, both the actual and ideal self-image need to be positive. This must occur, however, on the individual level.

Porter and others[43] designed a study to evaluate the public's perception of the nursing profession. The study included three groups (registered nurses, physicians, and the general public) who were asked to describe their image of nursing in one word. Analysis of the data indicates that the nurse group demonstrated the lowest percentage of positive responses (72%) in comparison with physicians (100% positive) and the general public (84% positive). Subjects most commonly used the following adjectives to describe their image of nursing:

- Caring
- Empathetic
- Nurturing
- Compassionate
- Warm
- Concerned
- Sensitive
- Patient

Twenty-three percent of physicians labeled nurses as "efficient, competent, professional, responsible, and organized." In sharp contrast, only 11% of the nurses used similar terms to describe themselves. In addition, 23% of the physicians characterized nurses as "superlative, indispensable, essential, valuable, and admirable," whereas only one nurse employed analogous terms. The nurse respondents used words such as "overworked, chaotic, harried, overstressed, moody, underestimated, ignored, underrated, underpaid, disillusioned, indifferent, and oppressed."

A study by Martin examined job characteristics responsible for nursing prestige as perceived by practicing health care professionals: registered nurses ($n = 30$), hospital administrators ($n = 154$), and physicians ($n = 300$).[33] The respondents' perceptions of nursing were compared to their perceptions of other health care professionals. The results revealed the following:

1. Physicians ranked nursing education significantly higher than did nurses and administrators
2. Administrators rated nursing income higher than did nurses or physicians
3. Administrators and physicians ranked nursing authority and prestige significantly higher than did nurses
4. Administrators rated nursing importance significantly lower than did nurses and physicians
5. Nurses viewed their occupation as one with great social expectations and requirements (importance, complexity, difficulty) but with few social compensations (income, authority, general prestige); this view was consistent among the nurse respondents

Mendez and Louis reported a study of the image of nursing among college students.[35] The responses of 163 nonnursing students were compared to those of 93 nursing students. The findings indicated that the image of nursing as a career choice among nonnursing students correlated with their ideal career ($r = .4072$). Nursing students correlated nursing with their ideal career more positively ($r = .5941$) than the nonnursing students. However, as we noted, even nursing students did not describe nursing as the perfect, ideal career.

■ NURSE—BEST TITLE FOR THE PROFESSION?

In past years various nursing organizations have discussed appropriateness and validity of the title *nurse*. Questions from these discussions include:

1. Does the title do justice to the profession?
2. Is the title sexist, a barrier keeping men out of the profession?
3. Would changing the title help the profession's image?

Before these questions can be adequately considered, the word *nurse* and its effect on the profession's image must be examined. Nurse is derived from the Latin word *nutricus,* meaning that which nourishes, fosters, and protects.[15] The average American dictionary will define *nurse* as (1) a person trained to care for the sick or disabled under the supervision of a physician; (2) a person employed to take care of a child, a nursemaid; and (3) a worker ant or bee that cares for the young.

Fagin and Diers suggest that *nursing* is a metaphor, and metaphors influence language, thought, and action.[15] They consider *nursing* to be a simile for mothering: therefore one associates nursing with nurturing, solacing, caring, the laying on of hands, and other maternal behaviors.

These behaviors are sometimes viewed in the context of current society's values and mores as humdrum and ordinary. The natural result is that too few of these nurturing characteristics are experienced in society, and many children and adults feel alone and unloved as a consequence. Fagin and Diers suggest that adults in contemporary society may not like to be reminded of the child within by having someone care for them in a maternal way.

Fagin and Diers[15] also note that *nursing* is a metaphor for equality. They believe that nursing not only symbolizes women's struggles for equality, but that the profession itself represents the typical figure of the "underdog" in its struggle to be heard, approved, recognized, and appreciated. This is, of course, a questionable situation because nursing composes the largest occupational group in the health care system.

Nursing is also closely associated with intimacy. By virtue of their work, nurses are involved in private, personal aspects of people's lives. Nurses do for others publicly what healthy persons do for themselves behind closed doors. Many clients are vulnerable and frequently depend on the nurse and the nurse's physical, emotional, and spiritual strength. After recovery the client may feel as if the nurse knows all of her or his secrets. It can be disconcerting for an individual to have been so intense and intimate with a virtual stranger.

Nurses see and touch the bodies of strangers during the course of their work. Unfortunately, somehow nursing as a role and an occupation became affiliated with the broad term of sex. Various circumstances were undoubtedly involved that altered a seemingly virtuous caring for human beings. Some individuals began to expand and to fantasize about the role, and what resulted was not an image of nurses as knowledgeable, willing, and capable caregivers but as experienced sexual partners. Although every occupation has individuals who fit this misinformed stereotype, most nurses are embarrassed by the development. This image is one perpetuated and encouraged by the mass media and by the sexist faction of our society.

The title *nurse* is presently all-inclusive, and incorporates many positions—registered nurse, licensed practical or vocational nurse, nurse assistant, nurse practitioner, and others. It does not discriminate between levels of educational preparation. Educational background usually creates differences in language, behavior, tastes, and thought processes. The lack of differentiation often contributes to the impression that "a nurse is a nurse is a nurse." One recommendation by Vann is to revamp the current system so that newly graduated nursing students can take an initial state-sponsored examination focused on nursing theory.[55] If successfully completed, this examination would entitle the graduate nurse to use the title "Nurse-in-Training." The individual would work under the direct supervision of professional nurses. After 4 or more years of clinical experience, she would be eligible to take a state-sponsored examination focusing on nursing practice. Successful completion of this final examination would result in the right to be called "Professional Nurse." This model is based on a concept employed by the engineering profession.

We conducted a study in California to determine the opinion of nurses regarding the proposal of changing the title *nurse.* Reactions were varied. Individuals opposing the name change believe that changing the name would do nothing to enhance the professional image of nursing. Suggestions from this group include (1) working to standardize the profession by elevating the entry level to the baccalaureate level and (2) increasing salaries. This group did not perceive that the title *nurse* excluded men from nursing, but one participant suggested that men could assume the title "Male Registered Nurse (M.R.N.)." Others felt that there are too many new titles in hospitals and that clients still have the most confidence in nurses.

Nurses approving of a name change believe that the title *nurse* is sexist and connotes subservience and passivity. One participant noted that the term *nurse* is "one of the most overworked, ill-defined terms in the English language"[7] and that it implies reference to the mammary glands. Also noted was "*nurse* implies that a client is going to be taken care of in an all-encompassing, infantile way. There is no recognition that he must do his part in getting well."[7] Others felt that the title *nurse* is stereotypical and archaic as well as sexist. The 48 suggestions for a title change included the following:

1. Clinical Coordinator
2. Health Care Professional
3. Medical Care Worker
4. Licensed Health Advocate
5. Patient Care Coordinator
6. Person Caregiver

7. Primary Health Care Specialist
8. Registered Health Care Facilitator
9. Trained Observer Patient Advocate

■ MEN AND THE IMAGE OF NURSING

The literature indicates that the nursing profession would benefit from a large influx of men into the profession.[2,31] But if a man decides to enter the profession, he is plagued by social stereotypes. Male nurses are often considered social misfits unable to fit into a "real man's" job. Again, the media is detrimental in its portrayal of men in nursing.

A fallacy about men in nursing is that men are new to the profession. When reviewing nursing history, one finds repeated documentation that men were the first nurses to experience large-scale conventional education in Western civilization. Men supplied half of the nursing care provided in the eleventh, twelfth, and thirteenth centuries. Until the late nineteenth century, nursing was considered as much a male profession as a female one. The profession was genderless.

Several circumstances led to the decline and near extinction of men in nursing. Ironically, Florence Nightingale was partly responsible, because she consciously defined nursing as female. She worked tirelessly to establish nursing as a worthy career choice outside the home for respectable women.[17]

The Industrial Revolution is also responsible for the lingering gender-specific stereotypes that exist within nursing today. Science, technology, and business became the accepted standards for aspiring men in the nineteenth century. Medicine was also a valuable vocation for males, causing further division of the health occupations into sex-specific roles. Men chose medicine; women chose nursing. This, and the restriction of men from the nursing profession, ultimately influenced the subordinate role that nursing assumed in relation to medicine.

In 1901 a single event resulted in making nursing gender-specific. The U.S. Congress created the Army Nurse Corps and designated it female. Seven years later the Navy Nurse Corps followed suit. As a result, a young man entering nursing became an oddity. The percentage of male nurses in the United States diminished from 7.6% in 1910 to 3.8% in 1920. In 1989 male nurses constituted only 3.1% of the nursing force in America.[36]

As previously mentioned, a reason often cited for the continued voluntary exclusion of men from nursing is the image of the profession as feminine and nurturing. This image creates difficulty for some men who might otherwise be attracted to the field. Holleran suggests that internal sexism keeps men out of nursing, whereas others suggest that changing the title *nurse* to a less female-oriented name might eliminate a barrier to the successful recruitment of men into nursing.[19,48]

During the 1990s, however, the increase in pay and prestige has influenced the public's attitude shift concerning men in nursing. In 1979 only one third of all women surveyed and one fifth of all men indicated it would be okay for their sons to become nurses. Today more than 40% of both groups would approve of nursing as a career choice for their sons.

Accompanying this view, society has begun to change its view concerning the care provider. The majority of the respondents (slightly more than half) did not mind whether they received care from a man or a woman.[5]

■ STRATEGIES FOR IMPROVING THE IMAGE OF NURSING IN THE 1990s

The nursing profession faces some difficult issues and challenges as it relates to image building. Many of these controversies must first be addressed and settled within the nursing community. Nurses need to assume responsibility and accountability for their profession and their professional image (see p. 406).

Collective Bargaining

Collective bargaining is the process by which unions participate in administrative decisions involving the terms of employment and the price of labor. Most nurses seek improvements in salaries, hours, and overall working conditions. Thus collective bargaining for a time became an attractive possibility as a positive and powerful organizational tool. Currently, approximately 120,000 R.N.s are represented and work under contracts arbitrated by state constituents of the ANA. These nurses, in conjunction with others represented by different labor unions, encompass a considerable percentage of the nation's 800,000 R.N.s employed in hospitals.

Labor groups who seek to represent R.N.s attempt to counteract the hackneyed image of the nurse as an acquiescent, powerless, and passive "handmaiden" in the work environment. Certainly, labor unions that are trying to expand and strengthen their position see nurses as a large, potentially strong, powerful group of professional people. However, nurses can also be vulnerable when they attempt to find fast solutions through this channel. Nursing must continue to foster a positive, powerful image and continue to organize. However, the question remains whether it is best done through means other than unions. Many promises by unions to potential members become idle after the contract is signed. Sometimes nurses find themselves in worse conditions than before they signed with a union.

Computer Technology

Experts are convinced that the development and implementation of computer technology enhances the management and delivery of health care and will continue to do so in the future. Nurses must become computer literate and more knowledgeable regarding computer use so that the profession will be in a proactive position to influence rather than be influenced by (reactive position) computer implementation.[22,58] An institution that does not invest in the costs of technology may become antiquated in a relatively short period of time. Nursing must be aware of this. Nursing simply cannot afford to lose this important opportunity to mainstream the profession.

The image of nursing can be influenced by the increase in computer technology. Documentation, care planning, "trending" of clients' laboratory values, quality management, committee work, and administrative records can be computerized. Nurses save time by accessing a computerized system. Nursing literature and daily developments in the nation and world affecting nursing can be accessed through the Internet on computer. This provides nurses with vast amounts of the most current knowledge available to impact practice and health care.

To acquire necessary clinical skills, nurses must become educated and proficient in computer technology. Hospital and nursing school libraries should maintain subscriptions to computer journals, especially those designed for nursing, so that nursing can keep abreast of current trends and knowledge. Nurses should develop their expertise in computers and participate in their institution's system. Nurses must be included in every aspect of the system, including the decision of which system to purchase, which software packages to acquire, and how programs should be used and implemented. Nurses can also enhance the image of nursing in the business community by marketing their expertise to leading computer-oriented companies. These companies need nursing input in the development, implementation, and marketing of health care packages. Nursing also needs the input and should seize this opportunity before someone unqualified speaks for the profession. The participants in our research survey were asked to reflect on how the explosion of technology affects the image of nursing.

Individuals who are interested in nursing are often people-oriented, as opposed to machine- or object-oriented. Consequently, the demand by technology to become involved can be unattractive and cause some not to enter the profession and others to leave it. The challenge is how to use the technology to enhance what nurses enjoy the most. This is one of the focuses to the newly created area of nursing research called *nursing informatics*.

Elimination of Internal Sexism

Halloran states, "It is ludicrous to think that the wholesale addition of men into nursing will make the nursing profession a better one."[17] It is suggested, however, that increasing the number of male nurses will make the profession a different one. Clients may experience a fuller range of professional interventions for their human responses.[30] The nursing profession and practice will also take on an improved public image by having more balance between men and women. In some occupations, the balance has already been improved with the admission of more women. Nursing will become balanced with the admission of more men.

Sexism—antifemale and antimale—must be eliminated from society and from the nursing profession. Sexism continues to harm and disrupt the professional image of nursing. It is time for each individual nurse, each nursing organization, and each nursing school to examine internal beliefs about each client, each member of the health care delivery system, and the general public. Nursing is not limited to one gender; it is a profession with room for all contributors of knowledge and client care delivery. Nursing is genderless, and its potential is equally as limitless.

Development of Internal Media Committees

Almost every health care institution and organization generates internal (in-house) media. Internal media, in the form of catalogs, brochures, newsletters, annual reports, program publicity, advertisements, films, and educational material, are important to the institution's relations but should be viewed as having equal importance to the image of nursing. Nursing, usually the largest group of employees in a health care facility or organization, often is not included in essential documents such as annual reports. This must end. Nurses are more cognizant of their role, their contributions, and what their services cost their clients than they were before; to be silent is unfair to consumers, as well as to nursing.

It is suggested that health care facilities have an internal media committee. Many have had such a group for years, though they have not always had the strong nursing representation that they should have. Nurses must become active in such committees and actively review all materials, paying special attention to the effect these materials have on the image of nursing. For example, the visual and verbal message of recruitment materials reflects the institution's beliefs and attitudes about nursing. Furthermore, means of communicating information that is generated should be examined and the following questions asked:

1. Is nursing included in all significant materials, including the annual report? If not, deficiencies should be noted and relevant recommendations forwarded to the appropriate people.
2. If nursing is referred to, are the references accurate and appropriate?
3. What pictures of nursing are included? Are nurses shown interacting with clients or are they shown following physicians?
4. What image of nursing is portrayed by the advertisements and recruitment of the institution? Do they illustrate nurses as cartoon characters or as professional, autonomous care providers?
5. Do the advertisements use professional language? Are there references to professional nursing practice?

Nursing must work with public relations (PR) committees to ensure that nursing is represented in a positive, professional manner to people and groups using the services of that facility or organization. Nursing can establish a PR liaison position to accomplish this. This PR liaison consultant can provide the PR department with accurate written materials and photographs when needed. Nursing must become proactive within the institution's marketing departments. To enhance the image of nursing, it is imperative that the profession receive acknowledgment for its many contributions to the health care delivery system.

Research indicates that internal marketing of a strong positive image of nursing improves nurses' self-perceptions, increases job satisfaction, and reduces turnover of nursing staff.[8]

External Media Committees

The mass media, print and broadcast, are the most pervasive influences on public attitudes and opinions in contemporary life. As previously discussed, this has not always been in the nursing profession's favor. Nursing has been and unfortunately still is misrepresented and often cast in an unfavorable light. Unfair portrayal of the nursing profession makes recruiting potential candidates difficult but also adversely affects the decision-making process of policymakers who decide what scarce resources the nursing profession will or will not have. One cannot expect the best individuals to aspire to a profession unless the members of that profession are consistently shown to be intelligent, competent, autonomous, and professional. External media campaigns are needed to profile the nurse of the 1990s.

What can nursing do to counteract and stop a seemingly pervasive negative image? Numerous nurses and groups of nurses suggest that external nursing media committees be organized within every hospital, every school of nursing, and at each level of every nursing organization. These media-watch groups must take responsibility for monitoring the media for all references to nursing. The groups must respond to the media for positive and negative referrals to nursing. It should be their responsibility to write letters to producers, television networks, and advertisers. Several groups already develop awards to give to journalists for accurate portrayals of nursing.

These media-watch groups can also offer technical assistance to the media. For instance, they can volunteer to review material before distribution, thus providing nursing with the opportunity to alter stereotypical and inappropriate images and replace them with positive and accurate portrayals.

Education

One area that has done little to unify the profession relates to educational levels. Entry into practice is remarkably controversial and divisive, both inside and outside the profession. Internally, the entry-into-practice question has divided the professional group. There are many educational differences among nurses; it is confusing for the public and often for future nurses themselves.[33] It may be inappropriate to lump all levels of education—nursing assistant (N.A.); licensed practical nurse (L.P.N.); diploma, associate degree (A.D.), and baccalaureate-prepared (B.S.N.) nurses—under one title, *nurse.*

It is becoming more and more common that a B.S.N. degree is the beginning educational level for entry into professional nursing practice. Donley suggested that nurses have let the lowest-common-denominator theory shape their present and forecast their future.[12] Persons trained for a period of time ranging from 3 months to 3 years should not be included under the same title. Otherwise it is detrimental to the profession. This has long been said, but no solid plan is yet in place to correct the problem as we face a new era in U.S. health care. Upward mobility programs for students and practitioners of technical and associate degree programs are at last making it possible for many nurses to earn the baccalaureate degree expeditiously.

Many well-educated, politically knowledgeable nurses practice in America in a variety of arenas. These nurses need to demand more attention within health care institutions. The public needs to be aware that endeavors such as nursing research exist and are important to patient health. Nursing is becoming more scholarly. It should be publicized as such.[7]

The 7 "C"s of Image Building

The foundation of nursing, its strategy for image building, and its vision for the future can be portrayed in the following seven Cs[3]:

To be:

- Compassionate—caring with one's whole being for another being
- Committed—giving of one's self for the total journey
- Collaborative—being open to share the responsibility, the rewards, and the criticism
- Creative—stepping out beyond the limits for the belief of what can be
- Change agent—willing to risk for opportunity, and learn through trial and error
- Competent—achieving the most with the least, relying on the knowledge of and belief in who you are

■ MARKETING

Historically, nursing, as a predominantly female occupation, has not perceived a need to market itself. This need has only recently become evident.[4] As the profession works to upgrade its image, marketing strategies are important. For an occupation to attain the status and power of a profession, the public must perceive it as such. The public can be informed by successful marketing. To change perceptions, a desirable image of nursing must be effectively and efficiently communicated. It is crucial that nursing services, nursing programs, and the nursing profession be strategically marketed to a wide range of audiences, to promote nursing excellence, and to project an achievement-oriented, professional image of nursing.

Stanton and Stanton suggest that the following important areas are critical in order to market nursing as a positive, powerful profession:[51]

1. Marketing of a more positive image
2. Marketing of the profession as a collective group
3. Marketing of nursing's unique role in health care delivery
4. Marketing of the profession in general to attract qualified candidates and to retain existing professionals
5. Internal marketing of the profession to ensure that all health care professionals and administrators realize how essential nursing is to the advancement and survival of health care institutions
6. Educating entry-level professionals to marketing strategies
7. Successful marketing of nursing products and services that have been used, tested, and evaluated
8. Conducting nurse-driven marketing research with networking and dissemination of results
9. Through research and education, evaluating marketing trends in relation to their effect on nursing

Before nursing can be marketed adequately, the profession must begin to "cost out" its services. It is impossible to market what one cannot measure in terms of dollars. Historically, nursing has been considered a cost center (in accounting terms) instead of a generator of revenue. The largest group of health care personnel is classified as "nursing." This may and usually does include all levels. To project a healthy internal, as well as public, image, it must be made obvious that consumers are getting what they are paying for. The health care organization must show that this group is not a liability but that it generates revenue/business. Nursing cannot afford to be a charitable, magnanimous profession. Health care is big business, with astronomical revenue turnover. To survive in such a highly competitive environment, nursing must also become profit oriented. With the current boom in home health care, new figures are arising regarding costs for service. Unfortunately, another establishment has learned that there is money to be made providing nursing care to people. Home health agencies are lauded by the public because of their meritorious goal of keeping people out of institutions. That praise comes along with significant profits for ownership of these agencies. The nurses working in this new system, however, are not reaping improved wages and benefits. In fact, in many cases, their wages are substandard to institutional nursing. Their biggest benefit may be increased independence.

DRESS FOR SUCCESS

In the business world there are dress-for-success rules. To be successful in business, one plays by the rules. Many nurses seem affronted by the dress-for-success prescription, but personal appearances certainly set the tone for the image portrayed. One's appearance must inspire confidence in one's ability, or the odds are automatically stacked against success. Dress is a powerful form of self-expression. Imagine being in a place where gum-chewing nurses wearing stained, drab uniforms are in charge of care. Regardless of how talented or how technically knowledgeable one is, professional image and credibility can be either strengthened or sabotaged by the image one projects to others. It is a simple rule, but one easily ignored or minimized by some members of all professional groups.

People derive images of nursing from a variety of sources, including personal acquaintances and contact during their own or someone else's illness or experience of nurses. Nurses need to present themselves as professionals to all with whom they come in contact. This is not limited to the client's room or nurses' station but includes the hallways, elevators, and cafeteria. It extends to the supermarket and social activities—any of the places where a nurse may come in contact with those who will influence the public or the media.

NURSING'S RESPONSIBILITIES FOR IMPROVING ITS OWN IMAGE

- Recognize that an image problem does exist and that each individual nurse has a responsibility to improve the profession's image.[52]
- Strengthen involvement in professional organizations; collectively, nursing is extremely powerful.
- Provide all nurses, including staff nurses, the opportunity to become salaried staff members rather than hourly wage earners.
- Become politically active and politically knowledgeable; nurses should run for office.[28]
- Document activities; it shifts the balance of power and allows nurses to state their case on a rational basis; documentation is also essential for third-party payment.[34,41]
- Write and submit feature stories on nurses for local media.[24,43]
- Demand that nurse authors be considered for editing health columns.[25,43]
- Provide technical assistance to the media.
- Provide ongoing public service announcements; focus attention on well-defined services created and controlled by nurses: case management, nurse-managed homeless centers, wellness centers, birthing centers.[14,38]
- Create public forums—"spend a day with a nurse."[14,47]
- Have nurses present educational talks at local shopping malls, public education series.
- Establish a speakers' bureau for local elementary, junior, and high schools.
- Improve the community image: volunteer for community-sponsored activities (Big Sister League, American Heart Association, AIDS Project).[9]
- Revise and update nursing career literature, especially books in schools and public libraries that introduce the profession to prospective nurses.[25,50]

- Improve and update health care texts to reflect the 1990s image of nursing.[50]
- Become more active as authors and as collaborators with established authors to receive accurate and quality literary portrayals.[27]
- Monitor the "get well" cards found in hospital gift shops and in local card shops; any adverse portrayal of nurses should be protested verbally and in writing.
- Establish schools of nursing as research and information centers for people experiencing critical health care issues, e.g., AIDS, homelessness.[38]
- Increase staff involvement in scholarly activities such as research.
- Never allow the nursing profession to be portrayed as physicians' handmaidens; instead insist that nurses be portrayed as physicians' peers.
- Be self-confident; self-confident behavior commands respect.[20]
- Be positive; complaining does not create a good impression and rarely solves any problems.[20]
- Share the positive aspects of the nursing profession with others.[16]
- Learn to describe nursing responsibilities in clear, nontechnical terms.[11,46]
- Continue to develop alternative nursing education programs designed for adult-learner nurses needing to advance their education.[46]
- Increase visibility; make sure that clients and their families know that the nursing staff is responsible for 24-hour care.[44]

NURSING'S IMAGE IS YOU

Since 1979 nurses have risen two places in the prestige ranking, according to a 1994 public opinion pole. Nurses are ranked third, behind engineers and physicians.[5] Over the course of the past two decades, and as a means of continuing this trend toward the year 2000, the public has perceived nurses less as handmaidens and more as professionals who are caring and knowledgeable individuals. This opinion has evolved not because of the media, but as a result of firsthand visits to hospitals and physician's offices. Nurses must continue to build on the existing strong foundation of clinical knowledge. Advancing this foundation will be implemented through effective public relations campaigns and built on the advancing level of educational preparation and the expanded complexity of functions and responsibilities performed by nurses.

Remember—nursing's image is you.

APPROACHING THE MILLENNIUM

As the year 2000 approaches, nursing is presented with one of the greatest crossroads for enhancing its image. Never before have we had to set the pace for new challenges, new opportunities, and new horizons. Never before have we faced the birth of a new era to advance and renew our image and to make a substantial difference for nursing, for ourselves, and for humanity. The vision is in our hands, and the door is wide open.

The value of seeking and enhancing leadership potential on the threshold of a bright, exciting image challenges our future in many ways. By incorporating new horizons, building new opportunities, and living new dreams, the following lights are available to illuminate our paths if we just seek them.

- **N**etwork with each other.

  Nurses are called to network with each other, with professional organizations, and with the health care community on a local, statewide, national, and internal basis for the enhancement of our image and the betterment of care.
- **E**ncourage the growth of partnership.

  The enrichment of our nursing image can be broadened as we integrate our partnerships with consumer payers and providers for the benefit of a cost-effective, integrated, broad-based, and reliable health care system.
- **W**atch carefully for the opportunity to expand educational endeavors in all phases of society.

  The profession of nursing has the challenge of expanding our educational horizons through advanced curriculum designs; strategic applied learning dimensions; political, economic, and business integration; mentoring opportunities; and entrepreneurial forecasting.
- **H**old fast to the highest standards possible and all greatest achievement in practice.

  Nurses are challenged to design, to create, and to implement the best and most appropriate practices for the achievement of quality care and education.
- **O**rganize the platform for collaboration among all facets of nursing.

  The leadership dynamics in nursing can be developed and integrated in conjunction with nursing organizations, institutions, corporations, and policy leaders.
- **R**esearch a plan for rewarding, acknowledging, and sharing the best of nursing.

  Recognizing the best in nursing is valuable in enhancing the image of nursing. To implement this concept, a plan is in order to recognize and reward all innovations in nursing, all scientific advancements, and social and community achievements in tandem with nursing, community, and political leaders.
- **I**nstitute a media means through web sites or the written word to share innovative tools, models, and research ideas.

  The enhancement of the nursing image can be documented, expanded, and publicized through various means of mass media.
- **Z**eal, reflection, motion, and enthusiasm: with these reach out to honor, credit, and celebrate one another's accomplishments.

  The value of sharing achievement and honor improves both the individual and the global image of nursing. Acknowledgment of all accomplishments within nursing through verbal presentations, physical tributes, and lasting memories are essential to sustaining an advanced and enhanced image.
- **O**pen forms of learning, sharing, and displaying innovations through conferences, gatherings, and open dialogue.

  Bringing leaders together, representing all dimensions of learning and growth; culture and ethnicity; status; and influences will enhance knowledge, sharing, and growth exchange.

- **N**egotiate ways by which all standards and achievements of excellence can be expanded and extended to all nurses.

  In this age of expansive media expansion, information and knowledge research and models can be synthesized and disseminated internationally.
- **S**pread nursing education and experience among all institutions and organizations.

  Beginning at the baccalaureate level, nursing education, faculty development, and research can be integrated in collaboration with other institutions and organizations.

CRITICAL THINKING *Activities*

1. **Provide specific examples of ways in which the image of nursing is positively or negatively influenced: for example, T-shirts with captions.**
2. **Discuss examples and then provide approaches and actions that the nurse can take when negative images are portrayed in written media, on television, and elsewhere.**
3. **List factors about "appearance" that nurses should consider when "on the job" and "off the job" to enhance public perception of nursing's status/image.**
4. **Describe a well-dressed, well-educated nurse who portrays the optimal image to others.**
5. **Describe how you would like the profession of nursing to be perceived by society, and what will be necessary to achieve that level. Compare your description with those of several of your friends or classmates.**

References

1. Alspach JG: Making an impact, *Critical Care Nurse* 9(10):2, 1989.
2. Alvarez AR: Selected characteristics of male registered nurses in New Jersey, *Nurs Forum* 21(4):166, 1984.
3. American Association of Critical Care Nurses: *Heart Lung* 19(3):31A-39A, 1990.
4. Auttonberry DS: The role of the master's-prepared nurse in marketing, *Nurs Manage* 19(9):40, 1988.
5. Begany T: Your image is brighter than ever, *RN* 59 (10):30-31, 1994.
6. Bille DA: The nurse's image—a mirror of the self, *Today's O.R. Nurse* 9(8):7, 1987.
7. Bower FL: Image making for nursing, *Calif Nurs Rev* 11(3): 10,29, 1989.
8. Bream TL and others: Beyond the ordinary nursing image. . . . *Nurs Manage* 23(12):44, 1992.
9. Curran CR: Effective utilization of the media. In McCloskey JC, Grace HK, eds: *Current issues in nursing,* ed 2, Palo Alto, 1985, Blackwell Scientific.
10. Curran CR: Shaping an image of competence and caring, *Nurs Health Care* 6(7):370, 1985.
11. Dickson GI: Nursing images and the nursing profession, *Imprint* 39(5):56, 1992.

12. Donley SR: Strategies for changing nursing's image. In McCloskey JC, Grace HK, eds: *Current issues in nursing,* ed 2, Palo Alto, 1985, Blackwell Scientific.
13. Deleted in proofs.
14. Evan D and others: A district takes action, *Am J Nurs* 83(1):52, 1983.
15. Fagin C, Diers D: Nursing as a metaphor, *N Engl J Med* 309(2) (1983):116.
16. Gallagher D: Promoting a positive nursing image, *Imprint* 36(5):5, 1989.
17. Halloran EJ: Men in nursing. In McCloskey JC, Grace HK, eds: *Current issues in nursing,* ed 2, Palo Alto, 1985, Blackwell Scientific.
18. Deleted in proofs.
19. Holleran C: Nursing beyond national boundaries: the 21st century, *Nurs Outlook* 36(2):72, 1988.
20. Hull M: Your nursing image: tending the flame, *Nursing 93* 23(5):116, 1993.
21. Jerwekh J, Clabom JC: *Nursing today: transition and trends,* Philadelphia, 1997, Saunders.
22. Johnson-Hofer P, Karasik S: Learning about computers, *Nurs Outlook* 36(6):293, 1988.
23. Kalisch BJ, Kalisch PA: Anatomy of the image of the nurse: dissonant and ideal models. In Williams C, ed: *Image making in nursing,* Kansas City, MO, 1983, American Nurses Association.
24. Kalisch BJ, Kalisch PA: Communicating clinical nursing issues throughout the newspaper, *Nurs Research* 30(3):132, 1981.
25. Kalisch BJ, Kalisch PA: Improving the image of nursing, *Am J Nurs* 83(1):48, 1983.
26. Kalisch BJ, Kalisch PA: Nurses on prime time television, *Am J Nurs* 82(2):264, 1982.
27. Kalisch BJ, Kalisch PA: The image of nurses in novels, *Am J Nurs* 82(8):1220, 1982.
28. Kelly LS: Agenda for tomorrow, *Nurs Outlook* 35(5):215, 1987.
29. Kelly LY: *Dimensions of professional nursing,* 1991, Pergamon Press.
30. Kus RJ: A challenge to nursing: eliminating anti-male sexism in American society. In McCloskey JC, Grace HK, eds: *Current issues in nursing,* ed 2, Palo Alto, 1985, Blackwell Scientific.
31. London F: Should men be actively recruited into nursing? *Nurs Admin Q* 12(1):75, 1987.
32. MacRae J: Nightingale's spiritual philosophy and its significance for modern nursing, *Image* 27(1):8-10, 1995.
33. Martin E: The prestige of today's nurse, *Nurs Manage* 20(3):80B, 1989.
34. Maxson-Ladage W: What image do you display? *A D Nurse* 3(2):26, 1988.
35. Mendez D, Louis M: College students' image of nursing as a career choice, *J Nurs Ed* 30(7):311, 1996.
36. Miller T: Men in nursing, *Calif Nurs Rev* 11(2) (1989):10.
37. Nauright L: Politics and power: a new look at Florence Nightingale, *Nurs Forum* 21(1):5, 1984.
38. Naylor MD, Sherman MB: Nurses for the future: wanted—the best and the brightest, *Am J Nurs* 87(12):1601, 1987.
39. O'Brien P: All a woman's life can bring: the domestic roots of nursing in Philadelphia: 1830-1885, *Nurs Res* 36(1):12, 1987.
40. Palmer IS: Origin of education for nurses, *Nurs Forum* 22(3):102, 1985.
41. Perry J: Creating our own image, *New Zealand Nurs J* 80(2):10, 1987.
42. Deleted in proofs.

43. Porter BJ and others: Enhancing the image of nursing, *J Nurs Admin* 19(2):36, 1989.
44. Reishstein J: Let's make nursing the visible profession, *Nursing '91* 21(11):148, 1991.
45. Reverby S: A caring dilemma: womanhood and nursing in historical perspective, *Nurs Research* 36(1):5, 1987.
46. Salvage J: Selling ourselves, *Nurs Times* 6(85):24, 1989.
47. Scherer P: When every day is Saturday: the shortage, *Am J Nurs* 87(10):1284, 1987.
48. Shiffer SW: California men in nursing, *Calif Nurs Rev* 11(2):6, 1989.
49. Sinetar M: *Do what you love, the money will follow: discovering your right livelihood,* New York, 1987, Dell.
50. Smith MK, Smith MC: What high school texts say about nursing, *Nurs Outlook* 37(1):28, 1989.
51. Stanton M, Stanton GW: Marketing nursing: a model for success, *Nurs Manage* 19(9):36, 1988.
52. Stewart-Amidei C: From bedpan to . . . ? *J Neurosci Nurs* 20(3):139, 1988.
53. Strasen L: Self-concept: improving the image of nursing, *J Nurs Admin* 19(1):4, 1989.
54. Tracy, B. *The psychology of achievement.* Chicago: Nightingale-Conant, 1984.
55. Vann DS: Essay on the title "professional nurses," *Nurs Forum* 23(2):69, 1987.
56. Deleted in proofs.
57. Zalar MK, Suter WN: Studying the image of nursing, *Calif Nurs Rev* 83(7):2, 1987.
58. Zeilstroff RD: Cost-effectiveness of computerization in nursing practice and administration. In McCloskey JC, Grace HK, eds: *Current issues in nursing,* ed 2, Palo Alto, 1985, Blackwell Scientific.
59. Deleted in proofs.

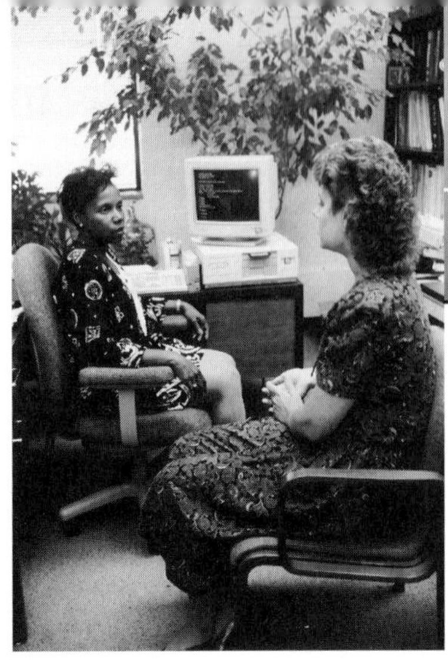

CHAPTER 16

Nursing as a Career

Grace L. Deloughery

OBJECTIVES After completing this chapter the reader should be able to:

- **Discuss some of the major socioeconomic dynamics that affect the nursing profession today**
- **List at least two pathways that nurses can utilize to attain the baccalaureate and higher degrees**
- **Discuss current trends in the employment of nurses**
- **List ways in which a nurse can personally help improve the status of both the profession and herself**
- **Understand steps to take when seeking a job**

For the nurse who is preparing to work in the health care field today, some complicated issues must be understood and reconciled to survive, not to mention be successful (survival is not synonymous with success). Funds for health care are extremely competitive, traditional health care organizations are toppling all around, and new health care–providing monsters are being created. Some would find it more comfortable not to look at the unpleasantness of the situation. The typical caring nurse would rather be in the center of alleviating human suffering, helping the elderly to live more fully, assist with the healing of human bodies after highly technical surgeries, keeping families together in their homes, and sharing the joy of new life made possible by recent scientific discoveries. The nurse has to come to terms with these and other highly complex and difficult issues before embarking on nursing as a career.

■ THE NURSING PROFESSION

The emphasis of nursing is on prevention of disease and health promotion, restoration, and maintenance. Humankind has approached healing from two distinct perspectives, and these must be understood if the nurse is to function professionally. First, people have sought healing through science and technology. If this approach is followed exclusively, only the physical components of disease are treated. This is not always successful, as demonstrated by a self-abusive or drug-dependent person who receives treatment only for his physical problems; if deeper causes of his behavior are not dealt with, then the problems will just recur. Persons through the ages have also sought healing through spiritual and psychologic reconciliation. At the extreme, followers of this approach believe that all disease ultimately has roots in the mind and, therefore, healing must be effected through mental influence and/or prayer. Examples of this approach are the teachings of Mary Baker Eddy and the tenets of the Church of Christ, Scientist, which she founded. Currently the extremes in schools of thought have moderated, causing the pendulum to stabilize in a more central position.

A synthesis of various approaches and ways of thinking must be achieved. Until then the nurse will be limited in her ability to effect sustained positive change. Literature contains a vast amount of theory and background on various schools of thought and approaches to change. The assimilation of this information into a useful framework is one of the goals of nursing education.

Vast changes are taking place in the health care industry today. Some geographic areas of the country have a surplus of physicians, especially the urban centers. Because of this, admissions to medical schools today are being limited in a manner somewhat similar to that of schools of nursing 10 years ago. There are unfilled places for practitioners in the less desirable chairs while the surplus exists. One needs only peruse the "help wanted" columns of newspapers of rural and central-city areas to find vacancies for "physician extenders," "physician substitutes," or physician assistants.

Nurses may not happily accept the role of "physician extenders" as their contribution for two reasons. First, the distinction between the medical and nursing professions is becoming increasingly blurred. Second, some nurses contend that the distinction was artificially drawn in the first place. In 1992 former U.S. Surgeon General C. Everett Koop predicted that 50% of physicians would soon be women. The number of women in medicine has almost doubled in 20 years (Table 16-1).

Generally speaking, women in any field who find themselves uncomfortable will give up that field. Practically speaking, it may fall on the nurse to help her female counterpart in medicine find her place. As primary caregivers, nurses can thus logically be the factor that makes the team—not as adjuncts, but as partners.[12] To be a part of this development challenges new graduates and practitioners of both professions. Unfortunately, professional partnership in a true sense does not appear in the current forecasts of health care reform and contrasts with the existing model of health care in America.

Dr. Melvin Konner, author of *Medicine at the Crossroads: The Crisis in Health Care,* suggests that an artificial health system has been created in which the human side of care is left to nurses, chaplains, psychologists, and social workers. The role of the physician, according to him, is to process people through automatic stages of diagnosis and treatment as quickly and efficiently as possible. Nurses, then, are given the role of ensuring that clients do not get scared to death in hospitals, and physicians then can be "just a very high-grade technician, a sort of physiological

TABLE 16-1

Percent of Female Workers in Selected Occupations, 1975-1994

	Women as percentage of total employed		
Occupation	**1975**	**1985**	**1994**
Airline pilot	—	2.6	2.6
Auto mechanic	0.5	0.6	1.0
Bartender	35.2	47.9	55.1
Bus driver	37.7	49.2	47.0
Cab driver, chauffeur	8.7	10.9	10.3
Carpenter	0.6	1.2	1.0
Child care worker	98.4	96.1	97.3
Computer programmer	25.6	34.3	29.3
Computer systems analyst	14.8	28.0	31.4
Data entry keyer	92.8	90.7	83.8
Data processing equipment repairer	1.8	10.4	18.0
Dentist	1.8	6.5	13.3
Dental assistant	100.0	99.0	96.6
Economist	13.1	34.5	47.4
Editor, reporter	44.6	51.7	48.8
Elementary school teacher	85.4	84.0	85.6
Garage, gas station attendant	4.7	6.8	5.2
Lawyer, judge	7.1	18.2	24.8
Librarian	81.1	87.0	84.1
Mail carrier (Postal Service)	8.7	17.2	34.0
Office machine repairer	1.7	5.7	2.1
Physician	13.0	17.2	22.3
Registered nurse	97.0	95.1	93.8
Social worker	60.8	66.7	69.3
Teachers, college and university	31.1	35.2	42.5
Telephone installer, repairer	4.8	12.8	16.8
Telephone operator	93.3	88.8	88.8
Waiter/waitress	91.1	84.0	78.6
Welder	4.4	4.8	4.4

From U.S. Department of Labor, Bureau of Labor Statistics, *Employment and Earnings* (monthly), January issues.

engineer, leaving the human dimension to other professionals."[10] The intent is to decrease the stress on physicians, but Konner proposes that this does not work. Seemingly absent from medicine is a culture of humans dealing with humans on a person-to-person basis. When there is teamwork between client and professional, suspicion and misunderstanding melt, and blame and lawsuits also decrease in frequency.

Changing Times

Nurses with advanced training and education are accepting increasing responsibility. In the operating room a surgeon may find it more helpful to call for assistance from an R.N. than to have a second physician work with him or her. Depending on what the chief surgeon allows, the R.N. may prepare the client, sew up incisions, and perform other assistant tasks; the difference between the R.N. assistant and the second physician is simply that R.N.s do not perform surgery. However, after the

Box 16-1 Wage Gap between Men and Women

On average, U.S. women earn 70.6 cents for every dollar earned by men. In most but not all job categories, women make significantly less than male workers do. The nursing profession is among the exceptions.

Average Pay in Several Occupations	Female	Male
Accounting	$ 26,936	$ 36,813
Internist (physician)	90,916	117,251
Orthopedic surgeon	152,841	286,654
Lawyers (average)	47,684	61,100
Mechanics and repair workers	27,196	25,792
Professor (private college/university)	59,970	70,180
Registered nurses	34,476	32,916

From Harris D: Does your pay measure up? *Working Woman*: 26-33, Jan 1994.

surgery the nurse can bill for services and receive third-party payment (be reimbursed by insurers). It is also becoming ever more common for advanced practice nurses to write prescriptions, as well as deliver babies (nurse-midwives), administer anesthesia (nurse anesthetists), and operate clinics (nurse practitioners). The regulations governing prescriptive privileges varies with state law; see State Board of Nursing (Chapter 9).

In today's information-based society, knowledge is often considered as powerful as capital. Physicians have been aware of the power of their knowledge for centuries. Now, however, that power is seriously threatened, and their attempts to retain control are seriously threatening to the nursing profession. This is most apparent in decisions made by hospitals and large medical conglomerates. Hospitals are controlled to a large extent by the physicians who work there. It is natural that physicians want the power associated with their medical knowledge to be solely theirs.

For this reason hospitals promote the training and hiring of L.P.N.s, nurses with 2-year degrees, and other ancillary staff. Perhaps physicians encourage this because such personnel are less threatening to their position, cheaper to train, and can be paid less. Leaders in nursing and the professional organizations representing nurses claim that hiring nurses with L.P.N. licenses or 2-year degrees is detrimental to the profession. Part of the reasoning behind this contention is that until nurses gain a level of expertise comparable to physicians, they must be satisfied with making minor decisions, earning lower wages, and holding lower status. Currently nurses earn roughly one quarter the salaries of physicians (Box 16-1). Of course, alternately, for many people seeking to enter the nursing profession, 2-year or shorter programs provide a more accessible approach to employment and can be used as a foundation for further education.

Nurses' roles at all levels are expanding. As this happens, nurses are beginning to perform tasks that have been jealously guarded by physicians for centuries. Simultaneously, the influence of physicians is being threatened as a result of several reasons: democratization of information, increasing use of alternative medicine (discussed in Chapter 1), and looming health care reform legislation.

New technology is democratizing medical knowledge. Now anyone can use a computer with a modem to access more information on any medical topic than the average physician ever reads. Further, computer and media sources report medical news before the physician even has a chance to read professional journals. This trend will probably continue and has the potential for being the source of increasing tension between the nursing and medical professions.

In spite of the development of various categories of ancillary personnel, a shortage of nurses continues to exist in some areas of the country, although the crisis of a few years ago has abated. Outside the larger cities it is possible to fill most positions and pay less than the norm for nurses. This is true in smaller cities of the Midwest, such as Rochester, Minnesota, and LaCrosse, Wisconsin. Technical schools produce graduates who remain in the area and work for lesser wages. However, cities not far away, such as Minneapolis-St. Paul, Minnesota, and Madison, Wisconsin, have temporary periods of nursing shortage, and their salaries are competitive with other large cities.[17]

As the United States is experiencing health care reform, nurses with advanced degrees or specialized certification are being given more responsibility. Studies have repeatedly shown that advanced practice nurses can perform 60% to 80% of all primary care just as well as physicians at a lower cost.[7] The next question might be whether advanced practice nurses are content to perform what was formerly the domain of well-paid physicians while earning less money. Keep in mind that physicians and their professional organizations are lobbying strongly to protect their own interests; nurses must likewise join forces to ensure that they will receive fair compensation.

In some states nurses continue to be excluded from receiving reimbursement from Medicare and Medicaid, writing prescriptions, and admitting clients to hospitals. Nurses and other alternative practitioners are repeatedly blocked from obtaining such authority because of the strong physician lobby, the weak nursing lobby, and an establishment that requires major effort to facilitate change.

Striving for Equality

Seeking to be in control of one's destiny makes for a rude awakening when one learns that what was hoped differs from reality. This has been so for many nurses.

Nurses, who have been predominantly women for over a century, have historically been underpaid for the work they perform. From medieval Europe to today, nurses have been the victims of "good business," which used them as cheap labor through several tactics: utilizing unpaid female members of religious orders, student nurses, less-skilled L.P.N.s, and nurses' aides when professional nursing care was required, and hiring nurses for less than male counterparts requiring similar skills. A recent salary survey indicates that the situation is not changing favorably for women going into nursing today (Table 16-2). The division of labor in hospitals was by sex-defined roles in the 1970s and continues as a form of systemic gender discrimination.[16]

Studies have shown that graduates of health professional programs tend to settle near where they are trained. For example, in an area where two private health care systems have monopolized the scene, there is now a mad scramble for ways to maintain "heap" manpower and have a surplus of workers to choose from. With need for cost-cutting and survival a reality, recently these two institutions have identified three other institutions (a private college with a school of nursing, a

TABLE 16-2

Average Annual Salaries of Registered Nurses

	1995[21]	1996[22]	1997[23]
Female	$35,776	$35,360	$36,036
Male	$35,256	$36,868	$37,180

branch of the university located in the area, and the area vocational-technical school) to form a consortium.[18] To fund this gigantic project they are applying for millions of state funds and conducting a major fund-raising drive. The goal is to provide a place where students in more than a dozen separate allied health fields "will learn and train."[18] The distinction made here is one between education and training. One implies independent thinking and decision making, and the other rote memory and behaviors.

From time to time attempts have been made to correct the inequality of reimbursement of nurses, but compensation for nursing continues to lag. The reason is not that women do not desire to receive equal pay for equal work, but rather that historically the inequality has existed and women as nurses accepted what came their way. Common strategies used by employers are making full-time positions part-time, lessening the number of hours available, capping salaries, putting people on unrequested leave, not recognizing stress-induced illnesses, and not being accommodating to working mothers (particularly single parents). All of these dynamics serve to lessen the nurse's leverage for social standing and perpetuate economic insecurity.

One reason that "women's work" has not commanded equality in pay for work done is that the nature of the work has complex facets such as human relation skills, emotional loading, balancing competing priorities, and having responsibilities for outcomes without commensurate authority to ensure completion.[16] Traditionally nursing has been viewed as having intrinsically female qualities rather than job-related qualities. It seems that nursing still has to prove its economic value.

As women move more competitively in the workforce with men, the problems that are common to women are beginning to parallel those of men. Even though the profession of nursing is still predominantly staffed by women, the stressors that are present in the field and in the surrounding environment continue to escalate in intensity. Concerns about unemployment, upward mobility, keeping up with the fast life of today, and the overall socioeconomic and political factors touch the lives of men and women alike. Nursing, as a part of the rapidly changing health care scene, is in the thick of the battle for its share of the potential trophies. An example of what this is doing to women is shown in the statistics: coronary heart disease is now the leading killer of both men and women in the United States, whereas it previously was the leading killer only of men.[20]

Professional job satisfaction is important to the nurse entering and remaining in the profession. Focus of control (perception of autonomy) has been identified as a vital ingredient in job satisfaction, and stress seems to be the major reason for dissatisfaction and burnout, especially in intensive care units. These two factors may in fact be appropriately linked.

Statistics can be deceiving, but it appears that the percentage of male to female nurses continues to increase; men made up 8.2% of nurses in 1989.[11] Men choosing nursing do so for various reasons. Many choose nursing to improve their economic and social status. Some use the process as a means toward upward movement into hospital administration, medicine, or specialty areas in nursing such as anesthesia, psychiatric nursing, and emergency and acute care. In contrast, women often enter specialties such as pediatrics, public health, medical-surgical nursing, and obstetrics. A previous study found that men entering nursing tended to be older, married, and to have previous work experience, often in health-related areas. Contemporary men entering nursing are more apt to be single. Though older and with previous health care employment, they are likely to go into 2-year programs and plan a career of upward mobility, having a means of earning a living as they move ahead. Men cite job security, career opportunity, and job flexibility as major reasons for entering nursing. Although it is valuable to recruit men and accept them solely for their interest, they could make major contributions in a practice setting traditionally associated with female nurses. This might be advantageous to women, who have typically been in a disadvantaged situation. Alternatively, it has also been proposed that recruiting more men into nursing may, in reality, *not* improve the lot of women in nursing.[14] The reason is that many men use nursing only as a stepping-stone to the career of their choice (not nursing) and really do not make efforts to elevate the status of the nurses they leave behind as they embark on their own futures.

Arriving at definite figures regarding the nursing profession is made difficult because of the various levels of preparation and uncertainty in defining who exactly is a nurse. The American Assembly for Men in Nursing, for example, reported in their Fall 1993 issue of *Inter Action* that 4% of the total number of registered nurses are male. The figure previously cited (8%) was probably arrived at by using a much broader definition of *nurse*.

The study by Blegen[2] of nurses' work satisfaction and its variables found no significant correlation between work satisfaction and pay. However, this does not mean that pay is unimportant to nurses. It may mean that nurses can like what they are doing and simply cut their standard of living or deal with the pay aspect in some other manner. Nurses may well tend to separate their job satisfaction from their pay. As a result, their clients are beneficiaries of an outwardly happy person, but the worry over financial affairs eats away silently at the nurse. Many nurses are single parents and have sincere concerns over money matters, yet they enjoy their work so much that they tolerate the stress of financial problems. It is likely that nurses as a whole have historically been very subtly indoctrinated to give freely of themselves and never grumble for financial rewards.

It is one thing to be a wide-eyed senior in high school making applications to colleges and then visiting before making a decision. It is another to get settled into one that had great appeal only to find that it mass-produces graduates for an employer or group of employers who are waiting to exploit them. This may paint a dismal picture of the situation, but I hope that putting this possibility before the reader in such a manner will erase the naiveté of the nurse-to-be.

Political Action

A number of concerns today can move nurses into political involvement. One could be a political activist without campaigning for public office. Many issues should be of political concern to each nurse both as a professional and as an American citizen.

Nurses moving into politics have been frustrated for decades by those contemporary feminists competing with them for political attention by seeking integration or assimilation into stereotypically male-dominated fields such as medicine, law, and engineering. These women resisted the establishment of ties with traditionally female groups. The issues related to sexism (such as pay equity and comparable worth, status, power, control, health, and social welfare benefits) cut across all occupations and social strata. As women began to recognize these dynamics, they become more determined; this serves as a catalyst to women from many groups to become active as a powerful new political force.

It is all too well known in American history that it is often the wife of the elected political official who actually is the moving force "behind her man." I apologize for bringing Hillary Rodham Clinton into this discussion, but it is only appropriate to ask whether this dynamic is not in fact true today. Women are entering the political world in ever-increasing numbers. The more they stick together and vigorously pursue their goals, the greater the chances of their success. Some are seated in Congress, and others at various state and local levels of government. Yet I would like to point out that not one woman is among the 20 best paid mayors in this country.[24]

One nurse—Eddie Bernice Johnson (D-Texas)—was elected to Congress in 1992.[4] Other nurses have run for state offices, and even though they have not been successful, they have greatly increased the visibility of nurses. In 1993, 20% of state legislators, 16.9% of U.S. senators, and 21.7% of U.S. representatives were women, and these percentages have not changed significantly.[25]

Because women perceive a multitude of issues differently than their male counterparts, they are influencing the definition of bills being introduced and passed. Their focus tends more toward addressing traditionally female concerns such as safety, domestic violence, and child care legislation. In a similar manner, nurses understand health issues differently than other groups, and they can be in the forefront when designing national health care policy.

Nurses who do not enter public office still have other ways of becoming involved. For instance, nurses collectively can have a powerful voice. Of the 2.5 million registered nurses in the United States, 82.7% are actively employed in nursing, including more than 100,000 with advanced degrees, compared with 615,00 actively employed physicians.[7] Nurses make up a significant segment of the voter population and have the potential for making significant changes in the health care system if they act collectively. It behooves each nurse to explore what she is doing to make significant changes in the health care system, thereby improving the status of care for herself, her family, and her community.

Nurses have been introduced to the potential of labor negotiations and union memberships. Strikes have hit some of the largest hospitals in the country during the last decades. Traditionally it has been the blue-collar worker groups that have been unionized but, as discontent grows among nursing staffs (and even physicians in certain situations), the potential of unions gaining power grows. The most common reasons that nurses walk off the job have been low wages, unfair working conditions, and shortage of nursing staff that put client safety in jeopardy. Historically nurse students were taught that striking was not ethical, the basic reason being that it signified the abandonment of clients who need care. However, an updated outlook on this dilemma has been raised before the audience of fellow nurses.[8] The American Nurses Association (ANA) Code of Ethics has been cited as a responsibility of the nurse who practices the profession to put forth efforts to maintain conditions of employment conducive to high-quality nursing care. Strikes then should be viewed as a last resort, but when there seems no way to resolve situations that bring about increased client risk it may be considered justified and the professional thing to do.

In response to proposals for a national health insurance program, nurses generally favor basic coverage, rather than having 100% of costs covered by a health insurance plan. Studies have suggested that nurses are concerned about waste in the health care system, so if waste is minimized, costs will naturally be less of an issue. For this reason, nurses have expressed less concern about health care costs than accessibility to basic coverage. These commonalities occur in spite of the diverse political persuasions of nurses: one study has identified that one third of nurses classify themselves as Democrats, one third as Republicans, and the remaining one third as independents.[3]

ANA, the nation's largest nurses' organization, has urged the adoption of a "health model" that promotes wellness and prevention rather than the traditional "clinical model" with its focus on expensive acute and high-technology treatments. Other nursing-related organizations in North America and around the globe support such a change in emphasis. A giant effort still to come is the joining of various fragmented forces to form a strong, united change movement working unrelentingly toward the goal of prevention and wellness.

On the Front Lines

Nurses have always found themselves in some situations where health and safety were not assured. War and epidemics serve as examples. The risk of contracting the HIV virus for nurses in emergency rooms and operating rooms is of current and real concern. With nurses' increased investment in professional education, increased responsibility and liability, and high risks to their own life and health should come salary and benefits that are commensurate.

It is hoped that one field learns from the mistakes of others. Athletics serves as an example of a field in which attempts to employ affirmative action programs many times had the outcome of destroying opportunities for the predominantly male programs without expanding them for women. Thus it is hoped that efforts made to expand opportunities for persons entering and working in the predominantly female field of nursing will truly reap the positive results of affirmative action and expanding possibilities that will truly assist them in their search for fairness and equality.[19]

Humanitarian aid. Nurses seeking to use their knowledge and abilities to help people in other parts of the world might consider obtaining experience in providing humanitarian aid abroad. Nurses working in war-torn and underdeveloped coun-

Box 16-2 AIDS/HIV Infections Reported in 1993 Through September in the U.S., Listed by Occupation

Occupation	Documented occupational transmissions	Possible occupational transmissions
Dental worker, dentist	—	6
Embalmer, morgue technician	—	3
Emergency medical technician/paramedic	—	8
Health aid/attendant	1	9
Housekeeper/attendant	1	6
Laboratory technician, clinical	15	14
Laboratory technician, nonclinical	1	1
Nurse	13	15
Physician, nonsurgical	5	8
Physician, surgical	—	2
Respiratory therapist	1	2
Technician, dialysis	1	1
Technician, surgical	1	1
Technician/therapist, other than those listed above	—	3

From Haddad A: Ethics in action: contract negotiations at your hospital, *RN* 60(5):17-19, 1997.

tries can relate multitudinous examples. A hospital that is modern and well-stocked can be destroyed in a moment's time, riddled by mortars and gunfire so that only a small portion or none of it can be used for its intended purpose. When electricity and water supplies are cut off, so is the mission of the hospital. The United Nations does provide food for staff and clients. Life-saving surgery can be accomplished even with a minimum of resources and, often, outdated drugs. A period of experience in such a setting makes the nurse realize she is in a vast, unexplored territory. It provides satisfaction to an exhausted staff nurse to do whatever can be done without worrying about conventional professional boundaries and jealousies that abound in the "calm" of peacetime, well-equipped, functioning hospitals or clinics.

One of the sad realities of working in underdeveloped regions of the world is the need to make very hard choices. For instance, it has been verified that HIV can be transmitted to infants through breast-feeding. Yet infants in some countries are exposed to still greater health risks from contamination associated with bottle-feeding, even when the mother is HIV-seropositive. Consequently, health officials are promoting breast-feeding in underdeveloped countries, even for mothers infected with HIV.[6]

Communicable diseases. The ideal image of nursing portrays nurses as giving their all for the benefit and comfort of their clients. At times this puts them at personal risk. As a result of nurses performing much of the "dirty work" in critical care and surgical settings, nurses and clinical laboratory technicians have a much higher risk of contracting AIDS than other health care professionals. One can wonder how it is that surgical physicians had no documented HIV transmissions listed (Box 16-2).

In light of these statistics, you must realize that *you* may ultimately pay for insufficient precautions. Always keeping a clear head and abiding by standard safeguards is a part of professionalism. Never knowingly put yourself or others at risk. It may seem irrational in light of all the attention on AIDS, but flagrantly unsafe practices still occur. Almost every nurse in practice today could give you at least one example she has witnessed of health care providers, in either rural or urban settings, who break sound infection control practices. Such carelessness only potentiates exposure to all kinds of infectious agents, including hepatitis B virus (HBV) and HIV.

The Lifestyle of a Nurse

As nurses expand their capabilities, their lives may also become more complicated. Odd work hours and long shifts place extra stresses on marriage and play a part in the comparatively high divorce rate among nurses. Single nurses (especially those employed in large institutions) may have little social life and few opportunities to refresh themselves by enjoying nature's bountiful beauty. Pressures on the job and access to medications are contributing factors in the relatively frequent incidences of chemical dependency among nurses. Various sources estimate that between 7% and 10% of nurses will be chemically dependent at some point in their career, compared to the 5% of the general public who face addiction. Those who are aware of such risks and can better handle stress have a better chance of avoiding problems.

Women make up roughly 85% to 90% of undergraduate nursing students at many schools and also constitute a majority of practicing nurses. As nurses they have unique sources of stress. Women in the workforce generally have a somewhat altered set of priorities from those of men—women generally try harder to balance work and family life. All married nurses must find a suitable balance between stresses and satisfactions in both areas to survive and thrive personally and professionally. Female nurses, however, feel a greater responsibility for their personal life responsibilities and are less apt to abandon family life for the job, as their male counterparts more typically do. One might therefore cautiously draw a generalized difference between women and men in the health care field.

To go into nursing is to acknowledge that professional activities involved require around-the-clock, everyday attention. To dream of a 9-to-5 job with weekends off is an unrealistic expectation if the reason for going into this occupation is to assist people. Perhaps some of the most urgent reasons for nurses to be engaged in the field are that the recipients of their care may need them at any time. During the early days of nursing it meant that nurses stayed with their clients for very long periods without respite and sleep. Present-day labor laws have changed the way people deliver goods and services, and shifts of varying lengths and various times of the day are the norm. Because people require nurses' care no matter what the hour or what the place, nurses, who are predominantly female, find themselves stressed by the increase in crime rates and safety as they come and go from their jobs. No statistics were found specifically addressing this issue, but it is no doubt of great interest to nurses that parking lots and ramps provide a sense of security and freedom from being attacked while they are on their way to or from work. Nurses may find this a challenging contribution to workers in all walks of life if they join citizen groups or provide leadership to find ways toward the improvement of this public problem.[20]

■ TRENDS IN NURSING SPECIALTIES

Nurse Entrepreneurs

Of all registered nurses in the United States, it is estimated that 6.3% have formal preparation to practice in advanced nursing positions. Among these are clinical nurse practitioners and nurse-midwives. These are nurses most apt to leave the stereotypical setting of the hospital or agency. They are entering a new era—one in which they are starting their own businesses. This may well take the form of a home care agency or a private practice based in the home. As such, all the resources and challenges that persons encounter when launching a start-up business apply. Small business consultants at local universities, state business guidelines, and regional programs are available to help persons develop their own businesses.

As with any business, there are certain basics. A business plan should first be developed. This helps delineate and establish the nature and boundary of the business and the steps necessary to implement all phases, including the development of a clientele base and building contacts with the community. In the geographic area where the business is to operate, it will be advantageous to join community and civic groups such as the Chamber of Commerce. Contacts in these organizations will help with the essential aspect of networking. Funding the necessities and meeting the criteria for third-party reimbursement will take time and patience. Financial and other records must be kept accurately so that income and expenses can be tracked and well-monitored on an on-going basis. This is essential to maintain good cash flow, as well as for reporting and tax purposes. Computers can help in the financial record-keeping process. In the case of nurses working in separate environments, a communication system must be established. This may require utilization of cellular or satellite phones, fax machines, and laptop computers. In addition to this new technology, client care equipment may need to be obtained for use in clinical situations. Most clinical equipment for individual clients can be rented and the cost reimbursed by insurance or other sources.

Before starting a private business, the nurse must remember that thinking about going into business is very different from the actuality of running one day to day. Before launching down the road toward being an entrepreneur, be careful to narrow the gap between dreams and reality by doing considerable preliminary work on areas of vision, planning, and action. To be successful, you must have a very clear vision of what your goals are and the inexhaustible commitment it will take to accomplish them. No longer will there be the safe 8-hour workday; sometimes the days will become exhaustingly long. Gone is the myth that the entrepreneur is not responsible to anyone. Clients are now the ultimate determinators; multiple licensing and funding sources must be satisfied.

Taking advantage of technology will make it easier for the nurse practitioner to be available to clients. Fax machines, satellite or cellular phones, voice-mail systems, secretarial services, and other advances can work to make the job easier and more rewarding but different from anything ever dreamed of before. Above all, the nurse entrepreneur cannot be afraid of the new challenges. Problem-solving skills learned earlier and optional utilization of a multitude of resources, experienced persons, and reading materials will get the job underway.

Gone must be the notion that to have a private practice is a way of getting rich quick. There will be unanticipated business expenses, so net revenue in the early phases will be small. Obtaining a carefully chosen but relatively inexpensive computer accounting program can facilitate good accounting. To keep track of profits and losses, it is essential to hire a knowledgeable bookkeeper or a CPA to review financial figures quarterly and explain their meaning.

Business will not just automatically be drawn to the private practitioner. You must market your services. It is necessary to listen to the needs of people and explain to them how their needs can be met. The entrepreneur must be as specific as possible about cost and the advantage this business has over other existing services. The only way to stay in business is to keep current both in the health care field (macroeconomic level) and the contribution that a nursing business as a private practice has economic advantages on without compromising quality (microeconomic level).

Remember, no new business will escape from politics and red tape. State and local agencies, government regulatory agencies, health care providers and agencies, and insurance programs demand a lot of paperwork.

Last, not every nurse is cut out to be a private practitioner—an entrepreneur. However, it offers great potential and personal fulfillment. Having spirit and a willingness to take risks is a prerequisite to starting a long planning process and working toward the goal. If becoming a private nurse practitioner is the decision made, the goal of having a private practice may be several years down the road. Because the licensing and start-up process takes a long time, the nurse who aims toward private practice/business will want to begin slowly, steadily, and expeditiously heading in that direction now.

Combination Careers

Variations on stereotypical nursing roles continue to evolve. As an example, clergy who become nurses or nurses who become pastors have combined those two roles in a holistic manner. Examples of such practitioners can be found in various parts of the United States. It is often a lifelong vocation.[13] No doubt numerous other careers combine the distinctive roles of two different professions. An individual with the ability to conceptualize a workable approach to meeting health needs along with other needs may be able to combine knowledge in two or more fields into a most unique and rewarding career.

Intercultural Nursing

For nurses finding themselves working with immigrant persons in the United States or abroad, a number of complex dynamics need consideration. Consideration needs to be given to the relationships among immigration, ethnic identity, and health. These factors, for example, were studied among people who were recent immigrants from Egypt, Yemen, Iran, Armenia, and Arabia. One conclusion was that although Armenians may be born and raised in several different countries, they socialize with Armenians, go to Armenian churches, have their own language at home, and so on.

Immigrants perceive themselves as being different from people of other ethnicities who live in the same region they do. It may seem laughable to the typical

TABLE 16-3

RNs with Current Licenses by Racial and Ethnic Background

	Number 1992	Percentage 1992	Number 1996	Percentage 1996
White (nonHispanic)	2,032,981	90.1	2,312,511	90.3
Black (nonHispanic)	90,611	4.0	107,527	4.2
Asian/Pacific Islander	75,785	3.4	86,434	3.4
American Indian/Alaskan Native	9,998	0.4	11,843	0.5
Hispanic	30,441	1.4	40,559	1.6

TABLE 16-4

Registered Nurse Population

	Number 1992	Percentage 1992	Number 1996	Percentage 1996
Total	2,239,816	100.0	2,558,874	100
Total employed in nursing	—	—	2,115,815	83

American young man to learn that his counterpart, a young Hmong prospective father, telephones his grandmother to make haste because his wife is in labor and he needs her experience to support him through the anticipated delivery. Situations such as these challenge the nurse who chooses to work in intercultural settings to be especially perceptive and not to make hasty assumptions.

A wide variation in cultural attitudes, social attitudes, family orientations, number of physical symptoms, number of psychologic symptoms, perceived health status, and morale exists among different ethnic groups. Ethnic groups vary greatly in terms of whether they maintain positive morale when suffering physical symptoms. This supports the need for nurses to consider ethnic identity as well as country of origin when providing care to people.

The quest for education, status, and retention of nurses representing ethnic minorities continues for the simple reason that a nurse from the particular culture often best understands the needs of minority patients. Tables 16-3 and 16-4 provide information about the sex and racial/ethnic background of the registered nurse population in the United States. States continue to increase funding for training of minority nurses who understand the language and culture of minority populations in the state. To emphasize this fact, 70% of Hispanic nurses are located in the west or south regions of the country, with 36% in the west and 33.5% in the south. Among all R.N.s, 18% were located in the west and 30% in the south.

Unique Needs for Nurses in Rural Areas

One career option becoming increasingly important is nursing in the rural setting. It can provide a variety of experiences. Nurses outside cities help provide access to health care by practicing as generalists rather than as specialists. Most often, clinical nursing education takes place in institutional settings in metropolitan areas,

TABLE 16-5

Total Nurse Population Employed By Sex

	Number 1992	Percentage 1992	Number 1996	Percentage 1996
Male	88,623	4.0	113,683	5.4
Female	2,149,398	96.0	2,002,132	95.6

and as a result graduates may not be aware of the variety of noninstitutional settings in rural areas, where they may find great personal and professional satisfaction.

A total of 161,711, or 6.3%, of the 2,558,874 registered nurses in the United States in March 1996 were estimated to have formal preparation to practice in advanced nursing positions. Among these, 7802 were estimated to be prepared to practice as either a clinical nurse specialist or nurse practitioner, 53,799 were clinical nurse specialists, 63,191 were nurse practitioners, 30,386 were nurse anesthetists, and 6534 were nurse-midwives.

In March 1996, 82.7%, or 2,115,815 of the 2,558,874 R.N.s, were employed in nursing. The proportion of the total registered nurse population who were working in nursing positions was the same in the March 1992 and March 1996 surveys. However, a larger proportion of the nurses were working full-time in the 1996 survey than in the 1992 survey; 59% of the 2.559 million in 1992, compared to 75% of the 2.240 million in 1996.

Among the 2,115,815 employed R.N.s in 1996, an estimated 113,683 were men, 5.4% of the total—a substantial increase over 1992. In March 1992 it was estimated that 79,557 out of the 1,853,024 persons who were employed in nursing were men, or 4.3% of the total (Table 16-5).

The average salary of an R.N. who was employed in nursing on a full-time basis in March 1996 was $42,071, an increase of 11% over the average salary of $37,738 in 1992. R.N.s in staff nurse positions averaged $38,567 in 1996, an increase of 9.5% since 1992.

The average age of all the registered nurses was 44.3 years. Among those who were employed in nursing, the average age was 42.3 years.

Based on 1992 samples, about 9% of the total United States population was Hispanic, whereas less than 2% of the R.N. population was Hispanic. Taking all nurses' education into account, both that which prepared them to become R.N.s and including all education acquired since that time, about 6% of Hispanic nurses had master's or doctoral degrees, compared to about 10% of the black nurses and 8% of white nurses.

By the turn of the century it is likely that 90% or more of women in the United States will be in the workforce. Already pointing in that direction in 1993, working mothers in Sioux Falls, South Dakota made up 84% of all women in the workforce.[1] A current counterforce to this trend is the development of more groups of concerned citizens speaking out against disintegration of the American family, the lack of opportunity for bonding with children, lack of family teamwork to meet family needs, and absence of economic stability as well as moral, ethical, and religious standards. The question remains as to whether the pressures of financial and personal needs to work outside the home will win out over the virtues of retaining traditional family lifestyles. It may be that both poles will equal out if women use their creativity in such ways as establishing their children in home-schooling programs, becoming successful bargain-hunters for necessities (and luxuries) in the marketplace, and developing their talents and earning ability through home-based businesses. The association between low income and poor health is common knowledge. When families attempt to improve the condition of their members, they readily turn toward working more hours, with children taking paper routes and mothers leaving the home to join the workforce. In the rural Midwest, with its strong egalitarian tradition, women formerly worked side by side with men on the farm. When agriculture continued to experience financial difficulty, it took more than working side by side to make ends meet. In the "tall corn state" of Iowa, the percentage of women in the workforce is among the highest in the nation. In 1993, 80% of all women in Des Moines had jobs, and Iowa had five cities in the top 25% of working mothers of children under age 18.[1] Rural America was earlier viewed as the wholesome "good life." Now all the problems of fragmented family life, depression and mental illness, and concern over safety and well-being of children present challenges. Many rural working women are in the health care field and in nursing. Moreover, it is the people who are products of this situation who must be helped. This is a dual challenge when the nurse is in a sense both victim and hero.

To emphasize the point further, although it is an unlikely location, Sioux Falls, South Dakota has the highest percentage of working mothers in the country—84%.[1] According to 1990 statistics, the other Midwestern states, basically rural, also have high percentages of women and mothers in the workforce. For those nurses who desire to work in a friendly, family-oriented environment, a career in rural areas such as the Midwest may fit the bill. For further discussion of rural nursing, see Chapter 13.

Preparation. In the past nurse students were very concerned about choosing a school of nursing that was accredited by the National League for Nursing (NLN). At this point even this question takes on a different slant. Since the U.S. Department of Education placed the NLN accreditation powers under study and threatened the withdrawal of their powers, students are currently uncertain what criteria should determine their choice of a school. It would behoove nurses to watch the dynamics and keep current on news regarding NLN. The Department of Education and the American Association of Colleges of Nursing is also exploring ways in which the profession itself will be best able to determine its own future education and graduation of nurses who are granted the right to practice.

There are various ways of achieving the nurse's educational goals, as discussed especially in Chapter 8. A major advantage of completing a baccalaureate degree in nursing first is that it provides the basic science, social science, and humanities foundation upon which subsequent professional knowledge and experience can be built. Such an education provides students inquiry and problem-solving skills that are necessary to function and pioneer in new and unexplored settings. Additional coursework in the humanities broadens their understanding of human history and heritage, thus making them better prepared to be active participants in their profession and society.

Part of the solution to inaccessibility of services in any area is innovation. Nurses with creativity can find settings in which services can be brought closer to the people who need them. For example, providing services for a constituency may be best performed in schools and churches instead of specially built clinics many miles away.

Changing specialties can be done in the course of a nursing career. Today it is wise to consider shifting from hospitals to clinics, surgery centers, home health care, and other outpatient and community settings. It is easier to make that shift than one from community settings to hospitals. That is because hospitals are requiring fewer and fewer personnel, while the shift to community treatment and maintenance is rapidly increasing.[15] Furthermore, technology and continued purchase of more specialized equipment in hospitals and medical centers create the need to learn intricacies of technology, the use of which may supersede the holistic care of persons.

School nursing. With society's increasing emphasis on prevention, discussion of health care and education provided to children in schools is especially relevant. For nurses who are involved in schools, new priorities seem to be constantly arising as a means of addressing changing needs and budgets. Diminishing funds for school district budgets across the country has caused major cutbacks over the past decade. Resulting layoffs have often hit schools first. This has occurred concurrently with the trend of "mainstreaming" (combining) children with disabilities into classes with nondisabled children. The result is often inadequate availability of health resources for all children in the school, since R.N.s who are school nurses or public health nurses cannot possibly provide direct nursing care in all of the schools to which they are assigned.

These nurses end up delegating nursing acts to auxiliary personnel such as L.P.N.s or unlicensed persons. In delegating responsibilities, the R.N. must be careful to comply with state rules, usually those of the state Board of Nursing. Usually only nursing acts may be delegated by a registered nurse; a medical act delegated to a nurse by a physician, podiatrist, or dentist may not be re-delegated to another person.

Nutrition and health. School nurses are increasingly stressing healthy diets for children. The U.S. Department of Agriculture, which administers the national School Lunch and Breakfast Programs, continues to study and supervise foods passing along the lunch line in school and criticize them for high fat content, saturated fat and sodium, and inadequate carbohydrates. The Wisconsin Dairy Council, as one example, is sponsoring special training for nutrition staffs in schools on how to "trim the fat."[9] The current requirements are that menus, on a monthly basis, contain 30% or less of their calories from fat.

For the dietary department to meet the Recommended Dietary Allowances, various standards and procedures are being recommended. To make school lunches healthy, all ground meat is drained and rinsed to remove excess fat; lower-fat and lower-sodium products are used; salt-free seasonings are used in place of salt; vegetables and bread are not buttered (butter is available for students to use if they choose). Low-fat mozzarella cheese and low-fat salad dressing are used. All potatoes are baked, not fried. Fruit is offered four times a week. A baked dessert is offered only once a week, and so on.

School nurses continue to be concerned about the nutritional status of children. A concern about inadequate intake of calories and unbalanced meals is being replaced. The focus is now on encouraging activity and muscular development of young children. Computers, videos, and other activities result in a sedentary lifestyle for young people. The current problem is an increase in obese children and young adults.[9] As a result, school nurses may need to educate children about the need for regular exercise.

School nurses are also in a good position to help prevent first-time use of tobacco by young children and adolescents. According to the Surgeon General's report *Preventing Tobacco Use Among Young People,* released in 1994, nearly all the first-time use of tobacco occurs before high school graduation. The suggestion is made that if people do not begin using tobacco in adolescence, most never will. Furthermore, tobacco is often the first drug used by adolescents who use alcohol, marijuana and other drugs.[5]

Sex education. School nurses in America have traditionally been involved in instructing elementary and secondary school students about issues relating to sex. Incidents have been reported in which children have contracted HIV from nonsexual contact with each other. Even more compelling is the fact that the under-18 population has become significantly more sexually active. As a consequence, the school nurse will be addressing issues such as use of condoms and HIV testing with more frequency. As more and more adolescents are voluntarily seeking HIV testing, denial and inability to fully comprehend the consequences of an HIV test may demonstrate the need for several counseling sessions. One of the main goals of counseling is to establish a rapport with the student who may never have discussed sexual issues with an adult. The purpose is to eliminate myths that youth tend to have, for instance, that a positive test result means immediate death, or only "bad" people get AIDS.[6]

With the increasing number of reported cases of tuberculosis, as well as the recurrence of other previously eradicated diseases such as typhoid fever, the nurse needs to be constantly on guard for these remote but actual possibilities. There is no place for the old band-aid image of the school nurse, nor of one who runs a "sick bay" for children who come to school but should have stayed home.

■ SEEKING EMPLOYMENT

This section discusses typical aspects of the job search that may be helpful to a nurse seeking employment. It is not intended to be comprehensive but rather to emphasize areas in which nurses as a whole often lack awareness. Every nurse seeking employment must develop a résumé. Libraries have numerous resources on preparing traditional formats of résumés that are standard in the health care field. University career placement services are a great resource for college students. These resources will also be helpful in learning about other aspects of the job search, such as writing cover letters, preparing for interviews, finding job-searching schools, and similar topics. A list of suggested materials is located at the end of this chapter.

Graduates in other fields may already recognize these strategies, but nurses tend to deal more on a one-to-one basis as they go through the process of finding the job they desire. They tend to take what is said and done more at face value than persons in some other fields. The subtle behind-the-scenes aspects, however, can make the difference between getting a job working for someone as an employee and taking a position working with someone as a dynamic force in an organization.

Before graduating and receiving the license to practice, each nurse will need to apply a significant amount of knowledge regarding general job-searching skills to obtain the position with the greatest potential for individual fulfillment. The advice presented here is based on current trends and is intended to give the job-seeking nurse the best opportunity to obtain the desired position. To ensure the best chance in getting the desired position, it is suggested that the guidelines in this chapter be followed closely to project the characteristics of a good employee.

The increased use of computers in settings where nurses work has also opened up a new option for nurses to work in places other than the clinical setting. Clinical experience is more important than knowledge about computers for the enterprising nurse marketing her skills and "going corporate" with computer companies.

Match Personality and Need with the Job

The first step is to define career goals as specifically as possible. A list of questions to ask include: "What do I enjoy doing? What do I do best? In what areas of nursing do I excel?" Include tasks, job characteristics, even general ideas that are most enjoyable. By answering these questions, you should be able to narrow your area of focus. Hopefully, many of the items on your list will coincide with your reasons for becoming a nurse in the first place.

Happiness often breeds success; conversely, discontentment can lead to problems. The appealing aspects of nursing are probably already obvious to the nurse who is looking for a job in the field. For example, the person who enjoys fast, high-energy work most likely will choose an area such as critical care nursing. The person who is extremely independent and can handle responsibility easily may well choose home health care, for example.

Research the Health Care Industry

If you have several types of work in mind, make an analysis of each to determine the fit between them and the position you most desire. Find out about the work pace involved. How much responsibility is entailed? Does this job stand by itself or does the position fit into a team? What is the work setting like, and what is the commuting distance to work? Learn about the specialty of interest. It is well to ask colleagues, nurse recruiters, or employers.

Making trade-offs is a realistic part of the job decision. The desired salary compensation may not exist in the specialty area where the position is being sought. For example, a clinic or nursing home position may offer better hours than are available in a hospital, but the pay may be 25% less.

Learn about Potential Employers

Whether you are applying for your first nursing position or are interested in moving into another position, your basic strategy will be the same. One of the most important principles in finding professional employment is to approach your job search from the employer's standpoint. There are at least three parts of the traditional job-seeking process:

- Identify the most important characteristics of the job being sought
- Explore opportunities for pursuing desired goals
- Obtain knowledge available about potential employers, résumé preparation, and preparing for the interview process

In preparing for an interview, research the possible employer by examining directories and annual reports if the health care provider is publicly held; otherwise request any literature that may be available. Educating yourself thoroughly about the potential employer is crucial and reflects the degree to which you desire the job—and, consequently, your likelihood of getting a position. Current or former employees are often good sources regarding job openings. Ask, for example, about the current demand for nurses with your background in the area and at the health facility. If the organization hires L.P.N.s, and perhaps admits doing so to save money, that gives a strong message. The person who is overqualified for the position will probably have to play down the level of preparation to land a job that calls for significantly less education or preparation. The placement office may be able to offer assistance to graduates of that particular school. The library, newspapers, and Internet provide information about potential job openings. Job openings are also posted on bulletin boards within health facilities. You might also check the want ads to see what positions the health facility posts.

Some jobs, particularly at the management level, are not advertised broadly. Professional search firms and recruiters can be helpful in identifying such positions.

Résumé Preparation

A potential employer's first impression of the job seeker is made by the professional résumé and cover letter. The person seeking the job reinforces this impression at the interview. If the professional résumé and cover letter do not sufficiently impress the person in charge of hiring, then the chances of even obtaining an interview are lessened. In fact, a résumé's main purpose is to persuade the future employer to schedule an interview with you. A résumé by itself will rarely land the job, but if it is clear, concise, and factual, it will go a long way toward selling the job candidate's abilities to a health care provider and lead to an interview. A good policy is to update your résumé frequently and keep extra copies in a file. Because the average person can expect to make several job changes throughout life, spending time now to develop a quality résumé will help facilitate career changes in the future.

The best policy is to use one of the conventional résumé formats that best exhibits the most impressive information first. Often more applicants than actual positions are available (depending on the supply of available nurses in any particular locality). Any specific résumé may receive only a cursory glance; if the reviewer does not know where to look for the important information, she or he may not be willing to spend the extra time reading that particular résumé.

The three standard résumé formats are chronologic, functional, and combination. Most libraries will have books on résumés, and these can be used for reference. An objective in a résumé gives focus to the particular interest that a candidate has in a given position. This prevents a deviation from the pursuit of career goals that may prove most beneficial the next time the person seeks a position in that particular specialty. Including objectives in a résumé makes it look more genuine.

The chronologic résumé should be used to emphasize a strong work history and may be the simplest to prepare. It documents work history in reverse chronologic order, including dates of employment. Highlighting past performance, the chronologic résumé leads an employer to believe that this candidate should be hired instead of others. If the objective of the applicant is to obtain a position that is different from the work history, it is advantageous to relate past history to the reason for seeking the present position; alternatively, fewer questions will probably be asked by omitting the history altogether.

The functional résumé highlights present abilities rather than past history. For this reason it may provide a better basis for the employer's decision; however, it is also much more time-consuming to write. After the applicant states the objective, it is necessary to document accomplishments, abilities, and transferable skills. It may be well to include a heading titled "Leadership" or "Team Skills," under which are listed offices held in community or academic organizations, projects you have worked on, and so on. Because the functional résumé is less dependent on work experience, it is the format often used by the new graduate.

In a way, the combination résumé incorporates the best attributes of the first two types. Abilities and skills are documented together with education and work history to provide a more complete picture. Placing the most impressive information first highlights it.

Regardless of what style of résumé you choose, word your résumé so that your history, career goal, and desired job project continuity. For example, it would seem odd to apply for a position in geriatrics when the primary interest is obstetrics.

Cover Letter

The cover letter should be just long enough to interest the reader in the résumé. It should begin by addressing the actual name of the health care recruiter. The cover letter should be clear, concise, and direct. The following format might be followed:

Paragraph One: Purpose and interest in the position must be stated. If the inquiry is made from an advertisement, reference to that document may be appropriate.

Paragraph Two: Potential contribution of the candidate to the facility should be emphasized and referenced in the résumé.

Paragraph Three: Initiative is demonstrated when the candidate indicates a plan for follow-up with an appointment. State that an interview is anticipated and when a follow-up contact will be made. This rather assertive approach will distinguish you from other applicants who simply ask for the recruiter to call.

Interviewing

Interviewing is a skill that can be developed by education and practice. Many books are available on the subject. In general, applicants must sell themselves. Each individual applicant should be clear about the reasons why the employer should make the choice in her favor. If potential negative aspects are present in a résumé or work history, they need to be turned into positive advantages. If the candidate has been unemployed for some time, that needs to be explained. (For example, if a job in a nursing home is being sought, it is important to explain that the candidate has been caring for a dying parent, for this lends support that the latter experience is relevant to the job). After looking through books on interviewing, the job seeker may benefit by enlisting a friend to practice a mock interview.

The Interview

Having proceeded through the previous steps, preparation for the interview is very important. Throughout the interview the nurse must project as much self-confidence and openness as she or he is comfortable with, but no more. It is natural to feel nervous, and it is best not to conceal the nervousness altogether. However, do not make an issue of it by explaining the nervousness or sitting on shaky hands.

The interviewer's first impression is in actuality a gut reaction. It is, however, often the factor that decides whether the individual lands the job. It is not rational, professional, or fair, but it is human. It has been said that most decisions are made for two reasons: a good one and the real one. Realize that some people click and some do not. The job may be right, but the factors in the hiring process may eliminate "landing" it.

A final suggestion is to try very hard not to be the last person being interviewed, or the last appointment of the day. Interviewers will tend to have other things in mind such as the drive home from work, concern about timing, a dinner engagement, or other things. When this happens, the last interviewee may be short-changed.

Physical appearance. Regardless of the dress that is acceptable on the job, the professional applying for a position should not assume that working attire is acceptable at the time of the interviewing process. Since a nurse aspires to be a professional equal with others, the universal standards in the process of job seeking must be accepted. The stereotype of conservative dress for interviews cuts across the entire professional world and influences what nurses can expect to comply with to be successful at the point of seeking the job of their dreams. The way the person walks into the room will create a reaction. Some of the factors that cause a particular response to your entrance are clothing, hair, makeup, and perfume. In the world of business and health it is expected that professionals dress appropriately, and it is assumed that professionals know what *appropriate* means. It means conservative and businesslike.

Nurses tend to have a special liking for soft, dressy clothing, perhaps because they spend so many hours a day in work clothing that is designed to be plain, nonrevealing, and allowing freedom of movement. It becomes a treat when they can put on special attire and look "dressed up." The temptation may be to do this for a job interview, but the result may be an unfavorable impression. There is a point between one in which a nurse looks ready to jump into the front lines of a clinical situation and one in which it appears that she or he is ready to attend a formal party. Neither is appropriate for the normal interview.

Specifically, in cool weather appropriate women's dress would be a tasteful, conservative suit with the length of the skirt at least to the knee. During very warm weather a classic style dress may be preferred—one- or two-piece attire preferable in solid conservative colors (definitely not gaudy). Shoes should appear classic and comfortable, avoiding very high or flat heels. Dress hose should be worn for any interview. Men would do well to go into an interview in a conservative suit in a weight appropriate for the climate. In certain situations, classic pants, shirt, tie, and conservative sport coat may be appropriate. It is definitely not appropriate to go in a short-sleeved sport shirt and casual pants. Both men and women should follow the same general dress guidelines; it is imperative to always avoid unorthodox styles and colors.

To put the finishing touches on a professional image, trimmed and attractive hair is appropriate for an interview. If hair is long, it needs to be arranged in a style that makes it look controlled and neat. There may be exceptions, but employers in most health care settings generally expect, or at least appreciate, a clean-cut appearance. Women should use makeup that makes the face look pleasant and natural (in other words, not bright and heavy). Perfume or cologne should be subtle, if used at all.

Voice. Speech must be clear and pleasing to hear. It is important to avoid projecting a voice that is grating, whiny, childlike, loud, or raspy-sounding. It is important to speak with ease and to be "natural."

Hands. Contrary to books of authority some years ago, the handshake today may be considered unisex. Earlier it was considered to be an acceptable gesture for men only. However, there are some considerations with regard to the shaking of hands, whether done by men or women. It is important to do it correctly if you choose to extend a handshake during a job search situation. If done carelessly, a handshake may reveal the nurse's insecurity, anxiety, or discomfort. To be positive in its effect, a handshake must be firm and timed in such a manner that it does not come across as hurried or as something done in passing. The hand grasp must not be limp and momentary. Professional nurses, of necessity, must concern themselves with hygiene, and hand washing is almost second nature to the job. For this reason, neat, clean fingernails are much more in character with professional expectation than are polished and/or simulated nails.

Because an interview is, by its very nature, stressful, the body will react physiologically and often cause hands to become cold and clammy. This is a normal response to such a situation, and the person receiving the handshake will easily recognize it for what it is.

First reactions. When entering the office or room where an interview is to be conducted, remember to sit down only when invited. This gives the interviewer the opportunity to sit where comfortable and also to seat other persons in the room as desired. The nurse who is there to discuss a professional position should come across as friendly but not too friendly. Sitting down immediately may be interpreted as being too familiar.

Personality. The personality of a nurse is considered very important in most situations. It is advisable to take stock of whether your personality reflects stiffness rather than warmth. It is also important to take stock as to whether you are frozen and barely able to speak; or whether the opposite may be occurring, with conversation being of a babbling nature, perhaps even with the body bouncing nervously like a yo-yo. A frequent error in a stressful situation is to stare at a given spot. When asked a question, the person not well in command of a situation may respond with words that are barely audible, or give simple "yes" or "no" answers to an interviewer's questions.

The interviewee may have some little quirk that can be a dead giveaway to the interviewer and eliminate the candidate in the interview process. For example, a candidate may be well groomed and dressed appropriately except that inappropriate socks or hose appear below the pant leg; a hair ornament may not be complementary to the remainder of the attire. These seemingly small factors may trigger the interviewer to wonder why everything else is so great with one such flaw. There may be a psychologic explanation assigned to such a faux pas: perhaps the nurse is unconsciously causing herself not to get the job. Not having an explanation for the inappropriate may well mean that the nurse does not land the position.

Do:

- Be on time
- Speak up and make eye contact
- Be prepared and honest when confronted with a difficult question
- Be friendly, but businesslike: do not linger after the interview is concluded
- Take along only what may be needed, such as two copies of a résumé, references, important-to-work samples (if appropriate), pen, pad; only those things that will fit into a purse or large envelope
- Act natural—no one likes a phony
- Apply makeup sparingly
- Definitely do not smoke or smell of smoke
- Avoid such detractors as heavy, clunky jewelry, low-cut blouses, or, in the case of men, hair tied in back, earrings, or any other unorthodox dress
- Advice for all nurses seeking the best position: do not use "sex" to get that job—or to obtain anything else in the professional world
- Let the interviewer bring up the subject of salary

Evaluate the Interview

Although it depends on the company, most people who conduct interviews are not professional or accomplished interviewers. It may happen that the interviewer is preoccupied with other things at the time of the interview. Some may not be trained to ask the questions that will allow the interviewee to shine or be herself, or to be her best. Occasionally the interviewer may be the type to put the interviewee through a "stress" test with the questions such as, "Why were you fired from. . .?" Since this person gauges the respondent's reaction under pressure, it is of utmost importance to remain calm. Opposite from the "stress" type is the "low-key" type of interview. Here the interviewee may actually wonder if the interviewer is listening. Easy questions may give much false assurance about having landed the job. Often the interviewee has no control over this aspect, but as stated before, it is best to try very hard if possible not to be the last person being interviewed. The last one in the day may be short-changed because the interviewer will have more on his or her mind at that time, such as rush-hour traffic, a dinner engagement, the kids, or other things.

A final reminder is to answer the questions that are not asked. Although the interviewer will depend on references for determining whether the person is reliable, he or she may have some questions in areas that are prohibited by law from being included in an application. It does not prevent the interviewer from wondering about these questions. It is always best to clear up any information that may be an obstacle in the interviewer's mind. They may not necessarily be mentioned, but the interviewee should address them before applying for the job.

- If single, will a career be interrupted by marriage?
- If married with no children, will pregnancy and children end a career?
- If there are children, will responsibilities at home interfere with the job?
- Will travel be refused because of husband or wife and children?
- Is child care stable so that it will not pose problems and cause absenteeism when one of the children gets sick?
- Does this candidate pose as a sure bet that when it comes to investing the employer's training monies and other expenses as a person of the other sex?
- Will this person be dedicated and be an asset to the company?
- If employed, does this candidate have positive work attitude, motivation, and a team spirit?

In Conclusion

It is important to be prepared by learning about potential employers and positions and to enter an interview prepared to answer—and question—intelligently. As discussed previously, the basic steps in contacting potential employers are:

1. Send a résumé and cover letter.
2. Follow up with a phone call or contact as appropriate.
3. Prepare to answer and ask tough questions.
4. Dress professionally for the interview and be poised; sell yourself for the job.
5. Follow up the interview with a thank-you letter indicating your eagerness to be hired for the position. This should be done within 24 hours of the meeting.

Never Quit Learning

Today's graduates can expect to make many position changes during their careers. Each time this happens, the applicant will probably have to be interviewed and selected from among other applicants. Also, as more responsibility is placed on nurses in the future, nurses will need to excel. This way they will promote increased respect and status for their profession, as well as the accompanying increased compensation. The purpose of continuing education programs is to ensure that nurses keep current and continue learning on their own.

Job Information Banks

One of the newest developments in the job search process provides updated information about job listings and employers nationwide, while taking less time and costing less money than traditional methods. One such electronic information clearinghouse is the MediMatch Health Care Job Information Bank, which provides a free job information service for health care professionals and employers. More information can be obtained by calling 1-800-562-7123. The sign-up process only takes about 5 minutes. Fees will be charged for résumé referral and custom searches.

■ SUMMARY

Deciding the first type of nursing position to seek is very important to beginning a successful career. However, one can reach success many ways, as long as key points are kept in mind along the way. Each experience adds knowledge, confidence, and poise. No career goes to the top in smooth increments. If a given situation does not provide satisfaction and increased morale and remuneration, the nurse must be honest with herself or himself, considering the job choice not as a mistake, but as a learning experience for the days ahead. Susceptibility to intimidation and lack of self-image are serious personal flaws, and they seem to be a more common handicap for professional nurses when they negotiate posts than are traits of arrogance and overconfidence. The nurse must evaluate the perceptions people have of her both on and off the job. Nurses internalize concern for their clients easily. However, a cool confidence and concern for self, as well as for the nursing profession, will go a long way toward opening doors during the years ahead.

CRITICAL THINKING *Activities*

1. **List ways that changes in the health care system will affect nurses and the nursing profession.**
2. **Identify two or three changes in health care organizations currently going on where you live. What possible "hidden agendas" might there be in advertising and news stories being publicized about these changes?**
3. **Determine and compare the expectations of nurse employees with those of employers in various health care settings such as a hospital, a nursing home, and a home health care agency.**
4. **What personal strengths and weaknesses are relevant to a career in nursing or in a given nursing specialty? Give examples.**
5. **Prepare a résumé and cover letter. In the process, refer to question #4. (Keep these on file and use them as a basis for future reference).**

References

1. Associated Press: *Post Bulletin,* Rochester, MN, Dec. 20, 1993, p 6B.
2. Blegen MA: Nurses' job satisfaction: a meta-analysis of related variables, *Nurs Research* 42(1): 36, 1993.
3. Caprino M: Industry fights for its health: hospitals hustle to mergers, *Post Bulletin,* Rochester, MN, Jan 8, 1994, p. 1E.
4. Cassetta RA: Texas nurse takes her place in Congress, *Am Nurse* 25(4): 19, 1993.
5. Department of Health and Human Services: *Preventing tobacco use among young people: a report of the Surgeon General,* Atlanta, 1994, Public Health Service, CDC, National Center for Chronic Disease Prevention and Health Promotion, Office on Smoking and Health.
6. Dodell D, ed: *The Health Info-Com Network Newsletter,* Scottsdale, Ariz, Internet address: "david@stat.com".
7. Galen M: Cheaper primary care: nurses may be the answer, *Business Week,* April 12, 1993.
8. Haddad A: Ethics in action: Contract negotiations at your hospital, *RN* 60(5): 17-19, 1997.
9. Halvorson L: Food service cooks up healthy menus, *School Update* 11(2): 12, 1994.
10. Konner M: *Medicine at the crossroads: the crisis in health care,* New York, 1993, Pantheon Books.

11. Perkins JL and others: Why men choose nursing, *Nurse Health Care* 14(1): 34, 1993.
12. R.N. update—Koop wants nurses to teach med school students, *RN:* 19, 1992.
13. Ratzloff T: A calling—parish nurses serve body, mind and spirit of congregations, *Minnesota Nurse,* Aug. 23, 1993.
14. Ryan S, Porter S: Men in nursing: a cautionary comparative critique, *Nurs Outlook* 41(6): 262, 1993.
15. Salzer D: Rural nurses, *Minnesota Nurse,* Aug 9, 1993.
16. Schreiber R: Pay equity and North American nurses, *Nurs Health Care* 14(1): 28, 1993.
17. *St. Paul Pioneer Press,* Nursing shortage and salary, Mar. 21, 1993.
18. Stoeffler D, ed: Health consortium offers economic boost to area, *LaCrosse Tribune,* April 22, 1997, p A4.
19. Will G: Washington Post writers group courts have erred on women's athletics, *LaCrosse Tribune,* April 25, 1997.
20. Winslow R: Women heart patient's cholesterol care should be more aggressive, study shows, *The Wall Street Journal,* April 23, 1997, p B8.
21. *Working Women:* Salary survey 1995, Jan. 1995, p 25ff.
22. *Working Women:* How does your pay stack up? Jan. 1996, p 27ff.
23. *Working Women:* Salary survey 1997, Jan. 1997, p 73ff.
24. Wright J, ed: *The universal almanac 1996,* p 193.
25. Yeakel L: Women's year? No, just the start, *U.S.A. Today,* March 31, 1993, p 11A.

Suggested Readings

Dehner M: *How to move from college into a secure job,* Lincolnwood, IL, 1994, VGM Career Horizons.

Jackson T: *Tom Jackson's interview express,* New York, 1993, Times Books.

Kirkwood C: *Your services are no longer required: the complete job-loss recovery book,* New York, 1993, Plume Books.

Martin ER: *Cover letters they don't forget,* Lincolnwood, IL, 1993, VGM Career Horizons.

Nursing opportunities, *RN* magazine, published annually.

U.S. Department of Labor, Employment and Training Administration, U.S. Employment Service: *Job search guide: strategies for professionals,* Washington, D.C., 1993, U.S. Government Printing Office.

Weinstein B: *Résumés don't get jobs: the realities and myths of job hunting,* New York, 1993, McGraw-Hill.

Yate MJ: *Knock 'em dead: the ultimate job seeker's handbook,* Holbrook, MA, 1994, Bob Adams.

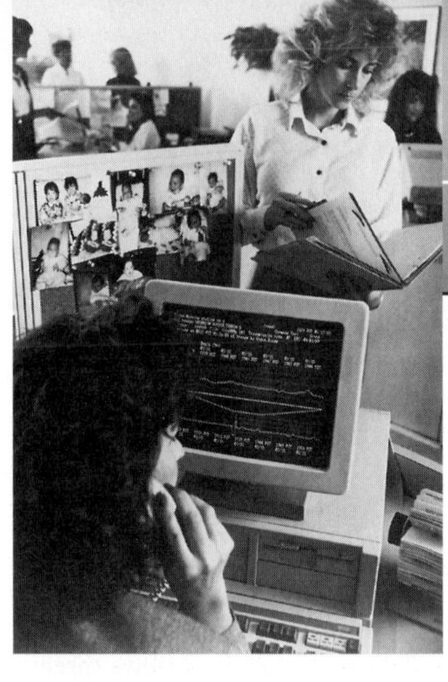

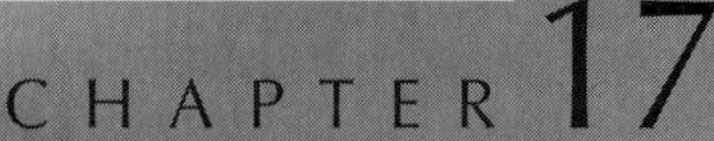

CHAPTER 17

Computers in Nursing: Navigating the Information Superhighway

Jack Yensen

Nurses as individuals and in groups, like many other disciplines, are being inundated, if not overwhelmed, with data and information that begs for their immediate attention. Furthermore, today, in the helping professions and occupations, there is an increasing emphasis on evidence-based practice coupled with increasing economic pressures to generate cost-benefit or cost-effectiveness measures. This means that nursing must embrace new strategies to deal with the large amounts of data and information necessary to respond to societal and economic pressures not just to survive, but to flourish. One of the overall strategies that is working well for medicine is the field of medical informatics. This has been followed by health and nursing informatics. The purpose of this chapter is to extract from the field of nursing informatics specific aspects of computer technology and applications that will help nurses and nursing to get more done with less time and less resources, while increasing their overall awareness of what is relevant and significant to the development of the discipline. This will be attempted by summarizing some of the current and widely available computer applications that have been found effective.

■ E-MAIL

Individual

Electronic mail may be text or multimedia messages (including text, graphics, sound, and video) sent from one computer to another via the Internet. Uses include communication and collaboration in clinically relevant ways. For example, nurses both at work and not at work can keep up to date with unit meetings, schedule changes, hospital or departmental news, and announcements. Nursing administrators can share news and views, policies and procedures, and management practices;

stay in touch with local, national, and international counterparts; and keep up to date with professional and union organizations. Educators use e-mail heavily to stay in touch with students and colleagues near and far and to share resources. Nursing researchers use e-mail to share research findings, databases, programs, and information about research grants, while in the community nurses use e-mail to stay in touch with their colleagues and with their administrative centers. As an example, I receive many e-mail requests for information through one of my Web sites, the Virtual Nursing College,[1] under the "Ask Cybernurse" category. I get anywhere from 10 to 20 requests a week on nursing topics across the spectrum. It is an amazing way for me to learn!

Push Technology

It is possible to use push technologies to constantly deliver customized news directly to your e-mail account or your computer screen. This means that automatically, at predetermined intervals, your e-mail address or your screen gets updated with the latest information about your personal interests. Examples of this would include the Pointcast[2] system and Netscape's In-box Direct.[3] As a personal example, I use Carl Uncover's Reveal,[4] which automatically sends the results of literature searches and the tables of contents of newly published journals directly to my e-mail box. This helps me to stay aware of what is current, although it is another thing entirely to be able to read and understand everything in order to actually be current.

Listserves

A *listserve* is software that will receive e-mail from a subscriber and automatically broadcast it to all other subscribers. Several well-known and heavily used listserves are specific to nursing interests, such as Nursenet,[5] Nrsing-l,[6] and RNMGR,[7] but many others are disease-or health-specific, which serve focused interests. For comprehensive listings of nursing and health-related listserves, see http://www.shef.ac.uk/~nhcon/nulist.htm for Rod Ward's Selection of Nursing and Health Mailing Lists.

Usenet

Another system that allows the general broadcast of topic-centered material is that of Usenet, which serves many different types of news groups. A *news group* is a collective of individuals who have subscribed to a broadcast system based on their common interests. When any member of the group posts to the news group, all subscribers can read that post and respond if they wish. There are several active nursing-related news groups, including news://sci.med.nursing, which is a general forum, and news://bit.listserv.snurse-1, which is specifically for student nurses. For a very comprehensive listing of nursing-related news groups, see http://www.shef.ac.uk/~nhcon/nunews.htm for Rod Ward's Usenet Newsgroups Relevant to Nursing & Healthcare.

■ VOICE MAIL

In this day and age it is sometimes difficult to reach people directly, and with limited resources it is inhibiting to try to telephone nursing colleagues using long distance. One of the ways to overcome this obstacle is to use voice mail and send the voice mail at very low cost across the Internet to the recipient's e-mail box. Once voice mail is received, it can be played by the appropriate e-mail software. An example of this would be Netscape Communicator version 4, which makes it possible to record voice or other sound sources to send to anyone. I was asked via e-mail recently for some specific heart sounds and was able to send back the actual heart sounds requested. It is now possible to send full video across e-mail, although video files are large and require considerable time and storage capacity for transmission and capture.

■ FILE SHARING

Most e-mail software allows files to be attached to e-mail messages, so it is very easy to share data and programs between e-mail accounts simply by designating for the outgoing e-mail message the name and location of the file to be attached and hence transmitted. The attached files may be text, data, or programs. This is one of the ways that nurses collaborating in national or international organizations are able to achieve efficient and cost-effective transfer of critical materials.

■ WEB BROWSERS

Much of the material published on the Internet conforms to hypertext mark-up language (HTML) specifications, which means that HTML browsers are able to read those materials. An HTML browser is a software program or client that runs on a personal computer that, if connected to the Internet, allows the browsing or reading of HTML documents at various sites on the Internet. Sites that are connected in this way form the basis of the World Wide Web (WWW). Each site has a specific electronic address, allowing any person with a Web browser to access that site and read, print, or capture that site's materials. This is of great significance for nurses and nursing, since more and more nurses and nursing organizations are publishing materials on WWW, making them freely accessible to nurses globally. The implications of this are enormous, since it is now possible for nurses anywhere to obtain electronic access to text, abstracts, articles, policies, procedures, critical pathways, clinical guidelines, new drug and treatment information, new clinical research, clinical multimedia sources, client and consumer health information, and a host of other material. Many web sites are now offering interactive pages, where it is possible for the browsing person to participate in electronic courses, surveys, examinations, continuing education, professional development, searching of databases, and research. Using web technology, nurses may interact with colleagues, students, or clients at a distance, which is known as *virtual nursing.*[8] It may be possible eventually to build a complete representation of nursing's knowledge base, which is globally distributed and maintained at multiple sites through interlinked concept-resource mapping, by using existing web technology. This hyperarchive would be constantly updated and remain current through the efforts of many groups of nurses throughout the world. It would help to reduce redundancy of resource use and replication of effort and greatly enhance health promotion, disease prevention, and nursing and consumer education.

Box 17-1 Memorable Moment Using A Search Engine

One gets what one searches!

At the 1996 Learning Resource Center Conference in Indianapolis, I was demonstrating the use of search engines and asked the audience to supply a nursing search term. After some coaxing, one nurse in the audience said that she was interested in the use of restraints. I typed in the search term "restraints" and carried on with my presentation while the computer was completing its task, using the Alta Vista search engine. Suddenly, the whole audience started to break up with laughter. I looked behind me at the video projection screen and saw that the most common documents retrieved related to sexual bondage and lingerie! However, the point was well made, namely that search engines will retrieve what is asked of them.

■ SEARCH ENGINES

Naturally, the idea of a huge, distributed knowledge base begs the question of how to find things accurately and easily. Electronic resources exist on most computers, and those that are connected to the Internet can make their resources available to other users and other computers by providing electronic addresses for these resources. In its simplest terms, I can locate a resource on my own computer by specifying its address, such as c:\Corel\Office 7\Personal\search.wpd. Unfortunately, all other Internet users cannot access this resource until I publish it at a Web or Gopher or Telnet site and give it an Internet address like http://www.langara.bc.ca/vnc/search.htm. If I am connected to a local network I can share these resources across my local network by providing network users with its local network address. However, once I publish its Internet address, anyone with access to Internet can access this resource. So if I want to see what is happening at the RNABC,[9] I can give the electronic address of the RNABC to my browser and retrieve any of its published resources. Similarly, I may wish to see what is available at BCNU[10] and can access its resources in the same way.

In excess of 400 million Web documents or resources are currently available, so the difficulty becomes one of knowing what is available and how to find it quickly. Search engines are software that index Web or other electronic resources and then maintain these indexes in a searchable form. A single search engine may have an index of 30 to 40 million Web documents and be able to retrieve any one of those document locations from a suitable search term or phrase. Different search engines have different capacities, indexes, and query methods, and it is worthwhile to spend enough time with each search engine to develop some familiarity with its strengths and weaknesses. Each search engine that is used should be bookmarked or filed in a favorites folder so that it can be accessed quickly as needed. I would encourage you to visit the Search Engines page at http://www.langara.bc.ca.vnc/search.htm and save the whole page to your own Bookmark file, so that you can explore each of these search engines and keep those that are most useful (Box 17-1).

Other search engines are known as *metasearch engines* because they search only the indexes of individual search engines rather than maintaining their own index of all of the WWW documents. When first conducting a search for nursing resources, it is worthwhile to submit the search term or terms to a metasearch engine, since

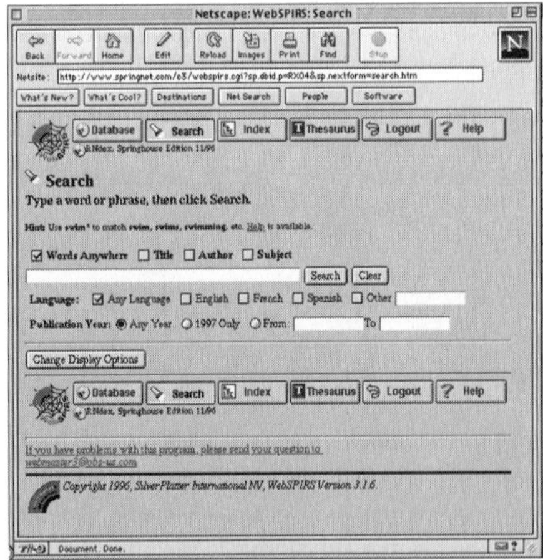

FIG. 17-1 Screen shot of the RNDex search form at SpringNet.

the yield is systematically higher and the time taken to search each of the individual search engines alone would be substantially more. Links for metasearch engines should be bookmarked, since they will be used frequently.

■ ACCESS TO TEXT ARCHIVES

Using web technology, nurses anywhere in the world are able to search literature databases such as CINAHL, RNDex, and Medline to support their nursing work. If I wanted to search the RNDex database, I would type in the address http://www.springnet.com/c3/webspirs.cgi?sp.dbid.p=RX04&sp.nextform=search.htm to my web browser, (if I had not already had it bookmarked so that I could just point and click). This would give me the screen shown in Figure 17-1, which would allow me to enter the search string of interest. Similar strategies are available for searching the Medline databases, so that any nurse, anywhere, can find out current information relating to her or his practice. Check http://www.langara.bc.ca/vnc/medline.htm for a list of some of the freely available sites for Medline searching. To access some databases, such as CINAHL, the user must subscribe and pay a yearly fee.

■ VIRTUAL OR COLLABORATIVE WORK

When nurses or nursing organizations are physically separate and distant from each other, it is still possible to collaborate using Internet or web technology. Some examples of collaborative software that works through Internet are ICQ, Netscape Conference, PowWow, and Teamwave. These applications allow users to collaborate on-line at the same time (synchronously) or at different times (asynchronously) and to use the same white board as each other, view applications, transmit files or WWW addresses (URLs), text chat, collaboratively browse the WWW, and audio or even video conference. This facilitates virtual community building, on-line seminars and conferences, shared bulletin boards, and all types of distance learning and teaching. The following figure shows one of the virtual offices of a graduate seminar in nursing informatics, hosted by Duke University. The course was conceptualized and structured by Dr. Linda Goodwin, faculty member of the Duke

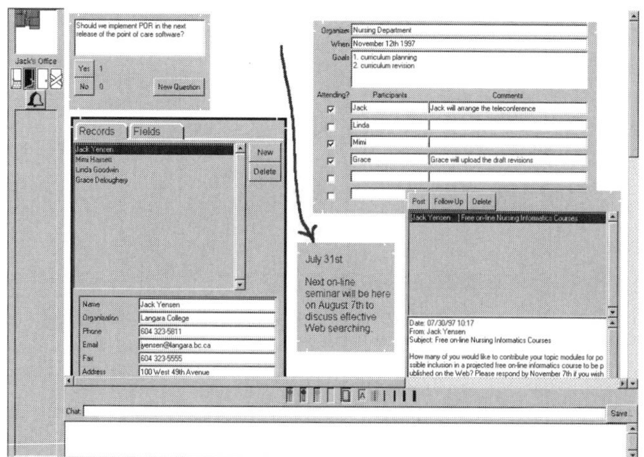

FIG. 17-2 Screen shot of a virtual office in Teamwave.

University School of Nursing and centered at Duke's web site, while the Virtual Work Issues module was developed and served from Vancouver, British Columbia, Canada, by the author, acting as a virtual faculty member. Members of the seminar from several states collaborated in both synchronous and asynchronous modes using Teamwave. Here is a typical screen shot of a work session in one of the virtual offices. It is evident that virtual or collaborative work using web technology has some exciting implications for the discipline and practice of nursing (Fig 17-2).

■ ELECTRONIC PRODUCTIVITY AND PERFORMANCE SYSTEMS (EPPS)

In her book *Electronic Performance Support Systems,* published in 1991, Gloria Gery defined EPSS as

> an integrated electronic environment that is available to and easily accessible by each employee and is structured to provide immediate, individualized on-line access to the full range of information, software, guidance, advice and assistance, data, images, tools, and assessment and monitoring systems to permit job performance with minimal support and intervention by others.

Another way of describing electronic performance support systems is any computer software program or component that improves employee performance by: (1) reducing the complexity or number of steps required to perform a task, (2) providing the performance information an employee needs to perform a task, or (3) providing a decision support system that enables an employee to identify an action that is appropriate or even optimal for a particular set of conditions. A typical EPPS for nursing service would be the on-line availability of all institutional policies and procedures in an easy-to-retrieve, highly indexed, hyperlinked format. This would mean that, with a few clicks and minimal keyboard entry, a nurse could find all policies and procedures relating to anything of interest. Many examples of tools and applications can be used to contribute to EPPS, including strategies for the management of information, current awareness profiling, and intelligent agents.

■ MANAGEMENT OF INFORMATION

So much information is available electronically that the nurse runs the risk of being overwhelmed by information. One way of dealing with large amounts of information requires the judicious use of bookmarks for important sources. Most web browsers have a means of storing, retrieving, and updating web site locations that have been stored by the user. Careful attention to the integrity and organization of a bookmark file can save many hours of fruitless searching for valuable nursing resources. It is possible to order bookmark entries by location, date last visited, or by date created in both ascending and descending order. This makes it easier to find resources. Another strategy is to use bibliographic management software as a database for storing web site locations, descriptions, and indexing terms. In this way it is possible to find sites based on keyword and index-term searching.

■ CURRENT AWARENESS PROFILING

Current awareness profiling is a method by which consumers of information can customize the supply of information from information providers and have that exact information delivered to their screens or e-mail addresses. Although the service is not yet generally available, software exists that could supply health, medical, and nursing customized information to any subscriber. Many of the current services are free, as they are supported by minimal advertising, or carry a nominal charge. It is possible to have continuous archivable updates on any topic refreshing your computer screen at predetermined intervals, or alternatively being delivered directly to your e-mail account.

■ INTELLIGENT AGENTS

Intelligent agents are software applications that can work in the background or while you, the user, are away from your computer, performing many tasks automatically. An example would be an agent that at predetermined times and days would conduct searches of some of the search engines for terms or phrases that are important to your work. It is possible to automate searching and updates in such a way that the agent database is continually being refreshed with new material and resources described by the search terms. This frees the user from having to spend time actually searching for such material and allows her or him, instead, to actually read and understand the updated material itself.

CRITICAL THINKING *Activities*

1. How many ways can you think of to use e-mail in your everyday work to lessen time spent on nonproductive or clerical tasks and maximize the currency of your knowledge base and your job satisfaction? When considering this issue it may be helpful to think of e-mail as embracing voice mail and multimedia mail and including access to general and specific nursing listserves and automated delivery of material.
2. How can you determine which individual or metasearch engines are best suited to your daily work habits and information needs? How would you establish an informal benchmark for comparison? What will determine

whether you use local metasearch engines from your own hard drive or Web-based engines directly?

3. **Can you find three free reliable sources for Medline searching? What happens when you compare the performance of each of these sources using a specific search string and the same search criteria?**
4. **What are the implications of using groupware in the service of your nursing work? List the ways that a groupware application like Teamwave might be useful in increasing group productivity and satisfaction and reducing the wear and tear of travel, attendance at meetings, and scheduling conflicts. How do you envision the future of groupware applied to nursing?**
5. **How many functions or applications can you identify in your current work environment that would be amenable to the appropriate use of Electronic Productivity and Performance Systems (EPPS)? Describe one such application where you can imagine clear and compelling benefits. How would you test the effectiveness of your ideas?**
6. **It is one thing to understand current awareness profiling and to seize its implications, but sometimes another to put it into practice. Given that it would support your work, how could you ensure that starting current awareness profiling for yourself would guarantee an increase in your knowledge of your field as it changes and expands?**

References

1. Yensen JAP. (1997, April 9th). Welcome to the Virtual Nursing College! [WWW document]. URL http://www.langara.bc.ca/vnc/index.html
2. Pointcast, Inc. -Front Door (1997, April 8th). Pointcast Network. [WWW document]. URL http://www.pointcast.com/
3. In-Box Direct (1997) In-Box Direct Registration - Netscape. [WWW document]. URL http://form.netscape.com/cgi-bin/forms/misc/ibd_form/html/ibd_services_frameset.html
4. UnCover Reveal Information (1996, Dece 4th) UnCover Reveal Information. [WWW document]. URL http://www.carl.org/uncover/revinfo.html
5. Nursing Issues (NURSENET) This is an open, unmoderated, global electronic conference for discussing diverse issues in nursing administration, education, practice, and research. To subscribe, send an e-mail message to: LISTSERV@LISTSERV.UTORONTO.CA In the body of the message (not the subject line), write only: SUBSCRIBE NURSENET yourfirstname yourlastname.
6. Nursing Informatics (NRSING-L) In this list, the primary discussion topics are those in nursing informatics. However, all topics related to nursing are welcome. To subscribe, send an e-mail message to: LISTPROC@LISTS.UMASS.EDU In the body of the message (not the subject line), write only: SUBSCRIBE NRSING-L Yourfirstname Yourlastname
7. Nurse Manager (RNMGR) is an unmoderated listserv for Nurse Managers that facilitates discussion about their role in delivering health services. Topics to be addressed include staff scheduling problems, downsizing issues, redefinition of jobs and responsibilities, dispute resolution, employment laws and regulations, and the use of new technology. To subscribe, send an e-mail message to: RNMGR-request@cue.com In the body of the message (not the subject line) write only: subscribe

8. Yensen JAP: Telenursing, virtual nursing, and beyond, *Computers In Nurs* 14(4):213-214, 1996.
9. Registered Nurses Association of British Columbia (1997, April 15th) [WWW Document]. URL http://www.rnabc.bc.ca
10. British Columbia Nurses' Union (1997, January 9th) Welcome to BC Nurses' Union [WWW Document]. URL http://www.bcnu.org

Suggested Readings

Gery G: Electronic performance support systems: How and why to remake the workplace through the strategic application of technology, Boston, MA, 1991, Weingarten Publications.

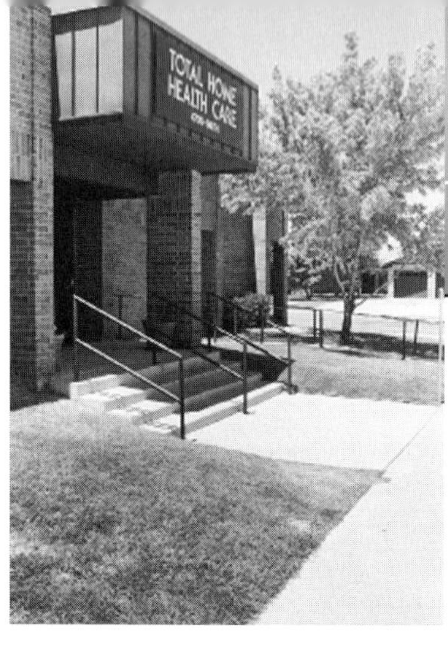

CHAPTER 18

The Future: A Challenge for Nurses and Nursing

Luther Christman

OBJECTIVES

After completing this chapter the reader should be able to:

- **Describe ways in which client care will be changed by technologic advances**
- **Identify new societal dynamics and problems that may create challenges to nurses and other health care professionals in the next couple of decades**
- **Propose changes in educational preparation for nurses that would provide greater congruency with educational levels of other highly respected professions**
- **Discuss how nurses are socialized into the profession through exposure in clinical settings and into nursing practice through interdisciplinary approaches**
- **Describe approaches to doctoral education that may be taken by nurses, and the emphases of these programs of study**

The future promises exciting and stimulating changes in the health care delivery system, and the nursing profession faces the challenge of taking an active part. The future image of nurses depends on how quickly and effectively nurses can lose the lethargy that is a major restraining force in their professional growth and development.

■ EXPANDING TECHNOLOGY

Every person involved in health care delivery is well aware of the economic, political, professional, scientific, and technologic forces that exert pressures on the system. For example, many nursing activities are already being done by technology. Vital signs will be monitored more accurately by machines than by clinicians.

Mechanisms will be built into monitoring devices to warn health care team members about deteriorating changes, alert them, and automatically effect changes in health status. Anxiety levels of clients will be assessed in a similar fashion. Software has been devised so that clients can perform much of their own psychotherapy without clinical assistance. Teaching machines will be available for clients to learn about their disease processes and how to manage them. Sensors will monitor therapeutic drug levels and automatically replenish them without clinician interface. All clinical records will be automated. Eventually all the scientific and clinical information generated by worldwide research will be online and available to clinicians of all types.[6,7]

The key to using this immense bank of knowledge will be the ability to ask the correct questions. Many persons will manage their personal health through home computers and access to this knowledge bank. As software becomes more sophisticated, each person will be able to have a highly individualized program for maintaining good health. Similarly, every clinician will have a personalized continuing education program tailored to knowledge deficits and to new and emerging knowledge needed to maintain competence. Another very important area of current research is the genome mapping project, which has the potential for introducing a very radical approach to both curing and preventing illness. Genetics may become the most studied field for the next few decades.

The Human Genome Project, funded at $3 billion, is moving ahead of schedule and will be completed by the year 2005 (or before). When finished, biology's periodic table will be produced. It will be composed of 100,000 genes. The resulting tree structure will depict ancestoral and functional affinities among human genes.[10] DNA and RNA applied knowledge utilization will be a major strand in client care. The genetic predisposition to states of health will be ascertained and closely monitored for each and every citizen as one means of reducing costs. Gene transplantation, and other applications of genetic research, will displace many of the present therapeutic modalities. Therapy in the womb may become commonplace.

The intense international cooperation in genetic research will catalyze the move to functional genomics.[14] Every clinician, of every type, will find it necessary to obtain an in-depth knowledge of genetics. Current students should be encouraged to ward off future obsolesence by taking a minor in genetics.

Ethical debates and the clarification of ethical approaches to the application of genetic therapy will become intensified and may last a long time before all the philosophical, religious, legal, racial, gender, ethnic, and socioeconomic issues are resolved.[3] The steady advancement of strong scientific understandings may enable the best ultimate use of all applied science for the human good.

■ COMPUTER ASSISTANCE

Microprocessors are in an astonishingly rapid state of change; a change many may find hard to realize and understand. Every 18 months microprocessors double in speed. Based on present trends, a scholar in this field has predicted that one desktop computer in the year 2020 will be as powerful as all of the computers in Silicon Valley today.[3] Ideas being investigated such as (1) quantum dots and other single-electron devices, (2) molecular computing, (3) nanomechanical logic gates, and (4) reversible logic gates all are indicators of rapid progress in this area.[9] Every clinician will have to be adept in informatics to participate in the care system. As computers become smaller and simpler to operate, they will be as common in homes as telephones presently are. Home care, in all likelihood, will dominate over all present types.

Computer-assisted client care can reduce error and give certitude to the clinical planning process. It also can be used to evaluate client care. It will be possible to develop methods to assess the quality of performance of each practitioner and the cumulative performance of the staff. A complete audit trail may be kept on each clinician. At the end of the year a performance score for each clinician of every type will be available. Licensure renewal will depend on performance based on national norms rather than some perfunctory protocols. All these developments will lead to the reorganization of hospitals into clinical and nonclinical entities. This approach will conserve considerable nurse time, increase productivity, require more competence, lower the costs charged against the nursing budget, and may reduce the total number of employees.

Increasing employment of computers for the maintenance of client records will eventually enable health care professionals in disparate locations to access this information and prevent problems such as conflicting prescriptions. Such individual records could either be carried by each person on a computer disk or be accessible by means of a magnetized card such as the "Health Security Card" that President Clinton promoted. Japan is using computers in a manner that may point to the future: big computer companies, telecommunications firms, and the government are trying to computerize two routine elements of hospital care—diagnosis and prescription.[16]

■ ROBOTS

Robots are also being used in clinical settings. At the beginning of 1994, the University of Virginia hospital was reported to have developed robots to conduct blood analyses.[4] The use of robots on intensive care units is not only time- and money-saving, but also cuts down on human exposure to bloodborne infections. The blood analyzers have mechanical arms that handle blood specimens so that health care workers have lower exposure. The robots also save time, taking only 2 or 3 minutes to perform analyses that normally take 20 minutes. These machines and other new forms of technology will be expensive, but they will pay for themselves in exactitude and in saved personnel time. Furthermore, they will have a 24-hour-a-day, 7-day-a-week availability. Artificial intelligence will emerge and be reliable and productive.[1] All these developments will put in place a strong framework to aid in reducing errors of both commission and omission. Each breakthrough in technology will stimulate further developments and refinements in a continuous panoply of technologic accrual.

Remote care will become a norm as devices for assessing clients from a considerable distance become commonplace. As an example, a school of engineering in a large state university has a federally funded project to develop a device that will enable clinicians to palpate clients some hundred or more miles distant as easily as if they were physically present. A fully cybernated system is in the offering.

■ NEW THREATS TO HEALTH

Some future forms of illness will require a multiprofessional approach. Possible examples are health problems that result from the environment. Depletion of the ozone layer may precipitate new forms of pathology. Problems secondary to waste disposal will inevitably arise. The disturbance created by disruption of natural ecologic balances may open significant avenues for future disease processes. An increasing density of the world's population may provide a built-in incubation medium for fostering new diseases. The air travel that facilitates movement of humans and animals around the world also circulates and transports vectors of airborne disease that are capable of creating massive health problems because of the other microorganisms they may contain. There is a reasonable possibility of more retroviruses emerging that are not dependent on sexual transmission. Longer lifespans may result in the manifestation of more genetically influenced diseases. The list of new impingements on good health is growing.

The ironic coexistence of loneliness and population density may cause new varieties of psychosocial/biologic stresses. People may work in more socially isolated environments that result from sophisticated technology. In an automated office, for example, a worker may have no other human contact. As the world's population nearly doubles, so does its social density. With this happening there may be many forms of sociologic pressures that are capable of creating concomitant disruption in human functioning. All of these suppositions are based on trends that are already in evidence.

Clients who experience disturbances of loneliness and population density have sociologic, anthropologic, and psychologic problems. Managing the client in his or her own setting then presents an opportunity to treat the holistic pattern of disarray instead of simply applying psychologic reductionism to every situation. Holistic care, properly managed, will require clinical training at the doctoral level to produce the best outcomes. Nurses who perform well in this role build confidence in clients, which enhances the image of the profession.

■ NURSES ENTER PRIVATE PRACTICE

Nurse-owned health care organizations also can deliver satisfactory and effective health care service to the public. A probable national health insurance, with all the bureaucratic controls inherent in such a system, may result in the curtailment or restriction of fees for service for all forms of clinicians. Contractual arrangements will be one of the chief means of reimbursement. Nurse-owned, home-based businesses such as home health care agencies are growing and becoming strong components of care.

The care of clients in hospitals of the future will be different. Only the acutely ill, who require all of the advantages of the automated hospital, will be hospitalized. As this new automated hospital is put into operation, nursing care may be a prime need for hospitalization. To keep pace with technology, nurses will have to perform far beyond the level of technology. In all likelihood, nurses will be able to manage only one client or very few clients under such intense conditions. The necessary closeness and constancy of interaction will change professional and public perceptions of the capability of nurses.

■ COLLEGIALITY AMONG HEALTH PROFESSIONS

Acceleration of technology and economic crises in the health care field requires the ability to positively shape and modify various pressures; this, in turn, depends on how much cohesion exists within each respective group of workers and clients within the system. Those groups with a strong public image can use their strength to influence the format of health care delivery and are better able to attract intelligent and career-oriented students, to be appointed to key policy-making commissions, and to foster collegial relationships with important power groups.

All clinical professions will find it increasingly necessary to function as multidisciplinary units. The movements toward doctoral preparation for all will result in a large overlap of knowledge content between them. There may ultimately be mergers of professions and a reduction in their number.[12] It is not possible to predict in which direction these mergers will go. What is certain is that the chief influence will be the state of scientific and clinical knowledge at the time these may occur.

As all the professions move into highly advanced preparation, a large overlap of scientific and clinical knowledge among all will ensue. The role expression of knowledge will be a distinguishing characteristic. The variations in time and space binding of each respective type across the diversity of clients will be a crucial factor as to the effectiveness of each and to their value to the health care system. Each different type, because of this vast sharing of knowledge, will have substantial respect and trust for others instead of the subtle undercutting often present in the current educational preparation system. Trust is very vital in helping to bring about constructive change.[5] Groups that will not commit to this scientific level of preparation will gradually lose membership on the health care team and slip out of professional existence. The exponential doubling of knowledge every 2 years will force this conclusion.

National registration will displace state regulation because remote care programs will cross state borders. Remote care will enable clients to be much more selective about obtaining the best possible care. National registration also will enable clinicians of all types to move freely when opportunities present themselves. Thus national norms are critical to progress by having standards that do not fluctuate. A single-payer system, or a similar means, will replace the hodge-podge disconnected system now in use.

It is reasonable to conceive that each citizen's health history will be charted on a microchip. A program for individual health maintenance will be encoded on it. Every individual who complies closely with the yearly requirements will get an income tax refund. Those who do not will have to pay an additional income tax charge. This will stimulate everyone to follow a health maintenance pathway. Thus a reduction in national health care costs across the entire population as a whole should ensue.

■ EDUCATIONAL PREPARATION: BUILDING TOWARD UNITY

Many studies about nursing are done by researchers outside the profession, and each study strongly recommends that preparation for nursing be in institutions of higher learning. Although some progress has been made, educational preparation continues as the major point of division. Nurses appear to insist on the weakest preparation of any of the members of the health professions; 70% have less than a baccalaureate education. The education process is crucial because it establishes the base around which a profession can rally its strengths and plan for advancement. To understand why it is currently a problem, it may be helpful to consider several significant factors.

The concept of nursing education was imported from abroad and lacked the predisposition to migrate to universities, a mark of the professions that developed out of higher education in this country. Customarily, nurses were trained in small neighborhood schools, where nursing students were kept in isolation from students of the various other health professions. This contributed to a lack of understanding, as nursing students gained only a rudimentary notion of the competencies of the members of the other professions. More serious, however, was the fact that members of other professions poorly understood nurses—a fact still evident in many situations. Thus the educational isolation of nurses is detrimental to all.

The pattern of an abundance of small schools tied to local communities continued with the advent of community college programs. Although the form of the preparation changed, the substance remained essentially the same. Community control and local employment opportunities continued to dominate. Career orientations were thwarted without further education. Employment histories of nurses displayed a series of jobs rather than a professional career. Hospitals and other local employers, in turn, were subject to local supplies of nurses. This relationship became a strong barrier to innovation and change, and the effect on nurses' incomes was profound. A few employers could quietly agree on nurses' salaries and mute the effect of supply and demand over a long period. These same employers paid nationally competitive salaries to persons in the other professional groups, since all had to recruit from the same university campuses. Thus the ground rules for professional income took different directions. This set of circumstances probably is a major reason for the nurse shortages that develop from time to time.

I, and others contributing to this text, believe that only on university campuses can students learn the political and organizational skills needed to effectively deal with the complexities of the world of health care. The power and influence of nurses has shrunk compared to other health care professionals as a result of the relative deprivation in education. Without a uniform educational base, it may be impossible to (1) inform the public about what nurses do, (2) stabilize colleagueships with other professionals, (3) set clear standards of care, and (4) ensure adequate funding of the profession.

As the various clinical professions increase their respective knowledge bases sufficiently to manage the rapidly enlarging scientific core, the differences between them may diminish. The merging of some, most, or all is one of the possible outcomes. The enlarging scientific core is used differently by each profession; this results in the total knowledge content that prepares individuals in a unique clinical profession. With a uniform educational base, nursing will be perceived as developing from a scientific core, shared with other clinical professions, into a profession in its own right with goals and skills that make it "nursing."

In the future, the Doctor of Nursing degree as pioneered at Case Western University may become the minimum background for entry into the profession. It is analogous to the Doctor of Dentistry or Doctor of Medicine degree. The clinical doctorate in nursing, as advanced preparation, is somewhat analogous to the clinical residencies. The combined D.N.sc./Ph.D. will give nurses equality with the M.D./Ph.D. and help them to be frontrunners. Adopting this pathway will enable nurses to keep pace with the expanding theory and content of science. Nurses, to be objective, must begin to compare nurses to other clinicians and not nurses to other nurses.

Changes in Role Image

Professional practice laws and licensure restrictions for any particular field are based mainly on the level of professional preparation required. This mode of recognition is deeply embedded in American culture. Significant changes in the level of recognition for nurses, notably a positive change in image and income, will come if the vast majority of nurses are rigorously educated.

Nursing has the stigma of inertia; part of this inertia results from the role-socialization process. Many nurses have not undergone the role-professionalizing process of the university-based professions. Role-socialization for these nurses occurs, for the most part, in isolation from other students because they are restricted by their educational and clinical commitments. Because of the paucity of instruction in fundamental sciences, moreover, their preparation is more task-oriented, with emphasis on motor skills rather than thoughtful analysis of the clinical scene. Heavily entrenched "ward routines" and procedure-book ideology help to condition them to almost automatic behavior with little variation at any time. Leo Simmons, the anthropologist who collaborated with Virginia Henderson on collating nursing research, once commented, "Nurses know more about *how* and less about *why* than any other profession."

Role empathy, or taking the role of the other person with all the insight that is required, is a means of assisting easy communication within the profession. It is, essentially, a form of social fit in which all the role dimensions are clear and each nurse can adjust with some degree of freedom instead of stereotyped preconceptions.

The heterogeneity of preparation by different routes lessens role empathy among nurses and saps their ability to mobilize for improvement. Thus several images of nurses and nursing practice have become indigenous to the profession. Clarification of the professional role image cannot result until nursing achieves a homogeneity of preparation.

Nurses with less than a baccalaureate degree have not had the advantage of enough time to comprehend the vast amount of knowledge necessary to become responsible health care providers. It is humanly impossible to acquire in just a few years the same knowledge base in chemistry, psychology, physiology, anatomy, and other natural and social sciences that other health care professionals have spent 10 years studying. Nurses are responsible for the accuracy and level of performance by practitioners with less educational preparation than they. Thus their very license is on the line when they must assume responsibility for the moment-to-moment activities of their team members. The lessening of role empathy that results kindles friction among nurses.

Examining professional preparation from an ethical perspective is one way to explore improvement of the nursing image. From that perspective, nurses must fulfill professional responsibility to the public. This does not happen when faculty members of schools preparing nurses hold less than university standing. Because of this situation, they are frequently out of the mainstream of knowledge about technical advancement, and the knowledge they do pass on to students is narrowed. Because nurses are sometimes the only interface between the most current health care and the client, the latter often loses. Nurses cannot maintain their ethical commitment to clients if they do not keep pace with the burgeoning output of science and technology.

By a mere matter of logistics, less than half the scientific content of university programs can be taught in 2-year programs. The advanced levels of science in the upper division are planned to be richer in content than introductory courses. Because one cannot use knowledge one does not have, no matter how highly motivated, graduates of nonbaccalaureate programs can provide care only from a restricted base. Education that narrowly restricts the knowledge base of graduates also restricts their ability to serve the best interests of clients. On these grounds, cranking out large numbers of graduates from "crash" training programs must be questioned in the growing ethical climate of the nation. The insidious comparison of a reduced scientific base for nursing education, compared to all other clinical providers, surely does pose an ethical and moral dilemma. Withholding scientific content through abbreviated curriculum offerings justifies an ethical probe into the ultimate outcome for clients. Rigorous examination reveals various ethical flaws.

Intertwined with these ethical problems are economic implications that result from increased overhead expenses incurred by maintaining large numbers of small schools. It appears that no one has seriously assessed this economic cost, because the pattern continues. Assessed and planned on a large scale, there could be enough saved on the overhead costs of maintaining so large a number of small schools that the savings could pay for most nurses to complete much or all of their graduate education. To project overall, only 150 large university schools may be needed to graduate more well-prepared nurses than can be done by the existing splintered system, which currently includes approximately 1150 accredited baccalaureate, associate, and diploma programs in the United States.

The nursing profession has a monopoly on its practice, granted by means of licensure or registration. It also has a concomitant obligation to supply high standards of service to the public. One cannot avoid the ethics of this position. Only professions that maintain high public trust can expect to wield strong social influence in the affairs of health. This influence is not a condition granted in perpetuity by society but must be continually earned and maintained through unstinting effort by those who make the profession a career. One of the easiest ways to spark this growth is to urge every new baccalaureate graduate to immediately enroll in graduate study. Within 5 years, an entirely new crop of nurse careerists could be in place. A new plateau would be a reality and act as catalyst to keep the flow of energy focused on high goals. The image of nurses as a superb public resource would be potentiated and recognized as a professional knowledge system able to keep current with the burgeoning of scientific knowledge and human needs.

Unification of Practice and Education

As discussed previously, nurses wishing to move to full professional status must strengthen their role. The full professional role for any of the clinical professions encompasses the activities generally listed under the concepts of practice, education, research, management, and consultation. When nurses adopt only one of these subroles and try to force that subrole into a full role activity, a diminution in quality occurs. Additionally, when large numbers of nurses make this decision, the profession is atomized. The growing edge of each part is narrowed and lacks stimulation. However, the growing edge has a far different quality when the full professional role is achieved. If all nurses were able to assume the full professional role, the profession would compare favorably with the progress identifiable in the other major clinical professions such as medicine and psychology.

The role induction or role socialization of students into the profession is in many respects as critical to their development as is their academic program. Students seem to experience less reality shock in settings where there is a smoothly operational unification of service and education. This role-induction process produces qualitative differences. Students experience qualitative differences that affect their role induction when they must learn in settings where aloofness, scapegoating, or any other forms of friction are present among nurses. This learning situation may be contrasted with settings in which service and education activities are mutually facilitative. In the first setting, students perform under wraps and must choose sides; in the other, the milieu encourages students to be expressive users of knowledge. Furthermore, the sensitive issues of ethical practice can be more thoughtfully examined when service and education are integrated components. The establishment of healthy learning environments for student nurses is a current challenge within schools of nursing, and the current status within each varies by degrees from what is most desirable.

If nursing education and practice become unified, an excellent means of socializing students is possible because behavioral models of excellence are in place. Commitment is fostered from a learned lifestyle dominated by values that stimulate growth and formulation of a professional conscience (in other words, an inner voice that guides and monitors behavior). This model of education and service provides mentors capable of stimulating students to think big about career choices and, in the final analysis, the way is paved for better interprofessional efforts to improve client care.

As stated earlier, the amount of scientific knowledge a practitioner possesses is set by the individual's level of educational preparation. Clinical behavior is a direct outcome of this background because the predispositions to act in the clinical situation are formed, limited, and defined by the quantity of knowledge possessed by each practitioner. Of course, one's ability to apply possessed knowledge in the practice arena differs among individuals. There can be no guarantee that individuals will use the knowledge they possess.

Structural variables used in organizing care also greatly influence the quality of care provided. An entirely different outcome is possible when the structure enables synchronized effort as opposed to settings where constraints are built in. In the first situation, service and education are not artificially limited and isolated entities, and the full use of knowledge can be mobilized. In the second situation, polarization of these entities hampers the innovative use of knowledge.

Full use of knowledge is an obligation the nursing profession owes to the public it serves. Artificial constraints on full professional competence result in disservice to the public. The academic enterprise cannot remain encapsulated from the empirical use of knowledge, and the service system cannot remain insulated from the source of most knowledge and still produce professional nursing services that will be highly valued by society. When the two elements of practice are melded together in a unified whole, the result is a rapid dissemination of new knowledge, for the examination of novel and more sophisticated practice issues, and for the growth of a rich medium to support more strength and vigor in clinical efforts. This unification is the absolute basic requisite for the creation of centers of excellence in nursing. Clinical research cannot thrive without easy entry to the care arena, for that is where the exciting research problems are to be identified.

Nurses in both service and education roles must work together to improve the nursing educational environment. Improvement may result in a higher percentage of nurses extending their education. Besides a low number of candidates for higher degrees as compared to all other clinical and scientific disciplines, nurses tend to further their education at a later period in life. The bulk of persons earning doctoral degrees in most other professions and disciplines generally do so by their late twenties. They launch their careers when they are young and energetic. The small percentage of nurses at the doctoral level is combined with an older age of attainment, a situation that is not conducive to building leadership strength. Clinical research as a means of enriching practice remains at low ebb, important positions in the profession are filled with less strongly prepared nurses, and collaboration with other major providers is hampered by inequalities in sophisticated knowledge. The reunification of education and practice is a powerful means of enhancing the strength of the profession.

Self-Governance

Self-governance is another means of consolidating professional pride, self-imagery, and clinical visibility.[6] Nurse faculty members generally function under self-governance. When self-governing concepts are used by nursing staff organizations, the potential to consolidate the strength of nursing management with that of the clinical vigor of the nursing staff may be enhanced to a considerable degree. The rights, responsibilities, and obligations of this pathway should enable nurses to serve through the standards emanating from a unified effort. Participation in this endeavor can result in new vistas of self-direction and augment the professional growth of each nurse.

Recruiting the Best Candidates into Nursing

A structural factor that affects nursing is its strong adherence to a single-gender profession. The recruitment of other-than-white women into schools of nursing is very noticeable. There especially has been an increase in the number of nonwhite women since President Johnson's administration and the advent of affirmative action legislation. Yet the incremental growth in the number of men seems to be influenced more by the admission decisions of individual schools rather than by a measured and united effort by the nursing profession. Continued democratization of health personnel and persistent effort by nurses to become a genuine two-gender profession will result in an improved image. It is awkward to insist on affirmative action for women and then not set a good example. A two-gender profession would have all the benefits of balance.

Relatively few studies examine variables related to what attracts and keeps men in nursing. In all probability, the characteristics listed as desirable nursing qualities are not possessed by all the women in the profession any more than all the needed qualifications to be a competent physician are limited to men. Job opportunity and potential for income growth are probably the two biggest basic attractions that must be present to recruit men. These two features will also attract more top-quality women candidates into nursing.

To ensure that nurses can recruit into the profession the most people with the highest attributes, the recruitment net has to be expanded. Men will have to be included, or those professions that recruit nondiscriminatingly by gender will have an advantage. The democratization of the profession to include minority populations and men will do much to change the image of nursing.

The increasing mass of scientific information is leading all of the clinical professions to enrich their respective preparations and to adopt a doctoral degree as the entry level of practice. Clinicians such as physicians, dentists, and veterinarians who have rich preparation are adding fellowships to their residencies. Clinical psychologists are emphasizing postdoctoral training. This movement to enrich basic preparation may be one of the reasons for the drop-off in nurse enrollments. Many parents want their children to attend colleges and universities because higher education for the professions is perceived by many to be the wave of the future. Because nursing education has not traditionally been an integral part of this movement, students may select those fields that are clearly in step with the future.

Nursing doctorates will need to have a strong background in the clinical aspect of the profession. Unless the Ph.D. programs offered by schools of nursing have rich content so that they become as strong clinically as those for the Ph.D. in clinical psychology, for instance, the gain will not be very substantial. Continuing to emphasize research methodology and functional content without a rich clinical base will not enable nurses to match the strengths of members of other health professions. The psychologist's model, for example, demonstrates that a strong clinical base and research competence can go hand in hand.

The clinical doctorate in nursing (D.Nsc.) comes closer to achieving this end than any other development in the graduate preparation of nurses. The essence of research is asking the right question. Without astute insight into practice there is less possibility of intuitively devising the discriminating question. The rigors of using the methods of science to transform theory and content of scientific knowledge into a social good called *clinical care* sensitizes the practitioner to the nuances of correct framing of clinical issues.

Professional degrees are usually regarded by the public as esteemed degrees and are given a higher social rating than academic degrees. Certainly, for the basic biologic and behavioral sciences, the academic degree is the major pathway. However, persons with professional degrees can be most useful when people need care, thus generating respect. Although it is not the only reason, this is a chief reason why physicians, lawyers, and ministers occupy the social status they are given. People who have the knowledge to assist the populace are given more recognition than those who are more remote, such as basic scientists, although basic scientists are as vital as applied scientists.

Lateral Mobility for Nurses

Another advantage of the clinical doctorate is that it permits the possibility of nurses earning combined doctorates in the manner of M.D./Ph.D. programs. The combination of a scientific doctorate with the professional one results in use of a wide range of content to develop interesting research problems and to participate with an enlarged contribution to multidisciplinary research. Futurists agree that research endeavors of the future will embrace several disciplines/professions in the research enterprise, because no one person will have a broad enough knowledge base to investigate the type of questions that have to be addressed. The first nurse to become a Nobel laureate might emerge from this background. The image of nurses as contributors to the scientific domain would be strongly enhanced by such an event.

■ SUMMARY

Unification of all elements of professional nursing is essential to survival as nurses face the burgeoning entirety of scientific knowledge. There is no longer time for division and boundary watching. No one is preventing nurses from obtaining superlative clinical skills except nurses themselves. Clarifying their educational preparation is the most important variable in changing the perceptions that society has of nurses. All the data collected about nurses show that nurses want respect, desire more input into the client care structure, and aspire to have more freedom of clinical decision making. All of these aspirations can be fulfilled by approximating the scientific and clinical preparation of those persons who already have these degrees of freedom. That knowledge leads to power has long been recognized.

The current mood of unrest makes the care system vulnerable to change. Developed plans that assist in mobilizing the imaginative qualities of nurses can become built-in catalysts that will surge as an electrifying current throughout the profession. Courage and desire to do what must be done must be demonstrated. The remarkable increase in the potential for improving the nursing care of clients has such social and moral mandates inherent in the concept that it can fan the flames of desire for change. Nurses have a splendid opportunity to move forward. Massive studies are not necessary. What is required is an aspiration to potentiate the competencies of nurses. Although the change will entail some disruptions in present lifestyles of many nurses, the benefits to clients will far outweigh existing rewards. These benefits will include improved client care, increased social value of the profession, increased financial renumeration for the individual nurse, and the self-actualization of each and every nurse.

Science is not self-limiting. It has a worldwide influence. The profession of nursing in every country will need to cope with the exponential increase in science, which is doubling about every 2 years. This increase challenges every scientist and every clinician, in all the various fields, to remain informed of changing theories and applications. If nurses throughout the world are to keep pace with this irreversible tide of expanding knowledge, they must thoughtfully plan a pattern of professional development that includes the ability to absorb and use scientific knowledge in a creative and socially useful manner.

As in other professions, basic preparation for nursing is being redefined as a result of the increasing knowledge base required for practice. Today only Iceland and Australia require university education for licensure, but this base may begin to spread to all other countries. Two states, North Dakota and Maine, have pioneered this approach in the United States, but there has not been as yet any movement by other states. If nurses in the United States accept the goal of increasing their educational base, they can become world leaders in the profession and stimulate international progress.

Some nurses in the United States have very sophisticated clinical and scientific backgrounds. They have the potential for being the behavioral models of preparation that will be emulated in the United States and worldwide. The lethargy that stymies the attainment of this sophisticated clinical competence must be overcome by concerted action of the various nursing professional organizations, educators, and nursing systems administrators. Many countries are developing small elite enclaves of nurses, but a widespread proliferation of numbers is key to the future of the profession.[2,7] Worldwide advancement is necessary to develop a strong and respected profession. Nurses can no longer be preoccupied exclusively with their own country of origin. Computer linkage throughout the world is making concerted action among nurses of various nations more feasible.

Nurses compose the largest number of all the health professions, with a huge potential to be enormously useful to society. If nurses individually dedicate themselves to a unity of purpose, commit themselves to adhere closely to the canons of true professionalism, shake off the doubts and misgivings that prohibit forward movement, give leadership to a worldwide strengthening of the profession, and develop scholarship and research at the Nobel laureate level, nursing *will* become a magnificent profession. The urge to serve, the deciding factor that caused each person to select nursing as a life work, can inspire all to unlimited progress. Striving in an organized and cohesive way, nurses can fulfill the desire to serve and do it gloriously. Now is the time to begin; each one who waits becomes guilty of wasting the greatest opportunity that nursing has ever had. The cumulative effect of moving in the direction of dynamic change is a stimulus to all.

CRITICAL THINKING *Activities*

1. **Discuss the pros and cons of having various levels/types of nursing education programs.**
2. **How does the socialization process for nurses take place? Give examples from experience.**
3. **What is meant by clarification of role image? How does it occur?**
4. **Explore the educational level of faculty in your school of nursing. How does it compare with other faculty on your college or university campus?**
5. **What are possible approaches to recruit the brightest and best candidates for nursing into the profession?**

References

1. Abu-Mostafa YS: Machines that learn from hints, *Scientific American* 272: 64-69, 1995.
2. Aiken LH, Fagin C: *Charting nursing's future: agenda for the 1990's*, Philadelphia, 1992, Lippincott.
3. Beardsley T: Vital data, *Scientific American* 274: 100-105, 1996.

4. Brown HN: Virginia hospital turns robots to handle risky blood work, *Philadelphia Inquirer* Jan. 4, 1994, p. 85.
5. Chapman M: Trust and its revelance to individuals and groups in institutions facing change, *Working Paper,* No. 10. The University of Lincolnshire and Humberside, 1996.
6. Christman L: The autonomous nursing staff in the hospital, *The National Joint Practice Commission Bulletin* 2(3), Oct, 1976. Reprinted in: *Nurs Admin Q* 1(1):37.
7. Christman L, Counte M: *Hospital organization and patient care,* Boulder, Colo.: 1981, Westview Press.
8. Deleted in proofs.
9. Editors, *Scientific American* 273: 67, 1995.
10. Lander EL: The new genomics: global visions of biology, *Science* 274: 536–539, 1996.
11. Deleted in proofs.
12. Misuse of R.N.'s spurs shortage, says a new study, *Am J Nurs* 89:1223, 1989.
13. Deleted in proofs.
14. Schuler GD and others: A gene map of the human genomes, *Science* 274: 540-545, 1996.
15. Deleted in proofs.
16. Tokyo: Science and technology: hospital hopes, *The Economist* Oct. 9, 1993.

Suggested Readings

Bridgeman, M: Collegiate education for nursing, New York, 1985. Russell Sage Foundation.

Cohen, B., and Jordet, C. Nursing schools: students' beacon to professionalism? *Nurs. Health Care* 9:38.

National Commission for the Study of Nursing and Nursing Education. *An abstract for action.* New York: McGraw-Hill Book Co., 1970.

News: R.N.s are stars of a multimedia campaign to mend their "Image." ASN 40 (April 1990):130.

News caps: Schools woo new students. AJN 40 (April 1990):130.

Royal College of Nursing. In L. Christman *In pursuit of excellence: A position statement on nursing.* London: 1987.

Sarvimaki, A. Knowledge in interactive disciplines (Research Bulletin No. 68). Helsinki, Finland: University of Helsinki, Dept. of Education, 1988.

Science, Genome Issue, October 25, 1996, Vol. 274.

Scientific American, Key Technologies for the 21st Century (150th Anniversary Issue), Sept. 1995, Vol. 273.

APPENDIX A

NURSING ORGANIZATIONS ONLINE

American Association for the History of Nursing (http://users.aol.com/nsghistory/AAHN.html)

This site provides general association information including membership benefits, awards programs, and annual conferences, as well as nursing history bibliographies and a preview of the table of contents for each upcoming issue of the journal *Nursing History Review.*

American Association of Colleges of Nursing (http://www.aacn.nche.edu)

AACN seeks to maintain high standards for baccalaureate and higher-degree nursing education programs. This resource contains information related to AACN affairs, nursing education, and nursing careers and also provides an interactive forum for members to discuss current issues in nursing.

American Association of Critical-Care Nurses (http://www.aacn.org)

AACN's site offers information on certification, specific chapters, publications, meetings and events, travel planning, teleconference programs, publications, research, and membership. Additional on-line resources are available for AACN members.

American Association of Neuroscience Nurses (http://www.aann.org)

Helpful information related to neuroscience nursing is included here, with such resources as the AANN newsletter (*AANN Synapse*), neuroscience registered nurse certification information, and abstracts from the most recent issues of *The Journal of Neuroscience Nursing.*

American Association of Occupational Health Nurses, Inc. (http://www.aaohn.org)

This site contains information on the AAOHN and its goals, mission, publications, and membership. Also included are links to information on employment, certification, and continuing education.

American College of Nurse-Midwives (ACNM) (http://www.acnm.org)

Information regarding ACNM, such as organization philosophy and membership, is provided at this site, as well as certification and education resources. A geographic index of nurse-midwifery practices is also presented with other hints for locating additional nurse-midwives.

American College of Nurse Practitioners (http://www.nurse.org/acnp)

This site reports the activities of the American College of Nurse Practitioners including conference information, and gives brief legislative updates affecting the nursing profession. Contact information is provided.

American Journal of Nursing Company Online Services (http://www.ajn.org)

Provides information relating to the online services available through AJN: company information, online publication and subscription information, the AJN Career Guide, continuing education courses, a multimedia catalog, and network services.

American Holistic Nurses' Association (http://ahna.org)

AHNA's site provides in-depth information about the organization, including their philosophy, membership information, events, and frequently asked questions. Additional services provided include a message board and a chat room.

American Nephrology Nurses' Association (http://www.inurse.com/~anna)

ANNA organizational information is presented at this site, which includes an in-depth upcoming conference events calendar.

American Nurses Association (http://www.ana.org)

This source, developed by the ANA, provides information about the organization, itself, as well as membership listings by state, credentialing information, and links to affiliated organizations. Also available at this site is access to ANA's intranet, some nursing publications, products offered by ANA and ordering information, information disseminated by the government affairs division of the organization, and other general nursing news links.

American Psychiatric Nurses Association (http://www.musc.edu:80/apna)

This source has information regarding the association and its goals while also providing general psychiatric, mental-health nursing resources such as the *APNA Journal*, mental health consumers' guides, and links to other related Web sites.

American Society of PeriAnesthesia Nurses (http://www.aspan.org:80/index.htm)

This society serves nurses who work in ambulatory surgery, preanesthesia, and postanesthesia care. This site contains the missions and goals of the group, as well as information on position statements, history, publications, membership, scholarships, research, conferences, and clinical practice.

AMIA Nursing Informatics Working Group (http://www.gl.umbc.edu/~abbott/nurseinfo.html)

This source represents the interests of nursing informatics and of the Working Group members. Included are links to annual and current activities, the 1996 slate of officers, recent newsletters, bylaws, and links to related sites and to the AMIA Homepage.

Association de Recherche en Soins Infirmiers, A.R.S.I. (http://perso.club-internet.fr/giarsi)

The French Nursing Research Association site contains information about the association's aims and activities plus links to other Internet nursing resources in French and English.

Association for Australian Rural Nurses (http://www.aarn.asn.au)

This site contains information about the Association of Australian Rural Nurses and its goals. Press releases, newsletters, and conference information are also available.

Association of Nurses in AIDS Care (http://www.anacnet.org/aids)

This association is dedicated to the professional development of nurses who are involved in the care of individuals with the human immunodeficiency virus. This site contains information on the group's goals, mission, membership, and activities.

Association of Operating Room Nurses, Inc. (http://www.aorn.org)

An association devoted to perioperative nursing related issues, AORN's site contains resources regarding current developments in perioperative nursing, education, and clinical practice. Information for further consultation assistance is also provided.

Association of Rehabilitation Nurses (http://www.rehabnurse.org)

Information on ARN membership, certification, continuing education, publications, networking opportunities, periodicals, grants/scholarships, the Rehabilitation Nursing Foundation, members of the board of directors, and general resources for the public are all provided at this site.

Australasian Neuroscience Nurses' Association (http://sydney.dialix.oz.au/~annaexec/anna_exe.html)

This ANNA resource provides information about membership, association events, the association's history, general meeting venues, contact information for the executive committee, its general meeting venues, and an in-depth discussion of ANNA's nursing standards. There are also additional links for nursing research and professional contacts.

Canadian Association of Critical Care Nurses (http://www.execulink.com/~caccn)

The CACCN site provides information on the association's mission, membership, chapters, conferences, and awards.

Canadian Council of Cardiovascular Nurses (http://ALUMNI.LAURENTIAN.CA/www/psyc/r/cccn)

The Canadian Council of Cardiovascular Nurses site provides information on membership, conferences, fellowships, and a link to the *Canadian Journal of Cardiovascular Nursing.*

Emergency Nurses Association (http://www.ena.org)

Describes the histories and goals regarding the following organizations: ENA, the ENA Foundation, Emergency Nurses Cancel Alcohol Related Emergencies (EN C.A.R.E.), and the Board of Certification for Emergency Nursing. Additional certification information such as application deadlines and examination schedules are also listed.

European Nursing Informatics Project (Nightingale) (http://www.dn.uoa.gr/nightingale)

This project works to educate and train nurses in the use of health care–related information systems. This site provides an overview and the objectives of the project, as well as information on the partners in the project, conferences, workshops, a newsletter, and links to related sites.

Hospice Nursing Association (http://www.Roxane.COM/HNA)

The association's purpose, mission statement, member groups, and other relevant links about this organization is provided here, along with information regarding national board certification for hospice nursing.

International Child Health Nursing Alliance (http://www2.ido.gmu.edu/ichna)

The goal of this organization is to improve the health care of children worldwide. This site contains membership information, task force reports, conferences, papers, and other resources related to pediatric nursing.

International Parish Nurse Resource Center (http://www.advocatehealth.com/sites/pnursctr.html)

This site describes the philosophy and organization of the International Parish Nurse Resource Center while also providing contact information, conference information, and access to their online newsletter.

Midwest Nursing Research Society (http://www.umich.edu/~nursing/mnrs)

The Midwest Nursing Research Society is an organization devoted to the development and utilization of nursing research in all health care service and educational settings throughout the 13-state region of the Midwest. The MNRS Web site provides information on nursing research, funding sources, publications, program meetings, and information about the MNRS.

National Association of Neonatal Nurses (http://www.ajn.org/ajnnet/nrsorgs/nann)

Membership information, ordering information for publications on practice standards and guidelines, conference schedules, and other Internet neonatal nursing resources are presented at this site.

National Council of State Boards of Nursing (http://www.ncsbn.org)

This site provides information on the National Council of State Boards of Nursing, NCLEX, ordering publications, events, programs, services, and an online library of publications.

National Institute of Nursing Research (http://www.nih.gov/ninr/index.html)

The National Institute of Nursing Research's mission is to promote science that strengthens nursing practice and improves health care. The National Institute of Nursing Research supports interdisciplinary research and research training in universities, hospitals, and research centers across the country and conducts intramural investigations at the National Institutes of Health.

Nursing Ethics Network (http://www.bc.edu/bc_org/avp/son/ethics.html)

Information is provided here about the Nursing Ethics Network (NEN), a regional organization of professional nurses. Purposes of the NEN, brief descriptions of the current advisory board members, and further contact information are presented.

Nursing Organizations and Publications with Electronic Mail Access (http://www.nursing.ab.umd.edu/students/~snewbol/sknorg.htm)

An alphabetical listing of approximately 40 nursing organizations and publications that have e-mail access. Contact information including names, addresses, phone numbers, and e-mail addresses is provided.

Nursing Specialist Interest Group Homepage (http://www.bcs.org.uk/siggroup/sg39.htm)

A British organization that is interested in the use of information management and technology and the nursing perspective of health care computing.

Oncology Nursing Society (http://www.ons.org)

This site contains information for oncology nurses, including current news topics, conventions, educational opportunities, awards available, membership benefits, employment news, position papers, and certification requirements. It also provides links to other Internet oncology-related sites.

Ordre des Infirmieres et Infirmiers du Québec (http://www.oiiq.org/ang.html)

OIIQ is composed of over 67,000 members, and this site seeks to address social, political, and professionals concerns of Québec nurses. Most of the site is in French, but English information is being added, including an excerpt from L'infirmière du Québec.

Royal College of Nurses (http://www.nursing-standard.co.uk/rcnl.htm)

A description of the Royal College of Nursing (RCN) based in the United Kingdom and information on Nurseline and RCN counseling and advisory services are available.

Southern Nursing Research Society (http://www.uams.edu/nursing/snrs/mainmenu.htm)

Founded in 1986, the SNRS works to promote nursing research in the southern United States. Included in this site is information related to the SNRS's membership, research interest groups, conferences, officers, newsletter, and awards.

■ Student Organizations

Colorado Student Nurses' Association's (http://WWW2.csn.net/~tbracket)

Sigma Theta Tau International: Honor Society of Nursing (http://stti-web.iupui.edu)

This site details information related to the society, including its program and people, its newsletter, and regional chapters. Also included is conference information and a demonstration of the online *Journal of Knowledge Synthesis for Nursing* (http://www.nursing.ab.umd.edu/students/~snewbol/sknstti.htm).

Contact information is available, including information for the (http://www.nursing.ab.umd.edu/students/~snewbol/sknpi.htm) *Pi Chapter Executive Board 1996-97.* Sigma Theta Tau International offers free online information that is accessible through the (telnet://visitor@stti-sun.iupui.edu) *Henderson Library* menu (login name and password: visitor and visitor).

WHO Nursing and Midwifery (http://www.who.ch/programmes/nur/NUR_Homepage.html)

This site provides links to the World Health Organization's bulletin board system (BBS) for nursing and midwifery. The BBS is a discussion space moderated by WHO and allows nursing professionals to share and answer questions. These bulletin boards are offered in several languages.

APPENDIX B

■ STATE BOARDS OF NURSING

Alabama Board of Nursing
P.O. Box 303900
Montgomery, AL 36130
Judi Crume, RN, MSN, *Executive Officer*
Phone: (334) 242-4060
Fax: (334) 242-4360

Alaska Board of Nursing
Dept. of Comm. & Econ. Development
Div. of Occupational Licensing
3601 C Street, Suite 722
Anchorage, AK 99503
Dorothy Fulton, RN, MA, *Executive Director*
Phone: (907) 269-8161
Fax: (907) 269-8156

American Samoa Health Services Regulatory Board
LBJ Tropical Medical Center
Pago Pago, AS 96799
Marie Ma'o, RN, MS, *Director, Nursing Services*
Phone: (684) 633-1222
Fax: (684) 633-1869

Arizona State Board of Nursing
1651 E. Morten Avenue, Suite 150
Phoenix, AZ 85020
Joey Ridenour, RN, MN, *Executive Director*
Phone: (602) 255-5092
Fax: (602) 255-5130

Arkansas State Board of Nursing
University Tower Building
1123 S. University, Suite 800
Little Rock, AR 72204
Faith Fields, RN, MSN, *Executive Director*
Phone: (501) 686-2700
Fax: (501) 686-2714

California Board of Registered Nursing
P.O. Box 944210
Sacramento, CA 94244
Ruth Ann Terry, RN, MPH, *Executive Officer*
Phone: (916) 322-3350
Fax: (916) 327-4402

California Board of Vocational Nurse and Psychiatric Technician Examiners
2535 Capitol Oaks Drive, Suite 205
Sacramento, CA 95833
Teresa Bello-Jones, RN, MSN, JD, *Executive Officer*
Phone: (916) 263-7800
Fax: (916) 263-7859

Colorado Board of Nursing
1560 Broadway, Suite 670
Denver, CO 80202
Karen Brumley, RN, BSN, MA, *Program Administrator*
Phone: (303) 894-2430
Fax: (303) 894-2821

Connecticut Board of Examiners for Nursing
Division of Health Systems Regulation
410 Capitol Avenue, MS # 12 HSR
Hartford, CT 06134
Wendy Furniss, RNC, MS, *Health Services Supervisor, Certification*
Phone: (860) 509-7624
Fax: (860) 509-7286

Delaware Board of Nursing
Cannon Building, Suite 203
P.O. Box 1401
Dover, DE 19903
Iva Boardman, RN, MSN, *Executive Director*
Phone: (302) 739-4522
Fax: (302) 739-2711

District of Columbia Board of Nursing
614 H. Street, N.W.
Washington, DC 20001
Barbara Hagans, *Contact Person*
Phone: (202) 727-7468
Fax: (202) 727-7662

Florida Board of Nursing
4080 Woodcock Drive, Suite 202
Jacksonville, FL 32207
Marilyn Bloss, RN, RNC, MSN, *Executive Director*
Phone: (904) 858-6940
Fax: (904) 858-6964

Georgia State Board of Licensed Practical Nurses
166 Pryor Street S.W.
Atlanta, GA 30303
Patricia Swann, *Executive Director*
Phone: (404) 656-3921
Fax: (404) 651-9532

Georgia Board of Nursing
166 Pryor Street S.W.
Atlanta, GA 30303
Shirley Camp, RN, JD *Executive Director*
Phone: (404) 656-3943
Fax: (404) 657-7489

Guam Board of Nurse Examiners
P.O. Box 2816
Agana, GU 96910
Teofila Cruz, RN, *Nurse Examiner Administrator*
Phone: (671) 475-0251
Fax: (671) 477-4733

Hawaii Board of Nursing
Professional and Vocational Licensing Division
P.O. Box 3469
Honolulu, HI 96801
Kathleen Yokouchi, *Executive Officer*
Phone: (808) 586-2695
Fax: (808) 586-2689

Idaho Board of Nursing
P.O. Box 83720
Boise, ID 83720
Sandra Evans, RN, MA, Ed, *Executive Director*
Phone: (208) 334-3110
Fax: (208) 334-3262

Illinois Department of Professional Regulation
James R. Thompson Center
100 West Randolph, Suite 9-300
Chicago, IL 60601
Jacqueline Waggoner, RN, MSN, *Nursing Act Coordinator*
Phone: (312) 814-2715
Fax: (312) 814-3145

Indiana State Board of Nursing
Health Professions Bureau
402 W. Washington Street, Suite 041
Indianapolis, IN 46204
Laura Langford, RN, *Executive Director*
Phone: (317) 232-2960
Fax: (317) 233-4236

Iowa Board of Nursing
State Capitol Complex
1223 East Court Avenue
Des Moines, IA 50319
Lorinda Inman, RN, MSN, *Executive Director*
Phone: (515) 281-3255
Fax: (515) 281-4825

Kansas State Board of Nursing
Landon State Office Building
900 S.W. Jackson, Suite 551-S
Topeka, KS 66612
Patsy Johnson, RN, MN, *Executive Administrator*
Phone: (913) 296-4929
Fax: (913) 296-3929

Kentucky Board of Nursing
312 Whittington Parkway, Suite 300
Louisville, KY 40222
Sharon Weisenbeck, RN, MS, *Executive Director*
Phone: (502) 329-7006
Fax: (502) 329-7011

Louisiana State Board of Practical Nurse Examiners
3421 N. Causeway Boulevard, Suite 203
Metairie, LA 70002
Terry DeMarcay, RN, BS, MS, *Executive Director*
Phone: (504) 838-5791
Fax: (504) 838-5279

Louisiana State Board of Nursing
3510 N. Causeway Boulevard, Suite 501
Metairie, LA 70002
Barbara Morvant, RN, MN, *Executive Director*
Phone: (504) 838-5332
Fax: (504) 838-5349

Maine State Board of Nursing
158 State House Station
Augusta, ME 04333
Jean Caron, RN, MS, *Executive Director*
Phone: (207) 287-1133
Fax: (207) 287-1149

Maryland Board of Nursing
4140 Patterson Avenue
Baltimore, MD 21215
Donna Dorsey, RN, MS, *Executive Director*
Phone: (410) 764-5124
Fax: (410) 358-3530

Massachusetts Board of Registration in Nursing
Leverett Saltonstall Building
100 Cambridge Street, Room 1519
Boston, MA 02202
Theresa Bonanno, *Executive Director*
Phone: (617) 727-9961
Fax: (617) 727-2197

State of Michigan
CIS/Office of Health Services
Ottawa Towers North
611 W. Ottawa, 4th Floor
Lansing, MI 48933
Brenda Rogers, *Assistant Administrator*
Phone: (517) 373-9102
Fax: (517) 373-2179

Minnesota Board of Nursing
2829 University Avenue SE, Suite 500
Minneapolis, MN 55414
Joyce Schowalter, *Executive Director*
Phone: (612) 617-2270
Fax: (612) 617-2190

Mississippi Board of Nursing
239 N. Lamar Street, Suite 401
Jackson, MS 39201
Maria Rachel, RN, PhD, *Executive Director*
Phone: (601) 359-6170
Fax: (601) 359-6185

Missouri State Board of Nursing
P.O. Box 656
Jefferson City, MO 65102
Florence Stillman, RN, MSN, *Executive Director*
Phone: (573) 751-0681
Fax: (573) 751-0075

Montana State Board of Nursing
111 North Jackson
P.O. Box 200513
Helena, MT 59620
Dianne Wickham, RN, MN, *Executive Director*
Phone: (406) 444-2071
Fax: (406) 444-7759

Dept. Of Health and Human Services
Regulation and Licensure Creditialing
Div.—Nursing/Nursing Support Section
P.O. Box 94986
Lincoln, NE 68509
Charlene Kelly, RN, PhD, *Section Administrator*
Phone: (402) 471-4376
Fax: (402) 471-3577

Nevada State Board of Nursing
1755 East Plumb Lane, Suite 260
Reno, NV 89502
Kathy Apple, RN, MS, *Executive Director*
Phone: (702) 786-2778
Fax: (702) 322-6993

New Hampshire Board of Nursing
Health & Welfare Building
6 Hazen Drive
Concord, NH 03301
Doris Nuttelman, RN, EdD, *Executive Director*
Phone: (603) 271-2323
Fax: (603) 271-6605

New Jersey Board of Nursing
P.O. Box 45010
Newark, NJ 07101
Margaret Howard, RN, MSN, *Field Representative*
Phone: (201) 504-6586
Fax: (201) 648-3481

New Mexico Board of Nursing
4206 Louisiana Boulevard, NE
Suite A
Albuquerque, NM 87109
Nancy Twigg, RN, MSN, *Executive Director*
Phone: (505) 841-8340
Fax: (505) 841-8347

New York State Board of Nursing
State Education Department
Cultural Education Center, Room 3023
Albany, NY 12230
Milene Sower, RN, PhD, *Executive Secretary*
Phone: (518) 474-3845
Fax: (518) 473-0578

Commonwealth Board of Nurse Examiners
Public Health Center
P.O. Box 1458
Saipan, MP 96950
Elizabeth Torees-Untalan, RN, *Chairperson*
Phone: (670) 234-8950
Fax: (670) 234-8930

North Carolina Board of Nursing
3724 National Drive
Raleigh, NC 27602
Polly Johnson, RN, MSN, *Executive Director*
Phone: (919) 782-3211
Fax: (919) 781-9461

North Dakota Board of Nursing
919 South 7th Street, Suite 504
Bismarck, ND 58504
Ida Rigley, RN, MS, *Executive Director*
Phone: (701) 328-9777
Fax: (701) 328-9785

Ohio Board of Nursing
77 South High Street, 17th Floor
Columbus, OH 43215
Dorothy Fiorino, RN, MS, *Executive Director*
Phone: (614) 466-3947
Fax: (614) 466-0388

Oklahoma Board of Nursing
2915 N. Classen Boulevard, Suite 524
Oklahoma City, OK 73106
Sulina Moffett, RN, MSN, *Executive Director*
Phone: (405) 525-2076
Fax: (405) 521-6089

Oregon State Board of Nursing
800 NE Oregon Street, Box 25
Suite 465
Portland, OR 97232
Joan Bouchard, RN, MN, *Executive Director*
Phone: (503) 731-4745
Fax: (503) 731-4755

Pennsylvania State Board of Nursing
P.O. Box 2649
Harrisburg, PA 17105
Mariam Limo, *Executive Secretary*
Phone: (717) 783-7142
Fax: (717) 783-0822

Commonwealth of Puerto Rico
Board of Nurse Examiners
Call Box 10200
Santurce, PR 00908
Beverly Dabula, *Executive Director*
Phone: (787) 725-8161
Fax: (787) 725-7903

Rhode Island Board of Nursing
Registration and Nursing Education
Cannon Health Building
Three Capitol Hill, Room 104
Providence, RI 02908
Carol Lietar, *Executive Officer*
Phone: (401) 277-2827
Fax: (401) 277-1272

South Carolina State Board of Nursing
110 Centerview Drive, Suite 202
Columbia, SC 29210
Barbara Kellogg, MN, RN, *Program Nurse Consultant*
Phone: (803) 896-4550
Fax: (803) 896-4525

South Dakota Board of Nursing
3307 South Lincoln Avenue
Sioux Falls, SD 57105
Diana Vander Woude, RN, MS, *Executive Secretary*
Phone: (605) 367-5940
Fax: (605) 367-5945

Tennessee State Board of Nursing
426 Fifth Avenue North
1st Floor - Cordell Hull Building
Nashville, TN 37247
Elizabeth Lund, RN, MSN, *Executive Director*
Phone: (615) 532-5166
Fax: (615) 741-7899

Texas Board of Nurse Examiners
P.O. Box 430
Austin, TX 78767
Katherine Thomas, RN, MN, CPNP, *Executive Director*
Phone: (512) 305-7400
Fax: (512) 305-7401

Texas Board of Vocational Nurse Examiners
William P. Hobby Building, Tower 3
333 Guadalupe Street, Suite 3-400
Austin, TX 78701
Marjorie Bronk, RN, MSHP, *Executive Director*
Phone: (512) 305-8100
Fax: (512) 305-8101

Utah State Board of Nursing
Division of Occupational and Professional Licensing
P.O. Box 45805
Salt Lake City, UT 84145
Laura Poe, RN, MS, *Executive Administrator*
Phone: (801) 530-6628
Fax: (801) 530-6511

Vermont State Board of Nursing
109 State Street
Montpelier, VT 05609
Anita Ristau, RN, MS, *Executive Director*
Phone: (802) 828-2396
Fax: (802) 828-2484

Virgin Islands Board of Nurse Licensure
P.O. Box 4247
Veterans Drive Station
St. Thomas, VI 00803
Winifred Garfield, RN, CRNA, *Executive Secretary*
Phone: (809) 776-7397
Fax: (809) 777-4003

Virginia Board of Nursing
6606 W. Broad Street, 4th Floor
Richmond, VA 23230
Nancy Durrett, RN, MSN, *Executive Director*
Phone: (804) 662-9909
Fax: (804) 662-9943

Washington State Nursing Care Quality Assurance Commission
Department of Health
P.O. Box 47864
Olympia, WA 98504
Patty Hayes, RN, MN, *Executive Director*
Phone: (360) 753-2686
Fax: (360) 586-5935

West Virginia State Board of Examiners for Practical Nurses
101 Dee Drive
Charleston, WV 25311
Nancy Wilson, *Executive Secretary*
Phone: (304) 558-3572
Fax: (304) 558-4367

West Virginia Board of Examiners for Registered Professional Nurses
101 Dee Drive
Charleston, WV 25311
Laura Skidmore Rhodes, *Executive Secretary*
Phone: (304) 558-3596
Fax: (304) 558-3666

Wisconsin Department of Regulation and Licensing
1400 E. Washington Avenue
P.O. Box 8935
Madison, WI 53708
Thomas Neumann, RN, MSN, *Administrative Officer*
Phone: (608) 266-2112
Fax: (608) 267-0644

Wyoming State Board of Nursing
2020 Carey Avenue, Suite 110
Cheyenne, WY 82002
Toma Nisbet, RN, MS, BSN, CS, *Executive Director*
Phone: (307) 777-7601
Fax: (307) 777-3519

INDEX

D

N

Q

R

Q